Pathology Exam Review

Editors

Atif Ali Ahmed, MD

Associate Professor of Pathology and Pediatrics
University of Missouri, Kansas City

Staff Pathologist and Director of Immunohistochemistry
Department of Pathology and Laboratory Medicine
Children's Mercy Hospitals and Clinics
Kansas City, Missouri

Ronald M. Przygodzki, MD

Director, Biomedical Laboratory Research and Development
Associate Director, Genomic Medicine
Office of Research and Development (121E)
Department of Veterans Affairs
Washington, DC

 Wolters Kluwer | Lippincott Williams & Wilkins
Health

Philadelphia · Baltimore · New York · London
Buenos Aires · Hong Kong · Sydney · Tokyo

Executive Editor: Jonathan W. Pine, Jr.
Managing Editor: Sirkka Howes
Project Manager: Alicia Jackson
Senior Manufacturing Manager: Benjamin Rivera
Senior Marketing Manager: Angela Panetta
Designer: Terry Mallon
Cover Designer: Joseph DePinho
Production Service: Maryland Composition/ASI

Printed in The People's Republic of China

Library of Congress Cataloging-in-Publication Data

Pathology exam review / [edited by] Atif Ali Ahmed, Ronald M. Przygodzki.
   p. ; cm.
Includes bibliographical references and index.
ISBN 978-0-7817-8514-3
1. Pathology—Examinations, questions, etc. I. Ahmed, Atif Ali. II. Przygodzki, Ronald M.
[DNLM: 1. Pathology—Examination Questions. QZ 18.2 P2968 2009]
RB119.P365 2009
616.07—dc22
                                2008052189

Care has been taken to confirm the accuracy of the information presented and to describe generally accepted practices. However, the authors, editors, and publisher are not responsible for errors or omissions or for any consequences from application of the information in this book and make no warranty, expressed or implied, with respect to the currency, completeness, or accuracy of the contents of the publication. Application of the information in a particular situation remains the professional responsibility of the practitioner.

The authors, editors, and publisher have exerted every effort to ensure that drug selection and dosage set forth in this text are in accordance with current recommendations and practice at the time of publication. However, in view of ongoing research, changes in government regulations, and the constant flow of information relating to drug therapy and drug reactions, the reader is urged to check the package insert for each drug for any change in indications and dosage and for added warnings and precautions. This is particularly important when the recommended agent is a new or infrequently employed drug.

Some drugs and medical devices presented in the publication have Food and Drug Administration (FDA) clearance for limited use in restricted research settings. It is the responsibility of the health care provider to ascertain the FDA status of each drug or device planned for use in their clinical practice.

To purchase additional copies of this book, call our customer service department at (800) 638-3030 or fax orders to (301) 223-2320. International customers should call (301) 223-2300.

Visit Lippincott Williams & Wilkins on the Internet: at LWW.com. Lippincott Williams & Wilkins customer service representatives are available from 8:30 am to 6 pm, EST.

10 9 8 7 6 5 4 3 2 1

We dedicate this book to our wives and children for their everlasting support and enduring patience during the process of this book.

Contents

Acknowledgments

The authors wish to acknowledge Dr. Enid Gilbert-Barness, Dr. Linda Cooley, Terencia Davenport, and others for providing images and other materials to be used in this book. We are grateful to Dr. Jack Moskowitz for his helpful suggestions and editorial assistance. We also wish to express our gratitude to Nancy Lathrom for her help in preparing and printing the manuscript. Many thanks are also due to the residents and staff at Children's National Medical Center who inspired us to write and pursue the publishing of this book.

Atif Ali Ahmed, MD
Ronald Przygodzki, MD

Foreword

Time in residency is limited with an overwhelming amount of information to learn. The field of pathology continues to advance with new concepts and expanding specialty fields. Acclimating to these changes, learning practical pathology, and preparing for examinations are necessary activities for a successful residency. *Pathology Exam Review* is here to help.

Active learning and rehearsing information are the keys to solidifying knowledge. *Pathology Exam Review* utilizes these learning keys by challenging residents to apply their knowledge toward answering multiple choice questions. This book contains comprehensive anatomical and clinical pathology board-style questions, written by a team of specialized pathologists. The strength of *Pathology Exam Review* includes thorough explanations and high quality images (about 540) covering a full range of pathological subjects. *Pathology Exam Review* is a tool that can be used early in training to enrich information presented in primary texts or can be used later as a stand-alone book for board preparation. Board preparation can never be started too soon and *Pathology Exam Review* is an efficient resource that emphasizes key facts, reinforces knowledge, and strengthens test-taking skills.

Jack Moskowitz, DO
Previous Pathology Resident and Board Exam Candidate

Preface

This book is mainly intended to help pathology residents and fellows prepare for and pass the American Board of Pathology Anatomic and Clinical Pathology examinations. Other residents preparing for in-service examinations and pathologists seeking re-certification might find it useful as well. These examinations can be difficult and require a lot of preparation. Studying large volume textbooks is sometimes brain-tasking. Residents and other trainees in pathology often feel the need for a review book like this one to emphasize solid facts. The book is not meant to replace classic textbooks but to strengthen the knowledge one gets from reading these textbooks. It is unique in the fact that it reviews the integrated principles of anatomic and clinical pathology in one single book.

The book is divided into two sections that cover all the major organ systems of anatomic and clinical pathology. The chapters are composed of multiple choice questions which are written by authors who are experienced in their fields. Most of the questions are formatted in a similar style to the questions in the American Board of Pathology examinations. The reader will find that the questions vary in degrees of difficulty similar to the board examination. Some questions are easy and simple and emphasize important facts in an ed-ucational style. Other questions are more difficult and require a focused study approach. Overall the questions are comprehensive and challenging. The reader may study this book in any way he or she likes. To maximize the benefit, however, the reader is encouraged to make an effort to answer the questions out of memory and then review the answers.

How to use the book

The chapter questions contain 4–5 answer choices. The reader is required to choose a single best answer. Few questions contain stem phrases that should be matched with the correct answer choices. Other questions are grouped to a common clinical scenario or an image. The chapter questions are followed by answers and short explanatory notes. A list of reference books is added at the end of most chapters to facilitate further reading.

We hope by providing a quiz study material this way strengthens the educational experience of pathology residents and other trainees. This book will be of tremendous value as a companion book to major textbooks in pathology as well as an indispensable tool that helps residents succeed in their board examinations.

Contributors

Jude M. Abadie, PhD, DABCC, FACB
Medical Director, Clinical Chemistry
Department of Pathology
Walter Reed Army Medical Center
Washington, DC

Atif Ali Ahmed, MD
Associate Professor of Pathology and Pediatrics
University of Missouri, Kansas City
Department of Pathology and Laboratory Medicine
Children's Mercy Hospital
Kansas City, Missouri

Fouad N. Boctor, MD, PhD
Director of Transfusion, Apheresis and Donor Service
Department of Laboratory Medicine
Geisinger Medical Center
Danville, Pennsylvania

D. Robert Dufour, MD, FCAP, FACB
Emeritus Professor of Pathology
The George Washington University Medical Center
Consultant
Department of Pathology and Hepatology
VA Medical Center
Washington, DC

Isam A. Eltoum, MD, MBA, MRCPath
Professor of Pathology
Director of Cytopathology
Department of Pathology
University of Alabama at Birmingham
Birmingham, Alabama

Valerie A. Fitzhugh, MD
Resident Pathologist
Department of Pathology and Laboratory Medicine
University of Medicine and Dentistry of New Jersey
New Jersey Medical School
The University Hospital
Newark, New Jersey

Bungo Furusato, MD
Assistant Professor
Uniformed Services University of Health Sciences
Department of Defense
Genitourinary Pathology
Armed Forces Institute of Pathology
Washington, DC

Joann Habermann, MD
Assistant Professor
Department of Surgical Pathology
University of Medicine and Dentistry of New Jersey
New Jersey Medical School
Newark, New Jersey

Debra S. Heller, MD
Professor of Pathology and Laboratory Medicine
Professor of Obstetrics, Gynecology, and Women's Health
Department of Pathology and Laboratory Medicine
University of Medicine and Dentistry of New Jersey
New Jersey Medical School
The University Hospital
Newark, New Jersey

Alison R. Huppmann, MD
Resident in Pathology
Department of Pathology
George Washington University Hospital
Washington, DC

Elmer W. Koneman, MD
Professor Emeritus
Department of Pathology
University of Colorado School of Medicine
Aurora, Colorado

Peter Kulesza, MD, PhD
Assistant Professor
Department of Pathology
University of Alabama at Birmingham
Birmingham, Alabama

Naomi L.C. Luban, MD
Professor of Pediatrics and Pathology
Division of Laboratory Medicine
George Washington University/Children's National
    Medical Center
Washington, DC

Steven D. Mahlen, PhD
Clinical Microbiology Fellow
Department of Laboratory of Medicine
University of Washington
Seattle, Washington

Christopher J. Papasian, PhD, D(ABMM)
Professor and Chair; Microbiology Consultant
Department of Basic Medical Science
University of Missouri-Kansas City, School of Medicine
Kansas City, Missouri

Ronald M. Przygodzki, MD
Director, Biomedical Laboratory Research and
    Development
Associate Director, Genomic Medicine
Office of Research and Development (121E)
Department of Veterans Affairs
Washington, DC

Elisabeth J. Rushing, MD
Professor of Neurology
Uniform Services University of the Health Sciences

Adjunct Professor
Department of Pathology
Georgetown University School of Medicine
Armed Forces Institute of Pathology
Washington, DC

Mariarita Santi-Vicini, MD, PhD
Associate Professor of Pathology and Laboratory Medicine
University of Pennsylvania Staff

Neuropathologist
Children's Hospital of Philadelphia
Philadelphia, Pennsylvania

Rangaraj Selvarangan, BVSc, PhD, D(ABMM)
Assistant Professor of Pediatrics
Department of Pathology and Laboratory Medicine
Children's Mercy Hospital
Kansas City, Missouri

Guanghua Wang, MD
Staff Pathologist
Department of Hepatic and Gastrointestinal Pathology

Chief, Division of Molecular Pathology
Department of Scientific Laboratories
Armed Forces Institute of Pathology
Washington, DC

Edward C.C. Wong, MD
Assistant Professor of Pediatrics and Pathology
George Washington University School of Medicine and
    Health Sciences
Director of Hematology/Associate Director of
    Transfusion Medicine
Division of Laboratory Medicine
Children's National Medical Center
Washington, DC

David L. Zwick, MD
Associate Professor of Pediatric Pathology
Department of Pathology and Laboratory Medicine
University of Missouri, Kansas City School of Medicine
    and The Children's Mercy Hospital and Clinics
Kansas City, Missouri

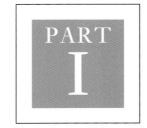

Anatomic Pathology

1

General and Autopsy Pathology

Atif Ahmed

■ Questions

1. All of the following agents and molecules are known causes of cell injury EXCEPT:
   a. Monoxyhemoglobin
   b. Alcohol
   c. Acetaminophen
   d. ATP
   e. IgG

2. Which of the following ultrastructural features of cell injury are considered irreversible?
   a. Myelin figures
   b. Swelling of endoplasmic reticulum
   c. Mitochondrial densities
   d. Cytoplasmic vacuoles
   e. Pyknotic nuclei

Questions 3 and 4:
This is a stomach biopsy taken from a patient who received a bone marrow transplant for myelodysplastic syndrome (Fig. 1.1).

3. All of the following statements concerning the process depicted in the gastric glands are true EXCEPT:
   a. It results from immunologic injury.
   b. It is triggered by decreased bcl2/p53 ratio.
   c. It can effectively be reversed by "Survivin."
   d. It occurs as sequence of the activation of caspase 3.
   e. It is an example of irreversible cell injury.

4. Biological events leading to the process seen in Figure 1.1 can occur through any of the following sequences EXCEPT:
   a. Fas, Fas-associated death domain, caspase 8, caspase 3
   b. TNF, death domains, procaspase 2, caspase 3
   c. P53, death receptors, caspase 3, caspase 9
   d. Bax, cytochrome c, APAF-1, caspase 9
   e. TRAIL, death receptors, caspase 8, caspase 3

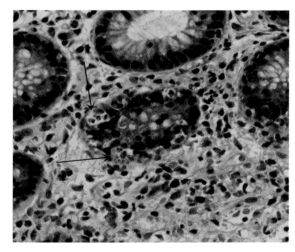

Figure 1.1

5. Ki-67 (MIB-1) index is increased in:
   a. Hypertrophy
   b. Metaplasia
   c. Hyperplasia
   d. Atrophy

6. This is a section of the mucosa of the trachea (Fig. 1.2). The process shown in this image can be induced by any of the following factors EXCEPT:
   a. Vitamin A deficiency
   b. Mechanical intubation
   c. Hypoglycemia
   d. Chronic inflammation
   e. Smoking

7. Calcification is a prominent component of which of the following pathologic entities?
   a. Psammoma bodies
   b. Sarcoid granuloma

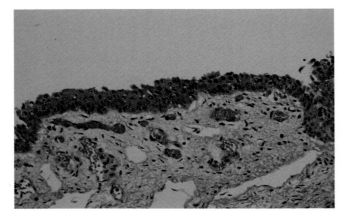

Figure 1.2

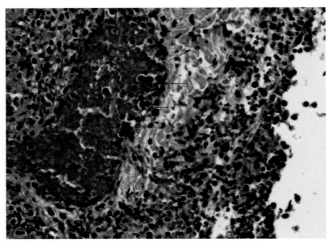

Figure 1.3

c. Corpora amylacea
d. Gamna Gandy bodies
e. Kimmelstiel-Wilson lesions

8. Which statement best characterizes telomerase?
   a. It shortens telomere length by removing nucleotides at the end of the chromosome.
   b. It is up-regulated in cancer cells.
   c. It is expressed in most somatic cells.
   d. It is important in cell apoptosis.
   e. It is activated during G1 phase of cell cycle.

9. Mutations in the DNA helicase gene result in:
   a. Formation of colonic polyps
   b. Apoptosis
   c. Accelerated aging
   d. Megalencephaly
   e. Cell hypertrophy

10. The earliest event in acute inflammation is:
    a. Vasodilatation
    b. Increased vascular permeability
    c. Endothelial contraction
    d. Leukocyte margination
    e. Increased hydrostatic pressure

11. The most common mechanism involved in increased vascular permeability is through:
    a. Histamine acting on venules
    b. Cytokine-mediated formation of endothelial gaps
    c. VEGF acting on endothelial cells
    d. Leukocyte-mediated endothelial injury
    e. Bacteria-mediated endothelial cell necrosis

12. Physiologic events depicted in this image (Fig. 1.3) are induced by mediators released in which of the following sequences?
    a. P-selectin, β-integrin, PECAM 1
    b. E-selectin, PECAM 1, integrins
    c. IL1, sLewis X, P-selectin

d. Redistribution of P-selectin, IL1, ICAM 1
e. L-selectin, P-selectin, VLA-4

13. Major chemotactic agents for leukocytes include all of the following mediators EXCEPT:
    a. Formyl-methionyl-leucyl-phenylalanine (fMLP)
    b. Complement 5a
    c. Leukotriene B4
    d. Interleukin 8
    e. Prostaglandin A1

14. Leukocyte "activation" results in:
    a. Increased surface expression of LFA-1
    b. Dephosphorylation of protein kinases
    c. Increased surface expression of P-selectin
    d. Phagocytosis
    e. All of the above

15. Injection of this molecule (Fig. 1.4) in laboratory animals directly leads to:
    a. Increased vascular permeability
    b. Proliferation of fibroblasts
    c. Activation of complement
    d. Bronchodilatation
    e. Blood clotting

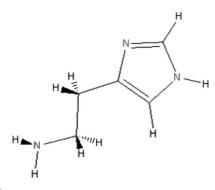

Figure 1.4

16. Primary defects in leukocyte phagocytosis and intra-cellular killing occur in all of the following conditions EXCEPT:
   a. Leukocyte adhesion deficiency
   b. Chediak Higashi syndrome
   c. X-linked gp91 phox deficiency
   d. Myeloperoxidase deficiency
   e. Glutathione reductase deficiency

17. All of the following mediators are considered inhibitors of acute inflammation EXCEPT:
   a. Prostaglandin E1
   b. Nuclear factor (NF) κB
   c. Bacterial leukocidin
   d. Alpha-1 antitrypsin
   e. COX-1 inhibitors

18. Serotonin differs from histamine in the fact that serotonin:
   a. Stimulates fibrosis via fibroblasts
   b. Is not released by platelets
   c. Causes increased vascular permeability
   d. Does not result in arteriolar dilatation
   e. Secretion is limited to carcinoid tumors

19. The lectin pathway of complement activation involves:
   a. C3a
   b. Collectins
   c. Properdin
   d. Peanut lectins
   e. Prekallikrein

20. Activated Hageman factor (factor XIIa) leads to:
   a. Bradykinin formation
   b. Fibrin formation
   c. Fibrin breakdown
   d. Activation of complement
   e. All of the above

21. Which of the following membrane protein receptors has the ability to "recognize" microbe–derived molecules?
   a. Seven transmembrane G-protein–coupled receptors
   b. Peroxisome proliferator-activated receptor
   c. Tyrosine kinase receptors
   d. Toll-like receptors
   e. Hormone receptors

22. In reference to the pathway in Figure 1.5, "??" mediators:
   a. Cause vasodilatation
   b. Cause vasoconstriction
   c. Result in increased vascular permeability
   d. Cause bronchospasm
   e. Inhibit neutrophil chemotaxis

23. Which of the following statements is NOT true about chemokines?
   a. They are large protein complexes.
   b. They bind to serpentine receptors.

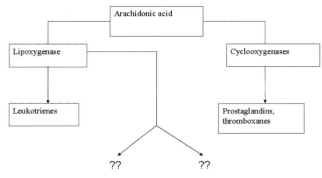

Figure 1.5

c. They are induced by interleukin-1.
d. They are caused by neutrophil chemotaxis.
e. They serve as receptors for HIV virus.

24. Defense against damage by free radicals employs all of the following factors EXCEPT:
   a. Catalase
   b. Superoxide dismutase
   c. Vitamin E
   d. Nitric oxide
   e. Peroxidase

25. The enzyme catalyzing the following reaction in the human body: $O_2^- + O_2 + 2H \rightarrow H_2O_2 + O_2$
   a. Is important in the elimination of free radicals
   b. Forms hydrogen peroxide, which is a natural antioxidant
   c. Uses an iron molecule as a catalyst
   d. Is part of the antioxidant system in the plasma
   e. Uses nitric oxide as a substrate

26. A scratch by a pen resulted in this skin response (Fig. 1.6). Inflammatory mediators released in this response include:
   a. Histamine
   b. Substance P
   c. Both histamine and substance P
   d. None of the above

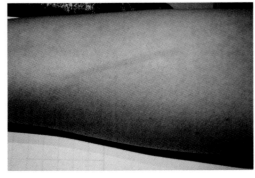

Figure 1.6 (Kindly provided by Judith Horn, National Cancer Institute, Bethesda, MD)

27. Fibroblasts differentiate into myofibroblasts through:
    a. Production of a fibronectin coating on the plasma membrane
    b. Forming intracytoplasmic bundles of fibers and dense bodies
    c. Acquisition of collagen-synthesizing enzymes
    d. Production of MyoD1 family of proteins
    e. Acquiring receptors for platelet-derived growth factors

28. Fibrosis is induced by all of the following mediators EXCEPT:
    a. Platelet-derived growth factor
    b. Heparin
    c. Transforming growth factor
    d. Fibronectin
    e. Fibroblast growth factor

29. Eosinophils accumulate in parasitic infections under the influence of:
    a. IgM
    b. Lymphotoxin
    c. Eotaxins
    d. Major basic protein
    e. γ-interferon

30. Factors involved in the formation of this colonic lesion (Fig. 1.7) include all of the following cytokines EXCEPT:
    a. IL-12
    b. γ-interferon
    c. Platelet-derived growth factor
    d. Chemokines
    e. Elastases

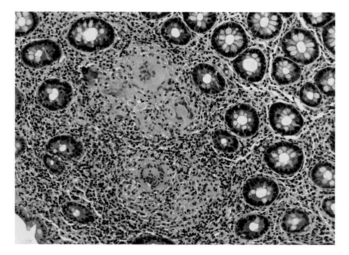

Figure 1.7

31. Systemic symptoms and signs of inflammation are mediated by all of the following proinflammatory cytokines EXCEPT:
    a. TNF
    b. IL-1
    c. IL-8
    d. IL-4
    e. IL-2

32. Match each of the following receptor descriptions with their common ligands listed below.
    i)   Receptors with intrinsic kinase activity
    ii) Receptors without intrinsic kinase activity
    iii) Seven-spanning receptors
    a. Growth factors
    b. Cytokines
    c. p53 protein
    d. Steroid hormones
    e. Nonsteroid hormones

33. Which of the following growth factors mediate the events involved in wound repair?
    a. Fibroblast growth factor
    b. Platelet-derived growth factor
    c. Epidermal growth factor
    d. Transforming growth factor
    e. All of the above

34. Match each of the following matrix proteins with their characteristic functions listed below.
    i)   Hyaluronic acid
    ii) Collagen
    iii) Fibrillin
    a. Is a member of intercellular adhesion molecules
    b. Accumulates in patients with thyroid hormonal dysfunction
    c. Accumulates in patients with cutis laxa
    d. Helps in the assembly of elastic fibers
    e. Defective cross-linking leads to homocystinuria

35. Factors that are important in the pathogenesis of this process (Fig. 1.8) include all of the following molecules EXCEPT:
    a. VEGF
    b. Angiopoietins
    c. Endothelin
    d. Platelet-derived growth factor
    e. Transforming growth factor

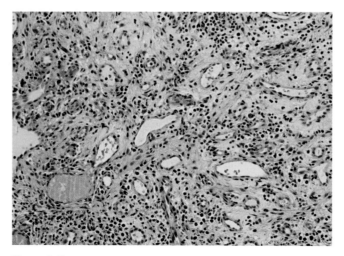

Figure 1.8

36. The extracellular material accumulation shown in this section of the glomerulus stained with H & E (Fig. 1.9) consists of:
   a. Basement membrane material
   b. Fibrin
   c. Collagen
   d. Glycosaminoglycans
   e. All of the above

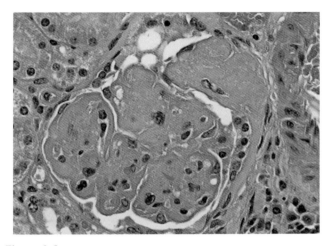

Figure 1.9

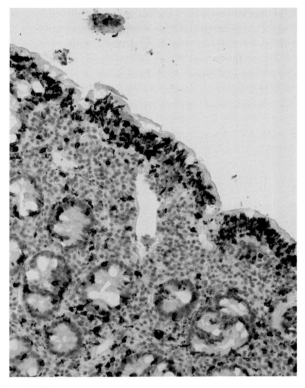

Figure 1.10

37. Diagnosis of systemic amyloidosis is commonly made through:
   a. Measurement of serum amyloid A and P proteins
   b. Performance of a rectal biopsy
   c. Kidney biopsy with congo red staining
   d. Radiologic imaging studies
   e. X-ray diffraction studies

38. Secondary AA amyloidosis is a complication of:
   a. Multiple myeloma
   b. Patients with rheumatoid arthritis
   c. Drug addicts
   d. All of the above
   e. Only options b and c are correct

39. This duodenal biopsy from a patient with celiac disease was performed before the institution of a gluten-free diet. There is a cellular infiltrate in the surface mucosa and the lamina propria, which is highlighted by the immunostain shown (Fig. 1.10). This immunostain is most likely:
   a. CD20
   b. CD4
   c. CD68
   d. CD8
   e. None of the above

40. Depletion of lymphocytes in the thymus is seen in which of the following immunodeficiency conditions?
   a. Severe combined immunodeficiency
   b. IgA deficiency
   c. Hyper IgM syndrome
   d. Common variable immunodeficiency
   e. Infection by human immunodeficiency virus

41. This glomerular lesion (Fig. 1.11) represents an example of:
   a. Complement-dependent cytotoxicity
   b. Delayed-type hypersensitivity
   c. Serum sickness
   d. Antibody-dependent cell-mediated cytotoxicity
   e. T-cell mediated cytotoxicity

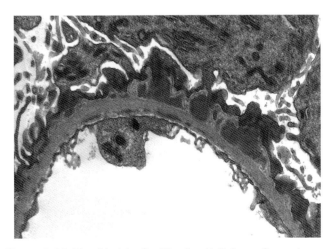

Figure 1.11 (Provided by Dr. Bhaskar Kallakury, Georgetown University, Washington, DC)

42. Hemolytic transfusion reactions occur through:
    a. Fc-mediated cell lysis without phagocytosis
    b. Assembly of the complement membrane attack complex
    c. Mast cell growth and differentiation
    d. Release of lysosomal enzymes
    e. Phagocytosis of antigen–antibody complexes

43. Defense mechanisms against parasites include all of the following immune reactions EXCEPT:
    a. Type I hypersensitivity reaction
    b. Immunoglobulin E-dependent eosinophil-mediated cytotoxicity
    c. Immunoglobulin E-mediated immune complex deposition
    d. Type IV delayed-type hypersensitivity

44. Match each of the following autoimmune diseases with their characteristic diagnostic serum antibodies listed below.
    i)   Systemic lupus erythematosus (SLE)
    ii) Systemic sclerosis
    iii) Sjögren syndrome
    iv) Mixed connective tissue disease
    v)   Inflammatory myopathy
    a. Anti-SS-A
    b. Anti-Sm
    c. Anti-Jo-1
    d. Anticentromere antibody
    e. Anti-U1RNP

45. Pathologic features characteristic of X-linked hypogammaglobulinemia (XLA) include:
    a. Hypertrophy of tonsils
    b. Absence of immunoglobulin gene rearrangement
    c. Susceptibility to infections caused by enteroviruses
    d. Mutation in tyrosine kinase receptor, c-kit
    e. Absence of T-cell receptor expression

46. Patients with DiGeorge syndrome usually present to their pediatricians with:
    a. Bacterial infections
    b. Aortic arch anomalies
    c. Neonatal hypocalcemia
    d. Physical limb deformities
    e. Small stature

47. Match each of the following viruses with the lymphocyte receptors that they bind with from the list below:
    i)   Human immunodeficiency virus
    ii) Human T-cell lymphotropic virus-1 (HTLV-1)
    iii) Epstein-Barr virus (EBV)
    a. CD21
    b. CD4
    c. CD8
    d. CD45
    e. CD3

48. Infections by double-strand RNA viruses usually result in:
    a. Myocarditis
    b. Upper respiratory tract infections
    c. Diarrhea
    d. Pneumonia
    e. Encephalitis

49. This is a section of a pulmonary cavitary lesion stained with GMS (Fig. 1.12). Proteins involved in the pathogenesis of this infection include:
    a. Chitinase
    b. Septin
    c. Restrictocin
    d. Mycolic acid
    e. M-protein

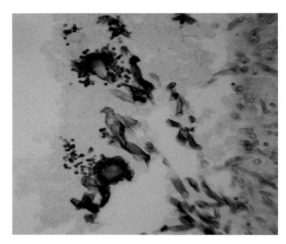

Figure 1.12

50. Hemolytic uremic syndrome is caused by:
    a. Hemolysin produced by *Escherichia coli* bacteria
    b. Toxins that block protein synthesis
    c. Bacterial antigens that cross-react with HLA-B27
    d. Invasins that bind host cell integrins
    e. IgA protease produced by Shigella bacteria

51. Infection caused by Yersinia organisms can result in any of the following pathologic manifestations EXCEPT:
    a. Mesenteric lymphadenitis
    b. Terminal ileitis
    c. Typhoid-like ulcers
    d. Pseudomembrane formation
    e. Erythema nodosum

52. Cryptococcosis is acquired through:
    a. Respiratory inhalation
    b. Blood transfusion
    c. Oral-fecal route
    d. Sexual transmission
    e. Close personal contact

53. Which of the following cells become infected by cytomegalovirus (CMV) in immunocompetent patients?
    a. Alveolar epithelial cells
    b. White blood cells
    c. Liver cells
    d. Renal tubular epithelial cells
    e. Intestinal epithelial cells

54. Which organism does NOT have an intracellular stage as part of its life cycle?
    a. Leishmania
    b. *Trypanosoma brucei*
    c. *Coxiella burnetii*
    d. Legionella bacteria
    e. Borrelia burgdorferi

Questions 55 and 56 (Fig 1.13):

55. This lesion arises as a result of:
    a. Mutation in chromosome 3p26
    b. NF1 gene mutation
    c. Deletion of a single copy of chromosomes 13
    d. Deletions of both copies of chromosomes 13
    e. N-myc amplification

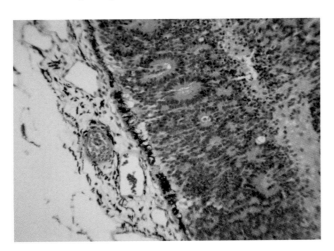

Figure 1.13

56. The protein primarily involved in the pathogenesis of the illustrated lesion plays a role in which part of the cell cycle, as shown in this image (Fig. 1.14)?
    a. A
    b. B
    c. C
    d. D
    e. E

57. Which statement is true regarding p53 protein?
    a. It is composed of 53 amino acids.
    b. The gene is mapped to chromosome 5p13.
    c. Mutations occur mainly as missense mutations.
    d. Mutations have the greatest effect when they occur in region 1 of the gene.
    e. The protein's function is to control the G_0 phase of the cell cycle.

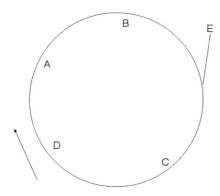

Figure 1.14

58. This is a section of a testis in a 21-year-old man with seminoma. The seminiferous tubules are stained with CD117 immunostain (Fig. 1.15). This result represents an example of a/an:
    a. In situ carcinoma
    b. Neoplastic process

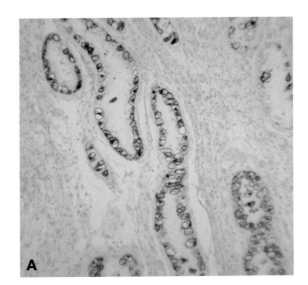

A

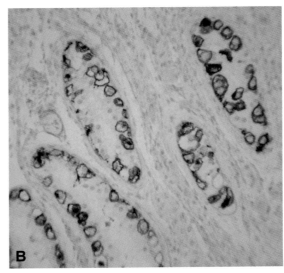

B

Figure 1.15

c. Precursor cell hyperplasia
d. Normal finding
e. Chronic inflammatory process

59. Mutations of the NF1 gene located on chromosome 17q11 can result in all of the following lesions EXCEPT:
    a. Lisch nodules
    b. Peripheral nerve sheath tumors
    c. Hyperpigmented skin lesions
    d. Retinal phakoma
    e. Renal artery stenosis

60. Which of the following statements regarding genomic instability is correct?
    a. It results in breaks and rearrangements of the chromosomes.
    b. It can be visualized by light microscopy.
    c. It can lead to cancer.
    d. It can result in an increased rate of sister chromatid exchange.
    e. All of the above.

61. "Anticipation" in genetics refers to:
    a. Predicting the mortality knowing the prognosis of the genetic disease
    b. Predicting the molecular test result with a given clinical phenotype
    c. Characterization of genes following the human genome data
    d. Increasing disease severity in consecutive family generations
    e. The process of counseling families affected by a genetically diseased child

62. All of the following methods are commonly used in clinical practice to detect gene mutations EXCEPT:
    a. Allele-specific oligonucleotide assay
    b. Ribonuclease protection assay
    c. Denaturing gradient gel electrophoresis
    d. Gene sequencing
    e. Chromosome immunoprecipitation

63. Which of the following statements in regards to mitochondrial DNA is true?
    a. It codes for peroxisomal enzymes.
    b. It contains less numbers of introns than nuclear DNA.
    c. It is transmitted through the sperm of the male.
    d. Mitochondrial DNA mutations affect the eye, muscle, and brain.
    e. It is a linear single-stranded molecule.

64. Chromosomal translocation t(14;18)(q32;q21) leads to follicular lymphoma through:
    a. Up-regulation of Bax and Bak proteins
    b. Inhibiting apoptosis

c. Arresting cell cycle
d. Inhibiting DNA repair
e. Activating *ras* oncogenes

65. Invasive ductal carcinoma of the breast differs from ductal carcinoma in situ (DCIS) in that the invasive tumor cells:
    a. Have more levels of metalloproteinase inhibitors
    b. Effectively suppress production of cathepsin D
    c. Have higher levels of collagenase IV
    d. Show overexpression of E-cadherin
    e. Lose expression of estrogen and progesterone receptors

66. Carcinogenicity of a chemical can be tested by its ability to:
    a. Block DNA repair
    b. Induce activity of cytochrome p-450–dependent pathways
    c. Enhance production of TGF-β
    d. Induce mutations in *Salmonella typhimurium*
    e. Induce p53 mutations in experimental cancer cell lines

67. Initiation of chemical carcinogenesis requires:
    a. Exposure to electron-rich carcinogens
    b. Presence of actively proliferating cells
    c. Conversion of the carcinogenic molecule to a pro-motor carcinogen
    d. Activation of cellular oncogens
    e. Activation of tumor suppressor genes

68. Radiation injury can cause all of the following EXCEPT:
    a. Melanoma
    b. Thyroid carcinoma
    c. Acute myelogenous leukemia
    d. Chronic lymphocytic leukemia
    e. Breast carcinoma

69. Increased susceptibility to radiation injury occurs in which of the following situations?
    a. Localized radiotherapy of glioblastoma multiforme
    b. Loss of DNA repair mechanisms
    c. Radiation to peripheral extremities with ischemic gangrene
    d. Radiated cells are in late S phase of the cell cycle
    e. Radiation particles have low linear energy transfer (LET)

70. Increasing incidence of skin cancers are attributed to which of the following environmental factors?
    a. Air pollution
    b. Global warming, "greenhouse effect"
    c. Depletion of the ozone layer
    d. Accumulation of radon
    e. Use of chlorofluorocarbons in household refrigerators

71. The LEAST hazardous habit of tobacco use is:
    a. Cigarette smoking
    b. Cigar smoking
    c. Chewing tobacco
    d. Snuff dipping

72. Mortality related to cigarette smoking is mostly caused by:
    a. Lung carcinoma
    b. Carcinoma of the esophagus
    c. Cerebrovascular lesions
    d. Chronic obstructive pulmonary disease
    e. Coronary artery disease

73. Nervous system changes primarily related to chronic alcoholism include all of the following EXCEPT:
    a. Hemorrhage and vascular changes in the paraventricular region of thalamus
    b. Loss of Purkinje cells in the cerebellum
    c. Recent memory deficit
    d. Loss of neurons in the basal ganglia and anterior horn cells of the spinal cord
    e. Demyelinating peripheral neuropathy

74. Vitamin A deficiency results in all of the following conditions EXCEPT:
    a. Squamous metaplasia of the urinary bladder
    b. Night blindness
    c. Hepatomegaly
    d. Follicular hyperkeratosis
    e. Kidney stones

75. Mental retardation due to abnormalities in chromosome 15 is a feature of:
    a. von Recklinghausen disease
    b. Beckwith-Wiedemann syndrome
    c. Proteus syndrome
    d. Angelman syndrome
    e. Ataxia telangiectasia

76. Which statement about Fragile X syndrome is true?
    a. It results from maternal folic acid deficiency.
    b. It is characterized by an abnormality in chromosome X inactivation.
    c. There is expansion of the "fraX" site by >200 CGG trinucleotide repeats.
    d. Low testosterone levels are found in affected boys.
    e. Testicular histology shows atrophic seminiferous tubules.

77. A 2-week-old baby developed acute onset of bloody diarrhea, abdominal distension, and subsequently died. Discoloration of the bowel was noticed at autopsy (Fig. 1.16). The most likely cause of death is:
    a. Ischemic colitis
    b. Necrotizing enterocolitis
    c. Blue rubber bleb nevus syndrome
    d. Intussusception
    e. Vitamin K deficiency

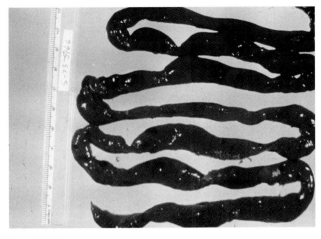

Figure 1.16

78. These are sections (Fig. 1.17) of a sacrococcygeal mass in a newborn infant. The diagnosis is most likely:
    a. Mature cystic teratoma
    b. Immature cystic teratoma
    c. Mixed germ cell tumor
    d. Mesenchymal hamartoma
    e. Teratoid cystic Wilms tumor

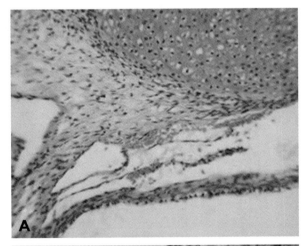

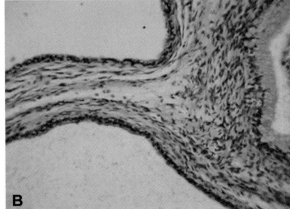

Figure 1.17 (continues)

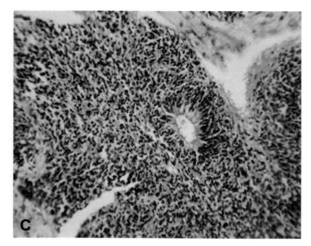

Figure 1.17 *(continued)*

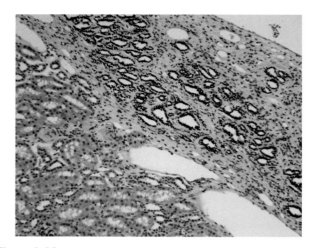

Figure 1.19

79. This adrenal tumor (Fig. 1.18) is best classified as:
    a. Undifferentiated neuroblastoma
    b. Poorly differentiated neuroblastoma
    c. Ganglioneuroblastoma
    d. Ganglioneuroma
    e. Schwannoma

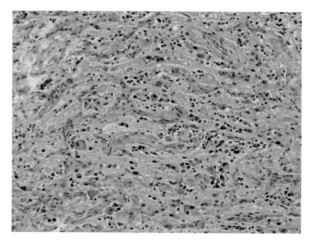

Figure 1.18

80. This lesion (Fig. 1.19) was found in a kidney of a 1-year-old baby with WT-1 gene mutation. The most likely diagnosis is:
    a. Epithelial-predominant Wilms tumor
    b. Renal dysplasia
    c. Nephrogenic rest
    d. Denys–Drash syndrome
    e. Mesoblastic nephroma

81. Characteristic features of Gaucher disease include all of the following EXCEPT:
    a. "Erlenmeyer flask deformity" on a bone x-ray
    b. Necrosis of the femoral head

c. Elevation of serum tartrate-resistant acid-phosphatase
    d. Autosomal dominant inheritance
    e. Beta-glucosidase deficiency

82. The pregnancy of this stillborn baby (Fig. 1.20) was complicated by maternal hypertension and oligohydramnios. The cause of death is most likely:
    a. Kernicterus
    b. Brain hemorrhage
    c. Congestive heart failure
    d. Lung hypoplasia
    e. Placental abruption

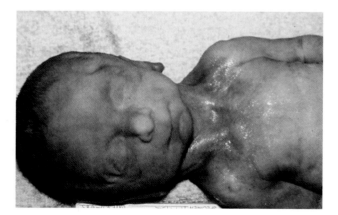

Figure 1.20

83. All of the following conditions are major causes of mortality in infants EXCEPT:
    a. Sudden infant death syndrome
    b. Pneumonia
    c. Malignant neoplasm
    d. Necrotizing enterocolitis
    e. Birth asphyxia

84. Children with fetal alcohol syndrome commonly present with all of the following anomalies EXCEPT:
    a. Atrial septal defect
    b. Microcephaly
    c. Low IQ scores
    d. Facial anomalies
    e. Short limbs

85. Infants born to diabetic mothers may have all of the following anomalies EXCEPT:
    a. Caudal regression
    b. "Vater" association
    c. Anencephaly
    d. "ADAM" complex
    e. Imperforate anus

86. This bilateral ovarian tumor (Fig. 1.21) in a 17-year-old African American female patient with mutation of the "patched" gene located on chromosome 9q22 is most likely:
    a. Juvenile granulosa cell tumor
    b. Leiomyoma
    c. Serous cystadenoma
    d. Fibroma
    e. Metastatic basal cell carcinoma

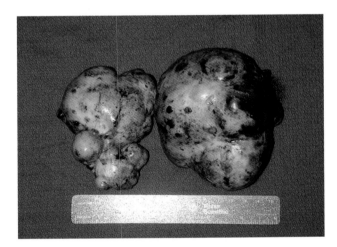

Figure 1.21

87. Which of the following statements is INCORRECT about this lung condition (Fig. 1.22)?
    a. It is related to surfactant deficiency.
    b. It is characterized by necrosis of alveolar epithelial lining cells.
    c. It may appear as early as 3–4 hours after birth.
    d. It does not occur in postterm infants.
    e. It may be complicated by bacterial infection.

88. The most common cause of hemolytic anemia in a newborn baby in the United States is:
    a. Congenital spherocytosis
    b. Drug-induced Coombs-positive anemia
    c. ABO incompatibility

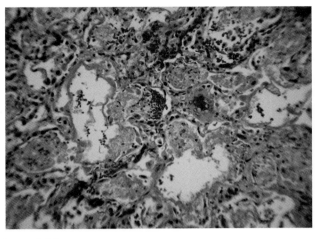

Figure 1.22

    d. Use of nursery warmers
    e. Rh incompatibility

89. An infant is born with profound mental retardation and congenital anomalies of the heart and brain. The diagnosis is most likely:
    a. Cystic fibrosis
    b. "NSAID" embryopathy
    c. Homozygous phenylketonuria
    d. Heterozygous phenylketonuria
    e. Turner syndrome

90. Major pathologic changes in patients with homozygous ΔF508 gene mutation include all of the following conditions EXCEPT:
    a. Meconium ileus
    b. Squamous metaplasia of the pancreatic duct
    c. Atrophy of pancreatic islets
    d. Bilateral absence of the vas deferens
    e. Hypovitaminosis A

91. Sudden infant death syndrome (SIDS) is a common cause of mortality in:
    a. The first month of life
    b. Premature infants between 2 and 6 months of age
    c. Infants between 6 months and 1 year of age
    d. Female infants born to white mothers
    e. Breast-fed infants

92. Which of the following findings is highly suspicious for child abuse?
    a. Retinal hemorrhage
    b. Periduodenal hematoma
    c. Metaphyseal fracture of the distal femur
    d. Posterior rib fractures
    e. All of the above

93. "Chain of custody" refers to:
    a. Documentation of continuity of custody of laboratory specimens

b. Enzymatic chemical reactions from substrate to product

c. Handling of children younger than 18 years of age by a care provider

d. Police obtaining custody of specimens involved in legal disputes

94. Which fluid is the best source for postmortem alcohol analysis?
    a. Intracardiac blood
    b. Vitreous fluid
    c. Urine
    d. Cerebrospinal fluid
    e. Bile

95. Which statement is true regarding heart measurements during autopsy?
    a. The left cardiac wall thickness should be measured at the heart apex.
    b. The left ventricular wall thickness correlates with septal hypertrophy.
    c. The cardiac wall thickness is not affected by formalin fixation.
    d. The left and right ventricular walls have similar thickness.
    e. The left ventricular wall thickness should be measured 1–2 cm below the mitral annulus.

96. Rigor mortis results from:
    a. Cross-linking of actin and myosin
    b. Falling levels of muscle glycogen
    c. Loss of body temperature
    d. Pooling of blood with gravity
    e. "Agonal" muscle contraction

97. Adipocere is:
    a. Dissolution of fat within the abdominal cavity
    b. Caused by *Clostridium perfringens*
    c. Related to insect activity
    d. An equivalent term to "maceration"

98. This wound (Fig. 1.23) is an example of a:
    a. Surgical incision
    b. Direct stab wound
    c. Blunt force
    d. Defense wound
    e. Motor vehicle accident

99. This wound (Fig. 1.24) is caused by a:
    a. Contact gunshot with the gun pressed against the skin
    b. Suicide gunshot

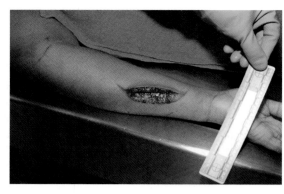

Figure 1.23

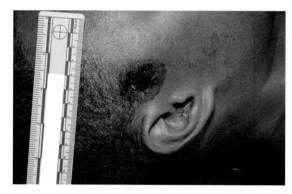

Figure 1.24

    c. Noncontact gunshot within 5 feet
    d. Pellet gunshot

100. This wound (Fig. 1.25) is caused by a:
    a. Suicide injury
    b. Gunshot within 2 feet
    c. Gunshot between 2–5 feet
    d. Distant gunshot (>5 feet)
    e. Bullet exiting the body

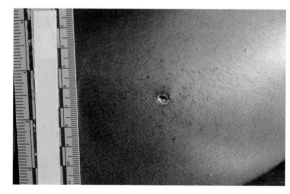

Figure 1.25

■ Answers

1. **d. Cell injury** can be caused by physical agents such as extremes of temperature, chemical agents such as drugs and toxins, infectious organisms, immunologic agents, and deficiency of nutrients and oxygen to the cells such as in monoxyhemoglobinemia. ATP is a natural substance that plays a role in energy, metabolism, and cell survival.

2. **e.** Cell death occurs by apoptosis or oncosis (cell swelling). **Pyknotic**, karyolytic, and karyorrhectic nuclei are examples of irreversible processes that occur with cell death. Other processes such as formation of membrane myelin figures, cytoplasmic vacuolization, swelling of endoplasmic reticulum, and mitochondrial densities can be found in reversible cell injury.

3. **c. Apoptosis** is an irreversible process that is triggered by increased TNF and a p53/bcl2 ratio and is not usually associated with inflammation. It can be blocked (but not reversed) by apoptosis inhibitor proteins such as **survivin**. It may occur as normal physiologic or pathologic processes as seen in hepatitis or graft-versus-host disease (immunologic injury).

4. **c.** Intracellular proteolysis is carried out by the caspases, which can be classified into procaspases such as caspase 8 or 9 and effector caspases such as caspase 3. Activation of caspase 3 is a late event in apoptosis.

5. **c. Hyperplasia** involves cell division, is part of the tissue response in wound healing, and may be accompanied by an increased MIB-1 proliferation index. On the other hand, hypertrophy occurs in nondividing cells and may show polyploidy. Both hyperplasia and hypertrophy are influenced by cytokines and growth factors.

6. **c. Squamous metaplasia** of the bronchial epithelium can be caused by intubation trauma, chronic bronchitis, vitamin A deficiency, and damage due to smoking.

7. **a.** Cells of certain carcinomas forming papillary structures tend to calcify, forming tiny gritty calcified bodies called **psammoma bodies**. Corpora amylacea is a glycogen-like material with attached phosphate and sulfate groups and occurs in aging brains and in the prostate. Hypercalcemia and metastatic calcifications can occur in sarcoidosis but sarcoid granulomas do not usually have central necrosis or calcifications. Gamna Gandy bodies are organized and fibrotic deposits of hemosiderin in the spleen caused by hemorrhage. Kimmelstiel-Wilson lesions contain basement membrane material deposited in the glomeruli of diabetic patients.

8. **b. Telomerase** enzyme adds nucleotides to the end of chromosomes and is important in cell aging. It is absent in most nondividing somatic cells but is **up-regulated** in cancer cells, stem cells, and dividing germ cells.

9. **c.** Mutations of the DNA helicase gene (WRN gene) occur in Werner syndrome, possibly accounting for the **increased cell aging**. Accelerated aging is also seen in Cockayne syndrome, Bloom syndrome, and progeria.

10. **a. Vasodilatation** leads to increased hydrostatic pressure and increased vascular permeability. Vasodilatation is induced by histamine, serotonin, and bradykinin, which can also cause increased vascular permeability.

11. **a. Histamine** and other mediators produce an immediate effect on venules, leading to vascular leakage. Vascular leakage can also occur by direct injury, in granulation tissue, and in diapedesis.

12. **a.** The image shows leukocyte adhesion and transmigration through a dilated vein in the wall of inflamed appendix. Selectins are involved in rolling and loose adhesion. Firm adhesion (or sticking) is brought about by linking of integrins (CD11a/CD18 forming a heterodimer called LFA-1) and ICAM-1 (member of the immunoglobulin family). PECAM 1 (platelet endothelial cell adhesion molecule 1) is essential for transmigration or diapedesis.

13. **e.** Chemotactic agents for leukocytes are diverse and include bacterial products such as endotoxin lipopolysaccharides and fMLP, complement components C3a, C4a, C5a, thrombin, fibrinolytic breakdown products, chemokines, and leukotrienes. **Prostaglandin A1** as well as several serum factors such as chemotactic factor inactivator (CFI) are actually inhibitors of chemotaxis.

14. **a.** Phagocytosis and chemotactic stimuli (antigen-antibody complexes, complement 5a, TNF) activate leucocytes, leading to increased surface expression of **LFA-1** integrin family and change in their configuration so that they can bind to endothelial ligand, ICAM-1.

15. **a.** This is **histamine** which, when injected, produces acute inflammation with pain and arteriolar dilatation and increased vascular permeability. Histamine is stored in mast cells and platelets.

16. **a.** Chronic granulomatous disease (resulting from X-lined mutation in the NADPH oxidase enzyme [gp91 phox deficiency]), myeloperoxidase deficiency, glutathione reductase deficiency, and Chediak-Higashi syndrome are all primarily defects of phagocytosis and intracellular killing. **Leukocyte adhesion deficiency syndromes** are autosomal recessive conditions characterized by recurrent infections, pneumonia, and sepsis in paradoxical association with neutrophilic leukocytosis. In type I of this disorder, neutrophils lack the cell surface glycoproteins CD11/CD18, resulting in decreased adhesion and motility.

17. **b. NF-κB** is a cytoplasmic molecule that locates to the nucleus to activate genes related to inflammation. PGE1 antagonizes the effect of histamine, serotonin, and other mediators and, unlike PGE2, is classified as an anti-inflammatory agent. Leukocidins produced by staphylococci and protease inhibitors such as alpha-1 antitrypsin also inhibit the effect of inflammation.

18. **a. Serotonin**, similar to histamine, is released by platelets and results in increased vascular permeability and arteriolar dilatation. Unlike histamine, serotonin stimulates fibroblasts and may result in **fibrosis**.

19. b. **Collectins** bind to carbohydrates on surfaces of bacteria and other organisms and activate the classic pathway. Complement components mediate many aspects of acute inflammation, including increased vascular permeability, leukocyte chemotaxis, phagocytosis by neutrophils, and degranulation of mast cells. C3a, C4a, and C5a are anaphylatoxins and can also cause vascular leakage. C3b is also involved in phagocytosis by opsonization.

20. e. Activated **Hageman factor** actives four enzyme cascades: the kinin system, clotting system, fibrinolytic system, and complement.

21. d. Toll-like receptors recognize microbial molecules, such as gram-negative bacterial lipopolysaccharides, peptidoglycans, and bacterial lipoproteins, and in turn activate innate immune response against microbial organisms.

22. e. **Lipoxins** are negative regulators of leukotrienes and inhibit neutrophils chemotaxis. On the other hand, leukotrienes can cause chemotaxis and vasoconstriction while prostaglandin E2 causes vasodilatation.

23. a. **Chemokines** are small, 8–10 KD proteins that include interleukin 8, C-X-C chemokines, and C-C chemokines. The group has chemotactic specificity for leukocytes and also serves as receptors for HIV virus.

24. d. **Nitric oxide** is produced by the enzyme nitric oxide synthase, which uses the substrate L-arginine. It is a free radical but also has important functions in inflammation. It reduces platelet aggregation and leukocyte adhesion and causes vasodilatation. Transferrin and ceruloplasmin are serum protein antioxidants that are also important in the O2-radicals scavenger system.

25. a. Superoxide dismutase, together with catalase, is part of the enzyme system that eliminates free radicals. Superoxide dismutase forms hydrogen peroxide, which is then eliminated by catalase. Superoxide dismutase is an intracellular enzyme found mainly in mitochondria and the cytosol.

26. c. Substance P is released by sensory nerve endings and degranulates mast cells. Mast cells secrete histamine, which causes local vasodilatation. In **triple skin response**, as shown in the picture, a red line appears first because of vasodilatation followed by a red flare spreading to several centimeters from the line. Skin swelling (a wheal) then forms after a few minutes and is caused by vascular leakage. Platelet-activating factor also has versatile function in acute inflammation with possible exception of vasodilatation. It is produced from neutrophils, eosinophils, platelets, vascular endothelial cells, vascular smooth muscle cells, monocyte-macrophages, renal epithelial cells, and mesangial cells.

27. b. **Myofibroblasts** have distinctive features not found in fibroblasts. These include expression of alpha-smooth muscle actin, cytoplasmic fibrils with dense bodies, and extensive gap junctions between cells. These features allow the myofibroblasts to have contractile properties, which are important in wound closure. Myo D1 is protein involved in myogenesis and is not found in myofibroblasts.

28. b. The list of cytokines that induce fibrosis is long and includes platelet-derived growth factor, insulin-like growth factor, fibroblast growth factors, and fibronectin. Fibronectin, although does not induce fibroblasts, plays a secondary role and forms, with fibrin filaments, scaffold, or footholds for epidermal cells and migrating fibroblasts.

29. c. **Eosinophils** are important in the defense against parasites. They differentiate in the bone marrow under the influence of interleukins 5 and 3. Eotaxins 1 and 2 are chemokines that act as chemotactic factors that cause eosinophils to migrate from blood vessels and accumulate in tissue. Eosinophils, similar to neutrophils, can phagocytize and kill bacteria and generate superoxide anions.

30. e. IL-12, produced by macrophages and dendritic cells, is crucial in T-helper lymphocyte response and induction of **delayed hypersensitivity**. γ-Interferon is also a key mediator of delayed-type hypersensitivity and is a powerful activator of macrophages. Platelet-derived growth factor stimulates fibroblast proliferation and collagen synthesis. Other cytokines that play a role in delayed hypersensitivity include IL-2, TNF, lymphotoxin, and chemokines such as IL-8.

31. d. Interleukin (IL) 1 and TNF are **proinflammatory cytokines** that produce fever, inflammation, and tissue destruction when administered to humans. IL-8 is a chemoattractant for neutrophils and causes degranulation. Interferon-γ is also considered a proinflammatory molecule because it augments TNF and induces nitric oxide. Major anti-inflammatory cytokines that control the proinflammatory response include IL-1 receptor antagonist, IL-4, IL-10, and IL-13.

32. i) a. Receptors with intrinsic kinase activity include growth factors such as TGF-alpha, PDGF, c-kit, and insulin. These activate receptor tyrosine kinase, which phosphorylates effector molecules such as phospholipase C-γ and PI-3 kinase.
ii) b. Receptors for many cytokines lack intrinsic tyrosine kinase activity.
iii) e. Seven transmembrane receptors are couples to G-proteins and include receptors for many physiologic peptides and hormones such as epinephrine and vasopressin as well as pharmaceutical drugs. These receptors also involve cAMP.

33. e. Epidermal growth factor, fibroblast growth factor, transforming growth factor, platelet-derived growth factor, and VEGF are major cytokines involved in **wound healing**.

34. i) b. **Proteoglycans** are components of connective tissue, retain water in the interstitial spaces, and are responsible for subcutaneous tissue turgor. Proteoglycans, especially hyaluronic acid, accumulate in patients with severe hypothyroidism "myxedema" and also in the pretibial spaces in patients with Grave

disease. They are also involved in the pathology of joints. ii) e. Interaction between collagen type IV, laminin, nidogen, and another proteoglycan protein named perlecan make up the molecular model of basement membranes. Abnormalities in collagen metabolism can result from defective hydroxylation, defects in cross-linking, digestion by enzymes, or calcification. Homocystinuria results from defective cross-linking of collagen and elastin molecules, which is caused by accumulation of homocysteine. iii) d. Elastin is a complex molecule produced by fibroblasts and smooth muscle cells and shares with collagen the molecular feature of "cross-linking." Fibrillin is a glycoprotein associated with elastin and is particularly abundant in the aorta, periosteum, and lens ligament. Marfan syndrome patients have defects in elastic fibers due to genetic defects in fibrillin synthesis.

35. c. The **angiogenesis** seen in this granulation tissue is formed by interaction of several mediators. Angiopoietins I and II and VEGF are important in early angiogenesis. PDGF and TGF are important in late stages of angiogenesis. Endothelin is a vasoconstrictor and is not mainly involved in angiogenesis.

36. e. Hyaline material in glomerular lesions can result from the accumulation of fibrin, packed collagen or basement membrane, glycosaminoglycans, or amyloid.

37. b. The gastrointestinal tract is commonly affected in **systemic amyloidosis** and hence the rectal mucosa has always been the biopsy site of choice for diagnosis. Several types of tissue can be obtained through rectal mucosa with little pain and minimal risk of infection.

38. e. These two categories of patients are responsible for the majority of **AA amyloidosis** seen nowadays. Other connective tissue disorders and inflammatory bowel disease can also result in secondary amyloidosis. Familial Mediterranean fever is an example of rare familial disease associated with AA amyloidosis. Certain amyloid proteins are found in various pathologic conditions. β-2 amyloid protein (Aβ) is primarily found in patients with Alzheimer disease. Mutated transthyretin molecule is deposited in patients with familial neuropathy, while normal transthyretin molecule is identified in patients with senile cardiac amyloidosis. Carpal tunnel syndrome patients have β-2 microglobulin as the main amyloid protein. Amyloid fibrils have a diameter of 7.5 to 10 nm. In comparison, collagen fibrils are 50 nm in diameter.

39. d. In **celiac disease**, as well as in transplant rejection, the majority of the lymphocytes are of the cytotoxic type, i.e., positive for CD8. Lymphocytic infiltrate, composed mainly of T lymphocytes, also is seen in granulomatous inflammation, type IV hypersensitivity reactions, and acute transplant rejection.

40. d. Severe combined immunodeficiency and other **immune deficiency states** are associated with thymic hypoplasia and lymphocyte depletion. Acquired thymic hypoplasia and involution are also commonly observed in severe infections, malnutrition, and debilitating diseases. In common variable immunodeficiency the thymic lymphoid tissue is hyperplastic and composed of B cells.

41. c. The electron micrograph shows electron dense immune complex deposits, which occur as result of **type III hypersensitivity** reaction. Immune complex-mediated hypersensitivity reactions can occur in "serum sickness," SLE, rheumatoid arthritis, polyarteritis nodosa, and hyperacute renal transplant rejection.

42. b. In hemolytic transfusion reactions, antibodies in the patient's serum react with red blood cell antigens causing activation of complement and assembly of membrane attack complex.

43. c. Immune complex lesions are induced by complement fixing antibodies such as IgG, IgM, and IgA and not by IgE. Although secondary glomerulonephritis can occur in parasitic infections from immune complex deposition, this is induced by other antibodies. Type I and IV reactions can occur as in ruptured hydatid cyst and formation of granulomas against parasites, respectively.

44. i) b. Antibodies against dsDNA and Sm antigen are diagnostic for SLE. By immunofluorescence Anti-ds DNA antibodies are commonly seen as peripheral nuclear staining.
    ii) d. Anticentromere antibody is found in up to 30% of systemic sclerosis patients, especially in cases with CREST syndrome.
    iii) a. Antibodies against SS-A and SS-B ribonuclear proteins are found in 90% of cases of Sjögren syndrome.
    iv) e. Mixed connective disease is characterized by high titers of antibodies to U1RNP.
    v) c. This antibody, against tRNA synthetase, is found in 15%–25% of cases.

45. c. Patients with **XLA** have mutation in BTK gene which is expressed in B lymphocytes and codes for tyrosine kinase (not the receptor). The genetic defect blocks differentiation of pre-B cells into mature B cells. Surface immunoglobulins are not expressed. However, there is normal immunoglobulin gene rearrangement and cytoplasmic immunoglobulins may be expressed in B cells. Patients have low levels of immunoglobulins in the serum and develop repeated bacterial pyogenic infections. The lymphoid tissue is hypoplastic because of absence of B cells. Thus, the tonsils could be atrophic or absent. Patients also do not make neutralizing antibodies against enteroviral infections and thus they may be susceptible to vaccine-associated paralytic poliomyelitis.

46. c. **DiGeorge syndrome** is characterized by T cell deficiency and hence bacterial infections are rare. Although patients have aortic arch anomalies, they are usually brought to medical attention because of hypocalcemic tetany.

47. i) b. ii) b. iii) a. Retroviruses infect T cells (through CD4 receptor). Retroviral *tax* gene is responsible for

viral replication and neoplastic proliferation of lymphocytes through IL-2 autocrine mechanism. EBV infects
B cells.

48. **c.** **Rotavirus** is a common example of dsRNA virus
and causes childhood diarrhea.

49. **c.** This is **aspergillus** with hyphae and fruiting bodies.
Restrictocin, mitogillin, and elastases are important in
the pathogenesis of aspergillus infections.

50. **b.** Shigella and *E. coli* produce a toxin that blocks protein synthesis by cleaving 28S ribosomal RNA. The
target cells of the toxin are glomerular endothelial cells
and tubular epithelial cells. The toxin does not cause
hemolysis of red blood cells.

51. **d.** **Yersinia** organisms are ingested orally and infect
the terminal ileum, causing ulcerative colitis-like ileo-
colitis with mesenteric lymphadenitis and secondary
manifestations of erythema nodosum, polyarthritis, and
septicemia. Pseudomembranes are not formed.

52. **a.** *Cryptococcus neoformans* is present in soil and bird
droppings, and infects through inhalation. This capsulated organism has particular tropism to the central
nervous system and the infection occurs in patients
with AIDS.

53. **b.** **Cytomegalovirus** infects and remains latent in
white blood cells. It causes a variety of conditions in
immunodeficient patients. CMV encephalitis is the
most frequent infection in neonates.

54. **b.** African trypanosomes are extracellular parasites.
Coxiella burnetii, Mycoplasma, and rickettsia are obligate intracellular organisms. Legionella can be intra- or
extracellular. *Borrelia burgdorferi* is a spirochete transmitted from rodents to people by the deer tick and is
the causative agent of Lyme disease.

55. **d.** The image shows a small round cell tumor with
rosettes, which is a **retinoblastoma**. The linear pigment identifies the choroids of the eye. Retinoblastoma
arises from two mutational hits in chromosome 13q14,
"the two-hit hypothesis." The Rb gene, located in this
region, is a tumor suppressor gene that codes for a
105-kDa protein that binds DNA and interferes with
the cell cycle.

56. **c.** Option E represents G_0, which occurs at some point
in G1 phase of the cell cycle. Option C refers to G1/S
phase transition in which Rb protein plays the main
role in cycle regulation. It inhibits mitosis by inhibiting
entry of the cycle into S phase. Option D corresponds
to the beginning of G2 phase, and option A is the beginning of M phase.

57. **c.** p53 protein is a 53-kD protein that controls entry of
the cell into the S phase. Mutations occur mainly as
missense mutations and have the greatest effect when
they occur in the conserved regions II-V of the gene.
APC is another example of tumor suppressor gene that
is normally involved in the regulation of beta-catenin.
Beta-catenin plays an important role in cytoskeletal
proteins. Mutations in APC gene result in familial adenomatous polyposis and colorectal cancer. DCC is an-

other cell molecule that is lost in colorectal cancers and
colonic adenomas.

58. **b.** This is an **intratubular germ cell neoplasia** (IT-
GCN), which is an example of an in situ cancer.
However, it should not be referred to as carcinoma because it is not an epithelial cancer. ITGCN is usually
seen in the testis in a patient with ipsilateral or contralateral germ cell tumor. It can progress to a germ cell
tumor and usually stains with CD117 and PLAP.
Normal adult testis should not stain with these immunostains.

59. **d.** The **NF1** protein has been given the name neurofi-
bromin. The protein is 2485 amino acids and shares
striking homology to rasGAP. Germ line mutations at
the NF1 locus result in multiple abnormal melanocytes
(café-au-lait spots) and benign neurofibromas. Some
patients also develop pheochromocytomas and CNS
tumors. Retinal phakomas are observed in patients with
tuberous sclerosis.

60. **e.** Several forms of **genomic instability** can be observed in general: (1) subtle sequence changes, including base substitutions, deletions or insertions, and
microsatellite instability; (2) alterations in chromosome number (aneuploidy, also termed chromosomal
instability or CIN); (3) chromosome translocations;
and (4) gene amplification. Genomic instability results in increased rate of tumors such as seen in
hereditary nonpolyposis colon cancer syndrome (HN-
PCC) and also in other hereditary cancer syndromes
caused by germline mutations in genes that regulate
DNA fidelity, e.g., Li-Fraumeni syndrome, Nijmegen
breakage syndrome, Bloom syndrome, and ataxia
telangiectasia.

61. **d.** **Anticipation** in genetics refers to the observation
that the severity of a genetic disorder increases with
each generation. This occurs in myotonic dystrophy (a
disease caused by expansion of the CTG repeats to
more than 50 nucleotides).

62. **e.** Allele-specific oligonucleotide assay, ribonuclease
protection assay, and denaturing gradient gel electrophoresis and microarray data can all be used to detect mutations that result in genetic diseases.
Chromosome immunoprecipitation and restriction
fragment length pleomorphism are two techniques that
are not usually used to detect genetic mutations.

63. **d.** **Mitochondrial DNA** is a circular molecule that
is maternally transmitted and codes for cytochromes,
transfer RNA, ribosomal RNA, and ATPase
molecules.

64. **b.** t(14;18)(q32;q21) translocation involving rearrangement of the bcl2 gene is present in 70–90% of
cases of follicular lymphoma. This translocation leads
to **bcl-2** overexpression, which in turn inhibits apoptosis.

65. **c.** Invasive tumors secrete **metalloproteinase** (like
collagenase IV) to degrade the extracellular matrix and
facilitate invasion. These proteins can be secreted by

tumor cells themselves, stromal fibroblasts, or macrophages.

66. **d.** This is the basis of the **"Ames"** test, which is positive in 70%–90% of known chemical carcinogens. The test is based on a strain of *Salmonella typhimurium* that carries a mutant gene making it unable to synthesize the amino acid histidine from the ingredients in its culture medium. The test is inexpensive, easy to use, and invaluable for screening substances in the environment for possible carcinogenicity.

67. **b. Initiation of carcinogenesis** requires proliferating cells so that DNA damage can become heritable and permanent. Initiator carcinogens are usually electron-deficient and hence are "reactive electrophiles" that bind to electron-rich regions of cellular DNA. Promotor carcinogens are chemical carcinogens that do not affect the DNA directly but rather act on initiated cells or cells exposed to initiating carcinogens. TPA, a phorbol ester, is an example of a promotor carcinogen and leads to activation of protein kinase C.

68. **d.** Chronic lymphocytic leukemia is not usually induced by radiation.

69. **b.** Bloom syndrome, ataxia telangiectasia, Fanconi anemia, and xeroderma are syndromes characterized by defective DNA repair that makes patients susceptible to the effect of radon, leading to the development of a variety of solid tumors and leukemias. Cells are more sensitive to radion injury in G2 and M phases and least sensitive in late S phase. Cells with low oxygenation status and low-dividing or non-dividing cells, such as brain and cartilage cells, are less susceptible to radiation.

70. **c.** The ozone layer prevents the sun's UV light from penetrating into earth. The incidence of skin cancer is directly related to sun exposure.

71. **b.** Cigar and pipe smoking are less hazardous than the other habits.

72. **e.** Coronary artery disease is the number one cause of deaths related to cigarette smoking.

73. **d.** Choice "a" refers to Wernicke encephalopathy, which can also occur in the hypothalamus, mammillary bodies, and periaqueductal brain. Memory loss is part of Korsakoff psychosis.

74. **c.** Hepatomegaly is seen in hypervitaminosis A. **Vitamin A deficiency** causes impaired maintenance of specialized epithelia with squamous metaplasia of transitional epithelium and columnar mucus-secreting surfaces. Deficiency of vitamin A and E occurs in conditions that cause fat malabsorption and steatorrhea.

75. **d. Angelman syndrome** is an example of uniparental disomy in which both chromosomes 15 are of paternal origin. The syndrome is characterized by severe mental retardation, seizures, abnormal gait with ataxia, and frequent paroxysms of laughter ("happy puppet syndrome"). Prader-Willi syndrome is another example of uniparental disomy and is due to deletion of the paternal chromosome in 15q11 and re-

sults in mental retardation, short stature, obesity, and hypogonadism.

76. **c. Fragile X syndrome** results from a fragile site in chromosome X. It requires folic acid-deficient lymphocyte culture for its demonstration, but is not commonly related to maternal folic acid deficiency. Prognathism with large ears is seen in adult patients with the disorder. Testicular histology is usually normal.

77. **b. Necrotizing enterocolitis** most commonly occurs in premature infants and can involve any part of the small or large bowel in a patchy or diffuse pattern. It can be complicated by gangrene and perforation of the bowel and is associated with high perinatal mortality.

78. **b. Sacrococcygeal teratoma** is the most common neoplasm of the newborn and is the most common germ cell tumor. Approximately 75% of sacrococcygeal teratomas are mature. Bone and cartilage are often present in both mature and immature teratoma. However, this is an immature cystic teratoma due to the presence of immature neuroepithelial tissue (as seen in Fig. 1.17). Immature teratomas are most likely to harbor malignant foci in the form of a yolk sac tumor.

79. **c. Neuroblastic tumors** represent the most common extracranial malignant solid neoplasms in children and account for 5%–10% of all childhood cancers. The presence of ganglion cells and nests of neuroblasts with neuropil indicate a better differentiated neuroblastic tumor, i.e., ganglioneuroblastoma. This tumor can regress spontaneously or after chemotherapy.

80. **c. Nephrogenic rests** are precursor lesions of **Wilms** tumor and are most commonly seen in bilateral Wilms tumor cases. They can be perilobar (subcapsular) or intralobar in location. Patients with unilateral Wilms tumor and nephrogenic rests are at increased risk of developing Wilms tumor in the contralateral kidney.

81. **d.** Gaucher disease is an autosomal recessive deficiency of the enzyme glucose cerebrosidase (or β–glucosidase). The disease has variable clinical manifestations and pathology. The diagnosis is suspected by identifying Gaucher cells in the reticuloendothelial system. Type 1 Gaucher disease is the most common and does not involve the brain.

82. **a.** The picture demonstrates the flattened facial features characteristic of **oligohydramnios (or Potter) sequence** and result from fetal compression due to oligohydramnios. Positional deformities of the hands and feet, hip dislocation, joint stiffness, and hypoplastic lungs are also seen. Internal anomalies include renal agenesis. Patients usually die of respiratory difficulty resulting from hypoplasia of the lungs.

83. **c.** Birth injuries, congenital anomalies, and infections are the main causes of mortality in infants and newborn children. Malignant neoplasms cause mortality in older children.

84. **e. Alcohol** is the most common and important teratogen in humans. Children with alcohol embryopathy have distinct facial appearance, mental and growth retarda-

tion, facial anomalies, and psychomotor abnormalities. Limb abnormalities occur with exposure to thalidomide.

85. **d.** Malformations emerge as the most important cause of mortality in infants of diabetic mothers and occur at an incidence rate of 6%–9%. Mothers with high HbA1c levels during pregnancy are more prone to give birth to babies with congenital anomalies. Diabetic embryopathy includes congenital heart defects, caudal regression anomaly, renal anomalies, and central nervous malformations. ADAM complex is association of amniotic deformities, adhesions, and mutilation caused by adherent constricted and swallowed amniotic bands.

86. **d.** Mutations in the "patched" gene in chromosome 9q22 are characteristic of **nevoid basal cell carcinoma (Gorlin) syndrome**. In this syndrome, patients have facial anomalies and develop multiple tumors, including basal cell carcinoma and medulloblastoma. Cardiac and ovarian fibromas also occur.

87. **d.** This is the typical histologic feature of **respiratory distress syndrome** with the formation of hyaline membranes. It occurs most commonly in preterm infants, infants of diabetic mothers, and infant delivered by cesarean section. There is also higher incidence in postterm infants.

88. **c.** ABO incompatibility usually results in group O mothers who have IgG antibodies against A or B antigens in infants. The incidence of Rh incompatibility has dramatically decreased in the United States, due to injection of "RhoGAM."

89. **d. Mothers with heterozygous phenylketonuria** may get pregnant and intrauterine damage to their fetuses occurs when high phenylalanine levels in the mother cause teratogenic effects on the brain and other organs of the fetus. Infants with homozygous phenylketonuria are born normal and the brain damage usually occurs later when the child is exposed to food with high phenylalanine content.

90. **c. Cystic fibrosis** affects the exocrine portion of the pancreas and other mucus-secreting glands, resulting in "mucoviscidosis." Damage to pancreatic islets does not develop until late in the disease.

91. **b. SIDS** affects mainly infants between the ages of 2–3 months and up to 6 months of age. It is common in premature black male infants and less common in infants born to white mothers. Overheating, overwrapping, and sleeping on the prone position are associated with high incidence of SIDS. Approximately 10% of SIDS cases are due to inborn error of metabolism.

92. **e. Abusive head trauma** can result in retinal hemorrhage, skull fracture with epidural hematoma, and even epidural hematoma without fracture of the overlying skull. Metaphyseal fractures, posterior rib fractures, scapular fractures, and sternal fractures in infants have high specificity for abuse. Blunt abdominal trauma leading to visceral hematoma is also a common cause of death in fatal child abuse.

93. **a.** Chain of custody refers to documentation of continuity of custody of laboratory specimens from the patient or deceased person to the lab. This is important to maintain in cases of forensic toxicologic specimens and in paternal testing.

94. **b. Vitreous fluid** is the best specimen for alcohol and drug analysis.

95. **e.** Cardiac wall thickness may increase with fixation and should be measured below the mitral annulus. Septal hypertrophy can occur without ventricular wall hypertrophy. The left ventricle is usually thicker than the right ventricle.

96. **a. Rigor mortis** is stiffening of muscle after death secondary to cross-linking of actin and myosin to form actomyosin as ATP levels fall. The process starts 3 hours after death.

97. **b. Adipocere** is postmortem saponification of body fat that happens with immersion. It allows preservation of body features and is due to *Clostridium perfringens*.

98. **d.** These wounds have clean edges and no tissue bridging and are examples of sharp force injury such as surgical incisions and stab wounds. However, the curved shape of the wound makes it unlikely to be caused by surgery. An attacker would not directly stab a victim in the arm. However, the victim while trying to ward off an attacker may incur such "defense wounds." Laceration caused by blunt force results in a wound with abraded edges and tissue bridging. Blunt force can also result in abrasion, contusions, and skin marks simulating the blunt instrument causing the injury.

99. **b.** This wound is a **contact gunshot** with the soot present around the wound and is caused by suicide. Close-contact gunshots with the gun pressed hard against the skin produce "muzzle stamp abrasions" that are not seen in this case.

100. **d.** Contact gunshot wounds, caused by suicide, produce stellate lacerations and "muzzle stamp abrasions" on the skin. Soot and tattooing are present in gun wounds inflicted within 2 feet. Stippling collars are present in wounds inflicted from more than 2 feet (intermediate range). Distant wounds may produce no marks or may have stippling depending on the distance of the gunshot.

■ Recommended Readings

Kumar V, Fausto N, Abbas A. *Robbins and Cotran pathologic basis of disease*, 7th ed. Philadelphia: Saunders, 2004.

Majno G, Joris I. *Cells, tissues, and disease: Principles of general pathology*, 2nd ed. Oxford: Oxford University Press, 2004.

Rutty G. *Essentials of autopsy practice: Current methods and modern trends.* New York: Springer, 2005.

Stocker JT, Dehner LP. *Pediatric pathology*, 2nd ed. Baltimore: Lippincott Williams & Wilkins, 2002.

2

Cytopathology

Peter Kulesza and Isam A. Eltoum

Questions

1. These nuclear changes (Fig. 2.1) are seen in thyroid papillary carcinoma and also in:
   a. Lung carcinoma
   b. Lymphoepithelial carcinomas
   c. Rhabdoid tumor
   d. Alveolar soft part sarcoma
   e. Ewing sarcoma

2. Conventional fluorescence in situ hybridization is useful in detection of all these conditions EXCEPT:
   a. Demonstration of the number of chromosomes
   b. Amplification of genes
   c. Gene translocation
   d. The number of cells in the S-phase of the cell cycle
   e. Detection of viral genomes

3. In DNA content analysis using flow cytometry, which of the following statements is NOT correct?
   a. Diploid content does not exclude malignancy.
   b. Aneuploid content indicates malignancy.
   c. Chromosomal translocations appear as a hyper-diploid peak.
   d. Routine flow cytometry will not detect change of DNA content that is less than 2%.
   e. DNA index reflects degree of tumor aneuploidy.

4. These cytologic changes (Fig. 2.2) are seen in all of these lesions EXCEPT:
   a. Thyroid carcinoma
   b. Ovarian carcinoma
   c. Benign mesothelial lesions
   d. Spindle cell melanoma

5. Which of the following cytologic changes is NOT a common feature of adenocarcinoma?
   a. Fine chromatin
   b. Nuclear hyperchromasia
   c. Prominent nucleoli
   d. Mitosis

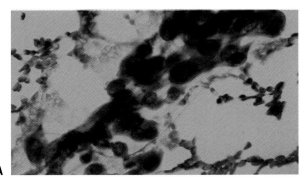

A

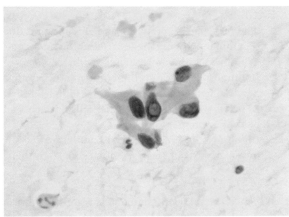

B

Figure 2.1

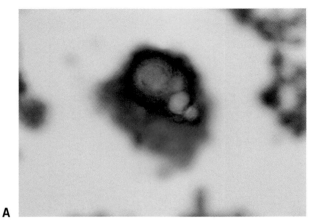

A

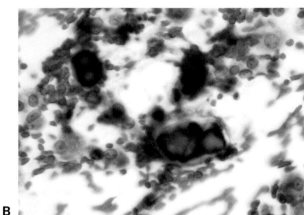

B

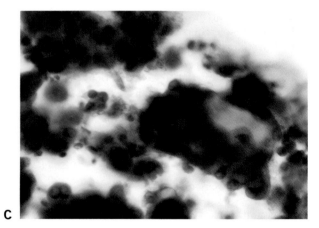

C

Figure 2.2

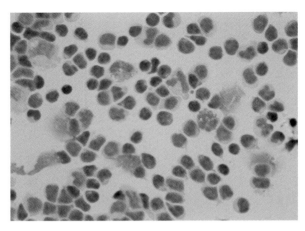

Figure 2.3

c. Prominent nucleoli
d. Hyperchromasia
e. High nuclear–cytoplasmic ratio

8. Increased numbers of lymphocytes in the pleural fluid are seen in:
   a. Empyema
   b. Pneumothorax
   c. Systemic lupus erythematosus
   d. Loeffler syndrome
   e. Parasitic infestation

9. Bronchial cells in pleural fluid may be seen in all of the following conditions EXCEPT:
   a. Bronchopleural fistula
   b. Trauma
   c. Price anomaly
   d. Teratoma
   e. Complication of bronchoscopy

10. All of the following are true about mesothelial cells EXCEPT:
    a. The presence of ectoplasm and endoplasm is due to accumulation of organelles around the nucleus.
    b. Windows are due to large microvilli.
    c. Immunostains for calretinin does not differentiate between benign and malignant mesothelial lesions.
    d. In pelvic washings, mesothelial cells have characteristically prominent nucleoli.
    e. Immunostain with HBME-1 parallels calretinin in sensitivity but lacks specificity for mesothelial cells.

11. Which of the following statements regarding fibrosarcomatous mesothelioma is true?
    a. It is more likely to be associated with asbestos exposure than with epithelioid mesothelioma.
    b. Diagnosis is more frequently established by fine needle aspiration than with fluid aspiration because it rarely presents as pleural effusion.

6. These cells (Fig. 2.3) are seen in pleural fluid in association with all of the following conditions EXCEPT:
   a. Pneumothorax
   b. Small lymphocytic lymphoma (SLL/CLL)
   c. Blood in the pleural space
   d. Hodgkin disease
   e. Acute pulmonary embolism

7. Radiation therapy is often associated with all of the following cellular responses EXCEPT:
   a. Vacuolated cytoplasm
   b. Nuclear pleomorphism

c. In spite of its name, the tumor is often formed of polygonal cells and is sometimes difficult to differentiate from metastatic non-small cell carcinoma.

d. The tumor is frequently CD34 positive and that helps differentiate it from other lesions that resemble it.

e. This tumor carries a better prognosis than epithelioid mesothelioma.

12. Mesothelioma is NOT known to occur:
    a. Following infection with SV40 in human
    b. As a familial disease
    c. Following occupational exposure
    d. In childhood
    e. In females

13. This lesion (Fig. 2.4) is likely to have the following staining pattern in a cell block:
    a. CEA+, EMA+, and MOC-31+
    b. Vacuoles in the cytoplasm stain positively with oil red O but not with mucicarmine
    c. Calretinin +, chromogranin +, and negative with synaptophysin
    d. Calretinin +, mucicarmine +
    e. Cytokeratin +, oil-red O +, and negative with calretinin

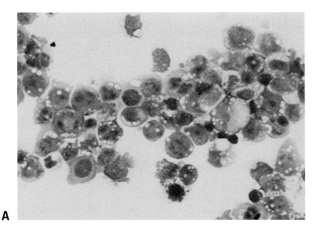

A

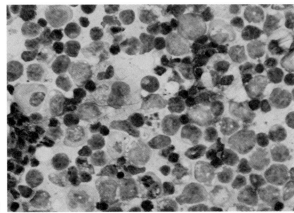

B

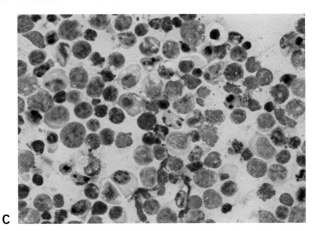

C

Figure 2.5

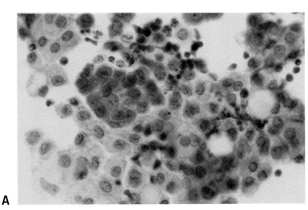

A

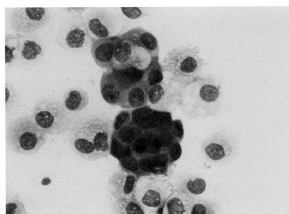

B

Figure 2.4

14. These are photomicrographs of a cytospin of a pleural fluid obtained from a 40-year-old man (Fig. 2.5). All the following viruses have been implicated in association with this lesion EXCEPT:
    a. HSV-8
    b. HIV
    c. EBV
    d. SV40

15. Which of the following statements regarding intrapleural small round cell desmoplastic tumor is true?
    a. Like Merkel cell tumors and small cell carcinoma, it often affects the elderly.

b. Desmoplasia is an essential element and needs to be present to differentiate this lesion from other small round cell tumors.

c. Individual cells are positive for desmin and cytokeratin.

d. Tumor cells are smaller than lymphocytes.

e. It has a characteristic EWS/Fli1 genomic translocation.

16. Features that are helpful to differentiate the above lesion from anaplastic large cell lymphoma include all of the following EXCEPT:
   a. Visible amount of cytoplasm
   b. Lymphoglandular bodies
   c. Nuclear protrusion or cleavage
   d. Prominent nucleoli

17. Anaplastic large cell lymphoma stains with all the following markers EXCEPT:
   a. CD45
   b. CD30
   c. ALK1
   d. CD15
   e. Epithelial membrane antigen (EMA)

18. This is a photomicrograph of a smear of peritoneal fluid obtained from a patient with ascites (Fig. 2.6). This lesion may be caused by all of the following tumors EXCEPT:
   a. Ruptured mucinous cystadenoma of the appendix
   b. Tumors of Meckel diverticulum
   c. Lobular carcinoma of the breast
   d. Mucinous tumor of the ovary
   e. Tumors that express MUC2

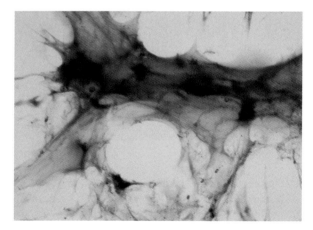

Figure 2.6

19. Features that are helpful in differentiating small lymphocytic lymphoma (SLL/CLL) from reactive lymphocytes in body fluid include all of the following, EXCEPT:
   a. Massive apoptosis
   b. High nuclear-cytoplasmic ratio
   c. Monotony of cells
   d. Conspicuous nucleoli

20. In addition to the above features, CLL/SLL is positive for all of the following markers EXCEPT:
   a. CD20
   b. CD5
   c. CD43
   d. CD23
   e. CD19

21. Which of the following statements about the cerebrospinal fluid (CSF) of neonates is true?
   a. Lymphocytes are more frequent than monocytes.
   b. The presence of choroid plexus is a normal finding.
   c. The specimen should be rejected when there are numerous neutrophils.
   d. Unlike in adults, cell block is the method of choice for processing CSF.
   e. Eosinophils should not be normally present.

22. All of the following statements are true about fine needle aspiration (FNA) procedure EXCEPT:
   a. Small-bore needle (high gauge) is better in obtaining specimens than large-bore needle.
   b. The most common reason for a false-positive diagnosis is an attempt to make a diagnosis in unsatisfactory specimen.
   c. The most common reason for a false-negative diagnosis is sampling error.
   d. The material that is examined through core-needle biopsy is five times that of the material that is examined using FNA.
   e. It can be performed under imaging guidance.

23. FNA is contraindicated in all of the following conditions EXCEPT:
   a. Carotid-body tumor
   b. Kaposi sarcoma
   c. Pheochromocytoma
   d. Echinococcus granulosus infection
   e. Bleeding diathesis

24. Which of the following statements about FNA procedure of the thyroid is true?
   a. Patients are typically asked to swallow while the needle is inside the thyroid to make sure that the needle is in the lesion.
   b. The needle is passed tangentially through the sternocleidomastoid muscle to avoid the great vessels.
   c. The use of a large-bore needle ensures proper sampling.
   d. In general, the best position for sampling is for the patient to lie flat without a pillow.
   e. A lateral approach minimizes the risk of hematoma formation.

25. FNA of the breast has been largely replaced by the core biopsy; however, it is still used:
    a. When the clinical and imaging suspicion is low
    b. For a assessment of chromosome 3 amplification using FISH
    c. For assessment of microcalcification
    d. For ER/PR hormone assessment
    e. When mammography shows a high-density lesion with spiculated appearance

26. This is a photomicrograph of an FNA of a subareolar nodule (Fig. 2.7). This lesion:
    a. Is a metaplastic carcinoma with squamous cell component
    b. Requires no further treatment
    c. Arises in a lactiferous duct
    d. Affects women only
    e. Is fibrocystic disease

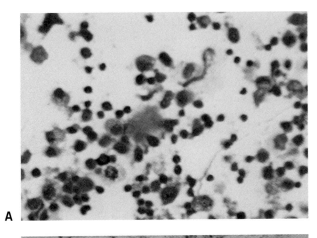

A

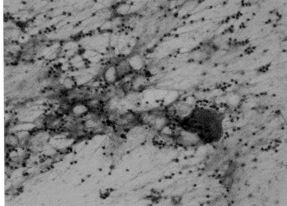

B

Figure 2.7

27. These are photomicrographs of a smear of an FNA of the breast (Fig. 2.8). Each of the following is true about this lesion EXCEPT:
    a. It increases the risk for developing breast cancer twofold.

b. It is frequently seen in a previous biopsy site.
c. Cells are positive for ER/PR but negative for Her2/neu.
d. It is can be clinically confused with cancer but the presence of foam cells is characteristic.
e. It occurs following trauma.

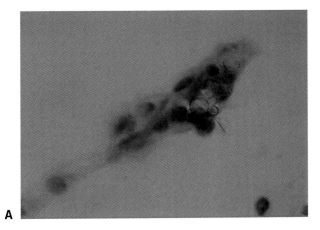

A

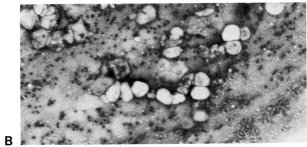

B

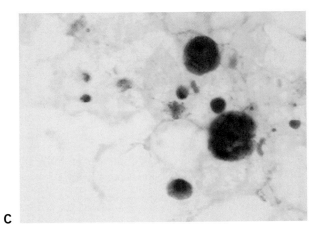

C

Figure 2.8

28. This is a photomicrograph of a smear of an FNA of the breast (Fig. 2.9). This type of tissue fragment is present in all of the following conditions EXCEPT:
    a. Fibroadenoma
    b. Fibrocystic change
    c. Lobular carcinoma
    d. Phyllodes tumor

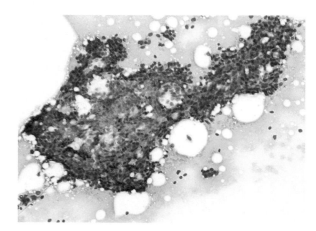

Figure 2.9

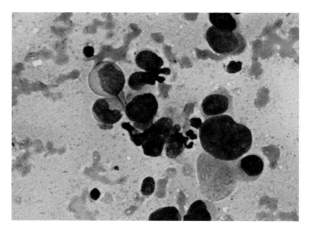

Figure 2.11

29. This is a photomicrograph of a smear of an FNA of the breast (Fig. 2.10). This lesion is most likely a:
   a. Fibroadenoma
   b. Fibrosis
   c. Fibromatosis
   d. Phyllodes tumor
   e. Lobular carcinoma

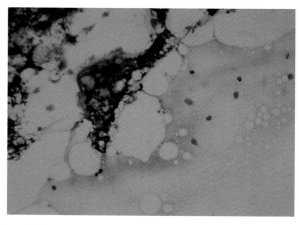

Figure 2.10

30. This is a photomicrograph of a smear of an FNA of the breast (Fig. 2.11). This lesion is most likely a:
   a. Tubular carcinoma
   b. Ductal carcinoma
   c. Lobular carcinoma
   d. Mucinous carcinoma
   e. Fibroadenoma

31. Which of the following will likely establish the malignant nature of a papillary lesion of the breast?
   a. The presence of columnar cells
   b. Excisional biopsy
   c. The presence of necrosis
   d. Needle biopsy
   e. The presence of papillary tissue fragments

32. Each of the following is true about the association of inflammatory cells and breast lesions EXCEPT:
   a. Inflammatory carcinoma and neutrophils
   b. Diabetic mastopathy and lymphocytes
   c. Duct ectasia and plasma cells
   d. Medullary carcinoma and T lymphocytes
   e. Fat necrosis and histiocytes

33. All of the following markers are associated with poor prognosis of breast cancer EXCEPT:
   a. High nuclear grade
   b. High S-phase fraction in DNA ploidy
   c. More than 20% of cells staining for Ki-67
   d. Lack of expression of Her2/neu
   e. Lack of expression of estrogen and progesterone receptors

34. This is a photomicrograph of a smear of an FNA of a thyroid nodule (Fig. 2.12). This lesion is most likely a:
   a. Benign nodular goiter
   b. Hashimoto thyroiditis
   c. Metastatic small cell carcinoma
   d. Small cell variant of anaplastic carcinoma
   e. Papillary carcinoma

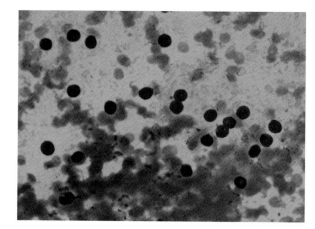

Figure 2.12

35. This is a photomicrograph of a smear of an FNA of a thyroid nodule (Fig. 2.13). This lesion is most likely a:
    a. Follicular variant of papillary carcinoma
    b. Follicular carcinoma
    c. Benign nodular goiter
    d. Endometriosis
    e. Hashimoto thyroiditis

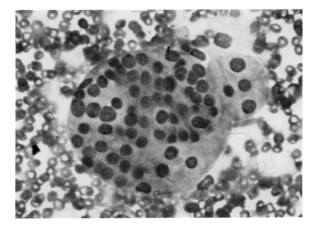

Figure 2.13

36. This is a photomicrograph of a smear of an FNA of a thyroid nodule (Fig. 2.14). These changes are likely to be present in:
    a. Hashimoto thyroiditis
    b. Acute thyroiditis
    c. Thyroid lymphoma
    d. Graves disease

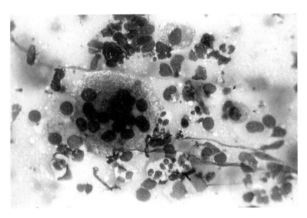

Figure 2.14 (Reproduced with permission from Koss LG, Melamed MR, eds. *Diagnostic cytology and its histopathologic bases*, 5th ed. Baltimore: Lippincott Williams & Wilkins, 2006.)

37. This is a photomicrograph of a smear of an FNA of a thyroid nodule (Fig. 2.15). All of the following statements are true EXCEPT:
    a. Less than 1% develops papillary carcinoma.
    b. More than 20% develop lymphoma.

c. Psammoma bodies have been reported in association with this lesion.
    d. There is a known association with multiple endocrine neoplasia-II.
    e. This lesion can present in children and adolescents.

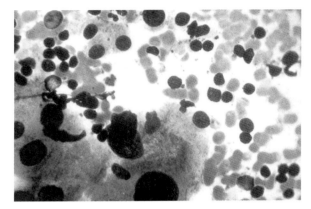

Figure 2.15 (Reproduced with permission from Koss LG, Melamed MR, eds. *Diagnostic cytology and its histopathologic bases*, 5th ed. Baltimore: Lippincott Williams & Wilkins, 2006.)

38. Spindle cells of stromal or epithelial origin can be identified in all of the following thyroid lesions EXCEPT:
    a. Rhabdoid tumor
    b. Papillary carcinoma
    c. Benign nodular goiter
    d. Riedel thyroiditis
    e. Subacute thyroiditis

39. According to the recent NCI guidelines on reporting of thyroid FNA, each of the following statement is true EXCEPT:
    a. FNA diagnosis of benign lesion is associated with <1% rate of malignancy.
    b. FNA diagnosis of malignancy is associated with 100% malignancy.
    c. FNA diagnosis of indeterminate lesion is associated with 10%–15% malignancy.
    d. FNA diagnosis of follicular neoplasm is associated with 80% malignancy.

40. Which of the following thyroid lesions can be differentiated based on cytologic material without much difficulty?
    a. Follicular carcinoma versus follicular adenoma
    b. Hürthle cell carcinoma versus Hürthle cell adenoma
    c. Hashimoto thyroiditis versus lymphoma
    d. Follicular variant of papillary carcinoma versus classic type papillary carcinoma

41. This is a photomicrograph of a smear of an FNA of a thyroid nodule (Fig. 2.16). This type of cell is classically seen in:
    a. Papillary carcinoma of the thyroid
    b. Medullary carcinoma of the thyroid
    c. Hürthle cell carcinoma
    d. Undifferentiated carcinoma
    e. Hurtle cell adenoma

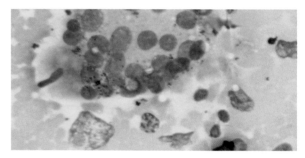

Figure 2.16

42. The following are known features of papillary carcinoma of the thyroid EXCEPT:
    a. Three-dimensional papillary formation
    b. Zymogens granules
    c. Dense cytoplasm
    d. Intranuclear cytoplasmic inclusions
    e. Nuclear grooves

43. In Hürthle cell neoplasm versus Hashimoto thyroiditis, which of the following is INCORRECT?
    a. In Hashimoto thyroiditis, Hürthle cells vary in shape and size and show considerable nuclear changes.
    b. Plasma cells are seen more frequently in Hashimoto thyroiditis.
    c. Presence of transgressing blood vessels favors Hürthle cell neoplasm.
    d. Antithyroid antibody is present in both conditions.
    e. Features of chronic thyroiditis are not seen Hürthle cell neoplasms.

44. All of the following are known variants of thyroid papillary carcinoma EXCEPT:
    a. Small-cell variant
    b. Follicular variant
    c. Columnar variant
    d. Warthin tumor-like variant
    e. Oncocytic variant

45. All of the following statements about thyroid carcinomas are true EXCEPT:
    a. Functioning adenoma is associated with constitutively active adenylcyclase.
    b. Papillary carcinoma is associated with constitutively active MAPK pathway.
    c. Her2/neu amplification is a common event in sporadic papillary carcinoma.

    d. Ret/PTC signaling is a common pathway in radiation-induced papillary carcinoma.
    e. BRAF mutations are detected in 50% of anaplastic carcinoma.

46. Localized amyloidosis in the thyroid gland is known to be associated with:
    a. Hürthle cell neoplasm
    b. Functioning adenoma
    c. Medullary carcinoma
    d. Papillary carcinoma
    e. Follicular carcinoma

47. These are photomicrographs of a smear of an FNA of a neck lesion (Fig. 2.17). This lesion is LEAST likely to be:
    a. Thyroglossal duct cyst
    b. Benign nodular goiter
    c. Branchial cleft cyst
    d. Squamous cell carcinoma

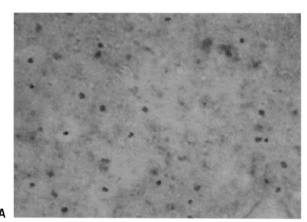

A

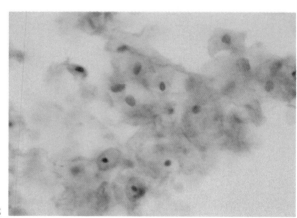

B

Figure 2.17

48. These are photomicrographs of a smear of an FNA of an enlarged lymph node (Fig. 2.18). Differential diagnosis may include all of the following EXCEPT:
    a. Reactive lymph node
    b. Sinus histiocytosis with massive lymphadenopathy
    c. Small cell lymphoma (SLL/CLL)
    d. Classical Hodgkin lymphoma
    e. Castleman disease

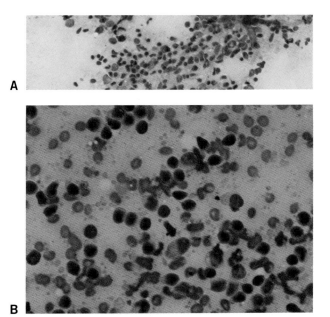

Figure 2.18

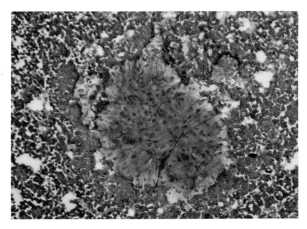

Figure 2.20

49. This is a photomicrograph of a smear of an FNA of an intra-abdominal nodule (Fig. 2.19). Which of the following staining pattern is likely to be positive if this lesion is a plasmacytoma, as compared with lympho-plasmacytic lymphoma?

a. High molecular weight keratin
b. S100
c. CD19
d. PLAP
e. CD138

51. This is a photomicrograph of a smear of an FNA of an enlarged lymph node (Fig. 2.21). Which of the following is true about this lesion?

a. Electron microscopy shows Birbeck granules.
b. It regresses spontaneously.
c. CD-1a is frequently positive.
d. Mycobacterium species can be demonstrated using sensitive methods such as polymerase chain reaction (PCR).
e. It is seen in postvaccinal lymphadenitis.

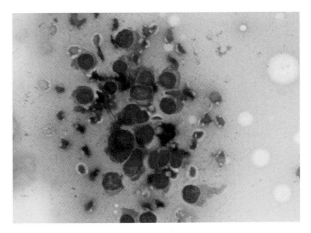

Figure 2.19

50. This is a photomicrograph of a smear of an FNA of a submandibular nodule (Fig. 2.20). The most likely diagnosis is:

a. Lymphoepithelial lesion
b. Epithelioid granuloma
c. Epithelioid sarcoma
d. Warthin tumor
e. Reactive lymph node

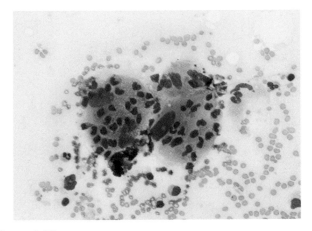

Figure 2.21

Questions 52–54:
This is a photomicrograph of a smear of an FNA of an enlarged lymph node (Fig. 2.22).

52. The differential diagnosis includes all the following EXCEPT:

a. Mantle cell lymph node
b. Small cell lymphoma
c. Follicular lymphoma, grade 2 of 3
d. Lymphoplasmacytic lymphoma
e. Lymphoblastic lymphoma

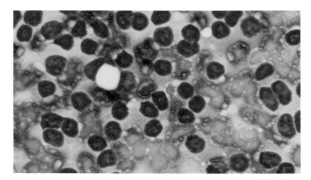

Figure 2.22

53. All of the following immunostaining patterns are likely EXCEPT:
    a. CD19+, CD5+, CD23−
    b. CD19+, CD5+, CD23+
    c. CD19−, CD5−, CD10−
    d. CD19+, CD5−, CD10−

54. This is a photomicrograph of FISH staining for 11q13 (red) and 14q32 (blue) (Fig. 2.23). The diagnosis is:
    a. Lymphoplasmacytic lymphoma
    b. Small cell lymphoma
    c. Mantle cell lymphoma
    d. Follicular lymphoma, grade 2
    e. Lymphoblastic lymphoma

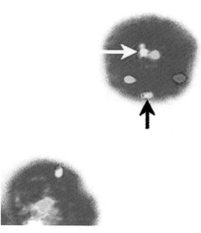

Figure 2.23 (Reproduced with permission from Koss LG, Melamed MR, eds. *Diagnostic cytology and its histopathologic bases*, 5th ed. Baltimore: Lippincott Williams & Wilkins, 2006.)

55. This is an FNA of mediastinal lymph node from a 25-year-old man (Fig. 2.24). This lesion is positive for all the following markers EXCEPT:
    a. Tdt
    b. Low molecular weight cytokeratin
    c. CD45
    d. MIC-2 (CD99)
    e. CD20

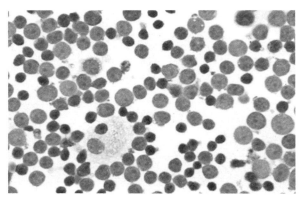

Figure 2.24 (Reproduced with permission from Koss LG, Melamed MR, eds. *Diagnostic cytology and its histopathologic bases*, 5th ed. Baltimore: Lippincott Williams & Wilkins, 2006.)

56. This is an FNA of mediastinal lymph node from a 41-year-old woman (Fig. 2.25). This lesion is likely to be positive for:
    a. MOC-31
    b. MART-1
    c. Calretinin
    d. CD38
    e. CD30

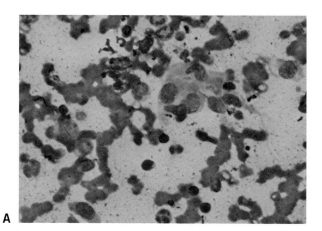

A

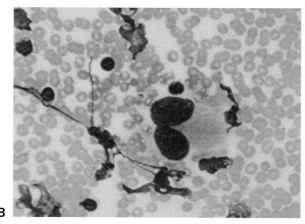

B

Figure 2.25

57. This is an FNA of mediastinal nodule of a 70-year-old woman (Fig. 2.26). All of the following statements are true about the pattern of staining EXCEPT:
    a. CK7+CK20− pattern supports the diagnosis of metastatic breast carcinoma.
    b. CK7+CK20+ pattern supports the diagnosis of metastatic pancreatic carcinoma.
    c. CK7+CK20+ pattern supports the diagnosis of hepatocellular carcinoma.
    d. CK7−CK20+ pattern supports the diagnosis of metastatic colon carcinoma.
    e. CK7+CK20− pattern supports the diagnosis of serous ovarian carcinoma.

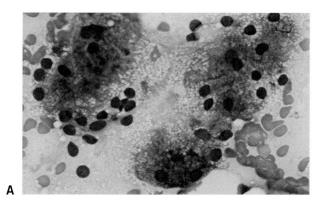

A

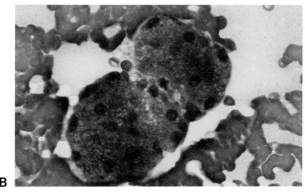

B

Figure 2.27

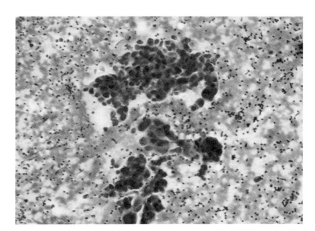

Figure 2.26

58. This is an FNA of a nodule in the upper right side of the neck (Fig. 2.27). The most likely diagnosis is:
    a. Normal salivary gland
    b. Metastatic renal cell carcinoma, clear cell type
    c. Granular cell tumor
    d. Warthin tumor
    e. Tuberculous lymphadenitis

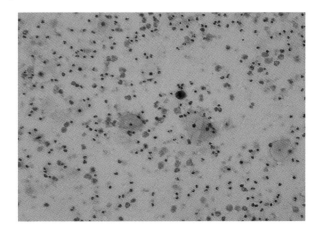

Figure 2.28

59. This is a fine needle aspiration of a bilateral cystic lesion at the angle of the jaw of a 27-year-old man (Fig. 2.28). This lesion most likely is:
    a. Sjögren disease
    b. HIV-related change
    c. Mumps
    d. Mucoepidermoid carcinoma
    e. Branchial cleft cyst

60. This is a fine needle aspiration of a submandibular lesion (Fig. 2.29). The most likely diagnosis is:
    a. Pleomorphic adenoma
    b. Acinic carcinoma
    c. Basal cell adenoma
    d. Adenoid cystic carcinoma
    e. Rhabdomyosarcoma

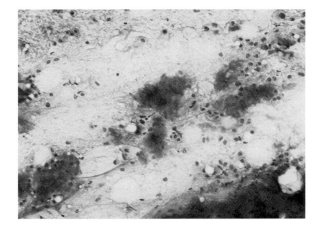

Figure 2.29

61. This is a fine needle aspiration of a submandibular lesion (Fig. 2.30). The most likely diagnosis is:
    a. Pleomorphic adenoma
    b. Acinic carcinoma
    c. Salivary gland large duct carcinoma
    d. Adenoid cystic carcinoma
    e. Mucoepidermoid carcinoma

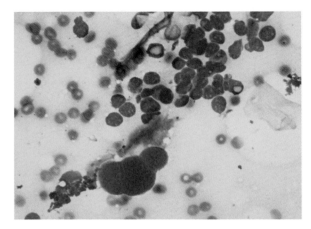

Figure 2.30

62. This is a fine needle aspiration of a submandibular lesion (Fig. 2.31). The most likely diagnosis is:
    a. Pleomorphic adenoma
    b. Acinic carcinoma
    c. Mucoepidermoid carcinoma
    d. Adenoid cystic carcinoma
    e. Dermoid cyst

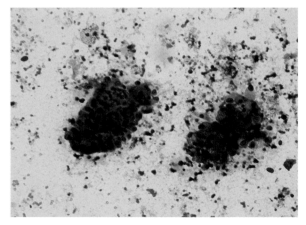

Figure 2.31

63. Lymphoid background is frequently seen in all of the following conditions EXCEPT:
    a. Warthin tumor
    b. Epithelial-myoepithelial carcinoma
    c. Acinic carcinoma
    d. Sjögren disease
    e. Lymphoepithelial cyst

64. Granulomatous inflammation can be seen in all of the following conditions EXCEPT:
    a. Hodgkin lymphoma
    b. Seminoma
    c. Subacute thyroiditis
    d. Melanoma
    e. Scrofula

65. Soft tissue tumors that show chromosomal translocations involving the EWS gene include all of the following EXCEPT:
    a. Desmoplastic small blue cell tumor
    b. Rhabdomyosarcoma
    c. Extra-skeletal myxoid chondrosarcoma
    d. Clear cell sarcoma
    e. Ewing sarcoma

66. In cytology of small blue cell tumors, all of the following are true EXCEPT:
    a. The presence of large cells favors rhabdomyosarcoma.
    b. The presence of small cytoplasmic fragments favors lymphoma.
    c. The presence of melanin pigment favors Merkel cell carcinoma.
    d. The presence of cytoplasmic vacuoles favors Ewing sarcoma.
    e. The presence of karyorrhexis and pyknosis favors neuroblastoma.

67. This is a micrograph of an FNA of intra-abdominal lesion in a 37-year-old man (Fig. 2.32). This lesion is characterized by:
    a. Inactivation of CDKN2
    b. t(x:18) translocation
    c. Strongly positive C-kit immunostaining
    d. Positive immunostain for muscle-specific actin (MSA)
    e. Positive staining for myogenin

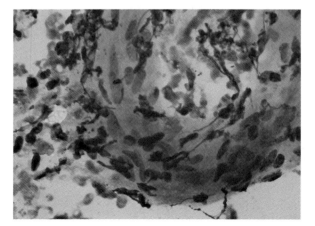

Figure 2.32

68. This is an FNA for the distal femur of a 20-year-old man (Fig. 2.33). Possible predisposing factors in this case include all of the following EXCEPT:
    a. Chronic osteomyelitis
    b. Paget disease of bone
    c. Fibrous dysplasia
    d. Radiation

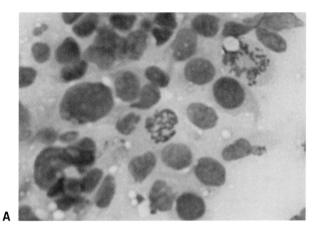

A

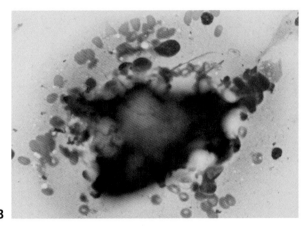

B

Figure 2.33

69. A 25-year-old woman had an osteolytic pelvic bone lesion with a sharply demarcated edge. A smear from the lesion yielded predominantly blood. This lesion is most likely:
    a. Osteosarcoma
    b. Aneurysmal bone cyst
    c. Chondroblastoma
    d. Chondromyxoid fibroma
    e. Chondrosarcoma

70. This is an FNA from a 60-year-old man with an osteolytic lesion in the femur (Fig. 2.34). This lesion is:
    a. Osteosarcoma
    b. Chondrosarcoma
    c. Chondromyxoid fibroma
    d. Chondroblastoma
    e. Giant cell tumor

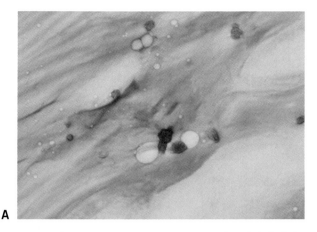

A

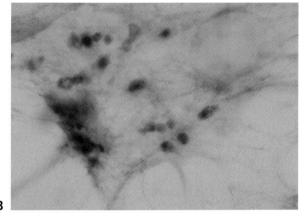

B

Figure 2.34

71. This is an FNA from a 30-year-old man with a well-demarcated osteolytic lesion in the upper part of the tibia (Fig. 2.35). This lesion is:
    a. Chondroblastoma
    b. Aneurysmal bone cyst
    c. Osteoid osteoma
    d. Giant-cell tumor
    e. Langerhans cell histiocytosis

72. This is an FNA from a 3-year-old man with an ill-defined tibial lesion (Fig. 2.36). Electron microscopy will show:
    a. Interdigitating axonal process
    b. Primary melanosomes
    c. Myosin filaments
    d. Microvilli
    e. Whorls of intermediate filaments

73. This is an FNA of a peri-esophageal lesion from a 70-year-old man (Fig. 2.37). Special stains that are likely to be positive are:
    a. HMB45
    b. CD34
    c. CD68
    d. CD99
    e. Cam 5.2

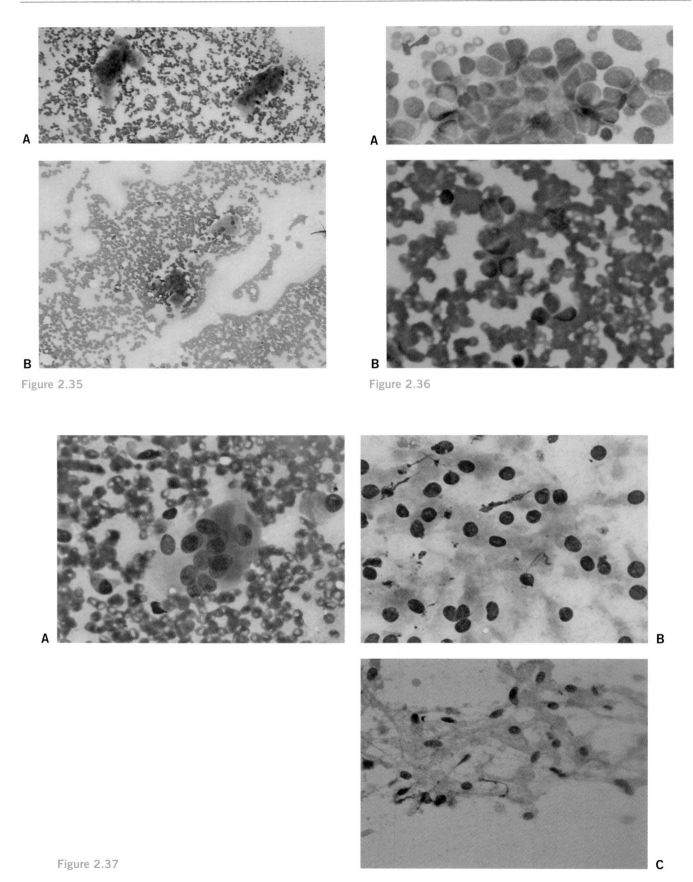

Figure 2.35

Figure 2.36

Figure 2.37

74. This is an FNA from a 40-year-old woman with a mediastinal mass, muscle weakness, and a long history of tobacco abuse (Fig. 2.38). The most likely diagnosis is:
   a. Small cell carcinoma
   b. Hodgkin disease
   c. Thymoma
   d. Benign lymph node
   e. Squamous cell carcinoma of the lung

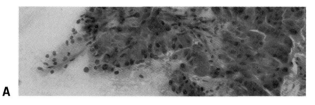

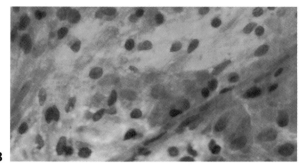

A

B

Figure 2.39

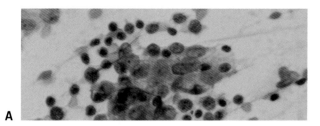

A

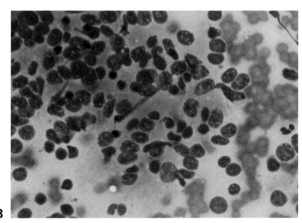

B

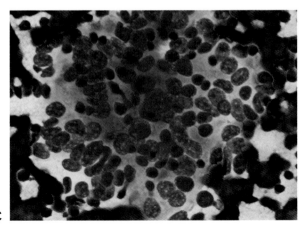

C

Figure 2.38

76. This is a cellblock from a spleen FNA from a 35-year-old man with HIV from Mississippi (Fig. 2.40). The FNA shows:
   a. Histoplasma duboisii
   b. Toxoplasma gondii
   c. Leishmania donovani
   d. Candida albicans
   e. None of the above

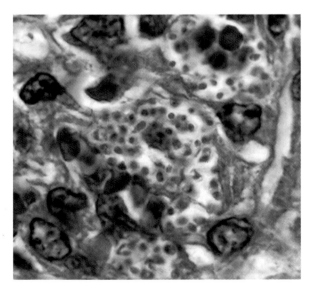

Figure 2.40 (Reproduced with permission from Koss LG, Melamed MR, eds. *Diagnostic cytology and its histopathologic bases*, 5th ed. Baltimore: Lippincott Williams & Wilkins, 2006.)

75. This is an FNA from a 70-year-old man with a liver mass (Fig. 2.39). This patient most likely has elevated levels for:
   a. Serotonin
   b. CEA19
   c. Alpha-fetoprotein
   d. Placental alkaline phosphatase

77. Which of the following statements about lymphocytic pancreatitis is true?
   a. The pathognomonic features can be demonstrated on routine cytologic smears.
   b. It may be associated with ulcerative colitis.

c. It is often associated with high levels of IgG2a.

d. It presents with marked uniform dilation of the main pancreatic duct.

e. Lymphocytes are mainly B-cell type.

78. Which of the following statements about intraductal papillary mucinous neoplasm is true?

a. Immunostains for trypsin is positive.

b. The main duct and side branches are frequently spared.

c. The presence of mucin in the background is diagnostic.

d. Correct diagnosis can only be made when the cytologic findings are correlated with imaging.

e. It compromises 40% of all pancreatic cancers.

79. This is an FNA of pancreatic mass in a 60-year-old man (Fig. 2.41). The most likely diagnosis is:

a. Chronic pancreatitis

b. Pancreatic carcinoma

c. Intraductal papillary mucinous neoplasm

d. Acinar carcinoma

e. Pancreatic cyst

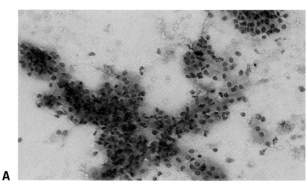

A

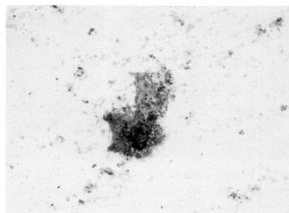

B

Figure 2.41

80. This is an FNA of pancreatic mass in a 50-year-old woman (Fig. 2.42). The most likely diagnosis is:

a. Acinic carcinoma

b. Ductal carcinoma

c. Pancreatoblastoma

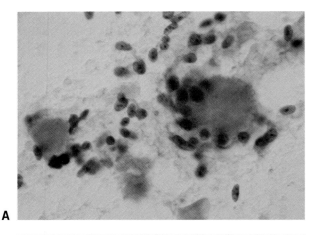

A

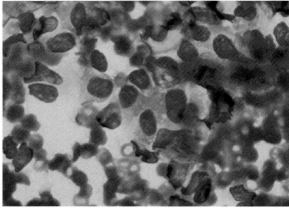

B

Figure 2.42

d. Neuroendocrine neoplasm

e. Intraductal mucinous tumor

81. This is an FNA of a renal mass in a 70-year-old man (Fig. 2.43). The most likely diagnosis is:

a. Chromophobe carcinoma

b. Clear cell carcinoma

c. Chromophil carcinoma

d. Medullary carcinoma

e. Angiomyolipoma

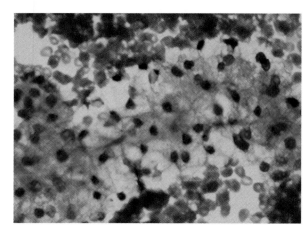

Figure 2.43

82. This is an FNA from a patient with a history of non-small cell carcinoma and an adrenal mass (Fig. 2.44). The diagnosis is:
   a. Metastatic melanoma
   b. Hepatocellular carcinoma
   c. Pheochromocytoma
   d. Myelolipoma
   e. Neuroblastoma

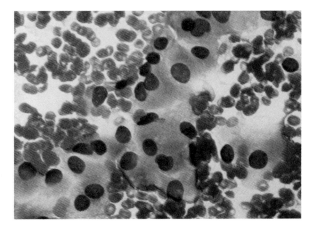

Figure 2.44

83. A 20-year-old man had a retroperitoneal mass with no lesions found elsewhere. An endoscopic ultrasound-guided FNA (EUS-FNA) revealed large pleomorphic cells with variable number of nucleoli and mitosis. A Diff-Quick air-dried smear revealed a characteristic mottling background in a "tigroid" pattern. The most likely diagnosis is:
   a. Primary retroperitoneal seminoma
   b. Intra-abdominal desmoplastic tumor
   c. Mesothelioma
   d. Ganglioneuroma
   e. Desmoid tumor

84. This is a fine needle aspiration of a peri-orbital mass in a 5-year-old boy (Fig. 2.45). The most likely diagnosis is:
   a. Retinoblastoma
   b. Granulocytic lymphoma

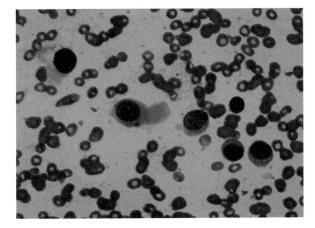

Figure 2.45

   c. Rhabdomyosarcoma
   d. Reactive intra-orbital lymphoid tissue
   e. Melanoma

85. This is an intra-operative smear of a frontal lobe mass form a 60-year-old man (Fig. 2.46). The most likely diagnosis is:
   a. Metastatic carcinoma
   b. High-grade astrocytoma
   c. Medulloblastoma
   d. Oligodendroglioma
   e. Ependymoma

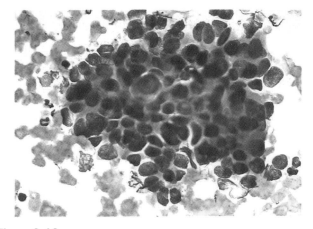

Figure 2.46

86. Which of the following is true about alcohol fixation?
   a. Laboratory needs a special license to use ethanol as a fixative.
   b. Alcohol fixatives are better for cytoplasmic details than air-dried specimen.
   c. Similar concentrations of methanol, ethanol, and isopropyl alcohol can substitute each other as fixatives.
   d. Fixation of smear more than 15 minutes will create excessive artifacts and render the specimen unsatisfactory.
   e. Alcohol fixatives contain oxidizing agents that cross-link proteins.

87. All of the following solutions can be used to get rid of red blood cells in cytologic preparation EXCEPT:
   a. Carnoy fixative
   b. RPMI
   c. Cyto-Rich-Red fixative
   d. 2 Molar urea solutions

88. The best diagnosis of this cervical smear (Fig. 2.47) is:
   a. Negative for intraepithelial lesion or malignancy
   b. Atypical squamous cells of undetermined significance
   c. Low-grade squamous intraepithelial lesion
   d. High-grade squamous intraepithelial lesion

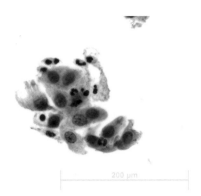

Figure 2.47

89. The best diagnosis of this cervical smear (Fig. 2.48) is:
    a. Negative for intraepithelial lesion or malignancy
    b. Atypical squamous cells of undetermined significance
    c. Low-grade squamous intraepithelial lesion
    e. High-grade squamous intraepithelial lesion

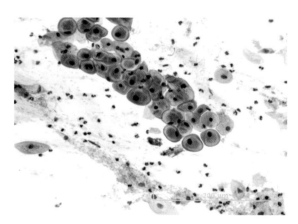

Figure 2.48

90. The best diagnosis of this cervical smear (Fig. 2.49) is:
    a. Negative for intraepithelial lesion, malignancy, or *Trichomonas vaginalis*
    b. Atypical squamous cells of undetermined significance
    c. Low-grade squamous intraepithelial lesion
    d. High-grade squamous intraepithelial lesion

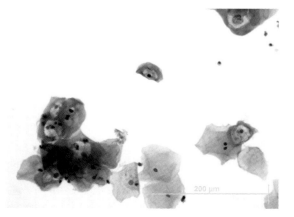

Figure 2.49

91. The best diagnosis of this cervical smear (Fig. 2.50) is:
    a. Negative for intraepithelial lesion or malignancy
    b. Atypical squamous cells of undetermined significance
    c. Low-grade squamous intraepithelial lesion
    d. High-grade squamous intraepithelial lesion

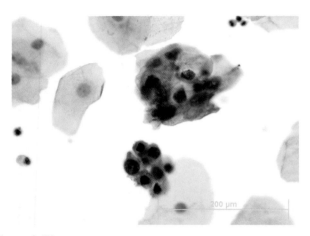

Figure 2.50

92. The best diagnosis of this cervical smear (Fig. 2.51) is:
    a. Negative for intraepithelial lesion or malignancy
    b. Atypical squamous cells of undetermined significance
    c. Low-grade squamous intraepithelial lesion
    d. High-grade squamous intraepithelial lesion

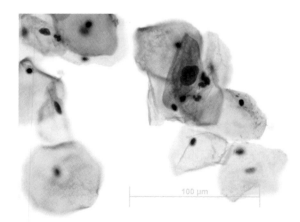

Figure 2.51

93. The patient had invasive squamous cell carcinoma of the cervix 6 months ago. The best diagnosis of this cervical smear (Fig. 2.52) is:
    a. Atypical glandular cells (AGS)
    b. Endocervical carcinoma in situ (AIS)
    c. High-grade squamous intraepithelial lesion (HSIL)
    d. Atypical squamous cells, cannot exclude HSIL (ASC-H)
    e. Negative for intraepithelial lesion or malignancy

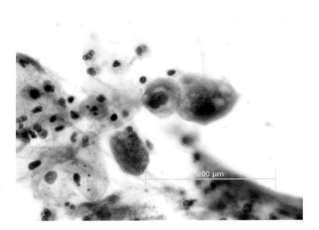

Figure 2.52

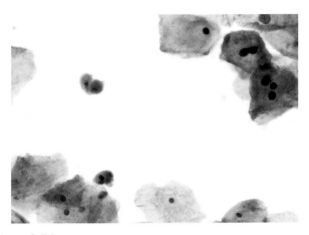

Figure 2.54

94. The best diagnosis of this cervical smear obtained 95 days after LMP (Fig. 2.53) is:
   a. Atypical glandular cells (AGS)
   b. Endocervical carcinoma in situ (AIS)
   c. High-grade squamous intraepithelial lesion (HSIL)
   d. Atypical squamous cells, cannot exclude HSIL (ASC-H)
   e. Negative for intraepithelial lesion or malignancy

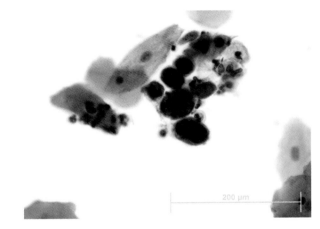

Figure 2.55

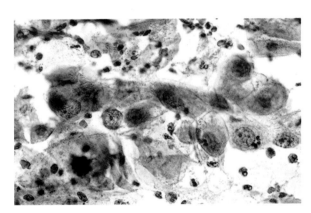

Figure 2.53

95. The best diagnosis of this cervical smear (Fig. 2.54) is:
   a. Candida albicans
   b. Chlamydia trachomatis
   c. Atypical squamous cells of undetermined significance
   d. Trichomonas vaginalis

96. The best diagnosis of this cervical smear (Fig. 2.55) is:
   a. High-grade squamous intraepithelial lesion (HSIL)
   b. C. trachomatis
   c. Herpes simplex
   d. CMV
   e. Atypical glandular cells (AGS)

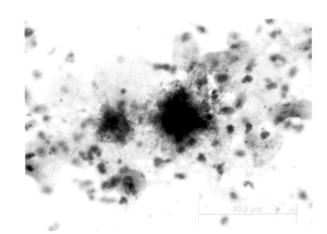

Figure 2.56

   c. Actinomyces
   d. Leptothrix

97. The best diagnosis of this cervical smear (Fig. 2.56) is:
   a. Nocardia
   b. Mucus strands

98. The best diagnosis of this cervical smear (Fig. 2.57) is:
   a. Atypical glandular cells (AGS)
   b. Endocervical carcinoma in situ (AIS)
   c. High-grade squamous intraepithelial lesion (HSIL)

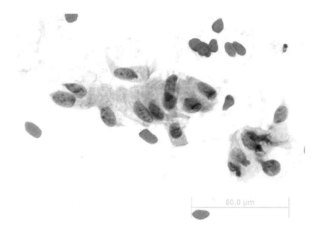

Figure 2.57

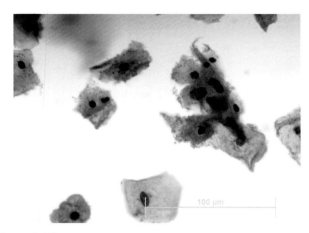

Figure 2.59

d. Atypical squamous cells, cannot exclude HSIL (ASC-H)
e. Negative for intraepithelial lesion or malignancy

99. The best diagnosis of this cervical smear (Fig. 2.58) is:
a. Negative for intraepithelial lesion or malignancy
b. Atypical squamous cells of undetermined significance (ASC-US)
c. Low-grade squamous intraepithelial lesion (LSIL)
d. High-grade squamous intraepithelial lesion
e. Squamous cell carcinoma

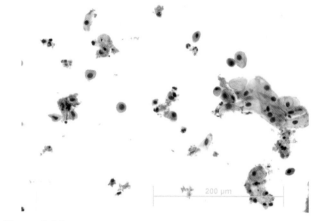

Figure 2.60

c. Low-grade squamous intraepithelial lesion (LSIL)
d. High-grade squamous intraepithelial lesion
e. Squamous cell carcinoma

102. The best diagnosis of this voided urine specimen (Fig. 2.61) is:
a. Negative for malignancy
b. Atypical urothelial cells, cannot exclude urothelial neoplasm

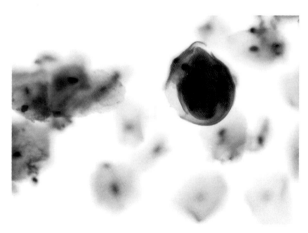

Figure 2.58

100. The best diagnosis of this cervical smear (Fig. 2.59) is:
a. Negative for intraepithelial lesion or malignancy
b. Atypical squamous cells of undetermined significance (ASC-US)
c. Low-grade squamous intraepithelial lesion (LSIL)
d. High-grade squamous intraepithelial lesion
e. Squamous cell carcinoma

101. The best diagnosis of this cervical smear (Fig. 2.60) is:
a. Negative for intraepithelial lesion or malignancy
b. Atypical squamous cells of undetermined significance (ASC-US)

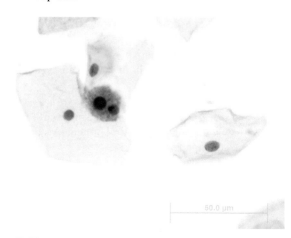

Figure 2.61

c. Low-grade urothelial carcinoma
d. High-grade urothelial carcinoma

103. The best diagnosis of this voided urine specimen (Fig. 2.62) is:
   a. Benign urothelial cells
   b. Atypical urothelial cells, cannot exclude urothelial neoplasm
   c. Low-grade urothelial carcinoma
   d. High-grade urothelial carcinoma

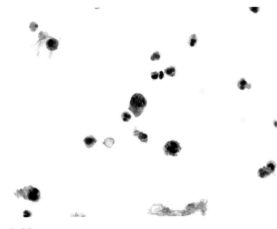

Figure 2.62

104. The best diagnosis of this voided urine specimen (Fig. 2.63) is:
   a. Benign urothelial cells, suggestive of cystitis glandularis
   b. Polyoma virus infection
   c. Urothelial papilloma
   d. High-grade urothelial carcinoma

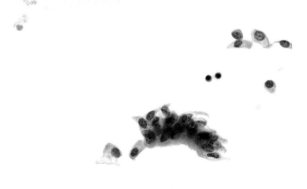

Figure 2.63

105. The best diagnosis of this voided urine specimen (Fig. 2.64) is:
   a. Benign urothelial cells
   b. Atypical urothelial cells, cannot exclude urothelial neoplasm
   c. Low-grade urothelial carcinoma
   d. High-grade urothelial carcinoma

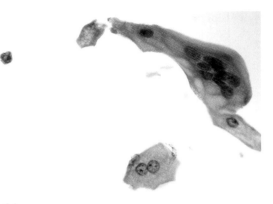

Figure 2.64

106. The best diagnosis of this voided urine specimen is (Fig. 2.65):
   a. Benign urothelial cells
   b. Atypical urothelial cells, cannot exclude urothelial neoplasm
   c. Low-grade urothelial carcinoma
   d. High-grade urothelial carcinoma

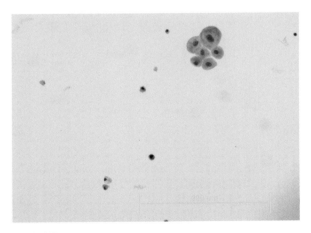

Figure 2.65

107. The best diagnosis of this bronchoalveolar lavage specimen (Fig. 2.66) is:

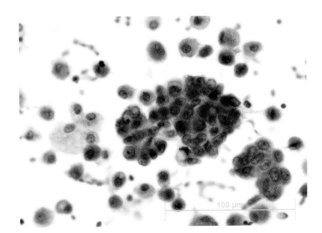

Figure 2.66

a. Lipid pneumonia
b. Specimen insufficient for diagnosis
c. Bronchioloalveolar carcinoma
d. Reactive type II pneumocytes
e. Aspiration pneumonia

108. The best diagnosis in this bronchoalveolar lavage specimen (Fig. 2.67) is:
a. Lipid pneumonia
b. Specimen insufficient for diagnosis
c. Pneumocystis carinii
d. Atypical epithelial cells, cannot exclude non-small cell carcinoma
e. Histoplasma capsulatum

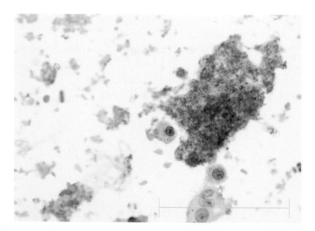

Figure 2.67

109. This specimen is a bronchoalveolar lavage from a lung transplant patient (Fig. 2.68). The best diagnosis is:
a. Lipid pneumonia
b. Specimen insufficient for diagnosis
c. Pneumocystis carinii
d. Atypical epithelial cells, cannot exclude non-small cell carcinoma
e. Histoplasma capsulatum

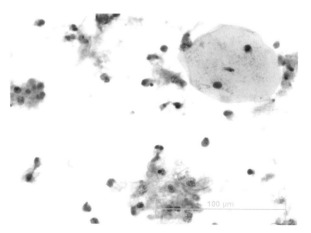

Figure 2.68

110. Which of the following should be performed on the cell block of this sputum (Fig. 2.69)?
a. pancytokeratin, CD3, CD20, CD45
b. S100, CD56, CD68, MART-1
c. CD56, CD45, pan-cytokeratin, chromogranin
d. chromogranin, synaptophysin, Tag72, MOC-31

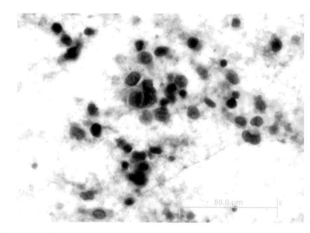

Figure 2.69

111. The most likely outcome of the patient with this lung FNA (Fig. 2.70; specimen shows air-drying artifact) is:
a. Surgery and cure
b. Surgery and recurrence
c. Palliative care, less than 5% survival at 5 years
d. Chemo-radiation, 75% survival at 5 years
e. Antibiotics and cure

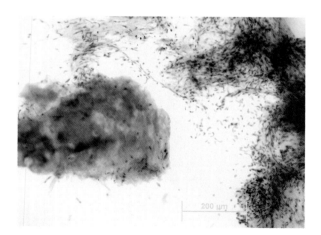

Figure 2.70

112. The most likely outcome of the patient with this lung mass FNA specimen (Fig. 2.71) is:
a. Surgery and cure
b. Surgery, chemotherapy, and recurrence
c. Chemotherapy, 40% survival at 2 years
d. Chemotherapy–radiation, 80% survival at 5 years

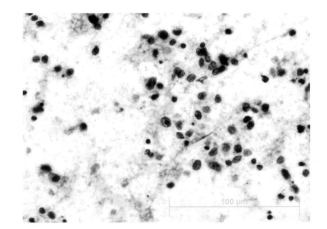

Figure 2.71

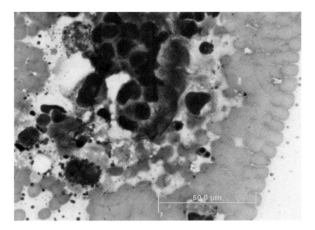

Figure 2.73

113. Which of the following statements is the best description for this transthoracic lung FNA specimen (Fig. 2.72)?
   a. Positive TTF-1, synaptophysin, and chromogranin (all three) are diagnostic for lung primary.
   b. This lesion is almost certainly malignant if necrosis and high mitotic index are present.
   c. The patient may be suffering from progressive leg weakness.
   d. Hodgkin lymphoma is in the differential diagnosis.

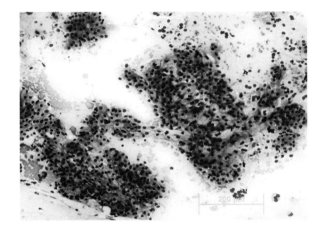

Figure 2.74

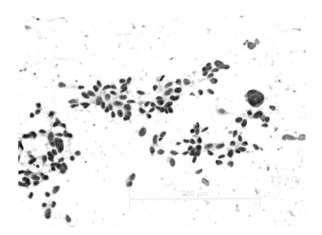

Figure 2.72

114. The best diagnosis for this transthoracic lung FNA specimen (Fig. 2.73) is:
   a. Benign, reactive changes
   b. Granulomatous inflammation, cannot rule out sarcoidosis or tuberculosis (TB)
   c. Non-small cell carcinoma
   d. Kartagener syndrome
   e. Atypical metaplasia

115. The best diagnosis of this pancreatic mass FNA (Fig. 2.74) is:
   a. Adenocarcinoma
   b. Atypical ductal epithelial cells, suspicious for adenocarcinoma

   c. Benign epithelial cells
   d. Small intestinal contamination

116. The best diagnosis of this pancreatic EUS FNA (Fig. 2.75) is:
   a. Small intestinal contamination
   b. Atypical epithelial cells, favor reactive

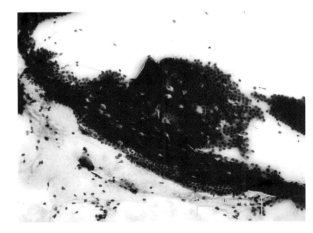

Figure 2.75

c. Adenocarcinoma
d. Chronic pancreatitis
e. Contaminating gastric epithelium

117. The best diagnosis of this cervical smear specimen (Fig. 2.76) is:
  a. Atypical glandular cells (AGS)
  b. Endocervical carcinoma in situ (AIS)
  c. High-grade squamous intraepithelial lesion (HSIL)
  d. Atypical squamous cells of undetermined significance, cannot exclude HSIL (ASC-H)
  e. Negative for intraepithelial lesion, malignancy, or tubal metaplasia

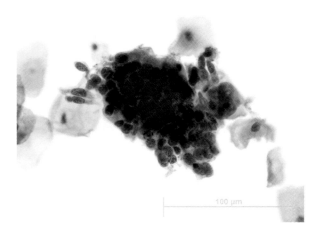

Figure 2.76

118. The best course of action after having reviewed this BAL specimen (Fig. 2.77) is:
  a. Perform Fontana-Masson to rule out melanoma
  b. Order cell block, and then order TTF-1 and Tag72 to rule out non-small cell carcinoma
  c. Perform PAS-D to make sure the structure is composed of mucin
  d. Page the clinician
  e. Perform iron stain to rule out remote pulmonary hemorrhage

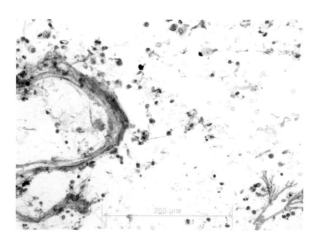

Figure 2.77

119. The best diagnosis of this bronchoalveolar lavage specimen (Fig. 2.78) is:
  a. Cytomegalovirus infection (CMV)
  b. Lipid pneumonia
  c. Alveolar proteinosis
  d. Atypical epithelial cells, cannot exclude non-small cell carcinoma
  e. Histoplasma capsulatum

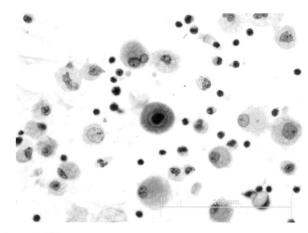

Figure 2.78

120. The best diagnosis of this biliary brushing (Fig. 2.79) is:
  a. Benign intestinal epithelium (contamination)
  b. Inadequate specimen
  c. Dysplasia in inflammatory background of primary sclerosing cholangitis
  d. Stent atypia
  e. Cholangiocarcinoma

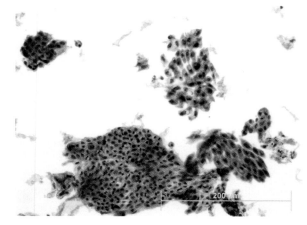

Figure 2.79

121. Which of the following statements is true?
  a. The chromocenter and the nucleolus are round structures.
  b. Multiple nucleoli occur only in malignant cells, but enlarged nucleoli can be found in both malignant and reactive cells.

c. The chromocenter includes mainly DNA, whereas nucleolus mainly RNA.

d. Due to tissue fragility, "bare nucleoli" are commonly seen in smears of hepatocellular carcinoma.

e. The chromocenter includes mainly RNA, whereas the nucleolus mainly DNA.

122. The feature most strongly indicative of malignancy in a discohesive cytology specimen is:
   a. Nuclear hyperchromasia
   b. Nuclear enlargement
   c. Nuclear border (membrane) irregularity
   d. Nuclear grooves
   e. Oval or spindle nuclear shape

123. The presence of "clue" cells in a cervical smear is important to note because:
   a. They are diagnostic of pathogenic bacterial vaginosis
   b. They have been associated with a 10-fold increased risk for LSIL
   c. They may prompt treatment for meningitis
   d. They require a follow up culture in postmenopausal patients

124. The molecular process responsible for malignant transformation in HPV-related cervical lesion is thought to be:
   a. E7 mediated stabilization of p53 leading to chromosomal instability
   b. E7 binding of bcl-2 leading to lack of apoptosis
   c. E7 binding of Rb protein leading to abrogation of cell cycle checkpoints
   d. E7 binding of T-cell cytokine IL-2 leading to immune tolerance

125. Which of the following statement is most appropriate regarding immunostaining for the tumor suppressor $p16^{INK4a}$?
   a. Increased staining for p16 indicates HSIL or carcinoma
   b. Increased staining for p16 is seen in squamous, but not adenocarcinoma of the cervix
   c. Negative staining for p16 means loss of tumor suppressor function, and is diagnostic of HSIL and carcinoma
   d. Increased staining for p16 supports HPV-related dysplasia
   e. Immunostaining for p16 is a marker for immature squamous metaplasia

126. Vaccines for prevention of cervical carcinoma have been more successful than for pancreatic carcinoma because:
   a. Adjusted for stage, pancreatic carcinoma has 5- to 10-fold shorter survival.
   b. Unlike cervical carcinoma, almost all pancreatic carcinomas have no expression of class I MHC.

c. Vaccines for cervical carcinoma rely on specific anti-viral responses.

d. Unlike the cervix, the pancreas is an immune-privileged site, such that T-cell cytotoxic response is limited.

127. The two widely used liquid-based methods for cervical smear preparation are ThinPrep (made by Cytyc) and SurePath or Autocyte (made by TriPath). Which of the following statement is true?
   a. Filter method (ThinPrep) may lead to clogging, and hypocellular slides in specimens containing blood and debris.
   b. SurePath samples cannot be used for HPV testing due to "open" container design.
   c. The "clustering" or "trailing" of abnormal cells is preserved on ThinPrep method.
   d. Both methods result in increase in cellular size compared to conventional PAP smears, leading to potential false increase in ASCUS diagnosis.

128. Maturation Index in cervical smears correlates to hormonal status of the patient. A change from 0:90:10 to 90:10:0 is most compatible with:
   a. Normal menstrual cycle
   b. Delivery
   c. Development of endometrial carcinoma in post-menopausal patient
   d. Hysterectomy

129. Which of the following features is most suggestive in differentiating HSIL from invasive nonkeratinizing squamous cell carcinoma in cervical specimens?
   a. Prominent nucleoli
   b. High N/C ratio
   c. Marked hyperchromasia
   d. Background of red cells

130. Which of the following is the most accurate statement about cervical screening tests?
   a. Because Pap smear is a cervical test, a pathologist cannot be liable for not detecting endometrial carcinoma.
   b. The current data indicate that liquid-based HPV testing is equivalent to morphologic analysis for normal, reactive, ASC-US up to and including LSIL diagnoses.
   c. It is more important not to miss HSIL than LSIL.
   d. It is more important not to miss LSIL than ASC-US.

131. Which of the following statements is INCORRECT?
   a. Cervical dysplasia samples are likely to be positive for more than one viral type in the same specimen.
   b. The hybrid capture II test detects HPV type 16.
   c. According to TBS2001, an adequate Liquid-Based cervical specimen should have an estimated minimum of at least 12,000 well preserved squamous cells.
   d. The main benefit of liquid-based preparations is a smaller area available for interpretation.

132. HPV types 16 and 18 have been classified as oncogenic, or "high-risk" viral types. Which of the following statements is most accurate?
  a. Type 18 is associated mainly with squamous cell carcinoma and type 16 mainly with adenocarcinoma.
  b. Koilocytosis is sufficient evidence of infection by high-risk HPV.
  c. Most of invasive cervical squamous carcinoma cells contain integrated HPV genome.
  d. Most untreated type 16 or 18 HPV infection will result in development of high-grade lesions (HSIL).

133. The hybrid capture test (commercially available as Digene II) relies upon:
  a. Hybridization of DNA probe to viral RNA, binding of antibody to the DNA-RNA hybrid, measurement of light emitted by the bound antibody
  b. Hybridization of antibody to viral DNA, washing of the unbound antibody, measurement of light emitted by the hybrid DNA-antibody
  c. Hybridization of RNA probe to viral DNA, binding of antibody to the RNA-DNA hybrid, measurement of light emitted by the bound antibody
  d. Denaturation of the specimen to form single-strand DNA, hybridization of labeled DNA probe, measurement of light emitted by the (viral-probe) DNA-DNA hybrid

134. The ALTS study offered support for which of the following statements?
  a. Hybrid capture assays should be performed on LSIL samples to rule out low-risk infection.
  b. The chance of HSIL in patients with negative HPV tests is very low.
  c. Positive HPV test in patients with ASCUS should prompt a re-screen for HSIL.
  d. HPV testing has higher specificity in women below the age of 30 compared to morphologic (cervical smear) diagnosis.

135. Which of the following statements best characterizes the consensus guidelines based on the Bethesda System 2001?
  a. Specimen with less than three ASCUS cells and less than 500 (total) squamous cells should be reported as "Unsatisfactory for evaluation due to scant cellularity."
  b. Patients with ASC-H, LSIL, and HSIL should undergo colposcopy.
  c. The presence of benign endometrial cells should be reported in all patients with history of abnormal uterine bleeding.
  d. The term HSIL encompasses moderate and severe dysplasia (CIN II and III) but not carcinoma in situ.

136. The most common differential diagnosis of a de novo AGC (AGUS NOS) diagnosis is:
  a. HSIL
  b. Adenocarcinoma

  c. LSIL
  d. Reactive squamous metaplasia

137. The strongest evidence of LSIL in a cervical smear is provided by:
  a. Numerous squamous cells with mild karyomegaly
  b. 5 to 10 squamous cells with moderate karyomegaly and hyperchromasia
  c. 5 to 10 squamous cells with dense, "hard" green cytoplasm
  d. 5 to 10 binucleated squamous cells

138. Endocervical adenocarcinoma in cervical specimens is characterized by:
  a. Frequent abnormal mitoses bodies and cellular debris
  b. Large, prominent nucleoli
  c. Palisading cells with large, hyperchromatic nuclei and apoptotic bodies
  d. Lack of rosetting and columnar glandular cells with loss of polarity.

139. In a patient with abnormal uterine bleeding, which cytologic finding on a routine cervical smear is most suspicious for endometrial carcinoma:
  a. Marked acute inflammation and debris
  b. Single cells with high N/C ratio, vacuoles, and prominent nucleoli
  c. Large clusters of polarized cells with enlarged nuclei
  d. Markedly enlarged squamoid cells with large hyperchromatic nuclei, and rare cytoplasmic vacuoles

140. Which finding is most worrisome for malignancy in peri-operative pelvic washings?
  a. Psammoma bodies
  b. Dense sheets of cells with small nucleoli
  c. Large three-dimensional clusters
  d. Small papillary clusters with occasional vacuoles

141. The adequacy of bronchoalveolar lavage is determined by the presence of:
  a. Neutrophils
  b. Type I pneumocytes
  c. Macrophages
  d. Ciliated bronchial cells
  e. Pigmented macrophages

142. Which of the following statements is most appropriate for a lymphocytic pleural effusion?
  a. If more than 90% of cells are CD20 positive, it should be regarded as lymphoma until proven otherwise.
  b. In a benign process, the majority of cells are CD20 positive B cells.
  c. T cell-rich effusions are not associated with occult carcinomas.
  d. T cell-rich effusions are rare, and occur almost exclusively in pediatric population.

143. The finding of multinucleated, polarized syncytial cells in bronchial washings is most consistent with:
    a. Sarcoidosis
    b. Reactive response of bronchial cells to injury
    c. Small cell carcinoma
    d. Bronchioloalveolar carcinoma (BAC)

144. Which finding in a sputum or bronchial washing specimen is most worrisome for carcinoma?
    a. Multinucleation
    b. Yellow or orange cytoplasm and evenly hyperchromatic nucleus
    c. Squamous pearls
    d. Intranuclear inclusions

145. The feature which best separates small cell carcinoma from lymphoma on smear specimens is:
    a. More pronounced crush artifact in lymphoma
    b. Minimal nuclear membrane irregularity of small cell carcinoma cells on PAP stain
    c. Absence of molding of lymphoma cells on DiffQuik stain
    d. Absence of nucleoli in lymphoma cells

146. Which finding in a voided urine specimen is most worrisome for malignancy?
    a. Multinucleated epithelial cells
    b. Urothelial fragments
    c. Small cells with high N/C ratio and hyperchromasia
    d. Large cells with dark, glassy nucleus

147. Eosinophilia is most closely associated with an allergic process in which of the following specimens?
    a. Pleural effusion
    b. Bronchial washings
    c. Pelvic washings
    d. Paratracheal lymph node FNA

148. In a sputum specimen of immunocompromised patients, which finding is of immediate clinical significance?
    a. Squamous pearls
    b. Oxalate crystals
    c. Curschmann spirals
    d. Corpora amylacea

149. Which of the following is the most accurate statement regarding sputum cytology?
    a. Specimens without macrophages are sufficient for evaluation.
    b. Finding of roundworms should prompt FLOW cytometric analysis of blood.
    c. Curschmann spirals are pathognomonic for an allergic process.
    d. Bronchorrhea is associated with primary lung adenocarcinoma.

150. Features which distinguish small cell carcinoma from atypical carcinoid include:
    a. Mitoses
    b. Necrosis

    c. Nucleoli and delicate cytoplasm
    d. Powdery "salt and pepper" chromatin

151. Which of the following statements is most appropriate for voided urine specimens?
    a. Urothelial fragments with irregular borders are diagnostic for low-grade carcinoma.
    b. Papillary urothelial fragments with fibrovascular cores are diagnostic for low-grade neoplasms.
    c. Urothelial fragments with increased N/C ratios, and eosinophilic cytoplasmic granules are indicative of intravesical therapy with Mitomycin C.
    d. Enlarged cells with coarsely vacuolated, fraying cytoplasm, prominent nucleoli, and indistinct nuclear outlines are suspicious for low-grade carcinoma.

152. Which of the following best describes the current state of detection of urothelial carcinoma?
    a. Urinary cytology for patients presenting with hematuria is effective in diagnosis of low-grade carcinoma.
    b. Cytoscopically-guided biopsy has higher specificity than voided urine cytology for diagnosis of flat high-grade carcinoma in patients presenting with hematuria.
    c. Papillary urothelial carcinoma can be detected with similar sensitivity and specificity in cytologic specimens as in biopsies.
    d. A cytologic diagnosis of high-grade carcinoma followed by a benign cystoscopically-guided biopsy should result in aggressive follow-up.

153. Which of the following statements is most accurate about diagnosis of pulmonary alveolar proteinosis?
    a. Sputum specimens show pathognomonic granular proteinaceous debris.
    b. BAL specimens show sterile, marked neutrophilic infiltrate.
    c. Foamy macrophages in BAL are usually PAS-D positive.
    d. BAL and sputum specimens show numerous desquamated type II pneumocytes.

154. The differential diagnosis of bronchioloalveolar carcinoma should NOT include:
    a. Creola bodies
    b. Clusters of type II pneumocytes
    c. Large single cells with vacuolated cytoplasm
    d. Small cells with fine chromatin and high N/C ratio

155. Which of the following statement is true about specimens obtained by endoscopic ultrasound-guided FNA?
    a. The sheathing of the needle effectively precludes contaminants from nonlesional tissue.
    b. Core biopsies can be procured at the time of the procedure with minimal increase in morbidity.
    c. It is useful for staging of patients with non-small cell lung carcinoma.
    d. It cannot be used for surveillance of patients with primary sclerosing cholangitis.

156. Which of the following features is most consistent with adenocarcinoma in biliary brushings?
    a. Loss of organization in large sheets of cuboidal epithelium
    b. Hyperchromasia and markedly prominent nucleoli
    c. Cleared chromatin on PAP stain and nuclear membrane irregularity
    d. Crowded glandular epithelial sheets with distinct cytoplasmic vacuoles

157. Which of the following statements is most appropriate about the differential diagnosis of gastric ulceration?
    a. Flat epithelial sheets and numerous single cells support a benign process.
    b. Nuclear and nucleolar enlargement favors a malignant process.
    c. Aspirin gastritis can be very easily misdiagnosed as carcinoma.
    d. Necrosis, nuclear atypia, and presence of single cells are diagnostic for carcinoma.

158. Features that are shared between biliary and pancreatic adenocarcinoma include:
    a. Marked hyperchromasia
    b. Atypical glandular formations on PAP-stained slides which are PAS-D negative
    c. Chromatin with clearing and clumping
    d. Presence of naked nuclei on smear slides from FNA

159. Which of the following statement about endoscopic ultrasound-guided FNA (EUS-FNA) of gastric masses is true?
    a. Spindle cell tumors are more common than in other anatomic sites.
    b. The finding of spindle cells is almost certainly diagnostic of Schwannoma if GIST and leiomyosarcoma have been ruled out.
    d. Differential diagnosis of GIST does not include infiltrating gastric adenocarcinoma.
    e. If a spindle cell lesion is S100 and c-kit negative, GIST can be ruled out.

▨ Answers

1. **a.** The presence of **cytoplasmic nuclear inclusions** is one of the features of papillary carcinoma but has been seen in other conditions of the thyroid, including Hashimoto thyroiditis and medullary carcinoma. It also has been reported in other non-thyroid diseases including lung carcinoma, melanoma, hemangioendotheliomas, hepatocellular carcinoma, pleomorphic adenoma, and other lesions as well.

2. **d.** Fluorescence in situ hybridization does not detect the S-phase of the cell cycle. S-phase can be determined using flow cytometry.

3. **c.** A quantitative method of **ploidy** expression is the DNA index (DI), which is the ratio of the mean tumor cells at G0/G1. The DNA content of normal diploid reference cells is 1. The greater the deviation of the DI from 1, the more "aneuploid" the tumor. Flow cytometry for DNA content does not detect chromosomal translocations. Translocations can be detected by FISH analysis or PCR for the chimeric gene or transcripts.

4. **d.** These are **psammoma bodies** which are laminated calcific concretions seen frequently in papillary carcinomas including that of thyroid, ovary, endometrium, and kidney. They are commonly seen in meningiomas and in benign mesothelial hyperplasia. They are not known to occur in melanoma. Osteopontin protein has been reported to be involved in formation of psammoma bodies. Nanobacteria, a new controversial class of organisms, have been suggested as a possible cause.

5. **b.** **Adenocarcinoma** generally shows fine chromatin and sometimes chromatin clearing. The other listed features are common in adenocarcinoma.

6. **b.** **Pleural fluid eosinophilia** is seen in pneumothorax, thoracentesis, pleural biopsy or surgery, introduction of blood in the pleural space (from infarction or trauma), and a few malignancies including Hodgkin disease. Pleural fluid eosinophilia is not a known feature of SLL/CLL.

7. **d.** **Radiation** can lead to numerous cellular changes including pleomorphism, nucleoli and hyperchromasia. Radiation is, however, associated with low nuclear- cytoplasmic ratio. This is one of the features that help differentiate it from dysplasia/neoplasia.

8. **c.** Systemic lupus erythematosus is associated with **pleural fluid lymphocytosis.** Empyema causes neutrophilia, while Loeffler syndrome, parasites, and pneumothorax cause eosinophilia.

9. **c.** **Price anomaly** is a congenital disorder in which there is sequestration of part of the lung. It does not usually communicate with the pleural cavity. The other conditions are known to shed bronchial cells in the pleura.

10. **d.** In pelvic washing the **mesothelial cells** nuclei and nucleoli are not particularly prominent as these sells are not shed in an effusion which generally induces reactive changes including prominent nuclei and formation of cell balls.

11. **b.** This is a true mesothelial lesion and does not generally express CD34. This type of mesothelioma has the worst prognosis of all other histologic types. It can be confused with metastatic non-small cell carcinoma. This lesion does not shed cells in fluid.

12. **a.** Mesothelioma association with SV40 beyond doubt has not been established in humans.

13. **b.** This is true **mesothelioma.** Vacuoles in mesothelioma are positive for oil red O (which stains fat) but not mucicarmine (which stains mucin). Currently, calretinin, thrombomodulin, WT1 gene product, and keratin 5/6 are considered the best antibodies for the identification of mesothelial differentiation. It is generally advised that, in addition to positive "markers," immunostaining panels should also include antibodies which should be negative in mesothelial cells and which may be positive in adenocarcinoma, particularly carcinoembryonic antigen (CEA), Ber EP4, Leu M1, MOC31, or B72.3

14. **d.** This is a body-cavity based **lymphoma.** All the viruses listed, except SV40, have been implicated in the lesion.

15. **c.** **Desmoplastic small round cell tumor** of the pleura resembles that of intra-abdominal desmoplastic small round cell tumor and is positive for desmin and cytokeratin.

16. **a.** Both have small but visible about of cytoplasm. The other features favor anaplastic large cell lymphoma.

17. **d.** CD15 does not stain anaplastic large cell lymphoma.

18. **c.** **Pseudomyxoma peritoneii** is caused by MUC2 mucin producing tumors, usually from the appendix or ovary. Lobular carcinoma of the breast is not known to be associated with pseudomyxoma peritoneii.

19. **b.** High nuclear cytoplasm ratio is present in both conditions. The other features suggest small cell carcinoma.

20. **c.** CLL/SLL is negative for CD10. **CD10** stains follicular lymphoma.

21. **d.** Cell block is not a routine method for CSF. The material is usually not sufficient to be processed for cell block.

22. **a.** To obtain a satisfactory specimen using FNA, small bore needle is better than large bore needle. Large bores (in excess of 23G) usually result in bleeding, which dilutes the specimen.

23. **b.** **Kaposi sarcoma** is not a contra-indication for FNA. Following FNA, carotid body tumor is known to be associated with thrombosis of carotid artery while pheochromocytoma may be followed by hypertensive crisis. Aspiration of an *Echinococcus* cyst (hydatid cyst) is known to be followed by anaphylaxis.

24. **d.** The best position for the thyroid FNA is to let the patient lie flat without the pillow.

25. **a.** FNA is helpful when the clinical suspicion is low. Core biopsy is the preferred methods in the other three conditions.

26. **c.** This is **subareolar abscess**. It affects both men and women and does no heal without excision.

27. **a.** This is **fat necrosis**. It affects elderly more than young women.

28. **c.** Smear of lobular carcinoma is usually associated with single cells. These are benign ductal cells and could be present in all of the other lesions.

29. **d.** This is a fragment of stroma with few cells in between the fibers. The stromal fragments in phyllodes tumor are characteristically cellular fragments.

30. **c.** This is **a lobular carcinoma** with characteristic small single cells, some of which show intracytoplasmic lumen.

31. **b.** Only excisional biopsy can establish the malignant nature of papillary carcinoma.

32. **a. Inflammatory breast carcinoma** is not associated with neutrophils infiltrate. This term is from the appearance of the lesion which appears clinically inflamed with warmth, erythema and edema.

33. **d. HER2/neu** expressing breast carcinomas behave poorly compared to HER2/neu-negative ones. However, the latter are more likely to respond to Herceptin. On the other hand estrogen receptor positive tumors are more likely to respond to antiestrogen therapy.

34. **a.** These are naked nuclei of follicular cells and not lymphocytes. The lesion is most likely a **benign nodular goiter**.

35. **c.** This is a spherule. It is frequently seen in benign nodular goiter.

36. **c.** The predominant cells in acute thyroiditis are neutrophils while in the rest of these lesions are lymphocytes.

37. **d.** This is **Hashimoto thyroiditis**. It is known to be associated with lymphoma (less than 1%) and papillary carcinoma (around 20%). There is no association between multiple endocrine neoplasia (MEN-II) and Hashimoto thyroiditis. Psammoma bodies have been reported in this disease.

38. **a.** Cells of rhabdoid tumor are generally epithelioid and not spindle in shape. Squamous metaplasia and/or fibrosis are seen frequently in benign nodular goiter. Papillary carcinoma variant with nodular fasciitis-like stroma has been reported. Any form of thyroiditis can be associated with fibrosis.

39. **d.** FNA diagnosis of follicular neoplasm is associated with 20%–30% rate of malignancy in resected specimens.

40. **c.** Compared to other pairs, it is easier to differentiate Hashimoto thyroiditis from lymphoma. Tissue examination is necessary to differentiate between the other entities.

41. **a.** Giant cells are classically seen in papillary carcinoma of the thyroid.

42. **b. Zymogens granules** are seen in the cells of pancreatic, salivary, or gastric epithelium. They are exocrine granules. The granules seen in thyroid cells (para vacuolar granules) are not zymogens granules.

43. **d. Hashimoto thyroiditis** is an autoimmune disease. An elevated antithyroid antibody is diagnostic feature of Hashimoto thyroiditis.

44. **a.** Small cell variant of papillary carcinoma has not been described.

45. **c.** HER2/neu amplification is not a common event in papillary carcinoma.

46. **c.** Amyloid deposition is a characteristic feature of **medullary carcinoma** of the thyroid.

47. **b.** Although **squamoid cells** may be present in benign nodular goiter with cystic changes, they are generally few in number. Cystic squamous cell carcinoma can easily be misdiagnosed as branchial cleft cyst or infundibular inclusion cyst.

48. **c.** There is a pleomorphic population of **lymphocytes** which is not seen in CLL/SLL.

49. **c.** CD138 stains plasmacytoma while CD19 stains lymphoplasmocytic lymphoma.

50. **b. Epithelioid sarcoma** is sometimes misdiagnosed as reactive/granulomatous process. It is usually located subcutaneously in the distal part of a limb.

51. **b.** This is a **macrophage with emperipolesis**, a characteristic feature of Rosai–Dorfmann disease. It has been linked to viral infection and it regresses spontaneously. CD1a-positive staining and Birbeck granules are seen in Langerhans cell histiocytosis.

52. **c.** This is a monotonous population of lymphocytes. It is unlikely to be a follicular lymphoma.

53. **c.** The pattern in "a" corresponds to mantle cell lymphoma, "b" pattern corresponds to SLL/CLL and choice "d" corresponds to lymphoplasmacytic lymphoma.

54. **c.** The yellow signal indicates fusion of the blue and red signal indication t(11;14) translocation. This staining pattern is characteristic of **mantle cell lymphoma**. PCR can also be used to detect the fusion of immunoglobulin heavy chain and bcl-1 gene which encodes for cyclin D1.

55. **c.** This is **lymphoblastic lymphoma** which is not cytokeratin positive. The other markers are known to be positive in this lymphoma.

56. **a.** This is a poorly differentiated carcinoma consistent with **embryonal carcinoma**. The tumor stains for MOC-31.

57. **c.** Hepatocellular carcinoma is CK7− and CK20−.

58. **a.** These are acini of a normal salivary gland.

59. **b.** This is a **lymphoepithelial cyst** which is seen frequently in HIV/AIDS.

60. **a.** This is a **pleomorphic adenoma**. The micrograph shows stromal and epithelial fragments.

61. **d.** This is an adenoid cystic carcinoma. The micrograph shows the characteristic metachromatic globule.

62. c. This is mucoepidermoid carcinoma. The micrograph shows the squamous differentiation and mucoid background.

63. b. Epithelial–myoepithelial carcinoma is not known to exhibit prominent lymphoid infiltrate like the other conditions.

64. d. Unlike other listed conditions, melanoma is not particularly associated with granulomatous inflammation.

65. b. Chromosomal translocations involving the **EWS gene** are found in Ewing sarcoma, clear cell sarcoma, extra-skeletal myxoid chondrosarcoma and desmoplastic small round cell tumor. EWG gene is not involved in rhabdomyosarcoma. Alveolar rhabdomyosarcoma is known to have PAX3-FKHR and PAX7-FKHR translocations.

66. c. Similar to melanoma, **Merkel cell carcinoma** is a malignant neoplasm of the skin. However, this lesion is not known to have a pigment. It is similar in morphology to other small blue tumor. It may stain positive for neuroendocrine markers, cytokeratin (dot-like staining) and c-Kit. Unlike small cell carcinoma of the lung it stains negative for TTF-1, a maker of lung and thyroid neoplasms.

67. a. This is a **neurofibroma** showing the classical slender long crooked nuclei. CDKN2 is inactivated in neurofibroma, especially in neurofibromatosis type II.

68. b. This is an **osteosarcoma** showing highly atypical polygonal cells and osteoid formation. All the conditions listed are known to be predisposing factor. However, Paget disease of bone is unlikely in the age group of this patient. It usually affects elderly patients.

69. c. **Aneurysmal bone cyst** aspirate consists predominantly of blood. Aneurysmal bone cyst may accompany other bone tumors or lesions and the aspirate should be reviewed carefully. X-ray findings are very characteristic.

70. d. This is a **chondroblastoma**. The lesion shows characteristic epithelioid cells with nuclear groves and calcification in the background. X-ray findings are also very characteristic.

71. d. This is a **giant bone tumor** with characteristic giant cells whose nuclei are similar to single cells in the background.

72. d. This is a **small round blue cell tumor of bone**. Differential diagnosis include: Ewing sarcoma, lymphoma, granulocytic lymphoma, metastatic rhabdomyosarcoma, or neuroblastoma. The vacuolated cytoplasm and absence of rosettes (neuroblastoma); lymphoglandular bodies (lymphoma); cytoplasmic granules (granulocytic lymphoma) or large cells (rhabdomyosarcoma); and the EM features support the diagnosis of Ewing sarcoma.

73. c. The cytologic features are those of **granular cell tumor**. A less likely diagnosis is melanoma which is positive for HMB45. CD99 stains Ewing sarcoma and other tumors. CD68 is a marker of lysosomes and stains granular cell tumor which has many large granular lysosomes.

74. c. This lesion is a **thymoma** which is known to be associated with myasthenia gravis. Small cell carcinoma may present similarly but the cytology of small cell carcinoma is different.

75. c. This lesion shows the features of **hepatocellular carcinoma** which is associated with high serum alpha-fetoprotein.

76. e. These are *Histoplasma capsulatum. H. duboisii* are generally larger. The presence of kinetoplast (the small dot near the nucleus) differentiates leishmania from the other organisms. Toxoplasma is either present as encysted form (bradyzoites) or single extracellular form with necrosis (tachyzoites).

77. b. The pathognomonic feature of **autoimmune pancreatitis** is intense periductal lymphoplasmacytic infiltrate. A biopsy is needed to demonstrate the periductal location of the inflammation. It is associated with high levels of IgG4 and marked acinar destruction along the pancreatic ducts. It is often associated with other autoimmune diseases.

78. d. It is difficult to differentiate this lesion from other mucinous neoplasm of the pancreas without correlating the cytologic finding with that of imaging studies.

79. b. This is the so-called "drunken honeycomb" pattern which is seen in well-differentiated **pancreatic ductal carcinoma**.

80. d. This is a neuroendocrine neoplasm.

81. b. Clear cell carcinoma.

82. c. Pheochromocytoma.

83. a. The question reveals characteristic features of **seminoma**. Neoplastic germ cells are large pleomorphic with clumped chromatin. In addition to the neoplastic cells, small lymphocytes, plasma cells, and histiocytes are admixed in a proteinaceous background.

84. c. The large cells among sea of small blue cells are a characteristic feature that differentiates **rhabdomyosarcoma** from other small blue cell tumors.

85. a. Metastatic carcinoma.

86. a. **Alcohol fixatives**, including methyl alcohol (methanol) and ethyl alcohol (ethanol), are protein denaturants and are very good for cytologic smears because they act quickly and give good nuclear detail. They are not used routinely for tissues because they cause too much brittleness and hardness. Ethanol is considered a controlled substance and laboratories need to have a license to use it. It is often substituted with other alcohols. When used however, the concentration of these alcohols needs to be adjusted to be equivalent to that of 95% ethanol to give similar fixation.

87. b. RPMI is a cell culture media and is not used for red cell lysis.

88. a. Negative for Intraepithelial Lesion or Malignancy. The cells are polygonal, with minimal elevation of N/C ratio, and round nuclei.

89. b. Negative for Intraepithelial Lesion or Malignancy. The yellow color is very typical of glycogen.

90. c. Low-grade Squamous Intraepithelial Lesion. There are many classical **koilocytes**; the cell in the upper right corner shows marked nuclear enlargement.

91. d. High-grade Squamous Intraepithelial Lesion. While the cells in the upper cluster may be considered ASC-H., the lower cluster has diagnostic hyperchromasia and high N/C ratio.

92. d. Atypical Squamous Cells of Undetermined Significance (ASC-US). The only abnormality is the nuclear size, approximately 2.5 times that of an intermediate cell.

93. e. Negative for Intraepithelial Lesion or Malignancy. Bizarre shapes, enlarged nuclei with relatively normal N/C ratio, squamous cytoplasmic features, and degenerative changes including cytoplasmic vacuoles are characteristic of **radiation effect**. Radiation is used in therapy of invasive squamous cell carcinoma, and its effects may persist for months.

94. e. Negative for Intraepithelial Lesion or Malignancy. The cells show nuclear enlargement and cytoplasmic clearing typical of **Arias-Stella reaction**.

95. d. The best diagnosis of this cervical smear is *Trichomonas vaginalis*. The finding of binucleated squamous cells is by itself not atypical. The organisms show diagnostic granular cytoplasm and pale, gray nuclei of *T. vaginalis*. Cilia are not necessary for diagnosis.

96. c. Herpes simplex. The glassy chromatin quality and multinucleation are diagnostic.

97. c. Actinomyces. Purple color, long strands, and large size of the clumps are diagnostic; PMNs in the background are merely suggestive.

98. e. Negative for Intraepithelial Lesion or Malignancy. The ciliated endocervical cells are diagnostic of tubal metaplasia.

99. a. Negative for Intraepithelial Lesion or Malignancy. The finding of squamous pearls is benign. The nuclei are too small to warrant a diagnosis of atypical parakeratosis.

100. b. Atypical Squamous Cells of Undetermined Significance (ASC-US). The finding of nuclear atypia in densely keratinized cells is diagnostic of atypical parakeratosis.

101. c. Negative for Intraepithelial Lesion or Malignancy. Many scattered cells show parabasal atrophy. The chromatin has a benign quality (identical to that seen in the more mature squamous epithelial fragment).

102. a. No malignancy. This is a completely degenerated urothelial cell, in a background of benign squamous contamination.

103. d. High-grade urothelial carcinoma. The well preserved hyperchromatic, high N/C ratio cell in the center is diagnostic; the degenerated cell scattered in the image are suggestive.

104. a. These are benign urothelial cells, suggestive of **cystitis glandularis**. The cells are small, with polarized, benign nuclei. Delicate cytoplasm with few vacuoles suggests cystitis.

105. a. These are benign urothelial cells. Multinucleated umbrella cells are always benign, they can occur with lithiasis.

106. a. Benign urothelial cells. The cells show round, small nuclei, and some missing fragments of cytoplasm. These are hallmarks of degeneration.

107. c. This is **bronchioloalveolar carcinoma**. The cells are markedly atypical, and form vague gland-like structures. There is loss of polarity or normal epithelial organization. While this specimen shows only mild nuclear enlargement, bronchioloalveolar carcinoma can appear indistinguishable from adenocarcinoma.

108. c. This is *Pneumocystis carinii*. The **pneumocystis** organisms appear as large, foamy clusters on PAP stain. On higher magnification, distinct, round, empty shapes can be seen.

109. b. Specimen is **insufficient for diagnosis**. BAL specimen should contain alveolar macrophages. The finding of mature squamous cells, debris, and background of neutrophils should raise the suspicion of oral contamination.

110. c. CD56, CD45, pancytokeratin, chromogranin. The cells are diagnostic of **small cell carcinoma**. The differential diagnosis includes lymphoma, and therefore the panel should include neuroendocrine differentiation markers (CD56, chromogranin, synaptophysin); lymphoid markers (CD45, possible CD20, usually not CD3). Pancytokeratin is confirmatory of epithelial origin.

111. a. The finding of benign-appearing stromal spindle cells and a fragment of cartilage is diagnostic of **hamartoma**. Most hospitals will elect to excise the lesion for complete histologic examination.

112. c. Chemotherapy, 40% survival at 2 years. **Small cell carcinoma** has very poor survival. It is almost never treated surgically.

113. b. This lesion is almost certainly malignant if necrosis and high mitotic index are present. Necrosis and high mitotic index are associated with malignant neuroendocrine phenotype. Paraneoplastic syndromes accompany at least 10% of such lesions, Lambert-Eaton being most common in small cell lung carcinoma.

114. a. These are **benign, reactive changes**. All cells are ciliated, benign bronchial cells. Ciliary motility cannot be assessed on ethanol-fixed material.

115. b. Atypical ductal epithelial cells, **suspicious for adenocarcinoma**. The specimen is very cellular, with large epithelial sheets, and occasional scattered single cells. While this pattern is worrisome, the disorganization of the epithelium is mild, and there is little nuclear atypia.

116. a. The "empty" holes in the benign epithelial fragment are goblet cells, and therefore represent a **small intestinal contaminant**.

117. b. Endocervical carcinoma in situ (AIS). The combination of abnormally condensed chromatin, high N/C ratios, and endocervical glandular morphology is diagnostic. Note absence of apoptotic bodies.

118. d. Page the clinician. The finding of *Aspergillus* in BAL specimen is urgent, especially in immunocompromised patients.

119. a. CMV. The "owl's eye" intranuclear inclusion is diagnostic for Cytomegalovirus.

120. d. Stent atypia. The epithelium shows completely normal, benign honeycomb pattern, and occasional nuclear enlargement.

121. c. The chromocenter includes mainly DNA, whereas nucleolus mainly RNA. **Chromocenters** are irregularly-shaped condensations of inactive chromatin, whereas nucleoli are round structures containing mainly ribosomal RNA. Multiple nucleoli are found in cells with increased protein synthesis (such as repair reactions) on terminal portions of chromosomes (13, 14, 15, 21, and 22). Prominent nucleoli are a feature of HCC; however they remain confined within the nucleus

122. c. The feature most strongly indicative of malignancy in a discohesive cytology specimen is nuclear border (membrane) **irregularity**. Nuclear membrane irregularity in well-preserved cells is almost always an indication of malignancy. All other features can be often seen in reactive cells.

123. c. The presence of **"clue" cells** in a cervical smear is important to note because they may prompt treatment for meningitis. Clue cells may represent Group B Streptococci. This may prompt antibiotic treatment of the mother during labor to prevent fetal meningitis or sepsis.

124. c. The process thought responsible for malignant transformation in **HPV**-related cervical lesions is: E7 binding of Rb protein leading to abrogation of cell cycle checkpoints. E6, not E7 has a major role in causing degradation of p53 (not stabilization), E7 does not directly affect neither bcl-2 nor cytokine receptors.

125. d. The statement that is most appropriate regarding immunostaining for the tumor suppressor p16^{INK4a} is that increased staining for p16 supports HPV-related dysplasia. Increase in **p16** does occur in dysplasias such as LSIL, and almost all HPV-related carcinomas such as endocervical adenocarcinoma. Very focal increase can be noted in reactive mucosa. Negative staining for p16 is usually seen in benign tissue due to rapid apoptosis of cells which degenerate too quickly to visualize p16-positive cells.

126. c. Vaccines for prevention of cervical carcinoma have been more successful than for pancreatic carcinoma because they rely on specific **antiviral responses**. Cervical dysplasia and carcinoma, unlike pancreatic counterparts (PanINs and adenocarcinoma) have a viral basis. The expression of foreign, viral peptides by the infected cells accounts for the effectiveness of the vaccine.

127. a. The two widely used liquid-based methods for cervical smear preparation are ThinPrep (made by Cytyc) and SurePath or Autocyte (made by TriPath). Filter method (ThinPrep) may lead to clogging and hypocellular slides in specimens containing blood and debris. Both methods can be utilized for HPV testing. Both methods use some form of disruption or mixing of the material such that only true epithelial tissue fragments are maintained, and both methods use an alcohol-based fixative which results in mild decrease of cell size.

128. b. Maturation Index in cervical smears correlates with hormonal status of the patient. A change from 0:90:10 to 90:10:0 is most compatible with **delivery**. While definitive methods replaced the Maturation Index for hormonal assessment, the pattern described is diagnostic of postpartum atrophy.

129. a. The features most suggestive in differentiation of HSIL from invasive nonkeratinizing squamous cell carcinoma in cervical specimens include the presence of **prominent nucleoli**. Nucleoli are almost never seen in HSIL.

130. c. It is more important not to miss HSIL than LSIL The natural history of LSIL is very similar to ASC-US, whereas HSIL carries much worse outcome than LSIL. This also has been recognized by the restructuring of old ASCUS category into two-tiered ASC-H and ASC-US to further separate low from high-grade lesions even in the face of equivocal morphologies. HPV testing in normal samples has very low specificity, whereas almost all LSIL samples are HPV positive. Pathologists can be liable for all diagnoses that bear their signature.

131. a. According to TBS2001, an adequate liquid-based cervical specimen should have an estimated minimum of at least 12,000 of well preserved squamous cells. The adequacy recommendation is for 5000 cells for Liquid-Based, and 8000 to 12,000 for conventional preparations.

132. c. HPV types 16 and 18 have been classified as oncogenic or "high-risk" viral types. Most invasive cervical squamous carcinoma cells contain integrated **HPV genome**. Koilocytosis is seen with both low- and high-risk HPV infection, and the vast majority of HPV infections regress without treatment. While HPV 18 is seen somewhat more frequently in adenocarcinoma and HPV 16 in squamous carcinoma, both types can cause either lesion.

133. c. The **hybrid capture test** (commercially available as Digene II) relies upon hybridization of RNA probe to viral DNA, binding of antibody to the RNA-DNA hybrid, and measurement of light emitted by the bound antibody

134. b. The **ALTS study** offered support for the fact that chance of HSIL in patients with negative HPV tests is very low. Almost all LSIL samples were high-risk positive and low risk subtypes were not studied. Positive HPV test in ASCUS diagnoses was thought useful in triage of subsequent clinical decision-making (colposcopy, repeat smear); re-screen decision is not based on ASCUS diagnoses. HPV testing has very low specificity in women under 30.

135. **b.** The consensus guidelines based on the Bethesda System 2001 state that patients with ASC-H, LSIL and HSIL should undergo colposcopy. As in the past, the diagnosis of atypical squamous cells precludes categorization of the sample as inadequate.

136. **a.** The most common differential diagnosis of a de novo AGC (AGUS NOS) diagnosis is **HSIL**. AGUS NOS cytologic diagnoses were shown to result in HSIL on follow-up biopsies in approximately 10%–39% of cases.

137. **b.** The strongest evidence of LSIL in a cervical smear is provided by the presence of 5 to 10 squamous cells with moderate **karyomegaly and hyperchromasia**. Binucleation and mild nuclear enlargement are often not related to HPV, and dense green cytoplasm is most often a consequence of cellular degeneration.

138. **c.** Palisading cells with large, hyperchromatic nuclei and apoptotic bodies are characteristic of **endocervical adenocarcinoma** in cervical specimens. Endocervical carcinoma in smears often displays rosetting, polarity is usually preserved, and cells usually lack prominent nucleoli. Abnormal (unlike normal) mitotic figures are usually not found.

139. **b.** In a patient with abnormal uterine bleeding, the cytologic finding on a routine cervical smear that is most suspicious for endometrial carcinoma is the presence of single cells with high N/C ratio, vacuoles, and prominent nucleoli. While inflammation and debris may represent tumor diathesis, choice "b" is superior as it describes the key features of most endometrial carcinomas. Choice "c" is most consistent with endocervical atypia, and "d" with radiation effects.

140. **c.** The finding that is most worrisome for malignancy in peri-operative pelvic washings is the presence of **large three-dimensional clusters**. Psammoma bodies are seen in benign washings; small papillary proliferations and sheets of small cells describe benign mesothelium.

141. The adequacy of bronchoalveolar lavage is determined by the presence of **macrophages**. Pigmented macrophages can indicate a pathologic process, but are not required for adequacy of BAL specimens.

142. **a.** If more than 90% of pleural effusion cells are CD20 positive, it should be regarded as **lymphoma** until proven otherwise. Benign lymphocytic effusions are composed of some B cells, and a majority of CD3 CD8 positive T cells. Such effusions have been associated with occult epithelial malignancies and tuberculosis infections.

143. **b.** The finding of multinucleated, polarized syncytial cells in bronchial washings is most consistent with **reactive** response of bronchial cells to injury. Multinucleated giant cells of macrophage origin are not polarized, and are very rarely seen in washings in sarcoidosis.

144. **b.** The finding in a sputum or bronchial washing specimen that is most worrisome for carcinoma is the presence of yellow or orange cytoplasm and evenly hyperchromatic nucleus. Squamous pearls are most often a consequence of a degenerative benign change. The answer describes the hallmarks of **keratinizing squamous cell carcinoma**. Multinucleation can occur in squamous carcinoma, but on its own is a nonspecific finding.

145. **b.** The feature that separates small cell carcinoma from lymphoma on smear specimens is that small cell carcinoma has minimal nuclear membrane irregularity on PAP stain.
Small cell carcinoma has predominantly smooth, oval outline, with rare acute angles. Lymphomas have frequent "blebs" and indentations in the nuclear membrane as well as prominent nucleoli. Both lesions show crush artifact, and molding on DiffQuik.

146. **c.** The presence of small cells with high N/C ratio and hyperchromasia in a voided urine specimen is most worrisome for malignancy. The answer describes hallmarks of **high-grade carcinoma**. While urothelial fragments can indicate low-grade papillary lesions, in absence of atypia they are often benign. Multinucleated umbrella cells can be seen in lithiasis, glassy nuclei in polyoma virus infection.

147. **b. Eosinophilia** is most closely associated with an allergic process in **bronchial washings**. Eosinophils in bronchial specimen are commonly seen in asthma. Eosinophilia in pleural or pelvis fluids is most often indicative of prior instrumentation; if seen in lymph node smears a consideration of Hodgkin lymphoma should be entertained.

148. **e.** In a sputum specimen of immunocompromised patients, the presence of **oxalate crystals** is of immediate clinical significance. Squamous pearls and *Corpora* are benign findings not related to a specific pathology, Curschmann spirals to chronic respiratory disorders. Oxalate crystals are associated with *Aspergillus*, and should prompt immediate attention.

149. **b.** Finding of roundworms should prompt flow cytometric analysis of blood. **Strongyloides infection** is very strongly correlated to acute T-cell leukemia-lymphoma. Curschmann spirals are seen in any chronic respiratory disorder. Bronchorrhea occurs in mucinous-type bronchioloalveolar carcinoma. Most sputum specimens without macrophages represent oral sampling only.

150. **c.** The features that distinguish small cell carcinoma from atypical carcinoid include the presence of nucleoli and delicate cytoplasm. **Nucleoli** are almost always absent in small cell carcinoma. In most smears, cytoplasm is either not seen, or appears as a thin blue rim around the nucleus. Carcinoid tumors usually show delicate, wispy cytoplasm, particularly inside rosettes.

151. **b.** Papillary urothelial fragments with fibrovascular cores are diagnostic for low-grade neoplasms. Mitomycin C effects are essentially identical to other

chemotherapy or radiation effects. Choices "a" and "b" describe differential diagnoses of degenerative changes.

152. **d.** A cytologic diagnosis of high-grade carcinoma followed by a benign cystoscopically-guided biopsy should result in **aggressive follow up**. Voided urine cytology has low sensitivity and specificity for low-grade lesions; it has however, very high specificity for high-grade carcinoma. Flat high-grade lesions are often not seen on cystoscopy.

153. **c.** Foamy macrophages in BAL are usually PAS-D positive. BAL is often the diagnostic and therapeutic procedure for **alveolar proteinosis**. The finding of proteinaceous debris in sputum is nonspecific.

154. **d.** The differential diagnosis of bronchioloalveolar carcinoma should not include small cells with indistinct chromatin and high N/C ratio. Bronchioloalveolar carcinoma, irrespective of type, does not show marked elevation of N/C ratios.

155. **a.** Endoscopic ultrasound-guided FNA is useful for staging of patients with non-small cell lung carcinoma. EUS FNA is a low-morbidity procedure which allows access to most paratracheal lymph nodes, as well as biliary epithelium. Core biopsies create additional risk, particularly in pancreatic sampling. Contamination with nonlesional cells originating from the GI tract is to date inevitable.

156. **c.** The presence of cleared chromatin on PAP stain and nuclear membrane irregularity is most consistent with adenocarcinoma in biliary brushings. While most carcinomas show loss of organization and crowding, these findings are often present in reactive processes, and unlike nuclear membrane irregularity cannot be regarded as diagnostic. Most biliary cancers show chromatin clearing, not hyperchromasia.

157. **c. Aspirin gastritis** can be very easily misdiagnosed as carcinoma. Single cells are worrisome, but not diagnostic for malignancy. Necrosis, nuclear atypia, nucleolar and nuclear enlargement are seen both in benign ulcers and gastric adenocarcinoma. Aspirin gastritis and adenocarcinoma share the described features.

158. **c.** The shared cytomorphologic characteristics of **biliary and pancreatic adenocarcinoma** include the presence of chromatin with clearing and clumping. While this feature is not seen on DiffQuik-stained slides, it is strikingly present on alcohol-fixed PAPs. Neither type of carcinomas typically shows hyperchromasia in cytologic specimens. Both carcinoma types are usually positive for mucin stains.

159. **a. Anatomic location** on ultrasound is uniquely relevant for spindle cell tumors. The radiologic resolution is almost always sufficient to ascertain sub-mucosal location of the mass. Benign smooth muscle originating from gastric wall is a fairly common contaminant in EUS-FNA. GIST tumors frequently contain epithelioid component, which can masquerade as adenocarcinoma. Although c-kit negative GIST is rare, it should be CD34 positive. Solitary fibrous tumor is exceedingly rare.

■ Recommended Readings

DeMay RM. *The art and science of cytopathology*, volumes I and II. Chicago: ASCP Press, 1996.

Koss LG, Melamed MR. *Diagnostic cytology and its histopathologic bases*, 5th ed. Baltimore: Lippincott Williams and Wilkins, 2006.

3

Skin

Atif Ahmed

▇ Questions

1. The histologic picture of spongiosis can be found in all of the following situations EXCEPT:
   a. Contact dermatitis due to poison ivy
   b. Skin eruption from thiazide diuretics
   c. Erythema nodosum
   d. Pemphigus vulgaris
   e. HIV patients with seborrheic dermatitis

2. A biopsy of a solitary nonitchy papule on the skin reveals the following picture (Fig. 3.1). The cellular bodies indicated by the arrows are formed from:
   a. Disintegrated collagen
   b. PAS-positive cytoplasmic inclusions

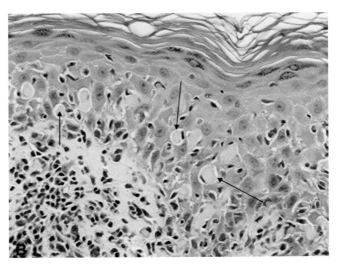

Figure 3.1 *(continued)*

   c. Colloidal iron
   d. Infiltrating IgM-positive histiocytes
   e. Apoptotic koilocytes

3. A 19-year-old HIV-positive man with a history of pneumocystis pneumonia developed erythematous, edematous macules symmetrically involving the skin of the arms, trunk, and legs, including the palms and soles. The diagnosis from this skin biopsy (Fig. 3.2) is:
   a. Psoriasis
   b. Seborrheic keratosis
   c. Arthropod bite reaction
   d. Erythema multiforme
   e. Urticaria

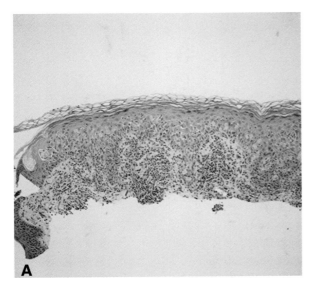

Figure 3.1 *(continues)*

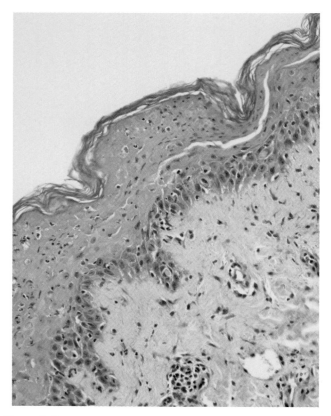

Figure 3.2

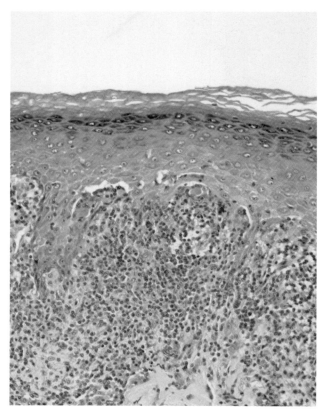

Figure 3.3

4. A 19-year-old African American woman with proteinuria and arthritis involving the knee and ankle developed a skin rash on the cheeks. Her serum was positive
for anti–dsDNA antibodies. The patient's skin biopsy is
shown (Fig. 3.3). The diagnosis can be confirmed with
any of the following tests EXCEPT:
   a. Acid-fast stain
   b. PAS stain
   c. Colloidal iron stain
   d. IgG and C3 immunofluorescence in biopsy from
      clinically normal skin
   e. IgG and C3 immunofluorescence in biopsy from
      clinically involved skin

5. Characteristic features of lymphomatoid papulosis include all of the following EXCEPT:
   a. Clinical course following an arthropod bite
   b. Perivascular lymphocytic inflammatory infiltrate
   c. CD-30 positive lymphocytes in the epidermis
   d. Clonal T-cell receptor gene rearrangement
   e. Benign disease with spontaneous regression

6. Lymphocytic cell infiltrate in the reticular dermis can be
reliably diagnosed as mycosis fungoides if the cells are:
   a. CD45+, CD30+, CD15+
   b. CD3+, CD4+, CD8−
   c. CD3+, CD4−, CD8+
   d. CD20+, CD45+, CD10+
   e. CD3−, CD8−, CD56+

7. The diagnosis (Fig. 3.4) is most likely:
   a. Staphylococcal scalded skin (SSS) syndrome
   b. Toxic epidermal necrolysis (TEN)
   c. Pemphigus vulgaris
   d. Systemic lupus erythematosus
   e. Pityriasis lichenoides et varioliformis acuta

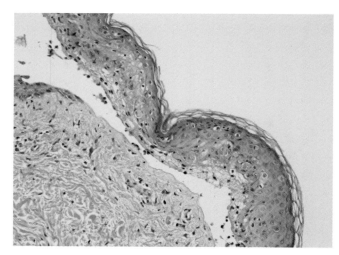

Figure 3.4

8. Which of the following is NOT associated with human
papillomavirus (HPV) viral infection?
   a. Epidermodysplasia verruciformis
   b. Condyloma acuminatum

c. Actinic keratosis
d. Bowen disease
e. Warty dyskeratoma

9. A 17-year-old girl developed macular erythematous skin eruptions in the face, neck, and upper chest. Two weeks earlier, she received bone marrow transplantation after finishing a course of ablation chemotherapy. Two skin biopsies of different sites are represented in the picture (Fig. 3.5). The diagnosis is:
   a. Pityriasis lichenoides et varioliformis acuta
   b. Viral infection
   c. Drug-associated linear IgA dermatosis
   d. Radiation dermatitis
   e. Acute graft-versus-host disease

11. A 45-year-old white HIV-positive woman developed a generalized skin rash characterized by erythematous scaly papules and plaques with sharp borders. The diagnosis from this skin biopsy (Fig. 3.6) is:
    a. Stevens-Johnson syndrome
    b. Pemphigoid
    c. Tinea corporis

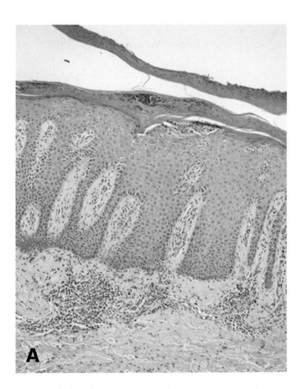

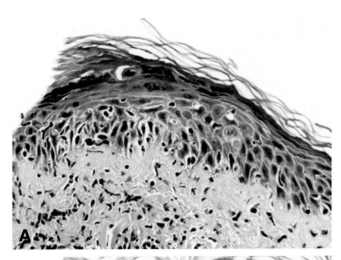

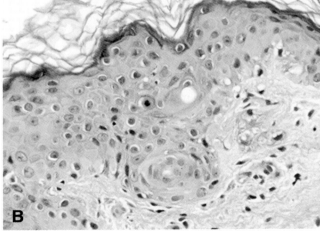

Figure 3.5

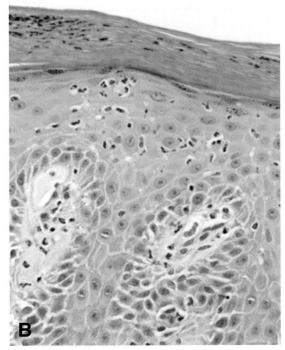

Figure 3.6

10. Tuberculosis of the skin may manifest as any of the following lesions EXCEPT:
    a. Lupus vulgaris
    b. Papulonecrotic skin lesions
    c. Erythema induratum
    d. Erythema nodosum
    e. Hidradenitis suppurativa

d. Psoriasis
e. Acanthosis nigricans

12. Which one of the following statements about lichen planus is true?
    a. It characteristically involves the palms and soles.
    b. Lesions show keratin-positive colloid bodies.
    c. It is characterized by the presence of atypical cells.
    d. It is differentiated from pemphigoid by absence of bullae.
    e. It shows a scleroderma-like fibrosis of the dermis.

13. Which of the following is true about granuloma faciale?
    a. It characteristically involves the face of young children.
    b. It is a form of vasculitis.
    c. Histology shows radial granulomas with necrotic centers.
    d. It is characteristically associated with mycobacterial infection.
    e. Histology resembles that of nodular panniculitis.

14. Erythema nodosum:
    a. Presents with ulcerated skin lesions
    b. Can progress to involve the muscles and bones
    c. Is a vascular neoplasm
    d. Is characterized histologically by nodular lymphoid infiltrate in the epidermis
    e. Results from streptococcal skin infection

15. A 37-year-old woman has a firm nonpruritic papule located on her hand. The lesion was excised (Fig. 3.7). GMS and an acid-fast bacilli stain are negative. What is the most likely diagnosis?
    a. Granuloma annulare
    b. Sarcoidosis
    c. Rheumatic nodule
    d. Atypical mycobacterial infection
    e. Epithelioid sarcoma

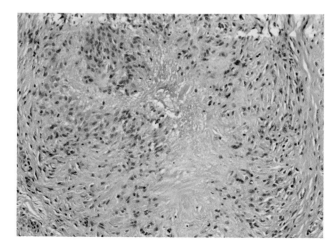

Figure 3.7

16. Reactions to drugs can manifest as any of the following skin lesions EXCEPT:
    a. Neutrophil-rich eccrine hidradenitis
    b. Erythema multiforme
    c. Photodermatitis
    d. Eosinophil-rich lymphocytic vasculitis
    e. Lichen simplex chronicus

17. Match each of the following pathologic findings (i–v) with their characteristic diseases listed below (a–e).
    i) Subepidermal unilocular bullae
    ii) Bullae with papillary microabscesses
    iii) IgG "fish-net" immunofluorescence pattern in the epidermis
    iv) Suprabasal epidermal bullae
    v) Granular IgA staining at the tip of the dermal papillae
    a. Dermatitis herpetiformis
    b. Bullous pemphigoid
    c. Erythema multiforme
    d. Linear IgA bullous dermatosis
    e. Pemphigus vulgaris

18. Skin lesions that are more common in patients infected with human immunodeficiency virus include all of the following entities EXCEPT:
    a. Seborrheic dermatitis
    b. Kaposi sarcoma
    c. Psoriasis
    d. Acrodermatitis
    e. Angioedema

19. Abnormalities in keratin synthesis occur in:
    a. Darier disease
    b. Psoriasis
    c. Epidermolysis bullosa simplex
    d. Hailey-Hailey disease

20. Pyoderma gangrenosum:
    a. Is a manifestation of Pseudomonas infection
    b. Is associated with inflammatory bowel disease
    c. Results from posttrauma infection with group A beta-hemolytic streptococcus
    d. Lesions are mainly found in the trunk and scalp
    e. Causes hemorrhagic bullae formation

21. The most common bacterial infection of the skin is:
    a. Dermatitis
    b. Impetigo
    c. Staphylococcal scalded skin syndrome
    d. Cellulitis
    e. Erysipelas

22. Nevus sebaceus of Jadassohn:
    a. Manifests as erythematous nodules
    b. Is the most common adnexal neoplasm in children
    c. Occurs with greater frequency in association with trisomy 21

d. Occurs in the scalp and face

e. Is preneoplastic for sebaceous carcinoma

23. An intraepidermal bullous disease with separation at the granular cell layer is:

a. Pemphigus vulgaris

b. Bullous pemphigoid

c. Darier disease

d. Pemphigus foliaceus

e. Hailey-Hailey disease

24. All of the following skin lesions are considered preneoplastic EXCEPT:

a. Actinic keratosis

b. Bowen disease

c. Acrochordon (skin tag)

d. Epidermodysplasia verruciformis

e. Xeroderma pigmentosum

25. The diagnosis is (Fig. 3.8):

a. Pseudoepitheliomatous hyperplasia

b. Poorly differentiated squamous cell carcinoma

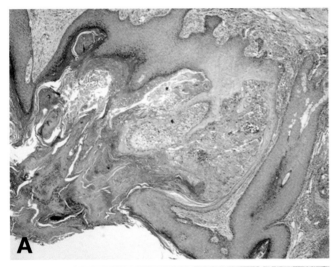

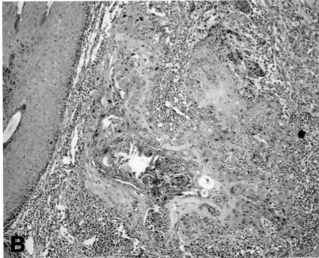

Figure 3.8

c. Bowen disease

d. Keratoacanthoma

e. Hyperkeratotic actinic keratosis

Questions 26 and 27 (Fig. 3.9):

26. This skin cancer:

a. Is a rare skin malignancy

b. Does not develop in areas protected from sun light

c. Is the most common skin cancer in African Americans

d. Shows immunoreactivity for S-100 and EMA immunostains

e. Develops after treatment of psoriasis patients with PUVA

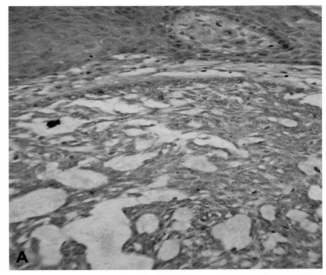

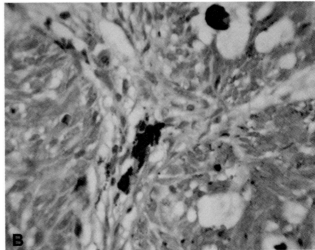

Figure 3.9

27. Increased incidence of recurrence of this lesion is related to:

a. Location of the tumor in the face

b. Nodular distribution of tumor cells

c. Overexpression of mucin

d. Degree of sebaceous differentiation
e. All of the above

28. The most common skin disease in children is:
    a. Seborrheic dermatitis
    b. Atopic dermatitis
    c. Impetigo
    d. Congenital nevus
    e. Freckles

29. Acanthosis nigricans is characteristically associated with:
    a. Insulin-resistant diabetes mellitus
    b. Acanthosis with elongation of rete ridges
    c. Hyperpigmentation
    d. Mutations of the ABCC/MRP6 gene
    e. All of the above

30. Which of the following is derived from apocrine ducts?
    a. Sweat gland carcinoma
    b. Hidradenoma papilliferum
    c. Syringoma
    d. Sebaceous adenoma
    e. Poroma

31. The best diagnosis for this lesion (Fig. 3.10) is:
    a. Sebaceous hyperplasia
    b. Follicular lymphoma

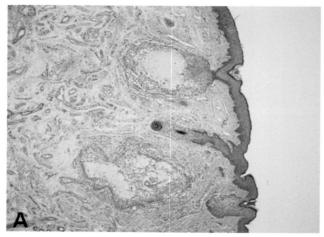
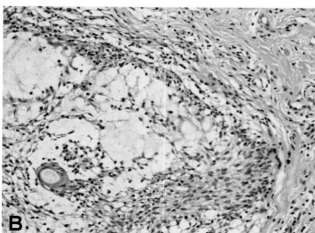

Figure 3.10

c. Follicular mucinosis
d. Mucocele
e. Alopecia areata

32. A 28-year-old woman has a small skin lesion in the lower lid of her left eye (Fig. 3.11). The most likely differential diagnosis is:
    a. Syringoma versus desmoplastic trichoepithelioma
    b. Sebaceous adenoma versus poroma
    c. Basal cell carcinoma versus seborrheic keratosis
    d. Cylindroma versus proliferating trichilemmal cyst
    e. Eccrine adenocarcinoma versus pilomatricoma

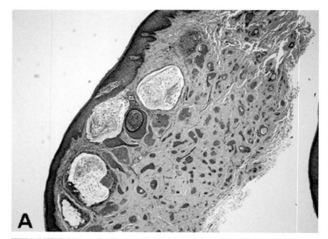
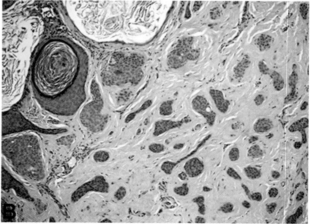

Figure 3.11

33. Neoplastic melanocytes are characteristically positive for all of the following markers EXCEPT:
    a. Tyrosinase
    b. S-100
    c. HMB-45
    d. Mart-1
    e. Synaptophysin

34. Congenital nevi differ from acquired nevi in the fact that congenital nevi:
    a. Do not show junctional activity
    b. Are characteristically associated with gastrointestinal hemangiomas

c. Do not give rise to melanoma
d. Show preferential nesting of melanocytes around and inside adnexal structures
e. Have higher incidence in childhood than acquired nevi

35. Spitz nevi can be differentiated from malignant melanoma by:
    a. The absence of mitotic figures
    b. Symmetric shape and circumscription
    c. The absence of intraepidermal pagetoid spread
    d. Their characteristic small size
    e. The absence of desmoplastic reaction around melanocytes

36. The most significant histologic finding in this lesion (Fig. 3.12) is the presence of:
    a. Dense desmoplastic reaction
    b. Invasive melanoma cells
    c. Pagetoid spread
    d. Nesting of melanocytes
    e. Pigmentation

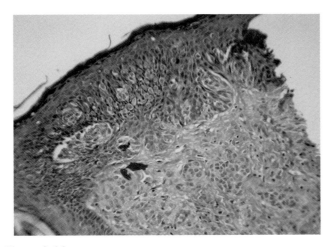

Figure 3.12

37. The pathologic name for "Hutchinson freckle" is:
    a. Acral lentiginous melanoma
    b. Lentigo simplex
    c. Superficial spreading melanoma
    d. Lentigo maligna
    e. Spindle cell melanoma

38. Which feature of melanoma indicates a better prognosis?
    a. Epithelioid histologic type
    b. Location in the scalp
    c. Amelanotic type
    d. Male gender
    e. Dermal inflammatory infiltrate

39. The most important prognostic parameter in melanoma is:
    a. Tumor stage
    b. Clark levels of dermal invasion

c. Presence or absence of ulceration
d. Ki-67 proliferation rate
e. Mitotic rate

40. Merkel cell carcinoma:
    a. Is commonly seen in children
    b. Usually occurs in the skin of the trunk
    c. Can present as metastasis in lymph nodes
    d. Is positive for TTF-1
    e. None of the above

41. This type of basal cell carcinoma (Fig. 3.13) is referred to as:
    a. Basosquamous
    b. Cystic
    c. Adenoid
    d. Sclerosing
    e. None of the above

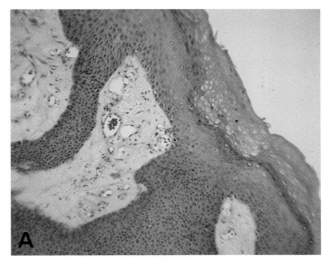

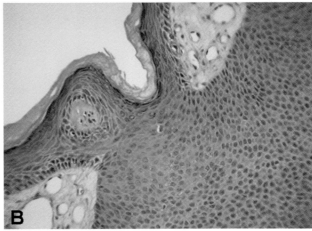

Figure 3.13

42. A small, firm, slowly growing, nipple-like nodule is identified on the chest of a 54-year-old man. Morphology of the biopsy is shown (Fig. 3.14). Additional factors supportive of the diagnosis include the presence of:
    a. Positivity for factor 13a
    b. COL1A1/PDGF gene fusion

c. Bizarre-appearing cells that are positive for CD99
d. Family history of facial trichilemmomas
e. Cytoplasmic whorls of intermediate filaments by electron microscopy

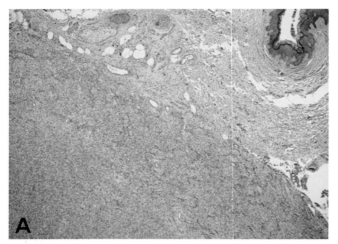

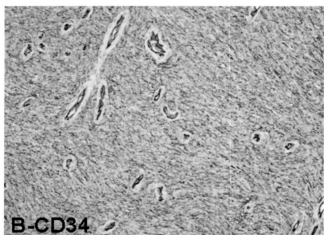

Figure 3.14

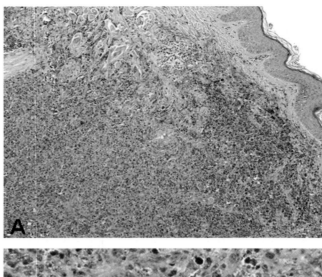

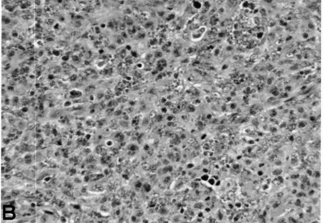

Figure 3.15

43. A blue-black papule is found on the arm of an 18-year-old white man that was not present at birth (Fig. 3.15). The most likely diagnosis is:
   a. Blue nevus
   b. Nevus of Ota
   c. Mongolian spot
   d. Pigmented Spitz nevus
   e. Melanoma

44. A biopsy of a small papule on the leg of a 33-year-old woman is shown (Fig. 3.16). The most likely differential diagnosis is:
   a. Atypical fibroxanthoma versus Bednar tumor
   b. Leiomyoma versus neurofibroma
   c. Dermatofibroma versus scar
   d. Keloid versus desmoid tumor
   e. Fibromatosis versus myofibromatosis

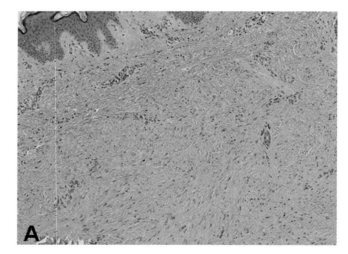

Figure 3.16 *(continues)*

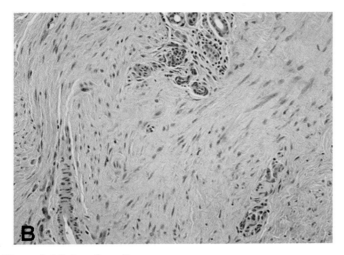

Figure 3.16 *(continued)*

45. A brown pruritic skin lesion on the scalp of an 8-year-old girl is shown (Fig. 3.17). Immunostains that may be necessary to confirm the diagnosis include all of the following EXCEPT:
    a. HMB-45
    b. S-100
    c. CD1a
    d. CD68
    e. Peanut agglutinin

46. An excisional biopsy of a small pink nodule found on a 10-year-old boy is shown (Fig. 3.18). The most likely diagnosis is:
    a. Amelanotic blue nevus
    b. Malignant melanoma

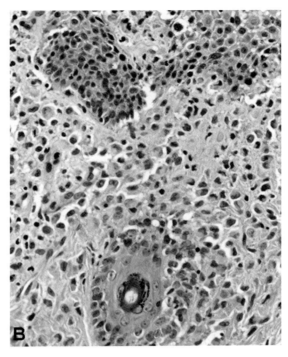

Figure 3.17 *(continued)*

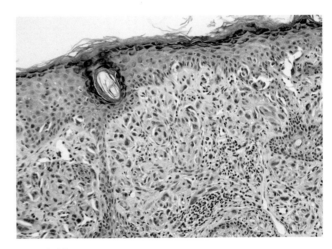

Figure 3.18

c. Dysplastic nevus
d. Congenital nevus
e. Spitz nevus

47. This subcutaneous cyst, found in the right orbital region (Fig. 3.19), is a/an:
    a. Epidermal inclusion cyst
    b. Dermoid cyst
    c. Pilar cyst
    d. Branchial cleft cyst
    e. Conjunctival cyst

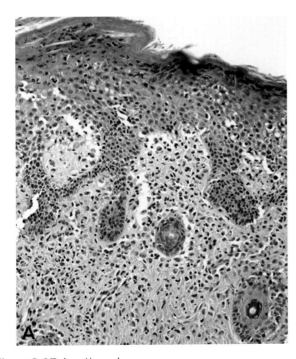

Figure 3.17 *(continues)*

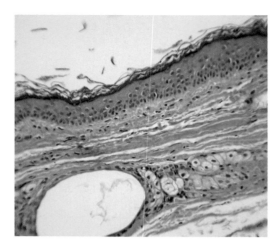

Figure 3.19

48. A red plaque on the scalp is biopsied (Fig. 3.20). The most likely diagnosis is:
   a. Syringocystadenoma papilliferum
   b. Cylindroma
   c. Trichoadenoma
   d. Hidradenoma papilliferum
   e. Pyogenic granuloma

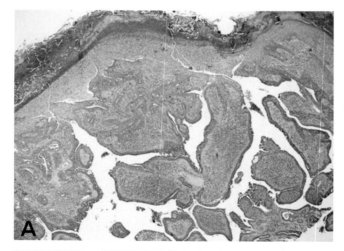

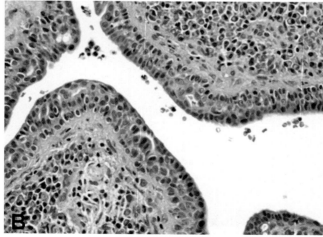

Figure 3.20

49. A 19-year-old woman has nodular lesions on the skin of the arm that becomes warm and pruritic upon palpation. A skin biopsy reveals a dermal infiltrate that was analyzed by H&E, Giemsa stain, and CD117 immunostain (Fig. 3.21). The most likely diagnosis is:
   a. Mast cell disease
   b. Langerhans cell histiocytosis

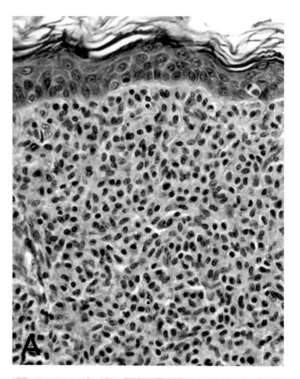

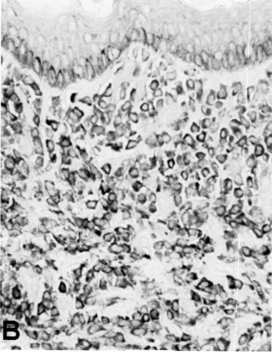

Figure 3.21 *(continues)*

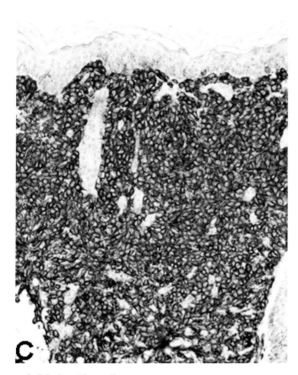

Figure 3.21 *(continued)*

c. Intradermal nevus
d. Metastatic ovarian tumor
e. Adnexal neoplasm

50. This subcutaneous mass (Fig. 3.22) is a:
a. Fibrosarcoma
b. Juvenile xanthogranuloma
c. Lobular hemangioma
d. Dermatofibroma
e. None of the above

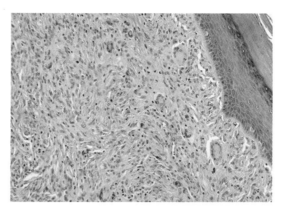

Figure 3.22

51. This epidermal lesion (Fig. 3.23) may be predisposed to by any of the following factors EXCEPT:
a. Sun exposure
b. Aging
c. Xeroderma pigmentosum
d. Arsenic poisoning
e. Mutations in the PTC gene on chromosome 9

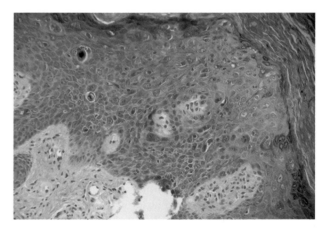

Figure 3.23

■ Answers

1. **c. Spongiosis** is an intracellular edema between keratinocytes in the epidermis. The edema may progress to spongiotic intraepidermal vesicles. Spongiosis is the hallmark of eczema but can be seen in other specific types of dermatitis. Erythema nodosum is characterized by a panniculitis-like picture with minimal epidermal involvement.

2. **b. Colloid bodies** are PAS-positive eosinophilic bodies found in the papillary dermis and lower epidermis in patients with lichen planus, drug eruptions, or lichenoid infiltrate. They consist of filaments and organelle remnants of apoptotic basal cells and appear as PAS-positive cytoplasmic inclusions. In lichen planus, they stain for IgM by direct immunofluorescence but they are not related to histiocytes.

3. **d.** The image shows **interface dermatitis**, which can occur in erythema multiforme, toxic epidermal necrolysis, dermatomyositis, SLE, and cytoxic drug eruption. **Erythema multiforme** and toxic epidermal necrolysis display marked keratinocyte necrosis. Blisters may develop in both disorders. The most frequent etiology of erythema multiforme is infection. However, drugs, particularly sulfonamides, can result in more severe form, termed Stevens-Johnson syndrome.

4. **a. Systemic lupus erythematosus** is characterized by hyperkeratosis, follicular plugging, colloidal iron-positive dermal mucin, dermal lymphocytic infiltrate, and granular deposits of IgG and C3 along the epidermal basement membrane in lesional skin as well as normal skin. PAS stain will demonstrate thickened basement membrane.

5. **a. Lymphomatoid papulosis** is a lymphoma-like lesion that is characterized by infiltrate of atypical CD30-positive, CD4-positive T-lymphocytes that may involve the epidermis. This lesion is benign but may progress to lymphoma or mycosis fungoides. An arthropod bite reaction does not give rise to lymphomatoid papulosis although the two entities may look similar in histology.

6. **b. Mycosis fungoides** may be considered a form of T-cell lymphoma of the T-helper phenotype. Cells express CD3 and CD4 and are negative for CD30 and CD7. The disease has a long course and appear as patches or plaques on the trunk that progress to infiltrative plaques. On histology, small cells with cerebriform or irregular nuclei infiltrate the dermis and epidermis.

7. **b.** The image shows epidermal necrosis and bulla, which can occur in both SSS syndrome and TEN. In TEN, subepidermal bullae are formed. In SSS syndrome, the plane of cleavage is at or above the granular area. **Toxic epidermal necrolysis** causes extensive sloughing of skin and may be life threatening. It is usually due to sulfonamides, phenytoin, and other drugs.

8. **e.** Despite histologic similarities to viral warts, warty dyskeratoma is not a manifestation of **human papilloma virus** infection. All of the other lesions are related to HPV infection. More commonly, verruca vulgaris occurs on the acral skin of the hands and feet as manifestation of HPV type 2 infection.

9. **e. Acute graft-versus-host** disease in the skin is characterized by spongiosis of the epidermis, vacuolization, and necrosis in the basal layer of the skin and subepidermal mononuclear cell infiltrate. Necrotic keratinocytes can also be seen in fixed drug eruption, pityriasis lichenoides, connective tissue disease, radiation dermatitis, and some viral infections. Thus, an appropriate clinical history in combination with histologic findings is needed for a proper diagnosis.

10. **e. Tuberculosis of the skin** is rare and can manifest in several forms. Lupus vulgaris presents as small red nodules in the face. Papulonecrotic tuberculid skin lesions show dermal necrosis, vasculitis, and edema. Erythema nodosum is subcutaneous panniculitis on the anterior surfaces of the legs. Erythema induratum occurs on the calves as subcutaneous nodules. Scrofuloderma results from extension to the skin of a tuberculous infection present in a lymph node or bone. All of these lesions may show granulomas with acid-fast bacilli. Hidradenitis is an adnexal inflammatory disease, not related to tuberculosis.

11. **d. Psoriasis** is a common inflammatory disorder that is characterized by scaly pink to red papules and plaques. It commonly involves the scalp, sacral region, and extensor surfaces of the extremities. It can extend to involve the entire skin. Histologically it is characterized by hyperkeratosis, parakeratosis, acanthosis, elongation of the rete ridges, and epidermal microabscesses (Monroe abscesses).

12. **b. Lichen planus** involves the extensor surfaces and is characterized by hyperkeratosis, acanthosis, band-like dermal infiltrate, and colloid bodies. Bullae may occasionally be seen. No dyskeratotic or atypical cells are seen in lichen planus.

13. **b. Granuloma faciale** is an idiopathic nonnecrotizing vasculitis forming dermal granulomas with eosinophils. The infiltrate is separated from the epidermis by a narrow band of uninvolved dermis. Typically it affects the face of adults as brown-red plaques. Streptococcal infections and radial granulomas are associated with erythema nodosum.

14. **e. Erythema nodosum** is a nonulcerative self-healing lesion that involves the anterior surface of the legs. The histologic changes are present mainly in the subcutaneous tissue with mild inflammatory infiltrate affecting the dermis and the dermal-epidermal junction. Although streptococcal infection is the most common cause, other bacterial, fungal, and protozoal infections can also be associated with erythema nodosum. It can also occur with some cases of leukemia, lymphoma, and other malignancies.

15. a. **Granuloma annulare** occurs on the dorsum of the hands and feet and shows well-demarcated area of disintegrated collagen surrounded by fibroblasts and histiocytes that stain with vimentin and lysozyme and not with CD68 (KP-1). It is not associated with any systemic disease. Differentiation of granuloma annulare from necrobiosis lipoidica or rheumatoid nodules can be difficult because these lesions show similar histologic features.

16. e. **Drugs** can cause various lesions in the skin, including maculopapular rashes, urticaria, vasculitis, erythema multiforme, Stevens-Johnson syndrome, toxic epidermal necrolysis, fixed drug eruptions, lichenoid drug eruption, spongiotic reaction, psoriasiform reaction, photodermatitis, hyperpigmentation, and lupus erythematosus. Eccrine hidradenitis can result from reaction to some chemotherapeutic reagents.

17. i) b. ii) a. iii) e. iv) e. v) a. **Intraepidermal bullae** occur in pemphigus, Hailey-Hailey disease, and Grover disease. **Subepidermal blistering** is seen in bullous pemphigoid, dermatitis herpetiformis, linear IgA bullous dermatosis, and epidermolysis bullosa. **Dermatitis herpetiformis** is an autoimmune disease occurring most commonly in middle-aged men presenting as papules and vesicles on the extensor surfaces and buttocks. **Neutrophilic microabscesses** are identified at the tip of the dermal papillae. Immunofluorescence shows linear IgA staining at the basement membrane.

18. e. **Human immunodeficiency virus** infection can also be associated with pruritic eruptions, drug eruptions, vasculitis, opportunistic skin infections, and folliculitis. Acrodermatitis enteropathica is related to defect in zinc absorption from the intestinal tract and may also be associated with AIDS.

19. c. **Epidermolysis bullosa** (EB) is a group of blistering disorders that start at birth or early childhood and are of different types. EB simplex is autosomal dominant and characterized by defects in keratin 5 and 14 (basal cell keratins). The blister occurs through the cytolytic basal cells.

20. b. **Pyoderma gangrenosum** is an uncommon inflammatory ulcerative skin lesion, frequently associated with systemic diseases such as inflammatory bowel disease. Most lesions occur in the extremities. Ecthyma is caused by group A beta-hemolytic streptococci. Ecthyma gangrenosum is a systemic manifestation of pseudomonas infection and causes hemorrhagic bullae.

21. b. **Impetigo** is a highly contagious superficial bacterial infection and can be complicated by acute glomerulonephritis. Impetigo can be classified as impetigo contagiosa, which is nonbullous, and bullous impetigo. It is usually caused by streptococci or staphylococci.

22. d. **Nevus sebaceous of Jadassohn** is a broad hamartomatous lesion characterized by epidermal hyperplasia, poorly formed hair follicles, and numerous sebaceous glands that give the lesions its characteristic yellowish color. Pilomatrixoma is the most common adnexal neoplasm in children.

23. d. **Superficial bullae** are found in pemphigus foliaceus, staphylococcal scalded skin syndrome, and pemphigus erythematosus. The other choices are characterized by suprabasal bullae. In bullous pemphigoid, dermatitis herpetiformis, erythema multiforme, epidermolysis bullosa, and porphyria cutanea tarda, there is separation beneath the epidermis resulting in subepidermal bullae.

24. c. **Acrochordon** is another name for fibroepithelial polyp (skin tag). Actinic keratosis, Bowen disease, erythroplasia, leukoplakia, HPV lesions, and xeroderma pigmentosa all predispose to invasive squamous cell carcinoma. Increased incidence of squamous cell carcinoma is also seen in patients with immunosuppression, draining dermal sinuses of osteomyelitis, burn scars, ingestion of arsenic, and skin irradiation.

25. d. **Keratoacanthoma** is a nodule or plaque that occurs on sun-damaged skin and can cause spontaneous regress. It is characterized histologically by a keratin-filled crater with atypical squamous epithelial cell proliferation forming keratin pearls or squamous eddies. This lesion can be considered as a subtype of squamous cell carcinoma.

26. e. This is **basal cell carcinoma** (BCC), characterized by nodularity, palisade arrangement of peripheral cels, accumulation of mucin between tumor cells, and presence of pigmented cells in between the nodules. BCC is the most frequent skin cancer and develops in both sun-exposed and sun-protected areas. It can develop after treating psoriasis patients with PUVA. The basosquamous type has a worse prognosis. Unlike squamous cell carcinoma, BCC does not express EMA or Ulex europaeus lectin.

27. a. Lesions in the face are difficult to excise with adequate margins and can extend easily to the meninges. The sclerosing histologic type has tightly clustered tumor cells (Morphea type) and shows high recurrence rate. **Increased recurrence** is also related to over expression of p53.

28. b. This IgE-mediated chronic skin condition may reach an incidence as high as 20%. **Atopic dermatitis** is characterized by areas of severe pruritus, erythema, scaling, excoriation, and other cutaneous changes due to chronic rubbing and scratching. Most cases are diagnosed in children and have female predominance. In acute phases, the lesion manifests histologically as parakeratosis, spongiosis, exocytosis of lymphocytes, and perivascular infiltrate. Secondary bacterial infection is common.

29. a. **Acanthosis nigricans** is associated with internal malignancies or conditions characterized by insulin resistance such as diabetes, obesity, and Cushing syndrome. It is characterized by papillomatosis and hyperkeratosis rather than acanthosis or hyperpigmentation. Mutations in the ABCC/MRP6 (ATP-binding

protein) gene are responsible for pseudoxanthoma elasticum.

30. **b. Hidradenoma papilliferum** occurs in the skin of the vulva, in the perineal or perianal region. Histologically, it is an adenoma with cystic and papillary projections that represent apocrine differentiation. It is located in the dermis, is well circumscribed and capsulated, and shows no connection to the overlying epidermis.

31. **c. Follicular mucinosis** refers to the degeneration of the follicular infundibulum with mucin deposition. The condition appears as erythematous papules and/or plaques and may cause alopecia. In adults, it can occur in association with lymphomas, particularly T-cell lymphomas. The deposited mucin consists predominantly of hyaluronic acid and is PAS-positive.

32. **a.** Both **syringoma and desmoplastic trichoepithelioma** commonly occur in the face of young women and may have similar histologic appearance. Syringoma is an adenoma of intraepidermal eccrine ducts. It is usually solitary but may multiply, and is composed of numerous small ducts embedded in dermal fibrous stroma. Keratin cysts may be present near the epidermis. Desmoplastic trichoepithelioma is an indurated lesion in the face that consists of narrow strands of basaloid tumor cells and horn cysts in desmoplastic stroma. However, trichoepithelioma lacks true ductal structures. Both lesions may need to be distinguished from eccrine carcinoma and basal cell carcinoma.

33. **e.** S-100 is very sensitive for neoplastic melanocytes and is almost always positive. HMB-45 and Mart-1 are more specific but less sensitive. In contrast, normal melanocytes are reactive for S-100, Fontana-Masson-Silver stain, and DOPA, but negative for keratin and HMB-45.

34. **d. Congenital nevi** can be intradermal, junctional, or compound and are less common than acquired nevi. They may progress to develop melanoma. Giant congenital nevi may be associated with leptomeningeal melanocytosis and neurologic disorders. Blue rubber bleb nevus is a syndrome of multiple cavernous hemangiomas in the skin and GI tract.

35. **b.** Melanomas are characterized by their large size, asymmetry, and irregular color and borders. In nevi, the melanocytes show good nesting pattern and maturation. **Spitz nevi** can also show mitotic figures, pleomorphism, and intraepidermal pagetoid spread, similar to melanoma.

36. **c.** Although the skin lesion as depicted in this picture demonstrates nesting of melanocytes and pigmentation, the most significant finding is spread of melanocytes into the epidermis (epidermotropism or **Pagetoid spread**). Pagetoid melanocytes are best known in melanoma, but can also be seen in benign melanocytic neoplasms such as Spitz nevus.

37. **d.** Hutchinson freckle is also called **lentigo maligna** and is commonly seen in the cheeks of elderly white people. It appears as a pigmented mottled, irregularly

outlined, slowly enlarging lesion, in which there are increased numbers of scattered atypical melanocytes in the epidermis. It frequently undergoes spontaneous regression but can give rise to melanoma. After many years, the dermis may be invaded and the lesion is then termed lentigo maligna melanoma.

38. **e.** The presence of tumor-infiltrating lymphocytes, among and in contact with tumor cells, has powerful independent prognostic significance. The prognosis is best in tumors where lymphocytes form a continuous band beneath the tumor or diffusely throughout the tumor. Tumors with no lymphocyte response have a bad prognosis.

39. **a.** All of these factors are important in determining the **prognosis** of the patient. Other important factors include vascular invasion, perineural invasion, microscopic satellitosis, infiltrating lymphocytes, and surgical margin. Depth of invasion is a very important prognostic indicator and can be measured by Clark levels or by measuring the thickness of invasion in millimeters from top of the granular layer to the deepest point of invasion (Breslow thickness). Tumor stage is calculated from the depth of invasion and presence or absence of ulceration and is the most significant prognostic factor.

40. **c. Merkel cell carcinoma** commonly occurs in the skin of the face and extremities of adults. Tumors can be found in lymph nodes (as metastasis) but with no apparent primary or after the primary tumor has regressed. The tumor cells are positive for CD20 and neurofilament but negative for TTF-1.

41. **e.** Basal cell carcinoma may show various histologic patterns including **nodular**, cystic, adenoid, superficial, sclerosing, and basosquamous. Basosquamous carcinoma has biologic aggressiveness intermediate between basal and squamous cell carcinomas.

42. **b. Dermatofibrosarcoma protuberans** (DSFP) is a relatively uncommon soft tissue neoplasm with intermediate- to low-grade malignancy. Although metastasis rarely occurs, DFSP is a locally aggressive tumor with a high recurrence rate. Cytogenetic studies may reveal reciprocal translocations of chromosomes 17 and 22, t(17;22), and supernumerary ring chromosomes composed from bands 17(17q22) and 22(22q12). These rearrangements fuse the collagen type I alpha 1 (COL1A1) and the PDGF-B chain genes.

43. **a.** The images show a heavily pigmented nevus, consistent with blue nevus. **Blue nevi** usually appear in the second decade of life and may be located in any location. Melanin pigment may be present in the spindle-shaped melanocytes or in the melanophages present in the dermis.

44. **c. Dermatofibroma** is the most common fibrohistiocytic proliferation in adults and has to be differentiated from a scar. A scar has epidermal atrophy and the fibroblasts are oriented parallel to the epidermis. Dermatofibroma has epidermal hyperplasia, and the fibroblasts often make whorls in the surrounding dermis.

Immunostains may also be necessary for correct diagnosis. Dermatofibroma, unlike DSFP, is positive for factor 13a and negative for CD34.

45. **a.** Langerhans cell histiocytosis is a proliferation of histiocytes that are immunoreactive with S-100 protein, peanut agglutinin and CD1a and contain Birbeck granules by electron microscopy. Cutaneous involvement is encountered most commonly in the acute disseminated form of the disease. Cutaneous lesions may appear as petechiae, papules, diffuse eruption, and often resemble seborrheic dermatitis.

46. **e.** Spitz nevi cells are usually large, spindle, or epithelioid in shape and show considerable pleomorphism. They may have pagetoid spread into the epidermis and frequently have mitotic figures. Thus, Spitz nevi can easily be confused with melanoma. However, they are usually symmetric and well-circumscribed. Kamino bodies, appearing as eosinophilic hyaline globules in Spitz nevi, may help in the diagnosis.

47. **b.** Keratin-containing cyst lined by squamous mucosa with adnexal structures is a **dermoid cyst.** It differs from trichilemmal cyst (pilar cyst) in that the squamous epithelium contains a granular layer. The cyst is commonly located on the lateral eyebrow.

48. **a.** The images show a cystic dermal neoplasm with papillary infoldings. **Syringocystadenoma papilliferum** is an adnexal neoplasm that often appears on the scalp as red papillomatous plaques. Histologically, the tumor connects to the overlying epidermis and contains cystic spaces and papillary proliferation lined by two layers of cells. The outer layer is squamous epithelium and the inner layer is sweat gland epithelium. Infiltrate of plasma cells is characteristically present around the tumor and in the papillary cores, and thus differentiates it from hidradenoma papilliferum.

49. **a. Mast cell disease** (urticaria pigmentosa) is a benign common infiltration of the skin by mast cells which exhibit cytoplasmic metachromatic granules (as seen with Giemsa stain). The mast cells are grouped together making a tumor aggregate and can also be highlighted with CD117 immunostain. The disease usually resolves spontaneously.

50. **b. Juvenile xanthogranuloma** is the most common form of non-Langerhans cell histiocytosis seen in children. Histologically, it appears as dense dermal infiltrate of variably lipidized histiocytes. The presence of "Touton" giant cells is characteristic. Juvenile xanthogranuloma is benign and rare forms may have systemic involvement. Other histiocytic or **fibrohistiocytic tumors** can also have giant cells, including dermatofibroma, reticulohistiocytoma, dermatofibrosarcoma protuberans, and fibroblastoma.

51. **e.** The histology demonstrates atypical keratinocytes with loss of polarity, loss of orderly maturation, dyskeratosis, pleomorphism, and increased mitoses, characteristic of **high grade dysplasia or squamous carcinoma in situ.** This disease occurs with sun exposure in the elderly but can occur in young individuals with xeroderma pigmentosum or arsenical keratosis. Mutations in the PTC gene in chromosome 9 (Gorlin syndrome) predispose to basal cell carcinoma in the affected patients.

■ Recommended Readings

Barnhill RL, Crowson AN. *Textbook of dermatopathology,* 2nd ed. New York: McGraw-Hill, 2004.

Caputo R, Gelmetti C. *Pediatric dermatology and dermatopathology: A concise atlas.* London: Martin-Dunitz, 2002.

Elder D, Elenitsas R, Jaworsky C, et al. *Lever's histopathology of the skin.* Philadelphia: Lippincott-Raven, 1997.

Rapini RP. *Practical dermatopathology.* Philadelphia: Elsevier Mosby, 2005.

Weedon D. *Skin pathology,* 2nd ed. Philadelphia: Churchill Livingstone, Elsevier, 2002.

Soft Tissue, Bone, and Joints

Atif Ahmed

■ Questions

1. Joint stiffness and decreased mobility of the joints are features of all of the following conditions EXCEPT:
   a. Gout
   b. Arthrogryposis
   c. Multiple pterygium syndrome
   d. Homocystinuria
   e. Osteoarthritis

2. An aspirate of a lytic bone lesion in the rib yielded the large cells shown (Fig. 4.1). These cells are:
   a. Myeloma cells
   b. Langerhans histiocytes
   c. Osteoblasts
   d. Osteoclasts
   e. Gaucher cells

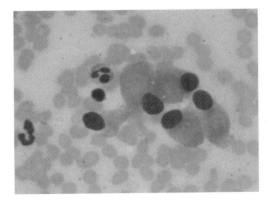

Figure 4.1

3. Short stature can result from of all the following metabolic conditions EXCEPT:
   a. Congenital hypothyroidism
   b. Hereditary fructosemia
   c. Congenital adrenal hyperplasia
   d. Hypoparathyroidism
   e. Pituitary adenoma

4. Rickets-like radiologic changes are characteristically seen in all of the following disorders EXCEPT:
   a. Vitamin C deficiency, "scurvy"
   b. Vitamin D deficiency
   c. Chronic liver disease
   d. Hypophosphatasia
   e. Hypophosphatemia

5. Fibrous dysplasia occurring in a patient with café-au-lait skin spots is a characteristic of:
   a. Xeroderma pigmentosa
   b. Tuberous sclerosis
   c. Peutz-Jeghers syndrome
   d. Neurofibromatosis
   e. McCune–Albright syndrome

6. Syndromes associated with "tall stature" include all of the following diseases EXCEPT:
   a. Klinefelter syndrome
   b. Homocystinuria
   c. Marfan syndrome
   d. Turner syndrome

7. This baby (Fig. 4.2) was born at 35 weeks of gestation and died a few days after birth with respiratory failure. The diagnosis is:
   a. Potter sequence
   b. Down syndrome
   c. Skeletal dysplasia
   d. Thalassemia major
   e. "Overgrowth" syndrome

8. This CD99-positive tumor (Fig. 4.3) is found in the metaphyseal region of the right femur of a 15-year-old

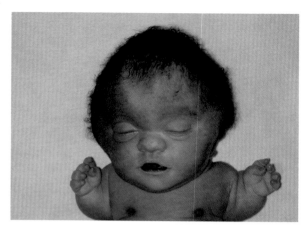

Figure 4.2

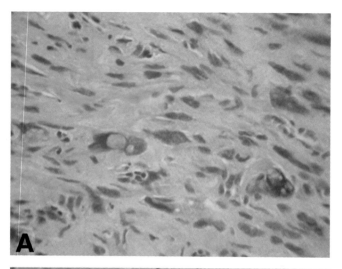

A

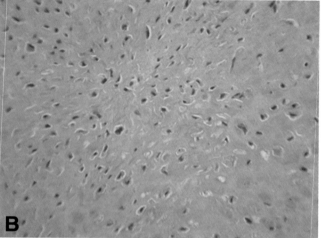

B

Figure 4.4

boy. The differential diagnosis should include all of the following EXCEPT:
a. Lymphoma
b. Ewing sarcoma
c. Osteosarcoma
d. Synovial sarcoma
e. Chondrosarcoma

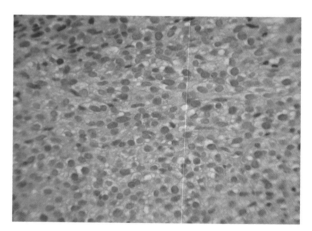

Figure 4.3

9. Which of the following statements best describes elastofibroma?
a. It is a well-circumscribed nodule occurring in the face of adults.
b. It is composed of alternating bands of collagen and elastic fibers.
c. It is found in the scapular region of young children.
d. It is related to injury associated with birth.
e. It is a rapidly growing tumor following trauma.

10. These are sections of a metastatic tumor in the lung of a 16-year-old boy (Fig. 4.4). The diagnosis is most likely:
a. Pleomorphic sarcoma
b. Chondrosarcoma
c. Osteosarcoma

d. Malignant fibrous histiocytoma with cartilaginous differentiation
e. Pulmonary hamartoma

11. Grading of soft tissue sarcomas depends on all of the following histologic features EXCEPT:
a. The degree of resemblance to normal adult mesenchymal tissue
b. The number of mitotic figures per 10 fields
c. The degree of tumor necrosis
d. Expression of P53
e. The histologic type of the tumor

12. A 25-year-old man developed a painless lump in his right arm (Fig. 4.5) that started to grow 3 weeks after playing in a football match. Which of the following statements apply to this lesion?
a. It needs to be reexcised with adequate margin because of its malignant potential.
b. Translocation t(12;15) is identified in most tumor cells.

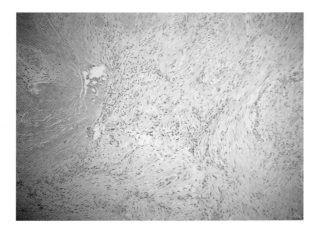

Figure 4.5

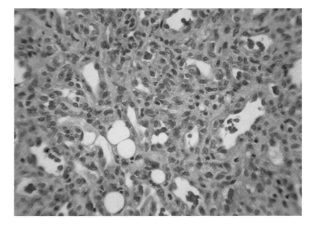

Figure 4.7

c. The tumor cells characteristically stain with CD34 and S-100.
d. It rarely recurs after excision.
e. It occurs chiefly in older individuals and the elderly.

13. Cytogenetic abnormalities identified in this type of neoplasms (Fig. 4.6) include:
    a. Abnormalities in chromosome 8q
    b. Chromosomal aberrations in 12q
    c. Translocation t(12;16)(q13;p11)
    d. Deletion of chromosomal region 1p
    e. Translocation involving chromosomes 17 and 22

c. Ewing sarcoma
d. Pleomorphic malignant fibrous histiocytoma
e. Myxoid malignant fibrous histiocytoma

16. These micrographs (Fig. 4.8) are from a section of radiolucent bony lesion in the distal fibula of a 23-year-old woman. The diagnosis is:
    a. Unicameral bone cyst
    b. Aneurysmal bone cyst
    c. Metaphyseal fibrous defect
    d. Giant cell tumor
    e. Benign fibrohistiocytic tumor

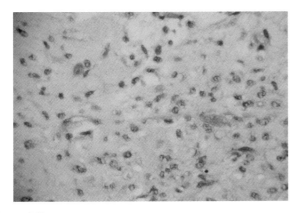

Figure 4.6

14. The nature of this neoplasm (Fig. 4.7) can be delineated by using any of the following immunohistochemical markers EXCEPT:
    a. D2-40
    b. Factor VIII
    c. *Ulex europaeus* lectin
    d. CD34
    e. CD31

15. The type of soft tissue sarcoma that develops most commonly in sites of prior radiation in adults is:
    a. Fibrosarcoma
    b. Extraskeletal osteosarcoma

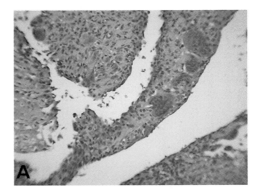

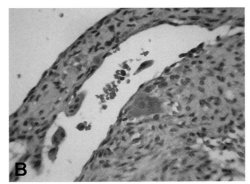

Figure 4.8

17. Criteria for the diagnosis of myositis ossificans include all of the following EXCEPT:
    a. Rapid growth rate
    b. Sarcoma-like histologic appearance
    c. Occurrence after trauma
    d. Radiologic films showing soft tissue mass with calcifications
    e. Absence of mitosis or atypia

18. This tumor (Fig. 4.9) has the EWS/WT1 fusion transcript. Which of the following statements about this tumor is true?
    a. It commonly presents as a bony lesion in long bones.
    b. It is more common in women than in men.
    c. Patients have a good prognosis.
    d. The tumor commonly occurs in the kidneys.
    e. The cells are positive for cytokeratin and desmin.

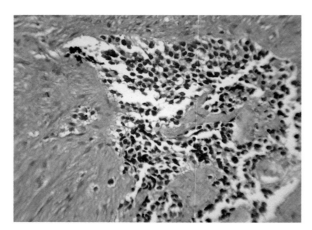

Figure 4.9

19. This tumor (Fig. 4.10) occurring in the wrist of a 32-year-old woman is most likely:
    a. Tendosynovial giant cell tumor
    b. Pigmented villonodular synovitis
    c. Tuberculous bursitis

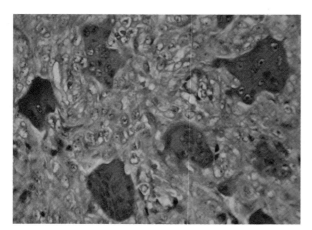

Figure 4.10

    d. Synovial chondrometaplasia
    e. Malignant giant cell tumor

20. Which of the following is a characteristic feature of desmoid fibromatosis?
    a. It occurs in blacks more than in whites.
    b. It can recur and metastasize.
    c. It commonly presents in the abdominal wall.
    d. Tumor cells do not show mitotic activity.
    e. Immunohistochemical expression of desmin and myogenin is characteristic.

21. The most important prognostic factor in patients with atypical lipoma/well-differentiated liposarcoma is:
    a. P53 gene mutations
    b. Amplification of MDM2 gene
    c. Foci of dedifferentiation
    d. Tumor location
    e. The presence of supernumerary chromosomes

22. Translocation t(12;16)(q13;p11) is the genetic hallmark of:
    a. Myxoid liposarcoma
    b. Atypical lipoma/well-differentiated liposarcoma
    c. Pleomorphic liposarcoma
    d. Pleomorphic lipoma
    e. Dedifferentiated liposarcoma

23. All of the following events are frequent occurrences in desmoid fibromatosis tumor EXCEPT:
    a. Inactivation of APC tumor suppressor gene on chromosome 5q
    b. Activating β-catenin mutations
    c. P53 gene mutation
    d. Gardner syndrome-associated genetic events
    e. Trisomy 8

24. The differential diagnosis of this soft tissue shoulder mass (Fig. 4.11) includes all of the following tumors EXCEPT:
    a. Epithelioid sarcoma
    b. Ewing sarcoma/PNET

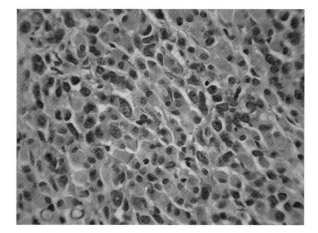

Figure 4.11

c. Rhabdomyosarcoma
d. Rhabdoid tumor

25. The most common location of rhabdomyoma is the:
a. Genital region
b. Heart
c. Skin
d. Head and neck region
e. Uterus

26. This intraosseous radiolucent lesion is eroding the skull of a 10-year-old boy (Fig. 4.12). The diagnosis is:
a. Hodgkin lymphoma
b. Langerhans cell histiocytosis
c. Giant cell tumor
d. Malignant fibrohistiocytoma
e. Rhabdomyosarcoma

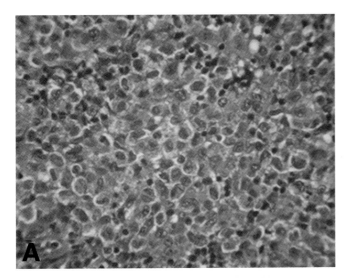

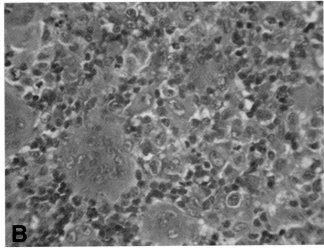

Figure 4.12

27. All of the following soft tissue tumors stain with cytokeratin EXCEPT:
a. Desmoplastic round blue cell tumor
b. Epithelioid sarcoma

c. Biphasic synovial sarcoma
d. Angiosarcoma
e. Granular cell tumor

28. Kaposi sarcoma occurs mainly in:
a. Elderly men of Mediterranean and eastern European descent
b. Non-HIV infected children in Africa
c. AIDS patients infected with human herpes virus (HHV8)
d. Immunosuppressed solid organ transplant recipients
e. All of the above

29. This is a polymerase chain reaction (PCR) study of a tumor located on a patient's left femur (Fig. 4.13). The patient's DNA (187R) and positive control (TC71 cell line with type 1 EWS/FLI1 fusion transcript) are tested with primers that can detect EWS/FLI1 (F) and EWS/ERG (F/e) transcription products. F/e is a consensus primer that can detect both EWS/FLI1 and EWS/ERG fusion transcripts while F is specific for EWS/FLI1. The result shows that the patient:
a. Is positive for EWS/ERG fusion transcript
b. Is positive for both EWS/FLI1 and EWS/ERG fusion transcripts
c. Is positive for EWS/FLI1 fusion transcript
d. Is indeterminate because of contamination
e. Should be tested by different set of primers

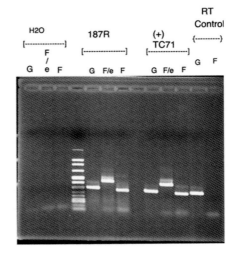

Figure 4.13

30. A clinicopathologic feature of alveolar soft part sarcoma that is important in the definitive diagnosis is:
a. Histologic appearance resembling alveolar rhabdomyosarcoma
b. Common presentation in the hand and wrist
c. Immunohistochemical expression of myogenin

d. The presence of PAS-positive granular eosinophilic cytoplasm in the tumor cells

e. The presence of intermediate filaments bundles in the cytoplasm by electron microscopy

31. This histologic appearance (Fig. 4.14) is compatible with a diagnosis of:
    a. Osteomalacia
    b. Osteopetrosis
    c. Hyperparathyroidism
    d. Pseudogout
    e. Myositis ossificans

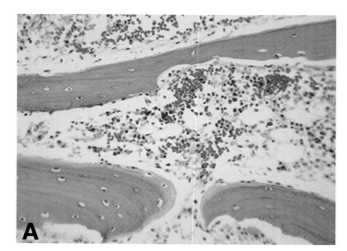

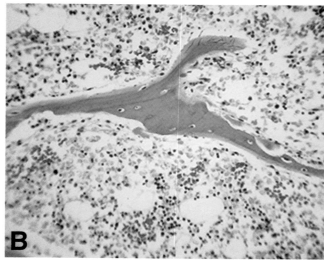

Figure 4.14

Questions 32 and 33:
This tumor occurred in the soft tissue around the knee (Fig. 4.15).

32. An immunostain that is most important in reaching the diagnosis is:
    a. Vimentin
    b. EMA
    c. Desmin

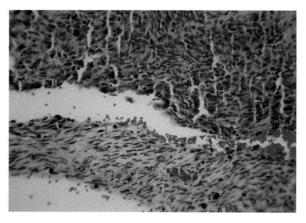

Figure 4.15

d. CD34
e. CD99

33. DNA from the tumor was tested by RT-PCR for specific translocations, using SX1 and SX2 primers that detect SYT-SSX1 and SYT-SSX2 fusion transcripts, respectively (Fig. 4.16). 194 R is the patient's sample, LAL is positive control containing SYT-SSX1 fusion transcript. Which of the following statements is most accurate?
    a. The tumor is positive for SYT-SSX1 fusion transcript.

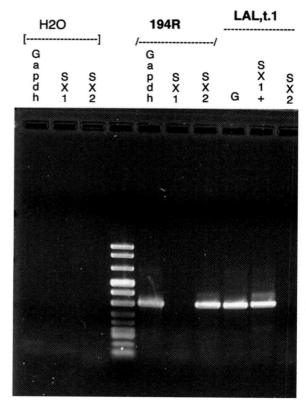

Figure 4.16

b. The tumor is positive for SYT-SSX2 fusion-transcript.

c. The test has to be repeated because of DNA contamination.

d. A positive control for SYT-SSX2 fusion transcript needs to be included.

34. This tumor occurred in a patient with NF1 gene mutation (Fig. 4.17). The diagnosis is most likely:
  a. Schwannoma
  b. Meningeal hemangiopericytoma
  c. Nerve sheath myxoma
  d. Malignant peripheral nerve sheath tumor
  e. Neurofibroma

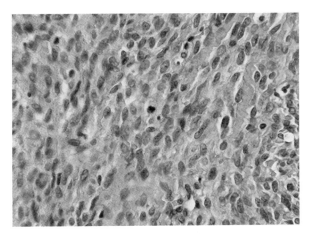

Figure 4.17

35. A small, round cell tumor immunoreactive to vimentin and CD99 is UNLIKELY to be:
  a. Ewing sarcoma
  b. Desmoplastic round cell tumor
  c. Synovial sarcoma
  d. Neuroblastoma
  e. Lymphoblastic lymphoma

36. Various histologic features seen in conventional osteosarcoma include the formation of any of the following mesenchymal elements EXCEPT:
  a. Thin arborizing lace-like osteoid
  b. Dense compact osteoid
  c. Large eosinophilic cells with cytoplasmic cross striations
  d. Fibroblastic spindle cells
  e. Cartilage

37. Which of the following types of osteosarcoma is considered a low-grade malignancy?
  a. Parosteal osteosarcoma
  b. Periosteal osteosarcoma
  c. Telangiectatic osteosarcoma
  d. Small cell osteosarcoma
  e. Conventional osteosarcoma

38. This is a soft tissue mass in the thigh of a 22-year-old man (Fig. 4.18). The diagnosis can be confirmed by demonstrating any of the following features EXCEPT:
  a. PAS stain positivity
  b. Nuclear immunoreactivity of TFE3
  c. Ultrastructural demonstration of cytoplasmic lysosomal granules
  d. Presence of chromosomal translocation t(X;17)
  e. RT-PCR showing ASPL/TFE3 fusion transcript

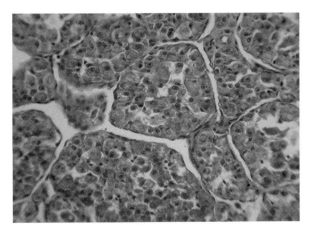

Figure 4.18

39. Deposition of refractile needle-shaped crystals in the joints occurs in which of the following conditions?
  a. Gout
  b. Pseudogout
  c. Oxalosis
  d. Ochronosis
  e. Amyloidosis

40. All of the following conditions can arise as a complication of osteoarthritis EXCEPT:
  a. Fibrillation
  b. Eburnation
  c. Tenosynovitis
  d. Chondrolysis
  e. Subchondral cysts

41. Which of the following statements apply to "exostosis"?
  a. It forms as a complication of osteoarthritis.
  b. It is an intramedullary cartilaginous neoplasm.
  c. It is an intramedullary body composed of mature compact bone.
  d. Exostosis is a cartilage-capped subperiosteal bony projection.
  e. Exostosis is a peculiar congenital anomaly of the thoracic wall.

42. Multiple enchondromas are a feature of:
  a. Ollier disease
  b. Maffucci syndrome

c. McCune-Albright syndrome
d. Both a and b are correct
e. Both a and c are correct

43. Necrosis of the femoral head can occur as a complica-
    tion of all of the following conditions EXCEPT:
    a. Sickle cell anemia
    b. Gaucher disease
    c. Paget disease
    d. Osteoarthritis
    e. Legg-Calvé-Perthes

44. Which of the following statements are correct concern-
    ing "Baker cyst"?
    a. It is commonly found in the popliteal fossa.
    b. It arises as a complication of congenital dislocation
       of the hip.
    c. It is commonly seen around the wrist joint.
    d. The cyst is lined by simple flattened epithelium.
    e. It is another name for ganglion cyst.

45. Which of the following statements is true concerning
    "dedifferentiated chondrosarcoma"?
    a. It is composed of small, round poorly differentiated
       cells with focal admixed areas of cartilaginous
       matrix.
    b. It contains numerous cells with clear cytoplasm.
    c. It is a low-grade malignancy.
    d. It comprises 10% of all chondrosarcomas.
    e. It commonly occurs in the epiphysis of long bones.

46. Which of the following bone conditions is considered
    neoplastic?
    a. Fibrous dysplasia
    b. Langerhans cell histiocytosis (eosinophilic
       granuloma)
    c. Brown tumor of hyperparathyroidism
    d. Nonossifying fibroma
    e. Intraosseous ganglion

47. Which of the following antibodies is helpful to differ-
    entiate chordoma from chondrosarcoma?
    a. S-100
    b. Cytokeratin

c. Desmin
d. Vimentin
e. Actin

48. Glomus tumors are most commonly located in the:
    a. Retroperitoneum
    b. Deep soft tissues of the extremities
    c. Liver
    d. Hand
    e. Lung

49. What is the most common location for
    chondrosarcoma?
    a. Pelvic bones
    b. Ribs
    c. Skull
    d. Short bones of hands and feet
    e. Long bones

50. A biopsy of a single bony lesion in the femur of a
    50-year-old man is shown (Fig.4 .19). All the following
    immunohistochemical stains are necessary to establish
    the diagnosis EXCEPT:
    a. HMB-45
    b. Cytokeratin
    c. Vimentin
    d. CD45
    e. Myogenin

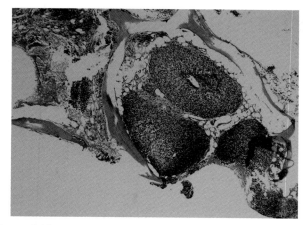

Figure 4.19

■ Answers

1. **d. Joint stiffness** can be congenital or acquired. Arthrogryposis refers to joint contractures observed at birth. Immobility interferes with limb development and causes joint fixation and formation of pterygia. Acquired inflammatory conditions such rheumatoid arthritis or osteoarthritis lead to joint pain and stiffness. On the other hand, patients with Marfan syndrome or homocystinuria have increased mobility of the joints.

2. **c.** These are osteoblasts with characteristic plasmacytoid cytoplasm. The nuclei, however, do not look like plasma cells. Osteoclasts can also be seen in bone aspirates but have multiple nuclei. Langerhans and Gaucher cells have characteristic morphology not observed in this smear.

3. **b. Short stature** with kyphosis and delay in ossification is a feature of congenital hypothyroidism. Pseudohypoparathyroidism is caused by defects in receptors and leads to obesity, short stature, and shortening of metacarpals, metatarsals, and phalanges. Hypoparathyroidism occurs in DiGeorge syndrome and also can be associated with short stature. Congenital adrenal hyperplasia, growth hormone deficiency, hypopituitarism resulting from adenomas can all lead to retardation of growth in children.

4. **a. Rickets** or osteomalacia results from conditions leading to impaired availability of vitamin D, decreased alkaline phosphatase, or increased loss of phosphates in urine. On the other hand, scurvy is characterized by inability to form extracellular collagen, which leads to osteopenia, demineralization, subperiosteal hemorrhage, and microfractures.

5. **e. McCune-Albright syndrome** compromises polyostotic fibrous dysplasia, skin pigmentation, and precocious puberty. Somatic mutations in the G signal transduction protein have been found in persons with this syndrome. The syndrome also causes variety of bony and endocrine abnormalities including hyperthyroidism.

6. **d. Tall stature** can result from growth hormone-secreting tumors, thyrotoxicosis, homocystinuria, and Klinefelter and Marfan syndromes. Patients with Turner syndrome are typically short females with broad chest, wide spacing of the nipples, and congenital lymphedema of the neck, and have 45XO chromosomal pattern.

7. **c.** Combination of short extremities, narrow thorax, and frontal bossing with cloverleaf-like skull configuration is consistent with a skeletal dysplasia. Patients with skeletal dysplasia usually die of respiratory failure due to lung hypoplasia.

8. **e. CD99** positivity is traditionally associated with Ewing sarcoma/PNET. However, some lymphomas, small cell osteosarcoma, and monophasic synovial osteosarcoma can all stain with CD99. Chondrosarcoma is rare in this age group and does not stain with CD99.

9. **b. Elastofibroma** is a benign, poorly circumscribed reactive tumor condition occurring exclusively in the scapular region of elderly people and is characterized by large numbers of prominent elastic fibers.

10. **c. Osteosarcoma** is the most likely diagnosis in this age group and can have cartilaginous differentiation. Thin osteoid can be seen in between the tumor cells in the left upper quadrant of the first image. Chondrosarcoma and malignant fibrous histiocytoma are rare in this age group.

11. **d. Grading of sarcomas** emphasizes tumor differentiation, number of mitotic figures, and tumor necrosis. For example, tumors with >5 mitosis/10 HPF and >15% necrosis are considered high grade or grade III. Certain tumors are by definition high grade, such as alveolar rhabdomyosarcoma.

12. **d. Nodular fasciitis** grows rapidly after trauma and usually affects children and young adults between 20 to 40 years of age. The tumor can have spontaneous regression and does not usually recur after excision. It can involve the skull bones but is considered a reactive nonneoplastic process.

13. **c.** The tumor is composed of lipoblasts in a myxoid background with delicate vasculature and is therefore a **myxoid liposarcoma**. Translocation t(12;16) is found in >90% of myxoid liposarcoma and leads to fusions of CHOP-FUS genes. In rare cases t(12;22)(q13;q12) has been described with fusion of CHOP-EWS ge

14. **a.** CD31, CD34, factor VIII, and *Ulex europaeus* lectin are **endothelial markers** that can be used to stain hemangiomas and other tumors. GLUT-1 is another endothelial marker that is specific for infantile hemangiomas. D2-40 stains lymphatic vessels and is not a general endothelial marker.

15. **d. Malignant fibrous histiocytoma** of the pleomorphic type is the most common postradiation sarcoma in adults and occurs after an interval of 10 to 12 years. It can also arise in chronic ulcers and scars. Other conditions can also develop in sites of prior radiation, including reactive spindle cell proliferation, fractures, osteosarcoma, and fibrosarcoma.

16. **b. Aneurysmal bone cyst** is usually seen in 1 to 20 years of age and occurs mainly in vertebrae and flat bones. Fibroblasts and giant cells in septa that separate cystic spaces are characteristic of aneurysmal bone cyst. On the other hand, solitary or unicameral bone cyst is lined by a slender fibrous membrane that appears different from that of aneurysmal bone cyst.

17. **e. Myositis ossificans** typically presents as a painful, rapidly enlarging mass after an episode of trauma. It occurs chiefly in the muscles of extremities in all ages but is more common in patients younger than age 35. Tumor cells may exhibit pleomorphism and mitotic activity but without abnormal mitotic figures.

18. **e.** A small, round blue cell tumor with EWS/WT1 fusion is **desmoplastic round cell tumor,** which is an aggressive tumor that frequently presents as an abdominal mesenteric or pelvic mass. The tumor occurs more commonly in men than in women. Characteristically, the tumor cells harbor EWS/WT1 gene fusion and are positive for cytokeratin and desmin.

19. **a.** The images show a tumor composed of medium-sized mononuclear cells admixed with giant cells. The histology and the location are more characteristic of tendosynovial giant cell tumor (**nodular tenosynovitis**). Mononuclear cells and the giant cells have similar appearing nuclei, a fact that is characteristic of giant cell tumors. Although pigmented villonodular synovitis can look similar, it is usually found in the knee. The reaming choices have different morphology and/or clinical presentation.

20. **c. Desmoid fibromatosis** occurs commonly in the abdominal wall in young adults. Extra-abdominal tumors can occur but chiefly in the pediatric population. Tumor cells express actin and β-catenin and not myogenin. These tumors can recur but do not metastasize.

21. **d.** The prognosis of **well-differentiated liposarcoma** depends on the degree of surgical excision. Tumors located in surgically accessible soft tissue (such as thigh) do not recur following complete excision with a clear margin. Tumors in deep anatomic locations such as retroperitoneum tend to recur and may dedifferentiate. Supernumerary ring chromosomes and amplification of MDM2 gene occur in both atypical lipoma/well-differentiated liposarcoma and dedifferentiated liposarcoma and are not related to prognosis. The presence of foci of dedifferentiation can affect the prognosis depending on their size but not as degree of surgical excision.

22. **a.** This translocation occurs in more than 90% of **myxoid liposarcoma** cases and results in fusion of CHOP (or DDIT3) and FUS genes. The presence of this fusion is highly sensitive and specific for this tumor.

23. **c. Desmoid tumors** occur more frequently in Gardner syndrome patients and show trisomies 8 and/or 20, inactivation of APC tumor suppressor gene, alteration of the Wnt pathway, and mutations of β-catenin that makes it resistant to the inhibitory effect of APC. P53 and RB1 mutations are infrequent.

24. **b.** The tumor shows cells with eosinophilic cytoplasm and eccentric nuclei. The differential diagnosis includes epithelioid sarcoma and rhabdoid tumor, which can rarely present as a soft tissue shoulder mass. The differential diagnosis also includes rhabdomyosarcoma with numerous eosinophilic rhabdomyoblasts that occur as a result of cytodifferentiation in response to treatment. Immunohistochemistry is helpful in reaching the accurate diagnosis.

25. **d.** The most common location for both adult and fetal **rhabdomyoma** is the head and neck region. It can, however, occur in all of the listed locations.

26. **b.** The image shows tumor cells with abundant cytoplasm and central large nuclei. The cells show nuclear grooves and giant cells, and the lesion is infiltrated by eosinophils. This is a classical example of **Langerhans histiocytosis** (histiocytosis X). Hodgkin lymphoma can have similar histologic appearance but rarely presents as a single radiolucent bony lesion. Giant cell tumor should have more abundant and characteristic giant cells. Immunohistochemistry is helpful as Langerhans histiocytes characteristically stain with S-100 and CD1a.

27. **e.** Desmoplastic round cell tumor, epithelioid sarcoma, and synovial sarcoma characteristically stain with **cytokeratin.** Ewing sarcoma, angiosarcoma, epithelioid fibrosarcoma, and, rarely, leiomyosarcoma can sometimes stain with cytokeratin as well.

28. **e. Kaposi sarcoma** is a low-grade endothelial proliferation that is often associated with immunosuppression. It also occurs sporadically in elderly people of the eastern Europe and Mediterranean region and is endemic in children in Africa.

29. **c.** A fusion transcript band is detected with both primers, indicating EWS/FLI1 fusion. If the patient's tumor had EWS/ERG fusion, only the consensus F/e primer would be positive. The position of the band indicates type 1 EWS-FLI1 fusion transcript, similar to the positive control. This result has to be confirmed with blotting techniques. EWS/FLI1 is the most common translocation found in patients with **Ewing sarcoma/PNET family of tumors.**

30. **d. Alveolar soft part sarcoma** is found in the lower extremities and has a bad prognosis. Cells express nuclear immunoreactivity for TFE3. No evidence of myogenic differentiation is identified in these tumors. The tumor cells show cytoplasmic PAS-positivity corresponding to rhomboidal crystals seen by electron microscopy.

31. **c.** The localized resorption of the bone surfaces resulting in "tunneling effect" is characteristic of **hyperparathyroidism.** Osteoporosis shows a similar histology with generalized thin bone trabeculae but without the concave surfaces.

32. **b.** A sarcoma occurring around the knee joint and showing slit-like spaces is most likely a **synovial sarcoma.** This diagnosis can be reached with positivity for cytokeratin or EMA, which is characteristic for synovial sarcoma. Desmin and C34 may also be helpful in excluding rhabdomyosarcoma and subcutaneous dermatofibrosarcoma protuberans, both of which do not have slit spaces.

33. **d.** A band is present with SX2 primer that has to be verified by including a positive control for SYT-SSX2 fusion transcript and to be further confirmed by southern blotting. Cytogenetic abnormalities, namely t(X;18)(p11;q11), in synovial sarcoma are present in more than 90% of cases. The presence of the genetic

translocation does not affect the prognosis of the patient. Up to 50% of synovial sarcomas recur and they commonly metastasize to the lungs, bones, and regional lymph nodes.

34. **d. NF1 gene** mutations are found in 60% to 70% of patients with multiple neurofibromatosis. However, the tumor in the picture is mitotically active and too cellular for a diagnosis of neurofibroma. Approximately 50% of patients with peripheral nerve sheath tumors have this mutation as well. The histologic picture is consistent with this diagnosis.

35. **d. Neuroblastoma** is reactive with synaptophysin and NSE and is not reactive to vimentin or CD99.

36. **c.** Osteoblastic, osteosclerotic, fibroblastic, and chondroblastic osteosarcomas commonly occur. **Osteosarcoma** is unlikely to have rhabdomyoblastic differentiation. Small cell osteosarcoma can also occur and is in the differential diagnosis of other small round cell tumors.

37. **a.** Parosteal and intramedullary **osteosarcoma** are low-grade tumors while telangiectatic, small cell, and conventional osteosarcomas are usually high grade. Periosteal osteosarcoma is of intermediate grade. Low-grade tumors have indolent growth pattern and high survival rate.

38. **c. Alveolar soft part sarcoma** characteristically occurs in the soft tissue of young adults and shows characteristic histologic, immunohistochemical, and genetic profiles. Translocation t(X;17) results in the fusion of TFE3 transcription factor with ASPL on chromosome 17. This can be demonstrated by nuclear immunoreactivity with TFE3. The tumor cells are positive for PAS, corresponding to the presence of rhomboidal crystals by electron microscopy.

39. **c. Oxalate crystals** appear needle-shaped on polarized microscopy.

40. **c.** Complications of arthritis include synovial hyperplasia. Damage to the articular cartilage is seen in the form of fraying and splitting (fibrillation); and necrosis (chondrolysis) with complete loss of cartilage. The underlying bone may undergo eburnation (superficial necrosis of the articular bone surface); osteophyte formation; microfractures; and subchondral cyst formation.

41. **d. Exostosis** is an osteochondroma that is subperiosteal bony projection capped by cartilage. Exostosis can be solitary or multiple. Option "c" refers to bone island which is an intramedullary island of compact bone. Option "a" refers to intra-articular loose bodies, which are formed of bone and cartilage and arise as a complication of arthritis.

42. **c.** Ollier disease is a developmental anomaly with multiple **enchondromas**. In Maffucci syndrome,

enchondromatosis occurs in association with hemangiomas. Enchondromatosis is more common with Ollier disease than with Maffucci syndrome.

43. **c. Necrosis of femoral head** can arise as common complication of osteomyelitis, radiation, sickle cell anemia, or degenerative joint disease. It can also occur in conditions in which the marrow is replaced by massive cellular infiltrates such as Gaucher disease, lymphoma, or other tumors. Legg-Calvé-Perthes disease affects children between 5 and 9 years of age and causes necrosis of the femoral head that results from interruption of blood flow to the epiphysis, resulting from trauma or increase in intra-articular pressure. Necrosis does not usually occur in Paget disease of the femoral head, unless it is accompanied by a degenerative joint disease.

44. **a. Baker cyst** is a synovium-lined cyst found in the popliteal fossa and may arise as complication of bursitis or arthritis.

45. **d.** Dedifferentiated **chondrosarcoma** is composed of highly malignant spindle cells resembling fibrosarcoma or fibrous histiocytoma and comprises 10% of all chondrosarcomas. It is a high-grade malignancy.

46. **b.** In **Langerhans histiocytosis**, the proliferating Langerhans cells are monoclonal, supporting the fact that it is neoplastic. None of the other conditions are considered neoplastic.

47. **b. Chordoma** is composed of physaliphorous cells that are immunohistochemically positive for S-100, cytokeratin, and epithelial membrane antigen. This immunostaining pattern helps distinguish chordoma from chondrosarcoma, which can focally have similar histologic appearance but is negative for cytokeratin.

48. **d. Glomus tumors** are typically located in the subungual region, the hand, and the foot. The tumor cells are usually positive for smooth muscle actin and type IV collagen.

49. **a.** The pelvic bones, particularly the ileum, are the most frequently involved sites in **chondrosarcoma**.

50. **e.** The differential diagnosis of this tumor include metastatic tumors such carcinomas, melanoma, lymphoma, and sarcomas. In this age group, rhabdomyosarcoma is very unlikely and myogenin is not necessary.

■ Recommended Readings

Fletcher CDM, Unni KK, Mertens F, eds. *World Health Organization classification of tumours: Pathology and genetics of tumours of soft tissue and bone.* Lyon, France: IARC Press, 2002.

Kempson RL, Fletcher CDM, Evans HL, et al. *Atlas of tumor pathology. Tumors of the soft tissue.* Bethesda, MD: AFIP Publications, 2001.

Weiss SW, Goldblum JR. *Enzinger and Weiss' soft tissue tumors*, 5th ed. St. Louis: Mosby, 2007.

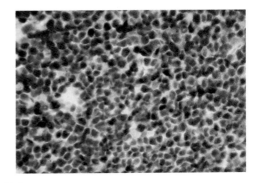

5

Hematopoietic and Lymphoid Tissues

Atif Ahmed

▌ Questions

1. All of the following cell types are found in increased numbers in cases of viral lymphadenitis EXCEPT:
   a. Immunoblasts
   b. Monocytoid B cells
   c. Atypical lymphocytes
   d. Reed–Sternberg cells
   e. Langerhans cells

2. Associated findings in patients with dermatopathic lymphadenopathy include all of the following EXCEPT:
   a. Peripheral blood eosinophilia
   b. Hyperplasia of Langerhans and dendritic cells
   c. Pruritus
   d. Oligoclonal B–cell proliferation
   e. Histiocytes laden with melanin pigment

3. Characteristic features of reactive lymphoid hyperplasia include all of the following EXCEPT:
   a. Lymphoid follicles of varying sizes
   b. Vascular proliferation
   c. Hyperplasia of dendritic cells
   d. Frequent mitotic figures
   e. Overexpression of bcl-2

4. PML-RARα fusion transcript characteristically results in:
   a. Undifferentiated leukemic cells without Auer rods
   b. Inv16(p13q22) translocation
   c. Chronic leukemia with prominent eosinophils
   d. Blast phase of chronic myelogenous leukemia
   e. Leukemia with marked coagulopathy

5. What is the immunostain used in this section of a bone marrow from a patient with acute leukemia (Fig. 5.1)?
   a. CD3
   b. CD20
   c. CD79a

Figure 5.1

   d. Tdt
   e. CD117

6. A most commonly observed feature in patients with Castleman disease is the presence of:
   a. CD1a-positive histiocytes
   b. Lymphoid hyperplasia with hyalinized germinal centers
   c. Lymphoid hyperplasia with numerous plasma cells
   d. Immunoglobulin rearrangement of gamma heavy chain
   e. Dermatopathic lymphadenopathy

7. Activation of the fusion gene AML1/ETO results in:
   a. t(9;11)(p21;q23) translocation
   b. Acute lymphoblastic leukemia
   c. Leukemic cells with Auer rods
   d. Leukemia with biphenotypic profile
   e. All of the above

8. Neoplasms associated with Castleman disease include all of the following EXCEPT:
   a. Hodgkin lymphoma
   b. Hemangioma

c. Kaposi sarcoma
d. Ewing sarcoma
e. Dendritic follicular tumors

9. Which population has the highest frequency of Rosai–Dorfman disease (sinus histiocytosis with massive lymphadenopathy)?
    a. White women
    b. White men
    c. Elderly African Americans
    d. Young African Americans
    e. Hispanic Americans

10. What is the most common lymphoma seen in children?
    a. Lymphoblastic lymphoma
    b. Classical Hodgkin lymphoma
    c. Nodular lymphocyte predominant Hodgkin lymphoma
    d. Diffuse large B-cell lymphoma
    e. Burkitt lymphoma

11. Of the following histologic types of Hodgkin lymphoma, which one has the WORST prognosis?
    a. Nodular sclerosis classical Hodgkin lymphoma
    b. Mixed cellularity
    c. Lymphocyte-depleted type
    d. Lymphocyte-rich
    e. Lymphocyte-predominant type

12. The most important prognostic parameter in Hodgkin disease is:
    a. Age
    b. Race and gender
    c. Clinical stage
    d. Location
    e. Histologic type

13. Classic CD 30+, CD15+ Reed-Sternberg cells are found in all of the following subtypes of Hodgkin disease EXCEPT:
    a. Fibrotic nodular sclerosis
    b. Interfollicular variant
    c. Fibroblastic
    d. Eosinophilic microabscesses
    e. Nodular lymphocyte predominance

14. Which of the following statements are correct regarding refractory anemia with ringed sideroblasts (RARS)?
    a. It is commonly caused by parvovirus infection.
    b. Bone marrow is hypocellular and shows depletion of the erythroid series.
    c. Abundant hemosiderin-laden macrophages are present in the bone marrow.
    d. Evolves to acute leukemia in 50% of cases.
    e. It characteristically occurs in children.

15. BCR/ABL gene fusion at the major breakpoint cluster region leads to all of the following events EXCEPT:
    a. Clonal hematopoietic cell proliferation
    b. Downregulation of tyrosine kinase activity
    c. Enhanced transcription of MYC and BCL-2 genes
    d. The formation of a p210 protein
    e. Chronic leukemia

16. Evolution of chronic myelogenous leukemia to a phase of worse prognosis is heralded by all of the following events EXCEPT:
    a. Presence of bone marrow blasts of lymphoid origin, >20% of cells
    b. Gain of additional chromosomal abnormalities
    c. Drop in absolute neutrophil count
    d. The appearance of pseudo-Gaucher cells
    e. Increase in the size of the spleen

17. Isolated deletion of chromosomal region 5q (5q- syndrome) typically leads to:
    a. Acute leukemia in children
    b. Essential thrombocythemia
    c. Worsening prognosis in chronic lymphocytic leukemia
    d. Myelodysplastic syndrome in elderly white men
    e. Refractory anemia

18. Progressive transformation of germinal centers is associated with which of the following conditions?
    a. Measles
    b. Toxoplasmosis
    c. Syphilitic lymphadenitis
    d. Nodular lymphocyte-predominant Hodgkin disease
    e. Castleman disease

19. A 21-year-old Hispanic woman developed a left-side neck swelling that was excised and a representative section is shown (Fig. 5.2). Which one of the following is the LEAST likely differential diagnosis?

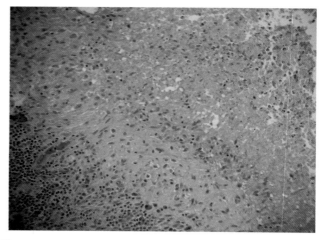

Figure 5.2

a. Cat-scratch disease
b. Kikuchi lymphadenitis
c. Toxoplasmosis
d. Mycobacterium tuberculosis
e. Tularemia

20. The type of cells shown in this Hodgkin lymphoma (Fig. 5.3) results from:
a. Apoptosis of neoplastic cells
b. Activation of NFκB
c. Release of cytokines
d. Immunoglobulin heavy chain rearrangement
e. Infection by Epstein-Barr virus

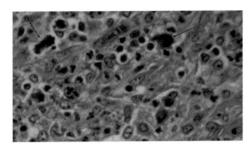

Figure 5.3

21. This phenomenon seen in the lymph node sinus (Fig. 5.4) is a histologic feature seen in all of the following conditions EXCEPT:
a. Sinus histiocytosis with massive lymphadenopathy
b. Castleman disease
c. Lymphoma
d. Familial histiocytosis
e. Epstein-Barr virus infection

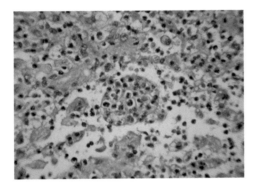

Figure 5.4

22. Lymph node changes seen in patients infected with human immunodeficiency virus include which of the following:
a. Reactive follicular hyperplasia
b. Epstein-Barr virus infection with B cell activation

c. Folliculolysis
d. Follicular involution
e. All of the above

23. A lymphoma with t(11;14)(q13;q32) translocation is most likely:
a. Mantle cell lymphoma
b. Lymphoblastic lymphoma
c. Burkitt lymphoma
d. Mucosa-associated lymphoid tissue (MALT) lymphoma
e. Follicular lymphoma

24. This lymphoma presented as subcutaneous nodules (Fig. 5.5) in a 34-year-old African American woman. Immunostains that are helpful in confirming the diagnosis include all of the following EXCEPT:
a. CD3
b. CD4
c. CD8
d. Granzyme B
e. Tdt

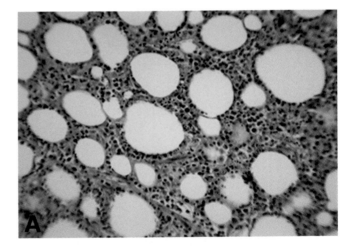

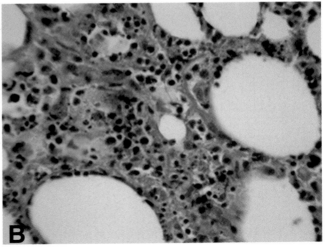

Figure 5.5

25. The features of chronic lymphocytic leukemia that are associated with a worse prognosis include all of the following EXCEPT:
    a. Diffuse bone marrow involvement
    b. Expression of CD5 and CD23
    c. Richter transformation
    d. Prolymphocyte count >10% of circulating lymphocytes
    e. Trisomy 12

26. "Smoldering myeloma" is designated as such because of:
    a. Absence of lytic bone lesions
    b. The presence of anemia with low erythropoietin level
    c. Plasma cells in the bone marrow do not have atypical or pleomorphic forms
    d. Characteristic M-protein spike in the serum
    e. Absence of Bence-Jones proteinuria

27. This is a section of spleen (Fig. 5.6) from a patient with:
    a. Idiopathic thrombocytopenic purpura
    b. Amyloidosis
    c. Rheumatoid arthritis

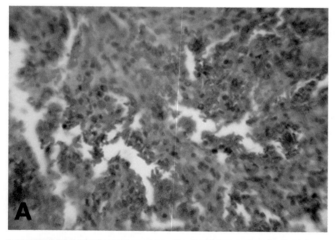

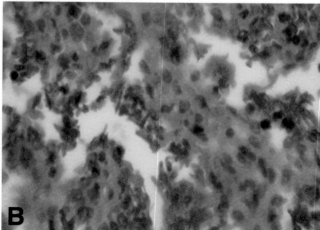

Figure 5.6

d. Chronic myeloid leukemia
e. Sickle cell anemia

28. Cells from this spleen (Fig. 5.7) reveal clonal rearrangement of TCR, gamma-delta type. The diagnosis is most likely:
    a. Small lymphocytic lymphoma
    b. Marginal zone B-cell lymphoma
    c. Anaplastic large cell lymphoma
    d. Hepatosplenic lymphoma
    e. T-cell lymphoma, unspecified

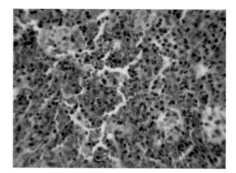

Figure 5.7

29. This intestinal lymphoma (Fig. 5.8) is most likely:
    a. Mantle cell lymphoma
    b. MALT lymphoma
    c. Large B-cell lymphoma
    d. Follicular lymphoma
    e. Immunoproliferative intestinal disease

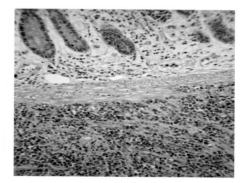

Figure 5.8

30. The term "lymphomatoid polyposis" is used to describe:
    a. Mantle cell lymphoma involving the skin
    b. Lymphoepithelial polypoid lesions in the pharynx
    c. Lymphoid polyps of inflammatory bowel disease
    d. Gastrointestinal polyps with lymphoma

31. The following statements regarding follicular lymphoma are true EXCEPT:
    a. It comprises 35% of non-Hodgkin lymphoma.
    b. It is rare in children and young adults.

   c. The lymphoma cells have rearrangement of
      BCL6 gene.
   d. The cells show BCL2/light chain rearrangement.
   e. Translocation t(14;18) is associated with a worse
      prognosis.

32. Adult T cell lymphoma results as a complication of:
    a. Epstein-Barr virus infection
    b. Human immunodeficiency virus state
    c. Infection by human retrovirus type 1
    d. Methotrexate therapy
    e. Translocation t(2;5)

33. Match each of the following types of lymphoma with
    their characteristic immunophenotype from the choices
    listed below:
    i)   Nasal NK/T-cell lymphoma
    ii) Enteropathy-type T-cell lymphoma
    iii) Intravascular lymphoma
    iv) Lymphomatoid granulomatosis
    v)   Primary effusion lymphoma
    a. CD19−, CD20−, HHV8+
    b. CD3+, CD7+, CD4−, CD8+
    c. CD20−, CD2+, CD56+, TIA+
    d. CD20+, CD79a+, CD19+
    e. CD20+, EBV+, CD30+

34. A 45-year-old man had a mediastinal mass and bilateral
    pleural effusion. Cells from the pleural tap are shown,
    stained with H&E and Tdt immunostain (Fig. 5.9).
    Unfavorable prognosis is expected in this patient
    because of presence of all of the following factors
    EXCEPT:
    a. Male gender
    b. High white cell count
    c. Polyploid tumor cells
    d. BCR/ABL fusion transcript
    e. Translocation t(1;19)(q21;q23)

35. A translocation involving these two normal chromo-
    somes (Fig. 5.10) is present in:
    a. Chronic eosinophilic leukemia
    b. Acute leukemia, M3
    c. Atypical chronic myeloid leukemia
    d. Precursor B-acute lymphoblastic lymphoma
    e. Precursor T-acute lymphoblastic leukemia

36. This lesion was excised from the mandible of an
    African child (Fig. 5.11). The diagnosis can be con-
    firmed with identification of:
    a. Positive staining with CD1a
    b. Translocation t(8:2)
    c. MIB-1 proliferative rate of 50%
    d. Clonal rearrangement of the T-cell receptor gene
    e. Expression of bcl-2

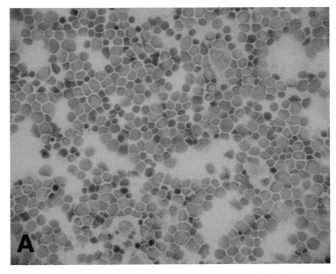
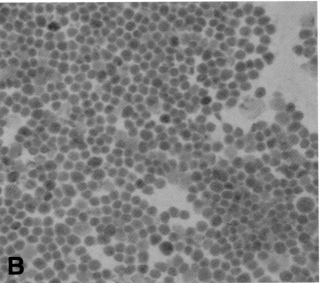

Figure 5.9

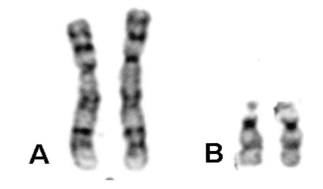

Figure 5.10

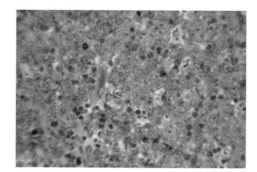

Figure 5.11

37. The blasts in this bone marrow of a 17-year-old patient with trisomy 21 (Fig. 5.12) will most likely stain with:
   a. Tdt
   b. Glycophorin A
   c. CD61
   d. Myeloperoxidase
   e. Sudan Black B

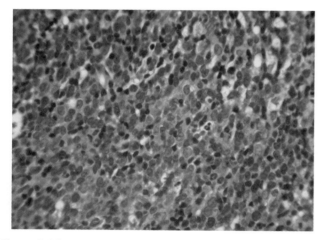

Figure 5.12

38. Epstein-Barr virus is present in all of the following lymphoma types EXCEPT:
   a. Primary effusion lymphoma
   b. Classical Hodgkin lymphoma
   c. Lymphomatoid granulomatosis
   d. Mediastinal large B-cell lymphoma
   e. Posttransplant B-cell lymphoma

39. Translocation t(9;14)(p13;q32) is identified in cases of:
   a. Splenic marginal zone lymphoma
   b. Extranodal margin zone B-cell lymphoma
   c. Mucosa-associated lymphoid tissue (MALT lymphoma)
   d. Lymphoplasmocytic lymphoma

40. Which of the following markers is specific for follicular dendritic cell neoplasms?
   a. CD25
   b. CD21

   c. Pax-5
   d. Vimentin
   e. HAL-DR

41. A hematology student was concerned because of the presence of increased granulocytes, promyelocytes, myelocytes, metamyelocytes, and blasts in the peripheral smear of a patient. Review of the hemogram revealed an elevated total white cell count of 55,000/mm^3. A FISH study was performed to rule out BCR/ABL fusion. Most of the cells had the result shown (Fig. 5.13). ABL is labeled with red probes and BCR with green probes. The diagnosis is:
   a. Chronic neutrophilic leukemia
   b. Leukemoid reaction
   c. Chronic myelogenous leukemia
   d. Acute leukemia
   e. Nonspecific myeloproliferative disorder

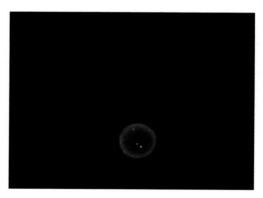

Figure 5.13 (Provided by Dr. Linda Cooley, Children's Mercy Hospital, Kansas City, Missouri.)

42. A 19-year-old patient with orbital mass had increased blasts in the bone marrow (15%). A cytogenetic preparation of the bone marrow was studied by in situ hybridization using probes from chromosome 21 and 8 (red and green, respectively). The result is shown (Fig. 5.14). The diagnosis is most likely:
   a. Acute myeloid leukemia
   b. Acute lymphoblastic leukemia/lymphoma

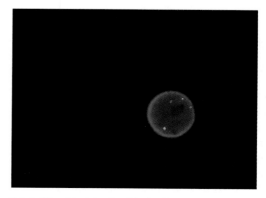

Figure 5.14 (Provided by Dr. Linda Cooley, Children's Mercy Hospital, Kansas City, Missouri.)

c. Myelodysplastic syndrome
d. Chronic idiopathic myelofibrosis
e. Nonhematologic malignancy

43. A 10-year-old girl had a mass in the right axilla that was subsequently resected and studied by histology and immunohistochemistry (Fig. 5.15: **A,B**: H & E; **C**: immunostain for ALKI; **D**: epithelial membrane antigen).

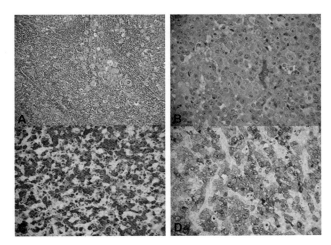

Figure 5.15

Which of the following statements is correct concerning the nature of this disease?
a. The presence of ALk1 positivity imparts a worse prognosis.
b. This tumor is associated with t(2;5) in 10% to 20% of cases.
c. This is a T-cell lymphoma.
d. This tumor has to be differentiated from inflammatory myofibroblastic pseudotumor.
e. A primary cutaneous tumor in the right arm is present in most cases.

44. Which of the following diseases is considered a disorder of T-helper lymphocytes?
a. Mycosis fungoides
b. Anaplastic large cell lymphoma
c. Subcutaneous panniculitis-like lymphoma
d. Large granular lymphocyte leukemia
e. Mantle cell lymphoma

45. What is the neoplastic cell line of Lennert lymphoma?
a. B lymphocytes
b. T lymphocytes
c. NK cells
d. Large granular lymphocytes
e. Epithelioid histiocytes

■ Answers

1. **e.** In **viral lymphadenitis** as in the case of infectious mononucleosis, there is follicular and paracortical hyperplasia with proliferation of immunoblasts, tangible-body macrophages, Reed-Sternberg–like cells, atypical lymphocytes, and monocytoid B cells. Necrosis and viral inclusions can also be seen. Langerhans cells and dendritic cells are not usually prominent. Their presence suggests dermatopathic lymphadenopathy.

2. **d.** **Dermatopathic lymphadenopathy** is a proliferation of histiocytes in patchy aggregates in the cortical or the peripheral areas of the lymph node. The paracortical areas are also expanded by Langerhans cells and interdigitating dendritic cells. 70% of patients with dermatopathic lymphadenopathy have cutaneous T-cell lymphoma or Sézary syndrome.

3. **e.** The size, shape, distribution, and density of the follicles, overexpression of bcl-2, and expression of CD10 in the compressed interfollicular zone in follicular lymphoma help differentiate it from reactive follicular hyperplasia. In **reactive hyperplasia**, there is proliferation of dendritic cells, histiocytes, tingible-body macrophages, and plasma cells.

4. **e.** This fusion transcript results in translocation t(5;17)(q22;q11–12), which is a feature of **acute promyelocytic leukemia**. Leukemic myeloid cells contain characteristic bundles of Auer rods in the cytoplasm, called "faggot cells." This type of leukemia has good prognosis if treated with transretinoic acid therapy.

5. **d.** Section shows diffuse proliferation of blasts that stain with markers of immature cells such as **terminal deoxytransferase** (Tdt). Of the list, Tdt is the only nuclear stain and is positive in lymphoblastic leukemia/lymphoma. All the other choices have antibodies that stain the cytoplasm.

6. **c.** **Hyaline-vascular Castleman disease** is more common than the plasma cell type, which is seen mainly in multicentric Castleman disease. This disease is sometimes associated with the clonal rearrangements of the T-cell receptor gene, and results in a clinical picture similar to that of angioimmunoblastic lymphadenopathy. It is also associated with herpes virus 8, Kaposi sarcoma, large cell lymphoma, and POEMS (polyneuropathy, organomegaly, endocrinopathy, M-protein, and skin changes) syndrome.

7. **c.** This translocation is one of the most common chromosomal aberrations in **acute myeloid leukemia** and occurs predominantly in younger patients. Leukemic cells have myeloid differentiation and show cytoplasmic Auer rods. This type of leukemia has good prognosis and good response to chemotherapy.

8. **d.** Vascular neoplasms, angiomyoid proliferative lesions, angiomatous hamartomas, and HHV-8 positive Kaposi sarcoma have all been reported to occur in patients with **Castleman disease**. Ewing sarcoma is not associated with Castleman syndrome.

9. **d.** **Rosai-Dorfman** disease is mainly seen in young African American children and adolescents. It presents as neck lymphadenopathy and also involves the extranodal areas in one fourth of cases. It is a benign histiocytosis characterized histologically by engulfment of lymphocytes. Phagocytic cells are reactive with S-100 but not with CD1a or Epstein-Barr viral markers.

10. **a.** **Lymphoblastic lymphoma** is the most common lymphoma type in children and is usually of the T-cell type. It presents with mediastinal mass with or without lymphadenopathy. It is a high-grade lymphoma that is typically positive for Tdt and not CD30.

11. **c.** The prognosis of **Hodgkin lymphoma** is best in nodular sclerosis type, followed by mixed cellularity. The overall 5-year survival rate for Hodgkin lymphoma is 75%, and is worst in lymphocyte-depleted type.

12. **c.** Clinical stage is the most important prognostic parameter. Stage IV has the worst prognosis. African Americans men, mediastinal tumor, splenic nodules, lymphocyte depletion, and age more than 50 years are other parameters associated with poor prognosis. Favorable prognostic features in **Hodgkin lymphoma** include female gender, white race, nodular lymphocyte-predominant, and nodular sclerosis histologic types.

13. **e.** Unlike other types of Hodgkin, **nodular lymphocyte-predominant Hodgkin lymphoma cells** are negative for CD30 and CD15 and stain with CD20, CD79a, and BSAP.

14. **c.** **Refractory anemia with ringed sideroblasts** (RARS) characteristically affects older individuals and shows evidence of iron overload in the bone marrow, spleen, and liver. It is an idiopathic disease that can only be diagnosed after excluding all other possible etiologies of erythroid abnormalities. It evolves to acute leukemia in 1% to 2% of cases.

15. **b.** In **chronic myelogenous leukemia**, the breakpoint in the BCR gene is in the major breakpoint cluster region (BCR exons 12–16) and a p210 protein is formed. The fusion gene leads to increased tyrosine kinase receptor activity. Inhibition of tyrosine kinase by Gleevec is a mode of treatment of chronic myelogenous leukemia.

16. **c.** Blast phase of **chronic myelogenous leukemia** resembles acute leukemia where the number of blasts exceeds 20%. The blast lineage is mostly myeloid but can be lymphoblastic in 20% of cases. There is gain of additional chromosomal abnormalities. Splenomegaly, thrombocytosis, and thrombocytopenia are seen in both accelerated and blast phases. The white cell count does not decrease.

17. **e.** **Monosomy 5q- syndrome** characteristically occurs in women and causes myelodysplastic syndrome with blasts <5%. The disease leads to refractory anemia and

increase in megakaryocytes with hypolobated nuclei. Isolated monosomy 5 syndrome is associated with good survival.

18. **d. Progressive transformation of germinal centers** describes an alteration of lymphoid architecture in which lymphoid follicles become enlarged and infiltrated by small lymphocytes. It occurs in association with nodular lymphocyte-predominant Hodgkin disease and other reactive lymphadenopathies.

19. **b.** The image shows a **necrotizing granulomatous lymphadenitis,** which can be caused by fungal, mycobacterial, and spirochetal infections. Cat-scratch disease is a necrotizing granulomatous lymphadenitis caused by *Bartonella henselae* introduced at the site of infection by a cat scratch. Similar to other infections, it can cause central stellate abscesses with palisading histiocytes. Kikuchi lymphadenopathy is a necrotizing lymphadenopathy that is more common in Asian women. Unlike this case, neutrophils and plasma cells are scanty or absent in Kikuchi disease.

20. **c.** The cells in the image, which have condensed cytoplasm and pyknotic nuclei, are called **mummified cells** and can be seen in all types of Hodgkin disease. They result from apoptosis of neoplastic cells. Activation of NFκB possibly protects Hodgkin cells from apoptosis and is not a known mechanism of inducing apoptosis. The inflammatory background in Hodgkin lymphoma results from release of cytokines by neoplastic cells and other reactive cells.

21. **b. Hemophagocytosis** is a characteristic of sinus histiocytosis with massive lymphadenopathy (Rosai-Dorfman disease) and is also seen in infection-associated hemophagocytic syndrome, familial hemophagocytic lymphohistiocytosis, and malignant lymphoma.

22. **e.** Reactive follicular hyperplasia with polyclonal B-cell activation is seen in early stages of infection by **human immunodeficiency virus.** In late stages of "follicular involution," the lymph nodes become atrophic and burnt-out, and the follicular dendritic network is disrupted.

23. **c.** t(11;14)(q13;q32) translocation is found in 70% of cases of **mantle cell lymphoma.** This translocation between immunoglobulin heavy chain and cyclin D1 gene leads to overexpression of BCL1. Additional genetic events in mantle cell lymphoma include deletion of the ATM gene, 13q14 deletion, trisomy 12, and mutations of the cell cycle regulatory proteins such as p53 and p16.

24. **e.** Images show neoplastic karyorrhectic lymphoma cells involving the subcutaneous fat, infiltrating the subcutaneous tissue septa and sparing the dermis. The history and histology are consistent with **subcutaneous panniculitis-like T-cell lymphoma.** The diagnosis is confirmed by positive immunostains with CD3, CD8, granzyme B, perforin, and TIA-1. Most cases have αβ phenotype. Staining for Tdt will not be helpful because the morphology does not look like lymphoblastic lymphoma.

25. **b. Chronic lymphocytic leukemia** is an indolent disease but not curable with chemotherapy. The overall median survival is 7 years. The disease is more aggressive in higher clinical stages with diffuse bone marrow involvement, increased percentage of prolymphocytes in the blood >10%, and presence of trisomy 12. Transformation to diffuse large B-cell lymphoma is called Richter syndrome and is associated with adverse prognosis.

26. **b. Smoldering myeloma** patients are asymptomatic, without bone lesions and are usually not treated until they develop symptoms. They have M-protein peak in the serum and plasma cells in the bone marrow and may have Bence-Jones proteins in the urine. They do not have anemia, hypercalcemia, or renal insufficiency.

27. **e.** Although **sickled red blood cells** are difficult to see in this magnification, the exclusion of other listed entities is the key to the right answer. Splenic lymphoid hyperplasia is seen in idiopathic thrombocytopenic purpura and rheumatoid arthritis. There are no amyloid deposits or infiltration by leukemic cells.

28. **d. Hepatosplenic T-cell lymphoma** presents with hepatosplenomegaly, fever, and weight loss. There is no lymphadenopathy. Infiltrating cytotoxic T cells are typically medium in size and monomorphic in appearance. Cells are usually positive for CD3 and cytotoxic protein TIA-1.

29. **c.** The image shows a lymphoma involving the submucosa and sparing the mucosa. The gastrointestinal tract is one of the most common extranodal sites of involvement by **diffuse large B-cell lymphoma.** Intestinal large B-cell lymphoma involves the mesentery and serosa first and may ulcerate through the mucosa. The remaining listed choices mostly involve the mucosa first and then extend to the submucosa.

30. **d. Lymphomatoid polyposis** is mantle cell lymphoma involving the gastrointestinal tract and presents as multiple polyps with lymphoma cells. The cells express surface IgM, cyclin D1 bcl-2, CD5, and FMC-7 and are negative for CD10 and CD23. Cells show chromosomal translocation t(11;14) between cyclin D1 and Ig heavy chain.

31. **e. Follicular lymphoma** comprises 35% of adult non-Hodgkin lymphoma and is very rare in children. It shows rearrangement of bcl2 and bcl6. Translocation t(14;18) is present in 70% to 90% of cases but is not associated with either better or worse prognosis.

32. **c. Adult T-cell lymphoma** is caused by human retrovirus type 1 and is endemic in Japan and Caribbean region. The cells express CD2, CD3, CD5, and CD4 but are usually negative for CD7. It presents as mediastinal mass and usually regresses spontaneously.

33. **i) c. NK/T-cell lymphoma** (angiocentric T-cell lymphoma) is usually extranodal and is more commonly seen in Asia, Central America, and South America and

causes atypical destructive infiltrate in the wall of the blood vessels.

ii) b. Enteropathy-type T-cell lymphoma is a tumor of intraepithelial lymphocytes and occurs in the jejunum or ileum of patients with celiac disease.

iii) d. Intravascular lymphoma is an aggressive large B-cell lymphoma that involves only the lumina of small blood vessels.

vi) e. Lymphomatoid granulomatosis is an angiocentric lymphoproliferative disease caused by Epstein-Barr virus. The cells have a B-cell phenotype and may be positive for CD30.

v) a. Primary effusion lymphoma is a large B-cell lymphoma presenting as serous effusions and characteristically associated with herpes virus 8 (Kaposi sarcoma herpes virus).

34. **c.** The image reveals an **acute lymphoblastic lymphoma,** which in the mediastinum is most likely of the T-cell type. Hyperdiploidy in acute lymphoblastic leukemia imparts good prognosis. Other poor prognostic features include hypodiploidy, age less than 1 year and more than 10 years, and translocation t(1;19).

35. **e.** The diminutive short arm of the smaller chromosome helps identify it as chromosome 22, which is a pair of t(9;22)(q34;q11) translocation that forms the Philadelphia chromosome der (22q). The **Philadelphia chromosome** is identified in chronic myeloid leukemia and 20% to 30% of acute lymphoblastic leukemia (ALL). It is found exclusively in CD10-positive precursor B-acute lymphoblastic lymphoma. Reports of its presence in T-ALL may represent chronic myeloid leukemia in lymphoid blast crisis rather than Philadelphia chromosome-positive ALL.

36. **b.** The location and the histology of monotonous population of medium-size cells suggest **Burkitt lymphoma.** Translocation of MYC at chromosome 8q24 to the immunoglobulin heavy chain gene at chromosome 14q32 [t(8;14)] or less commonly to the light chain region on 2p12 is found in all cases of Burkitt lymphoma and practically confirms the diagnosis. The starry star appearance is characteristic but not present in this image. MIB-1 proliferative rate is high (99%–100%). Bcl2 is not expressed.

37. **c.** Down syndrome patients develop **acute myeloid leukemia** of the megakaryocytic type. The blasts are usually MPO, SBB, and Tdt negative and are positive for CD61 (platelet glycoprotein IIIa) and CD41 (platelet glycoprotein IIb/IIIa).

38. **d. Epstein-Barr virus** is identified in several lymphoma types including Hodgkin lymphoma, primary effusion lymphoma, NK cell lymphoma, lymphomatoid granulomatosis, and posttransplant lymphoid proliferations. Mediastinal B-cell lymphoma is a subtype of diffuse large B-cell lymphoma that occurs mainly in women in the 3rd to 5th decade of life.

39. **d.** Translocation t(9;14)(p13;q32) and rearrangement of the PAX-5 gene are reported in up to 50% of lymphoplasmocytic lymphoma.

40. **b. Follicular dendritic cell tumor** is a neoplastic proliferation of follicular dendritic cells. They are specifically positive for markers of follicular dendritic cells, i.e., CD21, CD35, and CD23. They are also positive for vimentin and HLA-DR but these are not specific. CD25 is specific for hairy cell leukemia and Pax-5 is a nonspecific B-cell marker.

41. **b. Leukemoid reaction** is an excessive number of neutrophils and other myeloid precursors in the peripheral blood that results as a reaction to infection or stimulation of the bone marrow with growth factors. The white cell count can be very high and can exceed $50,000/mm^3$. Leukemoid reaction can sometimes be confused with chronic myelogenous leukemia and can be differentiated from it by elevation of leukocyte alkaline phosphatase and absence of BCR/ABL fusion (as seen in the image).

42. The image of an interphase nucleus shows fusion transcript of AML1 on chromosome 21 and ETO gene on chromosome 8. Translocation t(8;21)(q22;q22) with AML1/ETO gene fusion is a characteristic finding in **acute myeloid leukemia** and patients may be diagnosed with leukemia despite blast numbers of less than 20%. This type of leukemia predominantly occurs in young patients and may present with a myeloid sarcoma tumor.

43. The images show a lymphoid neoplasm that is positive for Alk1 and epithelial membrane antigen (EMA), thus consistent with **anaplastic large cell lymphoma.** This is a T-cell lymphoma that expresses CD30, EMA, and cytotoxic proteins. Most tumor cells are also positive for ALk1 and thus can be differentiated from the cutaneous large cell lymphoma which can metastasize to regional lymph nodes. Translocation t(2;5) is present in 70% to 80% of cases. ALk1 expression is associated with good prognosis. Inflammatory myofibroblastic tumor also shows ALk1 expression but has a completely different histology and presentation.

44. **a.** Mycosis fungoides is considered a disorder of mature T-helper lymphocytes. The cells express CD2, CD3, Cd5, and CD4 and are negative for CD8.

45. **b. Lennert lymphoma** is an aggressive epithelioid T-cell lymphoma that may be nodal or extranodal. Most cases are positive for CD4 and negative for CD8. Trisomy 3 is frequently present as well.

■ Recommended Readings

Jaffe ES, Harris NL, Stein H, et al, eds. *World Health Organization Classification of Tumours: Pathology and genetics of tumours of haematopoietic and lymphoid tissues.* Lyon, France: IARC Press, 2001.

Kjeldsberg CR. *Practical diagnosis of hematologic disorders*, 4th ed. Chicago: ASCP Press, 2006.

6

Digestive System

Guanghua Wang

■ Questions

1. A segment of esophagus lined by columnar epithelium:
   a. May be an incidental finding with NO clinical significance
   b. Changes to stratified squamous epithelium by 25 weeks of gestation
   c. May indicate Barrett esophagus
   d. May indicate heterotopic gastric mucosa
   e. All of the above

2. Normal findings in the lower esophagus and gastroesophageal junction include all of the following EXCEPT:
   a. The basal layer of the distal esophagus thicker than the rest of esophagus
   b. Abrupt transition between squamous mucosa and oxyntic mucosa
   c. Glycogenated squamous mucosa above the Z-line
   d. Squamous mucosa with submucosal mucous glands
   e. The presence of goblet cells

3. All of these statements are correct about esophagus EXCEPT:
   a. Esophagus length in adults varies with the height of the individual and ranges from 25 to 30 cm.
   b. Esophageal mucosa has three components: squamous epithelium, muscularis mucosae, and the lamina propria.
   c. It may be normal to find glands similar to those of the gastric cardia in the lamina propria of the distal esophagus.
   d. Submucosal mucous gland complexes in the esophagus are most prominent at the upper and lower ends of the esophagus.
   e. Heterotopic gastric mucosa known as the "inlet patch" often results in peptic ulcer or carcinoma.

4. A mediastinal cyst lined by columnar mucosa is a/an:
   a. Bronchogenic cyst
   b. Enterogenous cyst
   c. Gastrointestinal duplication
   d. Thymic cyst
   e. All of the above

5. Failure of the tracheal bud to develop normally from the primitive foregut during embryonic life results most commonly in:
   a. Esophageal web
   b. Tracheomalacia
   c. Esophageal atresia with tracheoesophageal fistula
   d. Duodenal atresia
   e. Zenker diverticulum

6. A 25-year-old man complains of epigastric abdominal pain. Which of the following statements about his biopsy shown in Figure 6.1 is NOT true?
   a. This disease is a frequent reason to be referred to a gastroenterologist.
   b. Patients with this disease often have decreased esophageal sphincter pressure.
   c. The presence of intraepithelial neutrophils indicates severe disease.
   d. It is often associated with hiatus hernia.
   e. The presence of eosinophils in squamous mucosa is a specific histological feature for the diagnosis.

7. All of the following about Barrett esophagus are correct EXCEPT:
   a. Barrett dysplasia is defined as a neoplastic change of the epithelium confined to the basement membrane of the glands with no evidence of invasion.
   b. High-grade dysplasia in a biopsy with Barrett esophagus indicates there is about 70% chance that carcinoma is already present.
   c. The metaplastic Barrett esophagus epithelium can be complete intestinal metaplasia or incomplete intestinal metaplasia.

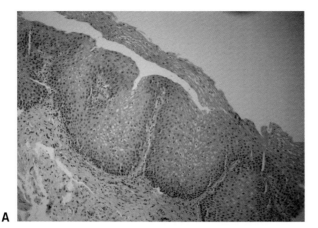

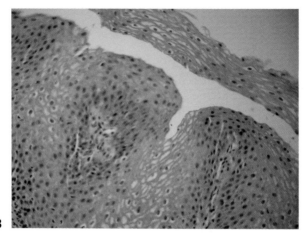

A

B

Figure 6.1

sented with dysphagia and esophageal mass. Genetic alterations implicated in the causation of this lesion include:
a. P53 mutations
b. Myc amplification
c. Microsatellite instability
d. K-ras mutations
e. All of the above

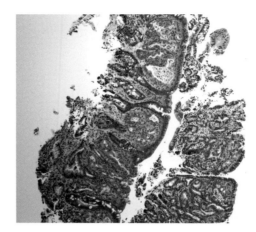

Figure 6.2

d. Incomplete intestinal metaplasia may be more prone to enter the dysplasia-carcinoma sequence than complete intestinal metaplasia.
e. Grading dysplasia in Barrett esophagus is based solely on cytologic features.

8. The diagnosis of Barrett esophagus is made through:
a. Barium swallow findings in a patient with a history of esophageal reflux disease
b. Characteristic endoscopic findings, and biopsy showing histology of esophageal reflux disease
c. Characteristic histologic findings of Barrett esophagus, such as goblet cells, present in the esophageal biopsy
d. Characteristic endoscopic findings of Barrett esophagus and evidence of intestinal metaplasia by biopsy
e. Characteristic endoscopic findings of Barrett esophagus and findings of dysplastic esophageal mucosa in biopsy

9. This esophageal biopsy (Fig. 6.2) was taken from a white male with a history of reflux esophagitis. He pre-

10. The most common cause of infectious esophagitis in AIDS patients is:
a. Bacterial esophagitis
b. Herpes simplex esophagitis
c. Cytomegalovirus (CMV) esophagitis
d. Candida esophagitis
e. Allergic esophagitis

11. This esophageal biopsy (Fig. 6.3) was taken from a 35-year-old man with intermittent dysphagia with food

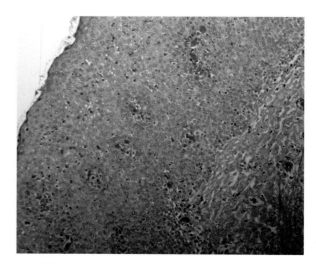

Figure 6.3

impaction. Endoscopy showed multiple esophageal rings. Which of the following statements about this lesion is NOT true?

a. The esophagus normally does NOT contain any eosinophils; their identification in esophageal biopsy represents a pathologic change.

b. The cause of this lesion is most likely associated with parasite infection.

c. The lesion is characterized by a prominent intraepithelial eosinophilic infiltrate.

d. The differential diagnosis in esophageal biopsy with eosinophils infiltrate includes reflux esophagitis, parasitic infection, drug reactions, or eosinophilic esophagitis.

e. Eosinophilic infiltrate in eosinophilic esophagitis is present in all parts of esophagus, while in reflux esophagitis, eosinophilic infiltrate is mainly found distally and taper proximally.

12. The best test to define esophageal reflux is based on:

a. Clinical symptoms of heartburn, regurgitation, and dysphagia

b. Characteristic appearance on upper GI endoscopy

c. Biopsy changes showing infiltration by eosinophils

d. Ambulatory pH monitoring

e. Response to medications

13. Which of the following statements is true about this esophageal mass (Fig. 6.4)?

a. This type of lesion is more common in women than in men.

b. When associated with Barrett esophagus, it has a better prognosis than when not associated with Barrett esophagus.

c. It is three times more common in Barrett esophagus than in the general population.

d. It is more common in whites than in blacks.

e. It is the most common esophageal cancer.

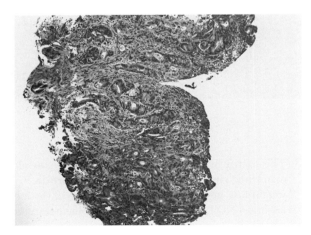

Figure 6.4

14. Which of the following is NOT considered as a risk factor in general for the development of squamous cell carcinoma of the esophagus?

a. p53 gene mutations

b. HPV infection

c. Smoking

d. Heavy consumption of alcohol

e. APC gene mutations

15. Which of the following concerning type of mucins in complete intestinal metaplasia complicating chronic gastritis is true?

a. The predominant mucin type is sialomucin.

b. There is over-expression of MUC-1 mucin.

c. There is over-expression of MUC5AC mucin.

d. There is co-expression of MUC-2 and MUC-6.

e. The predominant mucin type is neutral mucin.

16. Chronic atrophic gastritis caused by *Helicobacter pylori* is mainly associated with increased incidence of:

a. Diffuse-type gastric carcinoma

b. Intestinal-type adenocarcinoma

c. Squamous carcinoma

d. Hepatic-type adenocarcinoma

e. Carcinoid tumor

17. Mutation in E-cadherin gene or alteration of its gene expression predisposes to:

a. Hereditary diffuse gastric carcinoma

b. Intestinal-type adenocarcinoma

c. Squamous carcinoma

d. Hepatoid-type adenocarcinoma

e. Carcinoid tumor

18. Predisposing lesions for the development of gastric carcinoma include which of the following?

a. Gastritis and intestinal metaplasia

b. Gastric Ulcer

c. Hyperplastic polyp

d. Adenoma

e. All of the above

19. This gastric biopsy (Fig. 6.5) was from a 63-year-old woman with a history of chronic atrophic gastritis. All of the following statements are true about this lesion EXCEPT:

a. This type of lesion usually arises from Enterochromaffin-like (ECL) cells of the stomach.

b. Chronic atrophic gastritis is a predisposing factor.

c. This lesion is expected to be positive for chromogranin A and negative for serotonin.

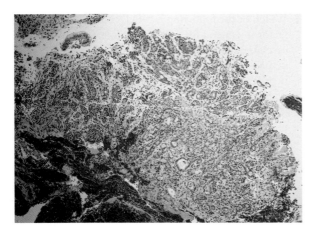

Figure 6.5

    d. This lesion occurs in association with multiple endocrine neoplasia type 2 (MEN2).

    e. Mutation and/or loss of heterozygosity (LOH) at the MEN1 locus is associated with the development of this lesion.

20. This section (Fig. 6.6) was taken from the stomach fundus. In addition to features of chronic gastritis, there is proliferation of cells that measure less than 0.5 mm and are positive for chromogranin immunostain (stain not shown). What is the best designation for this entity?

    a. Carcinoid

    b. Neuroendocrine carcinoma

    c. Neuroendocrine cell hyperplasia

    d. Gastrinoma

    e. Early carcinoid

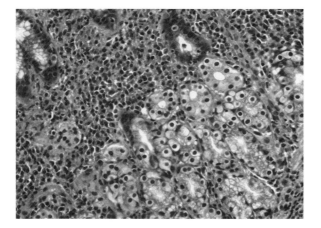

Figure 6.6

21. All following statements are true concerning gastrointestinal stromal tumor (GIST) EXCEPT:

    a. Most GISTs are sporadic, affecting individuals in age group of 50–60 years, and have a slight male predominance.

    b. The type or location of mutation in C-kit may determine the patient's prognosis and treatment response.

    c. PDGFR-α mutations are significantly associated with higher frequency of epithelioid or mixed morphology GIST tumors and impart a favorable prognosis.

    d. Gastrointestinal autonomic nerve tumor (GANT) is a variant of GIST and often stains positively for neuron-specific enolase (NSE), S-100, synaptophysin, chromogranin, and neurofilament protein.

    e. Tumors larger than 10 cm, with no detectable mitotic activity do not recur or metastasize.

22. A 45-year-old man presented with a gastric mass. Histology of the lesion is shown (Fig. 6.7). Immunostains show that neoplastic lymphoid cells are positive for CD20, CD43, and bcl-2 and are negative for CD3, CD5, and CD10. Which of the following is NOT true of this lesion?

    a. t(11;18) API2/MALT1, t(14;18)/IGH-MALT1, t(1;14)/IGH-BCL-10, and t(3;14)/IGH-FOXP1 translocations can all be found in this lesion.

    b. 60%–70% of patients with this lesion have t(11;18) API2/MALT1 translocation.

    c. It is associated with *H. pylori* infection.

    d. Patients with this lesion and t(11;18)(q21;q21) translocation do not respond to antibiotics treatment for *H. pylori* eradication.

    e. t(11;18) API2/MALT1 translocation is usually negative in gastric large B-cell lymphoma arising from this type of lesion.

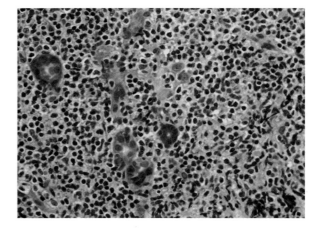

Figure 6.7

23. This gastric biopsy (Fig. 6.8) was from a 45-year-old man with symptoms of epigastric pain, anorexia, weight loss, and peripheral edema. Which of the following is NOT part of the clinicopathologic features described in this lesion?

    a. Clustered incidence in adult and middle-age men

    b. Marked foveolar hyperplasia

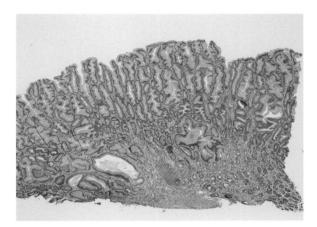

Figure 6.8

   c. Atrophy of oxyntic glands
   d. Prominent chronic inflammatory cell infiltrate
   e. Mucosal cysts

24. All following statements are true about gastric polyps EXCEPT:
   a. The majority of gastric polyps is nonneoplastic.
   b. Fundic gland polyps and hyperplastic polyps are two most common types of gastric polyps.
   c. Fundic gland polyp can occur sporadically or in the setting of familial adenomatous polyposis (FAP), and it can develop after a prolonged use of proton pump inhibitors.
   d. Most hyperplastic polyps develop on a background of chronic gastritis.
   e. Inflammotory fibroid polyps are most commonly found in children.

25. This section (Fig. 6.9) was taken from a 22-year-old man who was found to have multiple small intestinal polyps. All sections show similar histologic features as demonstrated in this image. Which of the following genes is involved in its pathogenesis?
   a. APC gene
   b. TP53

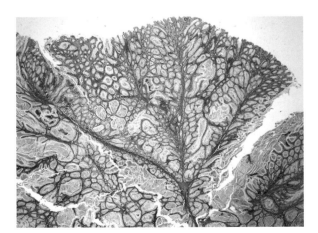

Figure 6.9

   c. STK11
   d. SMAD4
   e. PTEN

26. A 55-year-old male presents with abdominal pain, dysphagia, and gastrointestinal bleeding and abdominal mass. The histology of lesion is shown (Fig. 6.10). Neoplastic cells are positive for CD117, CD34, and S-100. This lesion may be associated with all of the following EXCEPT:
   a. Mutations in PDGFRA or C-KIT genes
   b. Ultrastructural features of neuronal cell processes
   c. Neurofibromatosis type I
   d. Extra-adrenal paraganglioma
   e. Familial trait in majority of cases

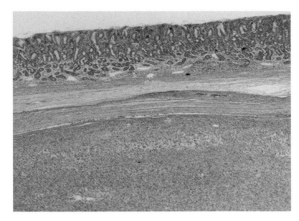

Figure 6.10

27. Which of the following statements is true about infantile hypertrophic pyloric stenosis HPS?
   a. It is more common in female children
   b. It is seen in 1 in 20,000 infants
   c. It has no recognizable pattern of inheritance
   d. Majority of patients present at birth with abdominal mass
   e. The outer longitudinal muscle fibers are hyperplastic and hypertrophic

28. Duodenal atresia is a feature of patients with:
   a. Cystic fibrosis
   b. Total colonic aganglionosis
   c. Turner syndrome
   d. Down syndrome
   e. Absent pancreas

29. This is a duodenal biopsy (Fig. 6.11) from a 25-year-old woman with a history of chronic diarrhea and anemia. The patient has a positive serologic test for transglutaminase antibody . Which of the following immunostains will be positive in the majority intraepithelial lymphocytes?
   a. CD20
   b. CD8

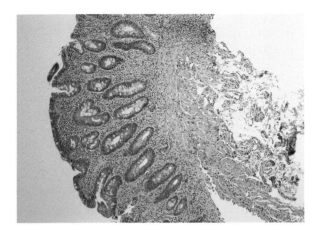

Figure 6.11

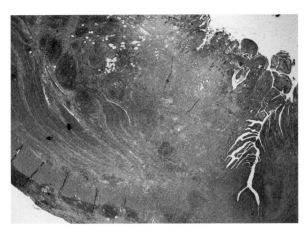

Figure 6.12

c. CD4
d. Anti-gliadin antibody
e. T-cell intracytoplasmic antigen (TIA-1)

30. Lymphoid depletion in the intestinal lamina propria is seen in patients with:
    a. Common variable immunodeficiency
    b. IgA deficiency
    c. Nezelof Syndrome
    d. Severe combined immunodeficiency (SCID)
    e. Adenoviral infection

31. Microscopic colitis is typically seen in patients with:
    a. Chronic watery diarrhea
    b. Nodular mucosa on colon endoscopy
    c. Male gender
    d. Bloody diarrhea
    e. Laxative abuse

32. Which of the following statements is true about the difference between Crohn disease and ulcerative colitis?
    a. Granulomas are only found in Crohn disease, not in ulcerative colitis.
    b. The rectum is not involved in Crohn disease, while it is commonly affected in ulcerative colitis.
    c. Crohn disease is not complicated by colorectal carcinoma
    d. The ileum is not involved in ulcerative colitis
    e. Ulcerative colitis has a higher incidence than Crohn disease

33. This section (Fig. 6.12) was taken from a 27–year-old woman with episodic diffuse crampy abdominal pain, diarrhea, anorexia, and weight loss. All of the following statements about this lesion are true EXCEPT:
    a. It affects whites at the same rate as African Americans.
    b. Patients with this lesion have a high risk of development of carcinoma.
    c. It most frequently affects the ileocecal region.
    d. It is associated with positive serology for anti-*Saccharomyces cerevisiae* antibody.

e. Patients with this disease typically require repeated operations.

34. Granulomas in inflammatory bowel disease:
    a. Occur in more than 80% of patients with Crohn disease
    b. Do NOT occur in ulcerative colitis
    c. Confer an increased risk for the development of carcinoma
    d. Are found more commonly in older patients
    e. Are found in grossly evident diseased areas as well as in grossly unremarkable areas

35. This colon (Fig. 6.13) was resected from a patient with positive p–ANCA serology. The diagnosis is most likely:
    a. Polyarteritis nodosa-associated colitis
    b. Crohn disease
    c. Low-grade dysplasia
    d. Ischemic colitis
    e. Lymphocytic colitis

36. Colon carcinoma complicating ulcerative colitis is mostly:
    a. Flat or ulcerative
    b. Polypoid
    c. Poorly differentiated
    d. Mucinous type
    e. Diffuse infiltrative type (linitis plastica)

37. All these statements are true about ulcerative colitis (UC) and Crohn disease (CD), EXCEPT:
    a. CD is associated with Th1 inflammation while UC is associated with Th2-like inflammation.
    b. CD affects the small bowel, colon, or both; UC affects the colon primarily.
    c. Hematochezia and abdominal mass are commonly seen in both UC and CD.
    d. Transmural granulomas are commonly seen in CD while superficial crypt abscesses and ulceration are more common in UC.

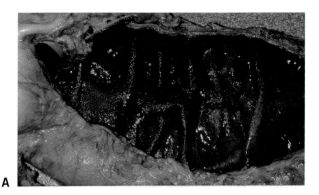

A

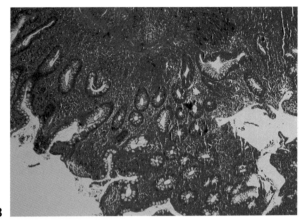

B

Figure 6.13

41. Poor prognostic features with the development of metastasis in carcinoid tumors of the appendix include all of the following EXCEPT:
    a. The presence of goblet cells
    b. Invasion of the muscle wall
    c. Tumors greater than 2 cm
    d. Concomitant presence of acute appendicitis
    e. The presence of signet ring cells

42. A 22-year-old man with a history of anemia, malnutrition, and abdominal pain had multiple polyps in the colorectal region. His older sister had a similar history. The histology of the lesion is shown (Fig. 6.14). Which of the following is true about this lesion?
    a. It is inherited as autosomal recessive pattern.
    b. It is limited to the colon and rectum.
    c. Hyperpigmentation around the mouth is commonly seen in patients with this lesion.
    d. There is increased risk for the development of colorectal cancer.
    e. Juvenile (retention) polyp is morphologically different from this lesion.

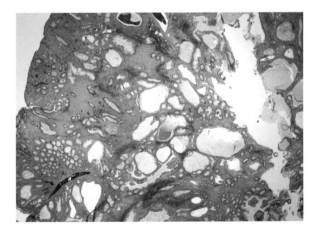

Figure 6.14

e. The risk of primary biliary cirrhosis (PSC) is higher in patients with UC than with CD.

38. Clinicopathologic features that distinguish colitis resulting from the use of non-steroidal anti-inflammatory agents (NSAIDs) include:
    a. Development of chronic watery diarrhea
    b. Sharp well-circumscribed ulcer, more common in right colon
    c. Increased number of intra-epithelial lymphocytes
    d. Presence of macrophages containing pigment in the lamina propria
    e. Mucosal damage limited to superficial layers

39. Pseudomembrane formation is seen in which of the following types of colitis?
    a. Ischemic colitis
    b. Infectious colitis
    c. *Clostridium difficile* colitis
    d. Neonatal necrotizing colitis
    e. All of the above

40. Acute appendicitis can be caused by:
    a. Adenoviral infection
    b. Diverticulitis of the cecum
    c. *Yersinia enterocolitis*
    d. *Enterobius vermicularis*
    e. All of the above

43. These sections were taken from the small intestine of a 41-year-old man who came for medical attention with an abdominal mass. Figure 6.15A shows low-power view of this lesion; Figure 6.15B shows tumor cells are positive for desmin stain. This lesion may be associated with all of the following EXCEPT:
    a. Gardner syndrome or familial polyposis
    b. CD117 positivity
    c. Beta-catenin immunoreactivity
    d. Carney triad
    e. Intestinal obstruction

44. Which of the following statements is true about anal carcinoma?
    a. It is most commonly of adenocarcinoma type.
    b. It does not develop in the anal transitional zone.

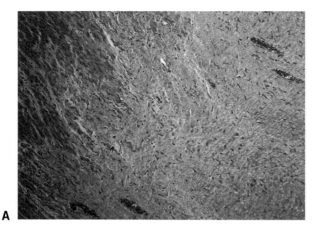

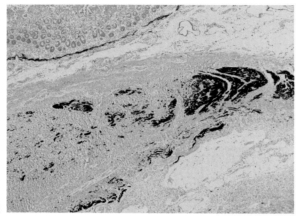

Figure 6.15

c. It frequently arises from Bowenoid papulosis.
d. It is frequently associated with chronic HPV infection.
e. It is frequently found in patients with hemorrhoids.

45. Which of the following statements regarding primary lymphoma of the gastrointestinal (GI) is true?
   a. Primary lymphoma of the GI tract occurs more often in the large than in the small intestine.
   b. The most common site of involvement in primary follicular lymphoma of the GI tract is the stomach.
   c. Mantle cell lymphoma can present as lymphomatous polyposis.
   d. Immunoproliferative small intestinal disease is a T cell lymphoma.
   e. Enteropathy-associated T cell lymphoma is of the helper T cell phenotype.

46. All of the following statements about serrated adenomas and sessile serrated polyps are true EXCEPT:
   a. Serrated adenomas can be found throughout the colorectum with a predisposition of involvement of the right colon.
   b. Histologically, serrated adenomas differ from hyperplastic polyps in that stratified cells lining the glands in serrated adenomas are dysplastic.

c. Sessille serrated polyps have a tendency to be right sided.
   d. Serrated epithelium extending all the way into the crypt base in sessile serrated polyps is the main feature that distinguishes it from hyperplastic polyps.
   e. Mutations in KRAS, APC, and p53 genes are common in the serrated adenomas.

47. All listed below are independent prognostic factors in primary colorectal carcinoma (CRC), EXCEPT:
   a. Tumor node metastasis (TNM) stage
   b. Venous and lymphatic invasion
   c. Tumor grade
   d. Expression of EGFR
   e. Microsatellite instability (MSI) status

48. All following statements about colorectal carcinoma are true EXCEPT:
   a. Colorectal carcinoma can be broken down into chromosomally unstable and microsatellite unstable molecular subsets.
   b. Microsatellite instability is found in about 11%–23% of all newly diagnosed colorectal carcinomas, including 10%–20% of sporadic colorectal carcinomas, and 1%–3% for hereditary nonpolyposis colorectal carcinoma (HNPCC).
   c. Sporadic colorectal carcinomas with microsatellite instability have worse stage-specific prognosis.
   d. Individuals with adenomas diagnosed at age <40 years should be screened for DNA mismatch repair (MMR) genes.
   e. The purpose of screening for MMR-defective colorectal carcinoma is to identify individuals at risk for inherited predisposition syndromes and predict the prognosis.

49. Which of the following statements is NOT true about molecular testing on colorectal carcinoma?
   a. V600E (exon 15) is the most common BRAF mutation, accounting for over 90% of mutations on BRAF.
   b. Finding BRAF mutation in a tumor indicates that tumor is of sporadic origin, as BRAF mutations are not found in HNPCC tumors.
   c. Methylation in MLH1 gene promoter region is an epigenetic event, which leads an alteration of gene expression activity without changing genetic structure.
   d. Detection of MLH1 promoter hypermethylation in colorectal carcinoma with MLH1 loss differentiates sporadic MSI-H colorectal carcinoma from HNPCC-associated colorectal carcinoma.
   e. Both BRAF and MLH1 genes are tumor suppressor genes.

50. Which of the following about Hirschsprung disease (HD) is true?
   a. It is much more common in females than in males.
   b. It involves the entire colon in about 50% of cases.

c. It has autosomal recessive inheritance in the majority of cases.

d. Various RET oncogene activating mutations are found in about 80% of familial HD cases.

e. HD is usually diagnosed through rectal suction biopsies.

51. Which of the following cystic lesions of the liver communicate with the intrahepatic biliary tree?
    a. Solitary (non-parasitic) cyst
    b. Hydatid (echinococcal) cysts
    c. Polycystic liver disease
    d. Caroli disease
    e. Cyst caused by Entamoeba hystolytica

52. The most common form of congenital extrahepatic bile duct dilatation is:
    a. Caroli disease
    b. Choledochal cyst
    c. Choledochocele
    d. Diverticulum of the common bile duct
    e. Cholangiectases

53. Characteristic histologic findings of mechanical bile duct obstruction include all following features EXCEPT:
    a. Portal edema and periportal inflammatory infiltrate, usually with more neutrophils
    b. Cholestasis and cholate stasis
    c. Ductule reaction
    d. Parenchymal and/or portal granulomas
    e. Cholangitis

54. A 45-year-old man had a long history of chronic liver disease including episodes of jaundice and cirrhosis. The patient died after an upper GI bleed. Autopsy revealed a nodular liver weighing 1900 grams. H&E stained sections showed a well-established cirrhosis. The image shown here is from a PAS-diastase stained section (Fig. 6.16). The diagnosis of this lesion is

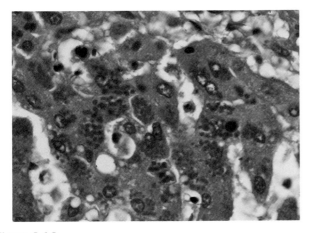

Figure 6.16

supported by all of the following pathologic findings EXCEPT:
    a. The demonstration of PASD-positive globules in periportal hepatocytes
    b. Positive immunohistochemical stain for alpha-1 antitrypsin
    c. The ultrastructural demonstration of electron-dense material inside the cisternae of the rough endoplasmic reticulum
    d. Serum electrophoresis of alpha-1-antitrypsin molecules
    e. The finding of macronodular cirrhosis with cholestasis

55. A 10-year-old girl was found to have hepatosplenomegaly and elevated liver function tests. Serum ceruloplasmin was 23 mg/dL (normal 18–45); serum copper 65 mg/dL (normal 66–145); and 24–hour urine copper level was 1135 mg (normal 15–50). H&E sections showed precirrhotic changes with extensive bridging fibrosis and incomplete nodules. A rhodanine stain for copper is shown (Fig. 6.17). All of the following are true about this disease EXCEPT:
    a. It usually presents with signs of liver disease during adolescence.
    b. Laboratory testing usually shows increased urinary copper and reduced serum copper and ceruloplasmin.
    c. Positive copper or copper associated protein stains are more prominent in zone 1 distribution in early phase and is more generalized in late phase.
    d. Characteristic mitochondrial abnormalities including dilatation of mitochondrial cristae and pleomorphic shapes are seen by electron microscopy.
    e. The disease is symptomatic before 3 years of age

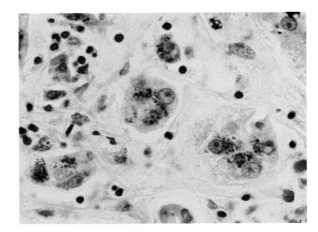

Figure 6.17

56. Clinicopathologic features of acute viral hepatitis include all the following EXCEPT:
    a. Liver biopsy is not usually indicated for the diagnosis of acute viral hepatitis.

b. Like chronic viral hepatitis, portal inflammation and interface hepatitis are dominant features in acute viral hepatitis.

c. Most characterized histologic feature in acute viral hepatitis is hepatocellular damage and inflammatory infiltrate (predominantly lymphocytic) in zone 3.

d. Hepatitis B is more prevalent than hepatitis C worldwide.

e. Nearly 100% of acute hepatitis A and E and most of hepatitis B are followed by complete resolution, while the risk of becoming chronic in hepatitis C is very high.

57. All following statements about chronic hepatitis are true EXCEPT:

a. Classical causes of chronic hepatitis include hepatitis B, hepatitis C, autoimmune hepatitis; drug-induced liver injury; and chronic hepatitis of unknown etiology.

b. Appropriate goals for the pathologist in evaluating liver biopsy with suspicion of chronic hepatitis include confirming the diagnosis, grading activity, grading fibrosis, and giving possible etiology on the basis of the histopathologic features.

c. Wilson disease, alpha-1-antitrypsin deficiency, steatohepatitis, primary biliary cirrhosis, and primary sclerosing cholangitis share some histopathologic features of chronic hepatitis.

d. Portal inflammation, interface hepatitis, and parenchymal injury are the main pathologic features of chronic hepatitis for all causes.

e. The mechanism of hepatic cell death in interface hepatitis is through necrosis.

58. Semiquantitative scoring system for chronic hepatitis is used to reflect all of the following parameters EXCEPT:

a. Interface hepatitis
b. Steatosis
c. Parenchymal inflammation (lobular necrosis)
d. Portal inflammation
e. Fibrosis

59. All of the following statements about drug-induced liver disease are true EXCEPT:

a. In intrinsic pathway, hepatotoxins cause liver damage in a dose-dependent manner, while in idiosyncratic pathway, drugs injure the liver unpredictably and only in susceptible individuals.

b. Idiosyncratic hepatotoxicity often has a latent period of many days or weeks, while intrinsic hepatotoxicity only needs a few hours or days.

c. Some drugs can produce autoimmune-like hepatitis.

d. Drug-induced liver diseases can essentially mimic any other type of liver diseases, including necroinflammatory, cholestatic, granulomatous, vascular, and metabolic liver diseases.

e. Zonal necrosis is usually caused by idiosyncratic drug injury.

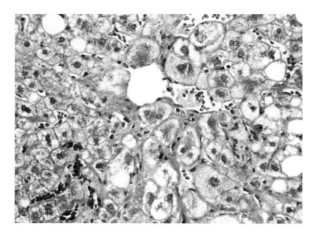

Figure 6.18

60. The liver biopsy stained with Masson trichrome in Figure 6.18 was from a 27-year-old woman with mildly elevated liver tests for approximately 1 year. There was no history of alcohol abuse, but the patient was obese. Which of following statements is true about the condition depicted in this biopsy EXCEPT:

a. This histopathologic process can be caused by alcohol, diabetes mellitus, obesity, or tamoxifen.

b. In pediatric cases, there is periportal pericellular fibrosis, while in adults the fibrosis is predominantly in zone 3 area.

c. Interface hepatitis is often present.

d. Mallory bodies are usually present in ballooned hepatocytes.

e. Mallory bodies surrounded by neutrophils are more often seen in alcoholic patients with this entity than nonalcoholic patients.

61. Nonalcoholic steatohepatitis can be caused by which of the following conditions?

a. Diabetes mellitus
b. Gastroplasty
c. Drugs
d. Weber-Christian disease
e. All of the above

62. All of the following are found in patients with autoimmune hepatitis EXCEPT:

a. Antinuclear antibodies
b. Smooth muscle antibodies
c. Liver-kidney microsomal antibodies
d. M2 mitochondrial antibodies
e. Hypergammaglobulinemia

63. The best method of distinguishing neonatal hepatitis from biliary atresia is:

a. The degree of liver enzymes elevation
b. Ultrasound
c. Hepatobiliary scanning
d. Liver biopsy
e. Cholangiography

64. Clinicopathologic features of acute rejection after allo-graft liver transplantation include all the following EXCEPT:
    a. Occurrence within the first month to 6 weeks after transplantation
    b. Inflammatory infiltrate in the portal tracts in which eosinophils are often abundant
    c. Endothelialitis of the portal vein branches, terminal hepatic venules, and sinusoid endothelial lining
    d. Bile duct damage
    e. Hepatocyte ballooning, lobular spotty necrosis, apoptotic bodies, and cholestasis

65. Clinicopathologic features of chronic rejection after liver allograft transplantation include the following EXCEPT:
    a. It occurs 60 days or longer after transplantation
    b. Obliterative vasculopathy in large and medium-sized arteries.
    c. Bile duct loss in more than 50% of portal tracts
    d. Ductular proliferative reaction is very common.
    e. Overlapping of histopathologic features of acute rejection

66. Findings of graft-versus-host disease (GVHD) in the liver include all of the following EXCEPT:
    a. Bile duct injury and cholestasis
    b. Portal inflammatory infiltrate
    c. Endosclerosis of blood vessels
    d. Lobular spotty necrosis and/or apoptotic bodies
    e. Endothelialitis of central vein

67. Clinicopathologic features of primary biliary cirrhosis (PBC) including all of the following, EXCEPT:
    a. Damage to the intrahepatic and extrahepatic bile ducts
    b. Presence of antimitochondrial antibodies (AMA)
    c. Presence of ruptured bile ducts surrounded by lymphocytes, plasma cells, and non-caseating epithelioid granulomas in portal areas
    d. Bile duct injury is mediated by CD8 and CD4 lymphocytes.
    e. Predilection to middle-aged and elderly women

68. AMA-negative cholangitis (autoimmune cholangitis) is characterized by all of the following EXCEPT:
    a. Presence of antibodies against the pyruvate dehydrogenase enzyme complex in inner mitochondrial membrane
    b. Portal lymphoid aggregates with germinal centers
    c. Granulomatous cholangitis
    d. Periductal fibrosis
    e. Progressive disease

69. All statements are about primary sclerosis cholangitis (PSC) EXCEPT:
    a. It occurs typically in patients with ulcerative colitis; about 70% of PSC patients have ulcerative colitis.
    b. Beading of the bile ducts demonstrated by cholangiography is characteristic.
    c. PSC usually affects the extrahepatic bile ducts and intrahepatic bile ducts.
    d. It occurs predominantly in women.
    e. Periduct edema and concentric fibrosis of medium-sized bile ducts are characteristic histologic features.

70. Cytoplasmic filaments in Figure 6.19 are composed of:
    a. intermediate filaments
    b. Cytokeratin
    c. Heat shock proteins
    d. P62-positive hyaline cytoplasmic globules
    e. All of the above

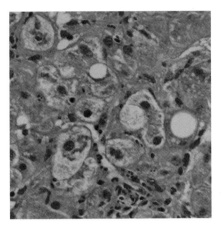

Figure 6.19

71. Delineation of the proliferating bile ductules in portal tracts is best accomplished by:
    a. Cytokeratin 7
    b. Hep-Par 1
    c. Cytokeratin 8
    d. PAS stain
    e. CAM 5.2

72. Bile ducts can be lost due to:
    a. Primary biliary cirrhosis
    b. Idiopathic ductopenia
    c. Allograft transplantation rejection and graft-versus-host disease
    d. Sarcoidosis
    e. All of above

73. Which liver lesion is associated with oral contraceptive use?
    a. Peliosis hepatis
    b. Periportal sinusoidal dilatation
    c. Acute cholestasis
    d. Hepatocellular adenoma
    e. All of the above

74. A 25-year-old primigravida woman developed a progressive fatigue, polydipsia, severe vomiting, and frequent brief loss of consciousness at her seventh month of pregnancy. 10 days later she became jaundiced. Thereafter she gave birth to a normal boy. Liver biopsy (Fig. 6.20) was taken two weeks after delivery. Which of the following diagnoses is most likely?
    a. Acute fatty liver of pregnancy
    b. Intrahepatic cholestasis of pregnancy
    c. Preeclampsia/eclampsia
    d. HELLP syndrome (hemolysis, elevated liver enzymes, and low platelets)
    e. Steatohepatitis

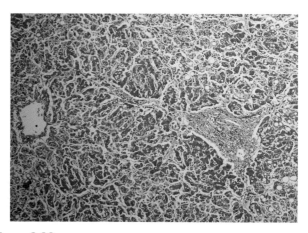

Figure 6.20

75. The histologic features shown in Figure 6.21 can be found in:
    a. Q fever
    b. Hepatitis A
    c. Hodgkin disease
    d. Cytomegalovirus and Epstein–Barr virus infection
    e. All of above

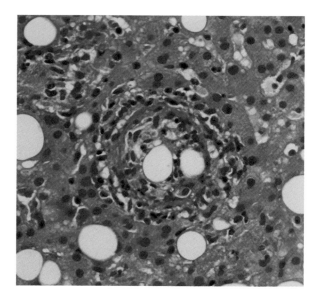

Figure 6.21

76. Which of the following statements about the typical histopathologic features of hepatitis caused by non-A, non-B, and non-C viruses is true?
    a. In Dengue fever, confluent focal necrosis with a predominantly midzonal distribution and abundant apoptotic bodies (Councilman bodies) are present.
    b. In cytomegalovirus infection, virus can be identified in hepatocytes, bile duct epithelium, and endothelial cells.
    c. Herpes simplex and herpes zoster viral infections cause irregular and randomly distributed areas of liver parenchymal coagulative necrosis.
    d. There are no specific hepatic lesions caused by HIV-1 infection.
    e. All of the above

77. A 2-year-old girl had hepatosplenomegaly, lymphadenopathy, cough swallowing difficulties since she was 2 months of age. She died from aspiration pneumonia. The liver section taken from autopsy for this patient is shown (Fig. 6.22). Which of the statements about this lesion is true?
    a. It is caused by deficiency in α-glucosidase A, mainly in macrophages.
    b. Affected cells are Kupffer cells.

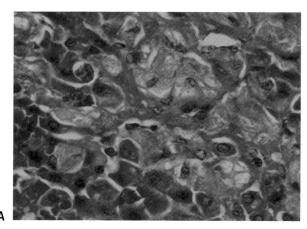

A

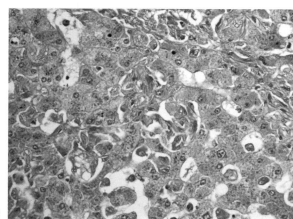

B

Figure 6.22

c. Affected cells are Kupffer cells and hepatocytes.
d. Among lysosomal storage diseases, this lesion is the least common type.
e. Genetic mutation is the sole factor responsible for the presentation of this lesion.

78. A 20-year-old woman with hepatosplenomegaly, ataxia, seizures, and remarkable atherogenic lipid profile developed portal hypertension. The liver biopsy is shown (Fig. 6.23). Lesional cells are positive for PASD, lysozyme stains, oil-red O, and filipin. Cultured fibroblast from this patient showed myelin-like figures and concentrically laminated membranous inclusions. Which of the following is true about this lesion?
a. It is an autosomal dominant disorder.
b. Various mutations on sphingomyelinase phosphodiesterase-1 gene in chromosome 11 account for all types of this disease.
c. Diastase-PAS positive lesional cells are Kupffer cells.
d. Diastase-PAS positive lesional cells are both Kupffer cells and hepatocytes.
e. Lipid lowering drugs can be successfully used for the treatment of this patient.

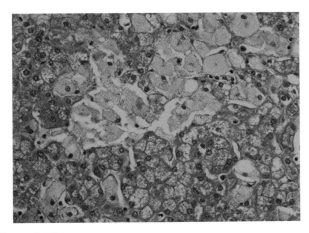

Figure 6.23

79. A 3-year-old girl was treated with aspirin at home for flu-like symptoms. After a few days, the patient became irritable. Shortly thereafter, the patient became lethargic and died in the hospital. The liver section taken from autopsy is shown (Fig. 6.24). All of the following are clinicopathologic features for this lesion EXCEPT:
a. Fatty liver and encephalopathy
b. Microvesicular fatty change with panacinar distribution
c. Severe decrease or absence of the enzyme succinate dehydrogenase
d. Swollen mitochondria with loss of matrix density and reduced number of cristae
e. Marked portal inflammation and cholestasis

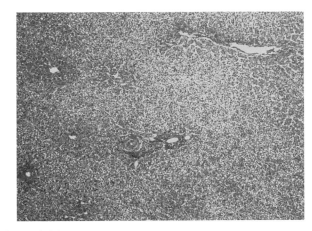

Figure 6.24

80. Common hepatic tumors in children include all of the following EXCEPT:
a. Hepatocellular carcinoma
b. Hepatoblastoma
c. Hemangioendothelioma
d. Rhabdomyosarcoma of the biliary tree
e. Mesenchymal hamartoma

81. A 4-cm nodule in the right hepatic lobe was accidentally found by a CT scan (for workup of kidney disease) in a 30-year-old female patient. The patient was taking oral contraceptives for the past 7 years and had normal liver laboratory tests. The mass was firm and well circumscribed, and contained a central scar. A microscopic section is shown (Fig. 6.25). Which of the following statements about this lesion is most likely to be true?
a. It is associated with myeloproliferative disorders.
b. It rarely presents with hemoperitoneum.
c. Contraceptive use is certainly associated with increased incidence of this lesion.
d. Chronic hepatic viral infection is identified in up to 50% of this lesion.
e. It is often associated with elevated liver enzymes and portal hypertension.

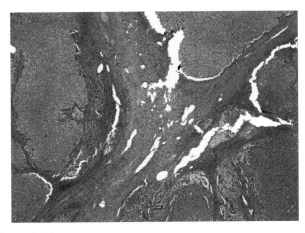

Figure 6.25

82. Increased incidence of hepatocellular carcinoma is seen in all of the following diseases EXCEPT:
    a. Congenital hepatic fibrosis
    b. Hereditary tyrosinemia
    c. Diabetes mellitus
    d. Hepatitis C
    e. Hepatitis E

83. A 2-year-old boy presented with a large mass in the right lobe of the liver and elevated serum alpha-feto-protein. A representative section from the mass is shown (Fig. 6.26). Good survival from this lesion is expected if the tumor:
    a. Is diagnosed at 1 year of age
    b. Secretes alpha-fetoprotein
    c. Shows a macrotrabecular pattern
    d. Is well circumscribed and surgically resectable
    e. Shows mutation or deletions of p53

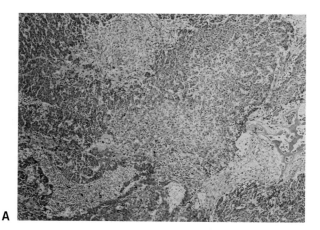

A

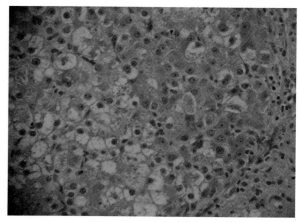

B

Figure 6.26

84. All following conditions are considered to be putative premalignant lesion of hepatocellular carcinoma (HCC), EXCEPT:
    a. Small-cell change
    b. Large-cell change
    c. Dysplastic nodules
    d. Focal nodular hyperplasia (FNH)
    e. Dysplastic foci

85. This section (Fig. 6.27) was taken from a 20-year-old woman with a 9-cm mass in the left lobe of the liver. All statements about this lesion are true EXCEPT:
    a. It is more common in young adults, rarely older than 40 years old.
    b. It is usually associated with cirrhosis.
    c. It has a better prognosis compared with other types of hepatocellular carcinoma.
    d. Characteristic tumor cells are large with eosinophilic granular cytoplasm separated by thick bands of hyalinized collagen and reticulin fibers.
    e. Is usually not associated with elevated alpha-fetoprotein.

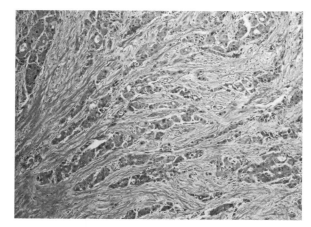

Figure 6.27

86. A 60-year-old man had a 5-cm liver mass detected by a CT scan. These sections (Fig. 6.28) were taken from the resection specimen. All of the following statements are correct about this lesion EXCEPT:
    a. Reticulin is often scanty or absent around tumor cells.
    b. Endothelial lining of the tumor trabeculae is usually positive for CD34, while in normal liver the sinusoidal endothelial lining is usually negative for CD34.
    c. Positive staining of bile canaliculi by polyclonal antibody to carcinoembryonic antigen (CEA) can help confirm tumor origin from the liver.
    d. Tumor cells are usually positive for cytokeratin 8 and 18 and always negative for cytokeratin 7 and 20.
    e. The cirrhosis associated with this tumor usually is macronodular.

87. All of the following statements are true about intrahepatic cholangiocarcinoma (ICC) EXCEPT:
    a. It occurs more often in older patients with no sex predominance.

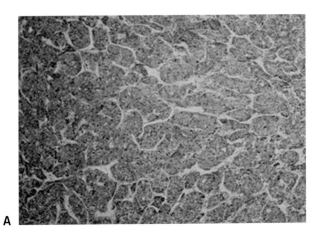

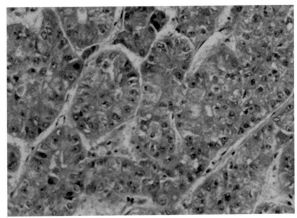

Figure 6.28

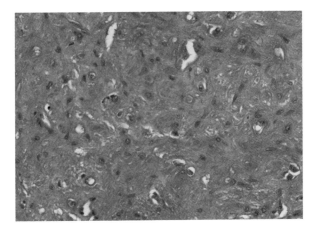

Figure 6.29

89. This liver section (Fig. 6.30) was taken from a 45-year-old woman during the procedure of cholecystectomy. Which of the following is true about this lesion?
   a. Lesions of this type are mostly single and often less than 1 cm in diameter.
   b. It is composed of small undilated ducts set in a fibrous stroma with no bile.
   c. It can be difficult to distinguish it from metastatic carcinoma in the liver.
   d. Main difference from von Meyenburg complexes is that von Meyenburg complexes is composed of irregular dilated bile duct that occasionally containing bile
   e. All of the above

   b. It often shows gray to gray-white, firm and solid appearance on the cut surfaces.
   c. Histologically, most ICCs exhibit tubular and/or papillary structures with mucin production.
   d. It has to be differentiated from metastatic carcinoma, especially from pancreas, lung, stomach, and esophagus
   e. Most ICC cases occur in cirrhotic liver.

88. A 40-year-old white woman with a history of jaundice, abnormal transaminases, right upper quadrant pain, and weight loss died in liver failure. The liver section from autopsy is shown in Figure 6.29. Characteristic immunostains for CD34, C31, and Factor VIII antigen were positive for neoplastic cells. Clinicopathologic features of this lesion include all of the following EXCEPT:
   a. Tumor cells are of endothelial origin
   b. Frequently occurs in infants
   c. Often misdiagnosed as adenocarcinoma because of its epithelioid appearance
   d. The prognosis of this lesion was considered to be much favorable than hepatocellular carcinoma.
   e. High cellularity of tumor cells is associated with unfavorable prognosis

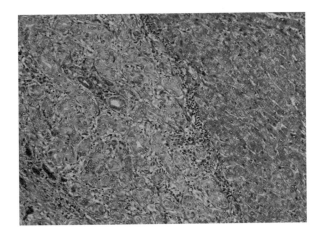

Figure 6.30

90. The H&E section (Fig. 6.31) was taken from a procedure of cholecystectomy for cholelithiasis from a 45-year-old woman. The incidence of this lesion shown in this photo is related to the presence of:
   a. Gallstones
   b. Congenital abnormal choledochopancreatic junction
   c. Porcelain gallbladder
   d. Genetic factors
   e. All of the above

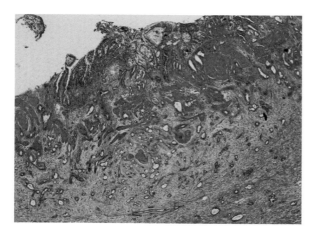

Figure 6.31

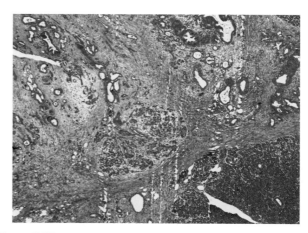

Figure 6.32

91. Which of the following statements regarding mucinous cystic neoplasms of the pancreas is true?
    a. Genetic alterations in K-ras, Tp53, and SMAD4/DPC4 genes play a role in pathogenesis of mucinous cystic neoplasms.
    b. These neoplasms have invariably bad prognosis.
    c. It occurs predominantly in males.
    d. It occurs commonly in the head of the pancreas.
    e. It occurs in patients with Von Hippel-Lindau disease.

92. A 69-year-old man presented with weight loss of 25 pounds, lower back pain, and jaundice. A CT scan revealed an ill-defined mass in the head of pancreas (Fig. 6.32). Which of following statements is true about this lesion?
    a. It is more common in smokers.
    b. K-ras mutation, p53 mutations and/or accumulation, and inactivation of tumor suppres-

sor genes SMAD4/DPC4 and p16 are common in this lesion.
    c. It commonly occurs in the head of the pancreas.
    d. It can be familial.
    e. All of the above.

93. Characteristic pathologic features of intraductal papillary mucinous neoplasms (IPMN) of the pancreas include all of the following EXCEPT:
    a. Activating K-ras point mutations and alterations of tumor suppressor genes of p53, SMAD4/DPC4, and p16/CDKN2A
    b. Survival rate worse than ductal adenocarcinoma
    c. More frequent occurrence in males than females
    d. Spectrum of biologic behavior from benign, borderline, to malignant
    e. Common location in the head of pancreas

■ Answers

1. **e.** Esophageal mucosa lined by columnar epithelium changes to stratified squamous epithelium by 25 weeks of gestation, and patches may persist in early infancy without any clinical significance. It has to be differentiated from ectopic gastric mucosa, which also shows glandular layer beneath the surface epithelium. Barrett esophagus is a possibility but requires demonstration of the presence of goblet cells and positive endoscopic findings.

2. **e.** The presence of **goblet cells** is not a normal finding in esophagus and may indicate Barrett esophagus. Cardiac mucosa may be found in the gastroesophageal junction and may have mild glandular distortion. Cardiac mucosa, however, is not normally found in children and in up to 30% of the adult population.

3. **e.** In most instances, the esophageal heterotopic mucosa is benign; it rarely results in peptic ulceration or carcinoma. The distance of the esophagogastric junction from the teeth averages 40 cm in adults.

4. **e.** All of these cysts can be lined by columnar mucosa. Bronchogenic cyst should have, in addition, cartilage and respiratory glands. The enterogenous cysts are lined by glandular mucosa without muscle coat. Gastrointestinal duplications have smooth muscle coat in addition to an alimentary mucosal lining. Thymic cyst can be located in the mediastinum or neck, and lymphoid tissue in the wall of thymic cyst is mainly of thymic origin and usually includes Hassall corpuscles.

5. **c. Esophageal atresia** occurs approximately 1 in 4000 live births, and it usually occurs together with tracheoesophageal fistula. Sometimes, a baby has atresia without fistula. The upper esophagus ends blindly, and there is a fistula between the lower portion of the esophagus and trachea.

6. **e.** Reflux esophagitis is caused by retrograde flow of gastric and, sometimes duodenal contents into the esophagus. It is histologically characterized by **intraepithelial eosinophils**, increased intraepithelial lymphocytes, basal cell hyperplasia, and elongated papillae. The presence of neutrophils reflects the acute erosive or ulcerative esophagitis. Infectious esophagitis and esophagitis caused by ingestion of caustic substances have to be excluded before the diagnosis of reflux esophagitis is made. Intraepithelial eosinophils are important for the diagnosis but can also be found in other diseases, such as allergic esophagitis.

7. **e.** Four mucosal features are needed to grade dysplasia in Barrett esophagus, including: surface maturation, glandular architecture, cytologic features, and inflammation around mucosa.

8. **d.** According to the American College of Gastroenterology, to make the diagnosis of Barrett esophagus, pathologists need to have both evidence of intestinal metaplasia in biopsy and positive endoscopic findings are needed.

9. **e.** The section shows glandular mucosa with intestinal metaplasia and glandular fullness and complexity of carcinoma in situ. These features are those of **Barrett esophagus** with high-grade dysplasia. All listed genetic alterations were suggested to be involved in the Barrett esophagus-dysplasia-adenocarcinoma sequence. In addition, EGFR, beta-catenins, erbB2, MCC, and DCC genes are also involved in this sequence.

10. **d. Candida** esophagitis causes most esophageal diseases in AIDS patients followed by CMV and herpesvirus infection. Candida esophagitis can also occur in other immunosuppressive disorders, diabetes and antibiotic therapy and may occasionally occur in immunocompetent individuals. Bacterial esophagitis is unusual and generally occurs in patients with granulocytopenia.

11. **b.** The figure exhibits features of eosinophilic esophagitis. The **food allergy** is a common cause of eosinophilic esophagitis. Most affected patients have clinical evidence of food and airborne allergen hypersensitivity. Many patients have a history of atopic disease. In contrast, parasitic infection is not a common cause of this disease

12. **d. pH dropping to less than 4** is a strong indication of reflux. Biopsy changes are not specific, and similar histology can occur in allergic esophagitis.

13. **d. Adenocarcinoma of the esophagus** is more common in white men and represents only 5%–10% of all esophageal cancers. Associated Barrett esophagus increases the risk of developing adenocarcinoma by 30–40 folds and worsens the prognosis of these tumors.

14. **e.** Esophageal squamous cell carcinoma develops as the result of a sequence of changes that include esophagitis, atrophy, mild to severe dysplasia, carcinoma in situ and finally, invasive cancer. Both genetic and environmental factors are involved in the pathogenesis of the esophageal squamous cell carcinoma. This type of cancer also shows great geographical diversity in its incidence. High incidence is noted in Northwest France, Northern Italy, East European countries, Iran, Central China, South Africa and Southern Brazil. In addition to the listed environmental risk factors, other factors include high intake of nitrosamines, thermal injury, and prior radiotherapy. Besides p53 mutation, other genetic alterations that are important in its pathogenesis include: (a) disruption of cell cycle control (inactivation of p16, via homozygous loss or promoter methylation, and amplification of Cyclin D1); (b) activation of oncogenes (FGFR and c-myc gene amplification); and (c) loss of tumor suppressor genes (such as loss of heterozygosity of RB gene). However, there is no convincing evidence that **APC gene mutations** play a crucial role in the development of esophageal squamous cell carcinoma.

15. **a.** In complete intestinal metaplasia (resembling small intestinal epithelium), the **predominant mucin type is sialomucin** with expression of MUC-2 and absence of expression of MUC1, MUC5AC, and MUC-6. In incomplete intestinal metaplasia (resembling colonic

epithelium), metaplastic cells may secrete, in addition to sialomucins, neutral mucins or sulfomucins. The cells strongly express MUC1, MUC2, MUC5AC5, and MUC6 mucin proteins.

16. **b.** It is true that infection with H. pylori is very common; the Centers for Disease Control and Prevention (CDC) estimates that about 20% of persons less than 40 years of age and about 50% of persons over 60 years of age are infected in the United States. However, most infected people do not have symptoms and only a small percentage develop disease. Gastric and duodenal ulcers can be caused by other reasons, but the most common cause is H. pylori infection. H. pylori infection is associated with a 1%-2% lifetime risk of stomach cancer and a less than 1% risk of gastric MALT lymphoma. *H. pylori*-associated chronic atrophic gastritis is the commonest precursor lesion for **intestinal type adenocarcinoma**.

17. **a.** Germline mutations in the gene coding for E-cadherin leads to an autosomal-dominant predisposition to **hereditary diffuse gastric carcinoma**.

18. **e.** Gastric carcinoma does not arise de novo from a normal mucosa. Chronic atrophic gastritis and intestinal metaplasia commonly precede and or accompany intestinal type adenocarcinoma. H. pylori associated gastritis is the commonest gastric precursor lesion to gastric carcinoma. Since gastric ulcer and gastric carcinoma share similar risk factors, patients with gastric ulcer are at greatly increased risk of developing gastric carcinoma. Gastric adenomas have a different frequency of malignant transformation, which depends on their size and histological grade. Gastric carcinoma may develop from gastric hyperplastic polyps with intestinal metaplasia and or dysplasia.

19. **d.** The section shows gastric lamina propria with small nests and gland-like lesion. The higher magnification (picture not shown) showed that tumor cells have uniform nuclei, diffuse chromatin and inconspicuous nucleoli. These features are those of **carcinoid tumor**. The formation of glands in gastric carcinoid tumor like this case can mimic adenocarcinoma. Five types of gastric carcinoid tumors are recognized, including ECL (enterochromaffin-like) cell tumor associated with type A chronic atrophic gastritis, ECL cell tumor with combined MEN-1 and Zollinger-Ellison syndrome, sporadic ECL tumor, Non-ECL tumors, and ECL cell tumor with achlorhydria and parietal cell hyperplasia. Hypergastrinemia, autoimmune chronic atrophic gastritis, MEN type 1, and Zollinger-Ellison syndrome are all predisposing factors for the development of gastric carcinoid tumor. There is no evidence that carcinoid tumor is associated with MEN type II.

20. **c.** If the collection of neuroendocrine cells is less than 0.5mm, it is best classified as **neuroendocrine cells hyperplasia**. The term "carcinoid" is usually applied to collection of neuroendocrine cells measuring more than 0.5 mm.

21. **e. Gastrointestinal stromal tumors (GIST)** are found mostly in the stomach and can be benign or malignant depending on the size and the mitotic rate. Tumors larger than 10 cm can recur and metastasize regardless of the mitotic rate. GANT tumors represent a GIST variant that have ultrastructural features of autonomic neurons, including cell processes with neurosecretory type dense core granules and arrays of microtubules.

22. **b.** t(11;18) API2/MALT1, t(14;18)/IGH-MALT1, t(1;14)/IGH-BCL-10, and t(3;14)/IGH-FOXP1 translocations are all associated with mucosa-associated lymphoid tissue (MALT) lymphoma. Only t(11;18) API2/MALT1 translocation is specifically associated with **MALT lymphoma**. Detection rate of t(11;18) API2/MALT1 translocation varies with different organ sites, but is only found in about 25%–30% of gastric MALT lymphomas.

23. **d.** The clinical presentation and histologic features are those of **Ménétrier disease**. Inflammation is usually minimal in Ménétrier disease. This disease is rare and usually occurs in men between 30–60 years of age. The disease is characterized by giant gastric folds. Large gastric folds are also found in Zollinger-Ellison syndrome, peptic ulcer, Crohn disease, eosinophilic gastritis, and gastric lymphoma. So, the presence of foveolar cell hyperplasia alone, which creates large gastric folds, is not sufficient to make a diagnosis of Ménétrier disease.

24. **e.** About 80%-90% of gastric polyps are nonneoplastic. Different genetic alterations are involved in pathogenesis of fundic gland polyp formation. Sporadic fundic gland polyps contain activating mutations of the β-catenin gene while fundic gland polyps in the setting of FAP contain APC gene mutations. Histologically fundic gland polyps show hyperplastic expansions of oxyntic mucosa with cystic dilatation. Most hyperplastic polyps develop on a background of chronic gastritis. Histologically, they exhibit foveolar hyperplasia with edematous stroma infiltrated with plasma cells, lymphocytes, eosinophils, mast cells, and neutrophils. Some hyperplastic polyps contain epithelial dysplasia that may have a potential for a malignant transformation. **Inflammatory fibroid polyps occur mainly in adults** and in general are considered as reactive in nature. Histologically, they are consisted of spindled fibroblast-like cells with inflammatory cells and abundant small blood vessels formed in the submucosa. Generally, they do not have epithelial proliferation.

25. **c.** The section shows a polyp with an infrastructure of arborizing smooth muscle dividing the nondysplastic glands into lobules, which is the characteristic histologic feature of **hamartomatous polyp**, Peutz-Jeghers type. Peutz-Jeghers syndrome is an inherited cancer syndrome with autosomal dominant trait. Mucocutaneous melanin pigmentation and hamartomatous intestinal polyposis are characteristic features. It is

associated with gene SKT11 (Serine/Threonine protein kinase), with nearly complete penetrance.

26. **e.** This patient has a **gastrointestinal stromal tumor (GIST)**. Constitutive activating mutations in C-KIT or PDGFRA genes can be found in approximately 85% and 4%–18% of GISTs, respectively. Approximately 12% of GISTs does not have C-KIT or PDGFRA mutation. In addition to mutations in C-KIT and PDGFRA genes, GIST is commonly associated with losses in chromosomes 14 and 22. Rare GIST tumors that show ultrastructural evidence of neuronal cell processes are termed gastrointestinal nerve tumors. Some GISTs occur in patients with neurofibromatosis type 1 or Carney triad (which includes GIST, pulmonary chondroma, and functioning extra-adrenal paraganglioma). GISTs in the setting of neurofibromatosis type I generally lack C-KIT or PDGFRA mutations. The mutation responsible for Carney triad is not yet identified. **Familial or autosomal dominant form of GIST can occur** but is rare, which develop due to germline activating mutations in C-KIT or PDGFRA gene.

27. **c.** It is true that there is **no recognizable pattern of inheritance** for this identity. HPS is more common in boys with a male to female ratio of approximately 4:1. The incidence is approximately 1 in 200 to 400 of live births. Majority of patients with HPS are asymptomatic till the first few weeks of life. Histologically, hyperplasia and hypertrophy of inner circular muscle fibers are the main histological features and, in contrast, the outer longitudinal muscle fibers appear to be unremarkable.

28. **d.** Duodenal atresia is associated with Down syndrome, not cystic fibrosis. Approximately 20%–40% of all infants with duodenal atresia have Down syndrome. Approximately 8% of all infants with Down syndrome have duodenal atresia. Cystic fibrosis is however associated with jejunoileal atresia.

29. **b.** The image exhibits a typical histologic feature of Celiac disease. Celiac disease is characterized by a marked intolerance to dietary gliadin. Intraepithelial lymphocytosis with villous atrophy and crypt hyperplasia are the main histological features of Celiac disease. A large infiltrate of **CD8+ T-lymphocytes** is usually found in the epithelium, while CD4+ T-lymphocytes infiltrate the lamina propria. The extensive infiltration of the small intestinal epithelium by CD8+ T cells of unknown Ag specificity is one of the diagnostic hallmarks of Celiac disease.

30. **d. Severe combined immunodeficiency** (SCID) represents a constellation of genetically distinct syndrome. They all have defects in both humoral and cell-medicated immune responses and have different inheritance patterns. SCID caused by mutation in the common gamma chain (γc) is inherited in an X-linked recessive pattern. Histologically, intestinal lamina propria is devoid of lymphocytes and plasma cells in SCID

patients. Instead, there are many vacuolated PAS-positive macrophages in the lamina propria. Lymphoid hyperplasia can be seen in IgA deficiency, common variable immunodeficiency, and adenoviral infection. Plasma cells are absent in common variable immunodeficiency. Nezelof syndrome (a form of thymic dysplasia) is an autosomal recessive congenital immunodeficiency condition due to underdevelopment of the thymus (but some children may exhibit an X-linked mode of inheritance). In general, lymphoid tissue is hypoplastic in Nezelof syndrome. However, GI biopsies generally show increased numbers of plasma cells and neutrophils in lamina propria.

31. **a.** Collagenous colitis and lymphocytic colitis are referred to collectively as microscopic colitis. Patients with microscopic colitis are usually women who present with **chronic watery diarrhea** and have normal appearing mucosa on endoscopy. Histology usually shows lymphocytic or collagenous colitis.

32. **e.** Both Crohn disease and ulcerative colitis are inflammatory bowel disease; they share many features clinically and histologically. Since the course of the diseases and treatments may be different, it is important to differentiate these diseases. Unfortunately, in some cases it may not be possible to differentiate one from the other. Histologic features can be seen in both lesions, although more often in one than other. The presence of focal active colitis, granulomas, and involvement of the upper gastrointestinal tract with skip lesions favor Crohn disease. Ulcerative colitis is generally confined to the colon. The ileum can be involved in ulcerative colitis (backwash ileitis). Ulcerative colitis affects the rectum in 95% of patients, while rectal involvement can occur in up to 50% in Crohn disease. Although ulcerative colitis has higher risk to develop colon cancer than Crohn disease does, patients with Crohn disease still have increased risk to develop intestinal cancer than in the general population. It is true that **ulcerative colitis has higher incidence than Crohn disease**. Ulcerative colitis occurs in 10–12 people for every 100,000 while Crohn disease affects about 5-7 for every 100,000 people in the United States.

33. **a.** The lesion depicted in the image is typical morphology in low magnification for **Crohn disease**. It affects whites more commonly than other racial groups, and also occurs more commonly in Jewish than non-Jewish populations.

34. **e.** Granulomas in Crohn disease occur in 50% of patients. They are found more in grossly diseased areas than grossly normal areas, and do not relate to any clinical differences. Mucin granulomas occur in ulcerative colitis.

35. **e.** The section shows features of **ulcerative colitis**. The diffuse nature of this inflammatory lesion is the key factor differentiating it from Crohn disease. Ulcerative colitis is associated with positive serology for p-ANCA.

36. **a.** Carcinoma complicating ulcerative colitis is mostly on the left side of the colon, tends to be ulcerative or flat, and is mostly well to moderately differentiated. Carcinoma associated with Crohn disease tends to be less differentiated and of the mucinous type.

37. **c.** Bloody diarrhea is common in ulcerative colitis and rare in Crohn disease. Patients with ulcerative colitis rarely present as abdominal mass while it is common in Crohn disease.

38. **b.** NSAIDs characteristically produce significant mucosal damage, resulting in sharp ulcers surrounded by ischemic histology. It can also induce diaphragm disease characterized by circumferential narrowing caused by concentric submucosal fibrosis, most likely resulted from ulceration of the top of mucosal folds. Patients present commonly with bloody diarrhea. Healing of ulcers by fibrosis can result in stricture formation. Epithelial lymphocytosis is seen in collagenous colitis and lymphocytic colitis but is not a prominent feature of NSAID colitis.

39. **e.** Pseudomembrane formation is a non-specific feature that can result from many types of mucosal damage. It is formed by necrotic epithelium embedded in fibrin, leukocytes, and erythrocytes.

40. **e.** Acute appendicitis can be caused by inflammatory conditions affecting the cecum such as diverticulitis or *Yersinia* colitis. Appendiceal lymphoid hyperplasia caused by adenovirus infection in children can cause intussusceptions and acute abdominal pain.

41. **d.** The presence of goblet cells, signet ring cells, invasion of the muscle wall, and tumors greater than 2 cm in diameter are associated with bad prognosis. Acute appendicitis, resulting from obstruction of the appendiceal lumen with tumor, probably leads to early identification and better prognosis.

42. **d.** The lesion in this figure depicts histologic features for **Juvenile polyp**. Similar histologic features also can be found in hyperplastic polyps, inflammatory polyps, and Cronkhite-Canada syndrome. In conjunction with the patient's history and his clinical presentation, most likely this patient had Juvenile polyposis coli. Juvenile polyposis coli is a rare autosomal dominant disorder characterized by germline mutations in SMAD4/DPC4 tumor suppressor gene on chromosome 18q21. Juvenile polyps may extend to the stomach and small intestine, may coexist with adenomatous polyps, and are associated with increased risk for colorectal carcinoma. It is not associated with the extraintestinal features seen in other hamartomatous polyposis syndrome. Juvenile (retention) polyp, also known as solitary sporadic juvenile polyp, is the most frequent colonic polyp in children. It may represent a hamartomatous or inflammatory process.

43. **d.** The section shows a uniform proliferation of spindle cells resembling fibroblasts in myxoid and collagenous stroma. A characteristic feature of neoplastic cell "melting insinuation" into the muscularis propria of the small bowel is seen in this case. Desmin stain highlights this melting insinuation feature on the tumor margin. These histologic features are those of **mesenteric fibromatosis**. Although the mesenteric fibromatosis is not commonly seen in regular surgical pathology practice, it is the most common primary mesenteric tumor with spindle cell morphology. It can sometimes mimic gastrointestinal stromal tumor (GIST) in many ways including its clinical, radiologic characteristics, histopathologic appearance, and immunophenotypes. Because there is specific therapeutic strategy for GIST and because they have different biological behaviors, it is important to discriminate between them. Carney triad comprises GIST, pulmonary chondroma, and extra-adrenal paraganglioma.

44. **d.** Squamous cell carcinoma is the most common type of anal carcinoma and **is frequently associated with HPV infection**. Most anal canal squamous cell carcinomas arise at or above the dentate line in the area of the transitional epithelial zone. Bowenoid papulosis occurs on the genitalia of both sexes in sexually active people. It is related to HPV infection, with majority of cases linked to HPV 16 infection. Many of the lesions spontaneously regress and do not progress to carcinoma. However about 2% of Bowenoid papulosis cases develop invasive carcinoma. Hemorrhoids are not considered as a predisposing factor to develop anal cancer.

45. **c.** Overall, **stomach is the most common site** of the primary lymphoma of the GI tract, followed by the small intestine. Primary extranodal follicular lymphoma in GI tract without peripheral lymphadenopathy is very uncommon. They constitute <7% of primary lymphoma of the GI tract. The small intestine is the most common site of involvement. The common B cell lymphomas include MALT lymphoma, diffuse large B cell lymphoma, Mantle cell lymphoma, IPSID, follicular lymphoma, and Burkitt lymphoma. Among them, MALT lymphoma is the most frequent lymphoma in GI tract. The most common T cell lymphoma occurring in GI tract is glutensensitive enteropathy-associated lymphoma. Postulated cell of origin is intraepithelial T-cell of intestine (cytotoxic T-cell phenotype).

46. **e.** Both serrated adenomas and sessile serrated polyps tend to occur in right colon. Since similar histological features are present among hyperplastic polyps, serrated adenomas, and sessile serrated polyps, it can be difficult to make a diagnosis. However, the accurate diagnosis is important, since they carry a different potential to develop colorectal carcinoma. Studies have shown that KRAS, APC, and TP53 mutations, which are traditionally seen in adenoma-carcinoma sequence, are absent in these lesions in general. Instead, BRAF mutations, microsatellite instability pathway, and DNA methylation abnormalities (such as in MLH1 gene methylation) are involved in their pathogenesis.

47. **d.** The TNM stage remains the main prognostic factor in CRC. The 5-year survival rate for patients with CRC is largely dependent on the TNM stage. Venous and lymphatic invasions are also independent prognostic factors. Tumor grade is an additional prognostic factor in CRC. Extensive studies have shown that analysis of MSI has both prognostic and predictive value. There is no consistent conclusion in the literature so far that the **status of EGFR expression** has prognostic or predictive value in CRC.

48. **c.** Sporadic colorectal carcinomas with MMR-defective genes tend to be larger, higher grade primaries, but lower stage at presentation, and have been shown in different populations to have a better stage-specific prognosis.

49. **e.** BRAF is classified as oncogene while HLH1 is a tumor suppressor gene. The most common mutation of BRAF (V600E) leads up to 500 folds activation and induces constitutive ERK signaling through hyperactivation of the RAS-MEK-ERK pathway.

50. **e.** Hirschsprung disease occurs in 1 in 5,000 to 30,000 liver births and is much more common in males than in females. Patients present with delayed passage of meconium, distal obstruction, abdominal distension, or constipation. Total colonic aganglionosis occur in 5% of cases. Hirschsprung disease is a genetic disease with a complex pattern of inheritance. Mutations in the RET proto-oncogene on chromosome 10 and the EDNRB gene located on chromosome 13 can lead to Hirschsprung disease. Point mutations in RET gene can cause HD, multiple endocrine neoplasia-II (MEN-II) and familial medullary thyroid carcinoma. The hallmark of Hirschsprung disease is absence of ganglion cells (aganglionosis) and the presence of hypertrophic nerves in both submucosal and myenteric plexus. **Rectal suction biopsies** can demonstrate the submucosal plexus and are commonly performed to document the presence of aganglionosis. Full thickness rectal biopsies are performed if the diagnosis cannot be made by rectal suction biopsy.

51. **d.** Hepatobiliary cysts can be parasitic, developmental, or undetermined origin. The most common type is solitary non-parasitic simple cyst. Cysts in Caroli disease communicate with the rest of the biliary tree. In other cystic lesions on the list, cysts do not communicate with the biliary tree in general. Ascending cholangitis can result from the communications between cysts and the biliary tract system. **Caroli disease** (congenital dilatation of the intrahepatic bile ducts) generally involves the entire liver. Microscopically, severe chronic inflammation, with or without superimposed acute inflammation, luminal inspissated mucin and bile are common findings in this disease.

52. **b. Choledochal cyst** is a congenital cystic dilatation of the extrahepatic biliary tree, intrahepatic biliary radicles, or both and commonly presents with the triad of pain, jaundice, and mass in the right upper quadrant. They are more prevalent in Asia than in the United States and other Western countries. Caroli disease is characterized by dilatation of the intrahepatic biliary tree. Caroli disease is sporadic, whereas Caroli syndrome is generally inherited in an autosomal recessive manner. The latter is often associated with congenital hepatic fibrosis and portal hypertension. This form of Caroli disease is also often associated with autosomal recessive polycystic kidney disease (ARPKD). Diverticulum of the common bile duct and choledochocele are less common than choledochal cyst. Cholangiectases are not congenital and usually are caused by inflammatory process.

53. **d.** Portal edema, periportal inflammatory infiltrates, cholangitis, cholestasis (bile thrombi in canaliculi, hepatocytes, and Kupffer cells) are usually seen in recent complete obstruction of bile ducts. If obstruction continues for weeks, chronic cholestasis (pseudoxanthomatous change, also known as cholate stasis, usually can be demonstrated by copper and or copper-associated protein staining), and portal and periportal fibrosis with ductular reaction are often seen. Giant cell transformation and cholestatic liver cell rosettes are also seen. Parenchymal and portal granulomas are features of primary biliary cirrhosis, and it is not a feature commonly seen in mechanical bile duct obstruction.

54. **e.** Cirrhosis associated with alpha-1 antitrypsin (AAT) deficiency is usually micronodular, but it may be macronodular or mixed type. Since many liver diseases can lead to cirrhosis, the finding of cirrhosis is not specific to this disease. The production of AAT is controlled by a pair of genes at the protease inhibitor (Pi) locus. The normal allele is M (PiM) and homozygous individuals (MM) produce normal amounts of AAT. The most common form of AAT deficiency is associated with allele Z, homozygous PiZ (ZZ). Serum levels of AAT in these patients are about 10%–15% of normal serum levels. Other genotypes associated with severe AAT deficiency include PiSZ, PiZ/Null, and PiNull. Patients with the null gene for AAT will not produce any AAT and are high risk for emphysema. But, patients with PiNull gene will not develop liver disease because they do not produce any AAT, thus no ATT accumulation in liver cell. Individuals with heterozygous MZ, MS or M/Null do not usually develop disease of AAT deficiency.

55. **e.** The lesion demonstrated here is **Wilson disease**. It is an autosomal recessive disease with mutations in gene ATPase that transports copper. Most Wilson disease patients have compound heterozygous mutation on the ATPase gene. The diagnosis should be considered in any patients with hepatocellular disease of unknown etiology, because histologic features of Wilson disease can mimic many varieties of parenchymal liver disease. Wilson disease should be ruled out in a young patient with the findings of fatty liver with chronic hepatitis. Fatty change in hepatocytes is the most common finding. Many patients may present with a chronic hepatitis-like histopathology with marked portal and periportal inflammation. Another notable finding is that

hepatocytes often have eosinophilic cytoplasm and contain Mallory bodies. Wilson disease rarely presents before 3 years of age. Kayser-Fleischer rings are diagnostic for Wilson disease, but it is only present in about 50% of adult patients with Wilson disease.

56. **b.** In general surgical pathology practice, a pathologist rarely has liver biopsy samples with acute viral hepatitis, because acute viral hepatitis is not indicated for liver biopsy. Although portal inflammation is often present in acute hepatitis with variable severity, zone 3 hepatocellular damage and lymphocyte infiltration are usually the dominant features for acute viral hepatitis.

57. **e.** The mechanism of cell death in interface hepatitis is mediated by **apoptosis**, not by necrosis. The term piecemeal necrosis was eliminated because of this reason. Cytotoxic T lymphocytes (CTL) are main players for virus clearance and hepatic cell death (Th1 pathway). Activation of CD4 T-helper cells (Th2 pathway) also plays a role in virus clearance and liver cell death via stimulating CTL responses and Fas-mediated cell death.

58. **b.** Since Knodell and Ishak proposed the first semi-quantitative scoring system (Knodell and Ishak score) for evaluating chronic hepatitis in 1981, several other scoring systems followed. Of these, popular ones are those of Batts and Ludwig, METAVIA, and modified Ishak scoring system. Interface hepatitis, parenchymal inflammation (lobular necrosis), portal inflammation, confluent necrosis, and fibrosis are components of scoring systems. The degree of steatosis, bile duct damage, dysplasia, or lymphoid follicles are not included in any scoring system.

59. **e.** Drug-induced liver disease may imitate any form of acute, chronic, vascular, and even neoplastic diseases caused by other etiologies. Hepatotoxic agents are classified into two categories, intrinsic and idiosyncratic hepatotoxins. Zonal necrosis is usually the result of intrinsic toxins, although some idiosyncratic hepatotoxins can also produce zonal necrosis. Zone 3 necrosis is the most common type of zonal necrosis and is the characteristic lesion caused by intrinsic hepatotoxins.

60. **c.** The picture shows pericellular fibrosis (chicken-wire fibrosis), steatosis, and ballooned hepatocytes with poorly formed Mallory bodies. **Steatohepatitis** is a histologic entity that is characterized by steatosis (can be macrovesicular or mixed macrovesicular and microvesicular steatosis); pericellular fibrosis (chicken-wire fibrosis); and/or Mallory bodies. Both alcoholic and nonalcoholic (diabetes, obesity, toxins, and drugs) causes are recognized. Interface hepatitis seen in viral hepatitis is not a feature of steatohepatitis.

61. **e.** Steatohepatitis could be related to alcohol causes (alcoholic steatohepatitis, ASH) or non-alcohol causes (non-alcoholic steatohepatitis, NASH).Diabetes mellitus and obesity are the most common causes of NASH. Rapid weight loss can be a cause of NASH. Some therapeutic drugs also can cause NASH, following are well documented ones: amiodarone, corticosteroids, difedipine, and tamoxifen. Steatohepatitis is a common finding in Weber-Christian disease which is a skin disease with features of relapsing fever and nodular panniculitis, especially found over the lower extremities

62. **d.** Three types of **autoimmune hepatitis** have been described; the most common one is type 1 that features the presence of antinuclear antibodies and/or anti-smooth muscle antibodies. Hypergammaglobulinemia, human leukocyte antigen (HLA) DR3, and/or DR4 also are usually present. Liver kidney microsomal antibodies are present in type 2 autoimmune hepatitis, which predominantly affects children (2–14 years of age). However, antimitochondrial antibodies directed against the inner mitochondrial membranes (M2 subtype) are considered to be specific for primary biliary cirrhosis, not to be found in type 1 or type 2 autoimmune hepatitis. Histologic features include bridging hepatocellular necrosis, liver cell rosettes, destructive bile duct lesions, and plasma cell infiltrates. Type 3 is the least common form with antibodies to soluble liver antigen/liver pancreas (anti-SLA/LP).

63. **d. Liver biopsy** is reliable in making the correct diagnosis in up to 95% of cases. Multinucleated hepatocytes and portal and lobular mononuclear cell infiltration are more prominent in neonatal hepatitis than biliary obstruction, while cholestasis and ductular reaction are more severe in biliary atresia.

64. **e.** Histopathologic triad of **acute cellular rejection** includes portal inflammation, bile duct injury, and endothelialitis. Banff grading scheme for acute rejection is based on these three histologic features. Liver cell ballooning in perivenular area, apoptotic bodies, lobular spotty necrosis, and cholestasis are features of preservation; reperfusion injury are features related to the process of graft preservation and reperfusion.

65. **d.** The distinction of acute and chronic rejection cannot be made based on histologic features only. The time to the onset of rejection and other clinical features are important. Usually, ductular reaction is not present in the presence of bile duct loss in the allograft transplantation rejection setting.

66. **c.** Graft versus host disease (GVHD) involvement in liver is most commonly seen in patients after bone marrow transplantation. Bile duct damage in the form of lymphocytic or mixed-cell cholangitis with degeneration and necrosis of bile duct epithelium is the most characteristic histologic feature of acute GVHD involvement in the liver. In chronic GVHD, bile duct loss with portal fibrosis becomes apparent. Nondestructive endothelialitis may be seen in acute but not chronic GVHD, and is not complicated by sclerotic changes like in chronic allograft rejection.

67. **a.** Primary biliary cirrhosis (PBC) is primarily a disease of the intrahepatic bile ducts with variable injury of hepatocytes. The image (Fig. 6.33) shows chronic inflammation and ill-defined granuloma surrounding a damaged bile duct. More than 50% of PBC patients

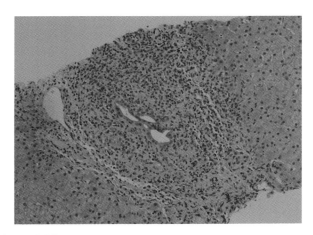

Figure 6.33

have some features of Sjögren syndrome. It has a strong female predominance of 9–10 to 1. It is a slowly progressive liver disease with final outcome of cirrhosis after many years of precirrhotic stages.

68. a. AMA-negative cholangitis is a variant of primary biliary cirrhosis (PBC). Its clinical, biochemical, and histologic features are those of typical PBC with exceptions of its autoantibody profile (negative for AMA and positive for ANA and anti-alpha smooth muscle actin antibody).

69. d. Primary sclerosing cholangitis (PSC) can involve any part of the biliary tract. It has to be distinguished from the secondary sclerosing cholangitis that may be caused by cholelithiasis, congenital biliary abnormalities, infections, ischemic, or neoplastic etiology. There is male preponderance of 2–3 to 1 for PSC.

70. e. Mallory bodies "alcoholic hyaline" are eosinophilic cytoplasmic structures that are characteristically seen in steatohepatitis. They are composed of **cytokeratin** intermediate filaments and can be detected by positive immunoassaying for ubiquitin and p62. Mallory bodies can be seen in wide varieties of liver diseases, including steatohepatitis (alcoholic and nonalcoholic), chronic cholestasis (any cause), focal nodular hyperplasia, Indian childhood cirrhosis, Wilson disease, and so on.

71. a. Hepatocytes are positive for cytokeratin 8 and 18. Bile ducts are positive for cytokeratin 7, 8, 18, and 19. Thus, cytokeratin 7 and 19 would stain bile ducts and would not stain hepatocytes.

72. e. Loss of interlobular bile duct can be evaluated only if a liver biopsy is adequate (at least containing several portal tracts). An interlobular bile duct is not necessary seen in all portal tracts. The bile duct hepatic artery ratio is greater than 1 in a normal liver (about 70%–90% of arteries are normally accompanied by a bile duct). To comply with the definition of bile duct loss, this ratio is reversed; bile duct to hepatic artery ratio is less than 1. In practice, some people use the criteria of bile duct loss in more than 50% portal areas to define the bile duct loss. The loss of bile duct is commonly seen in PBC and PSC, but it is not specific for them.

73. e. Oral contraceptives can also cause thrombosis of hepatic veins (Budd-Chiari syndrome), hepatic rupture, and are possibly related to the development of hepatocellular carcinoma and angiosarcoma.

74. a. The section from this patient shows diffuse steatosis, predominantly microvesicular, which is more severe in acinar zone 3 than in zone 1. The normal hepatic architecture is preserved, and portal areas are unremarkable. These histologic features are those of **acute fatty liver of pregnancy**. Fibrin thrombi in portal vessels and periportal sinusoids are seen in preeclampsia/eclampsia and HELLP syndrome. The canalicular cholestasis is seen in intrahepatic cholestasis of pregnancy. The features of steatohepatitis are not present here (see Answer 60).

75. e. The photo shows a **fibrin-ring granuloma**, central fatty vacuole surrounded by histocytes and a mesh of brightly eosinophilic ring of fibrin. It can be found in all listed diseases. It is a distinctive lesion, but is not specific.

76. e. A detailed clinical history and serologic testing are important to delineate all types of viral hepatitis.

77. b. The patient's clinical presentation and histology shown in this section is typical for **Gaucher disease**, type II. Gaucher disease is caused by a deficiency in acid β-glucosidase, mainly in macrophage. It is the most common type of lysosomal storage diseases. There are three types of Gaucher disease, including type I (chronic non-neuronopathic/adulthood); type II (infantile disease); and type III (juvenile disease). About 200 mutations in the gene responsible to β-glucosidase have been described; there is a poor genotype-phenotype correlation. The diagnosis of Gaucher disease is made by assay of acid β-glucosidase enzyme in blood. Enlarged cells with wrinkled tissue paper appearance in cytoplasm are affected Kupffer cells, not hepatocytes.

78. d. **Niemann-Pick disease** is an autosomal recessive disorder. There are three types of Niemann-Pick disease; type C Niemann-Pick disease is clinically, biochemically, and genetically different from type A and B. While type A and B are caused by mutations on sphingomyelinase phosphodiesterase-1 (SMPD1) gene in chromosome 11p15.4, the type C is caused by mutation in NPC-1 gene in chromosome 18q11-12. Sphingomyelin accumulates in reticuloendothelial and other cell types throughout the body. At the present time there is no effective treatment for Niemann-Pick disease.

79. e. Most likely, the cause of death for this patient was **Reye syndrome**. Incidence of Reye syndrome declined due to the decrease of usage of salicylates for children with viral illness. Usually there is only minimal portal inflammation, and cholestasis is rarely seen.

80. d. Hepatoblastoma, mesenchymal hamartoma, and infantile hemangioendothelioma are the most common tumors in children. Hepatocellular carcinoma can be seen in older children. Rhabdomyosarcoma of the biliary tree can occur but is a rare tumor.

81. b. The section shows that the liver parenchyma is subdivided into nodules by collagenous septa. The hepa-

tocytes appear normal but without any acinar architectural organization. There are numerous bile ductules and pseudoxanthomatous changes in the hepatocytes (chronic cholestatic feature) on the edge of nodules. These histologic features are those of **focal nodular hyperplasia** (FNH). Histologically, FNH can be difficult to differentiate from hepatocellular adenoma and inactive cirrhosis, particularly in biopsy specimens. Hepatocellular adenoma is a well circumscribed and encapsulated lesion associated with contraceptive use. It frequently presents with hemorrhage. FNH is well circumscribed but not encapsulated and rarely presents with hemorrhage. There is no convincing evidence that oral contraceptive use plays a role in its pathogenesis. It is well accepted that it develops from abnormal blood flow. Liver function tests are normal, and portal hypertension usually is not present in this condition. Myeloproliferative disorders are associated with nodular regenerative hyperplasia (NRH), not with focal nodular hyperplasia.

82. **e.** **Chronic hepatitis C** infection is responsible for the rising incidence of hepatocellular carcinoma in the United States. Hepatitis A and hepatitis E infections are usually acute infections that are not associated with the development of hepatocellular carcinoma. Congenital and metabolic conditions such as hereditary tyrosinemia, genetic hemochromatosis, and hepatic fibrosis pose an increased risk for the development of hepatocellular carcinoma. Diabetes mellitus is associated with 2–3 fold increase in the incidence of hepatocellular carcinoma.

83. **d.** The section shows a **hepatoblastoma**, mixed epithelial and mesenchymal type. Light and dark cells are seen in epithelial types of hepatoblastoma. The mesenchymal components consist of osteoid-like material and primitive fibrous stroma. Hepatoblastoma is the most frequent liver tumor in children less than 5 years old. Its survival correlates with a complete resection of the tumor. The stage of the tumor at the time of initial resection is an important prognostic factor. Except for the small cell undifferentiated variant, histologic patterns do not correlate with survival when adjusted for age, sex, and stage. Age and level of alpha-fetoprotein are not prognostic factors. Wnt signaling pathway involving mutation of the β-catenin and APC genes plays an important role in hepatoblastoma. Mutations in β-catenin can be found in about 50% of hepatoblastoma patients. Mutations and deletions of p53 are not common in this tumor.

84. **d.** Except for FNH, all lesions listed are considered as putative precursors of HCC. FNH is not considered a neoplastic lesion. X-chromosome inactivation studies show that the lesion is polyclonal with a very rare malignant transformation.

85. **b.** This is a **fibrolamellar variant of hepatocellular carcinoma** (HCC). It is rarely associated with cirrhosis or alpha-fetoprotein elevation. It is seen more commonly in young adults. However in children, classic hepatocellular carcinoma still predominates.

86. **d.** The section shows a hepatocellular carcinoma **(HCC)** with trabecular growth pattern, which is the most common pattern in HCC. Tumor cells in HCC are positive for CK8 and CK18. However, it is a wrong statement saying that CK7 and CK20 are always negative in HCC. In fact, about 50% of HCC cases are positive for CK7, and CK20 can be found in about 20% of HCC cases. Reticulin and immunostains with CD34 and polyclonal CEA are useful markers to establish a diagnosis of HCC in conjunction with morphologic evaluation. The absent staining of Reticulin around liver cell plates and positive staining of endothelial lining of hepatocytes by CD34 can help to distinguish benign from malignant lesion in the liver.

87. **e.** Most ICC patients occur in the fifth or sixth decade of life and there is no predominant sex distribution. Hepatocellular carcinoma (HCC) with pseudogland growth pattern can be difficult to be distinguished from intrahepatic cholangiocarcinoma. Mucin production in ICC and presence of bile in the tumor cells in HCC are helpful features for the differential diagnosis. Immunostains for HepPar-1, polyclonal CEA can help in the differential diagnosis as well. Metastatic carcinomas to the liver have to be excluded before the diagnosis of ICC is made. The exclusion is based on reliable clinical grounds and not on histology alone. Most ICC cases **occur in non-cirrhotic liver**.

88. **b.** The lesion presented in this case is **epithelioid hemangioendothelioma**, a rare neoplasm of vascular origin. This disease (unlike infantile hemangioendothelioma) occurs in older age group (20–80 years of age). Tumor cells often have pleomorphic nuclei arranged in clusters or singly embedded in a dense fibrotic stroma. Some tumor cells form capillary lumens with signet-ring appearance. In some cases, tumor cells have glandular growth pattern, which can mimic adenocarcinoma. Clinically, the tumor behaves as a low grade malignancy. The metastatic rate for this disease in one AFIP series was 27%, and about 20% of patients survived for 5 years.

89. **e.** The lesion shown here is the **bile duct adenoma**. In an AFIP series, 82.9% of patients have solitary lesion. The most important practical issue for this entity is that it may be misdiagnosed as metastatic carcinomas.

90. **e.** The picture shows a **well-differentiated adenocarcinoma** with invasion into the perimuscular connective tissue of the gallbladder. The incidence of carcinoma of gallbladder is higher in Native Americans, Hispanic Americans, and South and Central American Indians, which indicates that genetic abnormalities may be involved in its pathogenesis. It is well-known that more than 80% of gallbladder carcinoma patients have gallstones. Abnormal choledochopancreatic junction can cause pancreatic juice reflux into the common bile duct that may lead to carcinoma through the sequence of inflammation, metaplasia, dysplasia, and carcinoma. Porcelain gallbladder is defined as calcification of gallbladder wall. About 90% of porcelain gallbladders are

associated with gallstones, and in about 20% of cases are associated with gallbladder carcinoma.

91. a. Accumulation of genetic alterations in K-ras, p53, and SMAD4/DPC4 genes are associated with different grades of these neoplasms. Mucinous cystic neoplasms occur predominantly in women, commonly in the body or tail of pancreas and are not associated with Von Hippel-Lindau disease (unlike serous cystic tumors). Prognosis depends on the presence of invasive component, the depth of invasion, and resectability of the lesion.

92. e. The case presented here is the **ductal adenocarcinoma of the pancreas.** It was well documented that K-ras mutation, p53 mutation, and SMAD4 inactivation are involved in its pathogenesis and its prognosis. It can be familial in about 10% of cases. Patients with Peutz–Jeghers syndrome, caused by germline mutations in SKT11/LKB1 gene have 132-fold increased risk of developing pancreatic cancer. Other genetic susceptibility syndromes also can cause familial aggregation, including familial breast cancer with germline mutation of BRCA2, familial atypical multiple mole melanoma syndrome with germline mutation in the p16, hereditary nonpolyposis colorectal cancer with germline mutations in one of the DNA mismatch genes, and hereditary pancreatitis with germline mutation in the cationic trypsinogen gene.

93. b. Survival rate and prognosis of IPMN, including patients with adenocarcinoma arising from IPMN, are better than in ductal adenocarcinoma.

■ Recommended Readings

Burt A, Portmann BC, Ferrell LD. *MacSween's pathology of the liver,* 5th ed. Philadelphia: Churchill Livingstone/Elsevier, 2006.

Fenoglio-Preiser C, Noffsinger AE, Stemmermann GN, et al. *Gastrointestinal pathology, an atlas and text,* 3rd ed. Baltimore: Lippincott Williams & Wilkins, 2008.

Ishak KG, Goodman ZD, Stocker JT. AFIP Atlas of tumor pathology: tumors of the liver and intrahepatic bile ducts, series III. Washington DC, 2001.

Ludwig J, Batts K. *Practical liver biopsy interpretation diagnostic algorithms,* 2nd ed. Chicago: American Society of Clinical Pathologists, 1998.

Noffsinger A, Fenoglio-Preiser C, Maru D, et al. *Atlas of nontumor pathology, gastrointestinal diseases.* Washington, DC: AFIP, 2007.

Scheuer PJ, Lefkowitch JH. *Liver biopsy interpretation,* 7th ed. Philadelphia: Saunders, 2005.

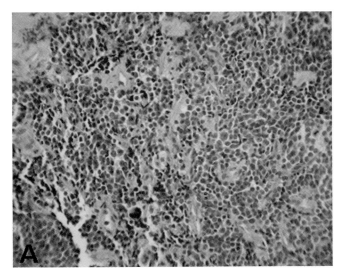

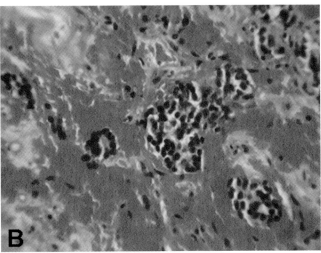

Figure 7.1

7

Head, Neck, and Endocrine Organs

Atif Ahmed

■ Questions

1. This tumor involved the kidney of a 2-year-old boy (Fig. 7.1). The tumor was negative for WT-1 mutations. This tumor will most likely show immunohistochemical staining with:
   a. Synaptophysin
   b. Myogenin
   c. Cytokeratin
   d. CD45
   e. CD99

Questions 2 and 3:
These are sections from a retroperitoneal periaortic abdominal tumor in a 35-year-old man who presented with hypertension (Fig. 7.2).

2. The most likely diagnosis is:
   a. Paraganglioma
   b. Renin-secreting tumor of the juxtaglomerular apparatus
   c. Renal cell carcinoma
   d. Hepatocellular carcinoma with neuroendocrine features
   e. Carcinoid tumor

3. S-100 immunostain was performed on the tumor in Figure 7.2. Which of the following applies to the cells highlighted by this immunostain (Fig. 7.3)?
   a. These cells are of myoepithelial origin.
   b. Similar type of cells is normally found in the skin.
   c. Their absence in this tumor correlates with more malignant behavior.
   d. These cells are also positive for CD21 and CD1a.
   e. These cells are only seen in this type of tumor.

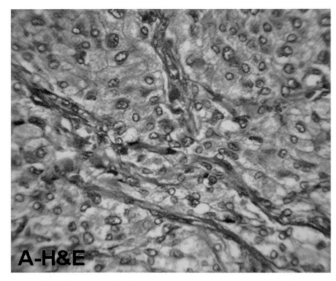

A-H&E

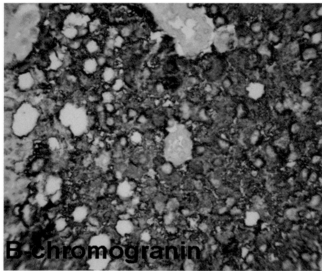

B-chromogranin

Figure 7.2

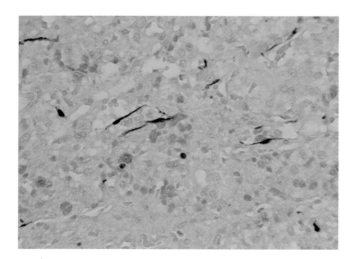

Figure 7.3

4. A large posterior mediastinal mass uniformly composed of elements seen in this image (Fig. 7.4) is most likely a:
   a. Neurofibroma
   b. Schwannoma
   c. Ganglioneuroma
   d. Gangliocytic paraganglioma
   e. Ganglion cell hamartoma

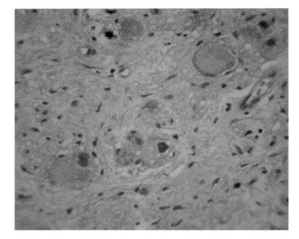

Figure 7.4

5. The best treatment of this encapsulated thyroid nodule (Fig. 7.5) is:
   a. Enucleation
   b. Hormonal therapy
   c. Surgical excision with adequate margins
   d. Lobectomy
   e. Radiotherapy

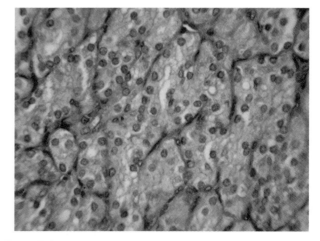

Figure 7.5

6. This thyroid lesion (Fig. 7.6) is associated with:
   a. Multiple endocrine neoplasia (MEN), type 1
   b. MEN type 2
   c. RET gene mutations
   d. No genetic abnormalities
   e. Cystic fibrosis

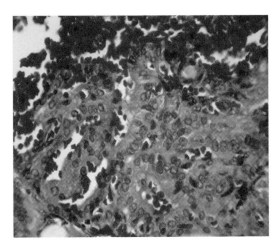

Figure 7.6

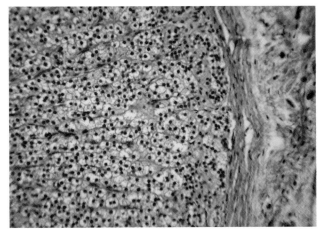

Figure 7.8

7. This lesion (Fig. 7.7) in the thyroid is seen mostly in patients with:
   a. Multiple endocrine neoplasia (MEN), type 1
   b. Cowden syndrome
   c. RET gene mutations
   d. Hyalinizing trabecular adenoma
   e. Goiter

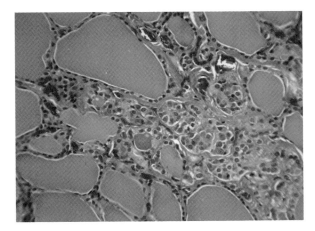

Figure 7.7

8. A nodule is incidentally found in a hernia sac specimen (Fig. 7.8). The diagnosis is:
   a. Adrenal rest
   b. Metastatic renal cell carcinoma
   c. Clear cell sarcoma
   d. Nodular mesothelial hyperplasia
   e. Adenomatoid tumor

9. A tumor that is LEAST likely to occur in patients with multiple endocrine neoplasia (MEN), type 1 is:
   a. Pheochromocytoma
   b. Thyroid adenoma
   c. Pancreatic gastrinoma
   d. Appendiceal carcinoid
   e. Growth hormone-secreting tumor

10. Pathologic features characteristic of hyalinizing trabecular adenoma of the thyroid include:
    a. Psammoma bodies
    b. Cytoplasmic inclusion bodies
    c. Histologic appearance similar to paraganglioma
    d. Expression of thyroglobulin
    e. All of the above

11. Seen in this image (Fig. 7.9) is a cytologic preparation from a nasal cavity tumor. All of the following test results are important in reaching the diagnosis EXCEPT:
    a. Positive staining for cytokeratin
    b. Positive immunostaining for synaptophysin and neuron-specific enolase (NSE)
    c. MYCN amplification
    d. Electron microscopy showing sparse dense core granules
    e. Flow cytometry positivity for CD45 (LCA)

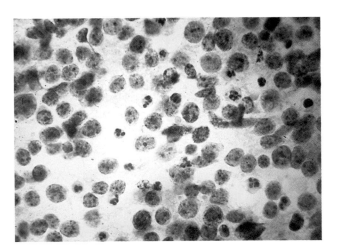

Figure 7.9

12. Tumor cells with this ultrastructural phenotype (Fig. 7.10) will most likely stain with all of the following immunostain markers EXCEPT:
    a. Chromogranin
    b. CD10
    c. Synaptophysin
    d. Neuron-specific enolase (NSE)
    e. CD56

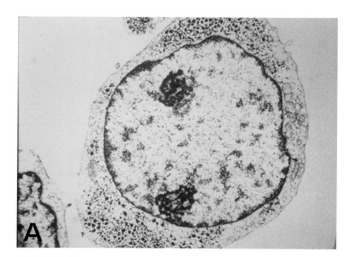

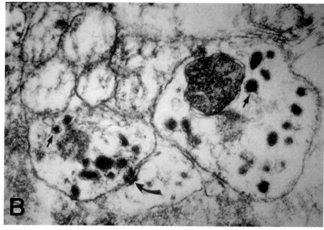

Figure 7.10

13. Favorable prognostic features in neuroblastoma include all of the following EXCEPT:
    a. Vanillylmandelic acid/Homovanillic acid (VMA/HVA) urine ratio of more than 1
    b. MYCN amplification
    c. Patient's age less than 18 months
    d. Ganglionic differentiation
    e. Aneuploidy

14. The term "black" adenoma most commonly refers to which one of the following tumors?
    a. Pituitary adenoma with old hemorrhage
    b. Vasoactive intestinal peptide (VIP)-secreting pancreatic adenoma

    c. Adrenal oncocytoma
    d. Adrenal adenoma with melanin pigment
    e. Colonic adenoma progressing to cancer

15. Additional stains that are required to establish the diagnosis of this adrenal tumor (Fig. 7.11) include:
    a. Chromogranin
    b. Vimentin
    c. Mucicarmine
    d. Melan-A (mart-1)
    e. Ki-67 (MIB-1) proliferative rate

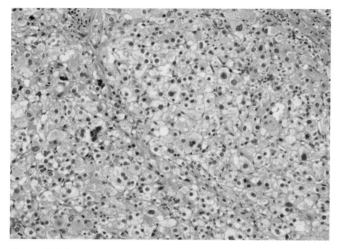

Figure 7.11

16. Features that strongly support the diagnosis of adrenocortical carcinoma versus adenoma include all of the following EXCEPT:
    a. Weight more than 500 gm
    b. Marked nuclear pleomorphism
    c. Nuclear positivity for P53
    d. The presence of necrosis
    e. High MIB-1 proliferation rate

17. Cushing syndrome is most likely caused by:
    a. Adrenal adenoma
    b. Adrenal carcinoma
    c. Diffuse adrenal hyperplasia
    d. Macronodular hyperplasia
    e. Functional neuroblastoma

18. A 60-year-old woman presented with swelling in the hard palate. Imaging studies revealed a large neoplasm eroding adjacent bony structures. Histology is shown (Fig. 7.12). The differential diagnosis should include which one of the following?
    a. Adenoid cystic carcinoma
    b. Polymorphous low-grade adenocarcinoma
    c. Carcinosarcoma
    d. Metastatic lobular breast carcinoma
    e. Basal cell adenoma

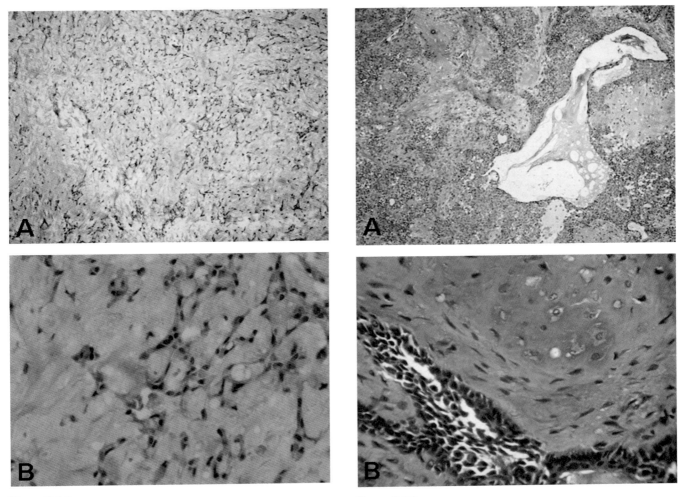

Figure 7.12

Figure 7.13

19. Which of the following statements correctly applies to this parotid gland tumor (Fig. 7.13)?
   a. It frequently presents as fast-growing painful mass.
   b. It is not seen in the minor salivary gland.
   c. It commonly involves the facial nerves, resulting in paralysis.
   d. Tumors with this histologic picture are frequently positive for S-100.
   e. It can recur after incomplete removal.

20. Which of the following lesions is NOT associated with human papilloma virus (HPV)?
   a. Fungiform schneiderian papilloma
   b. Inverted schneiderian papilloma
   c. Columnar cell (oncocytic) papilloma
   d. Juvenile laryngeal papilloma
   e. Verruca vulgaris of the nose

21. A 35-year-old immunocompetent white man has chronic complaints of nasal congestion and obstruction and nasal discharge. Endoscopic sinus surgery was performed. What are the organisms that are most likely responsible for causing this condition (Fig. 7.14)?
   a. Candida
   b. Dematiaceous fungi
   c. Mucor
   d. Mycobacterium tuberculosis
   e. Rhinosporidium

22. Granuloma in the meibomian glands is most likely caused by:
   a. Ruptured dermoid cyst
   b. Necrobiotic xanthogranuloma
   c. Granuloma annulare
   d. Chalazion
   e. Sarcoid granuloma

23. Which of the following statements is true regarding this parotid gland tumor (Fig. 7.15)?
   a. It is the most common malignant salivary gland tumor.

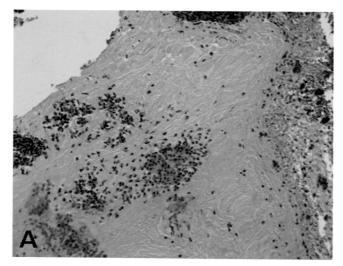

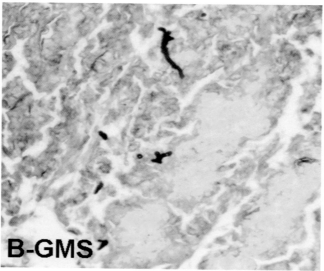

Figure 7.14

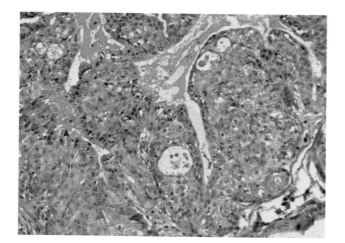

Figure 7.15

b. It arises from pleomorphic adenoma.

c. It is best designated as a low-grade mucoepidermoid carcinoma.

d. It is more common in men than in women.

e. It is locally aggressive but does not metastasize.

24. A 31-year-old human immunodeficiency virus (HIV)-positive woman has an enlarged lymph node in the posterior triangle of the neck. Histology is shown (Fig. 7.16). Which one immunostain is LEAST useful to delineate the nature of this lesion?
    a. Cytokeratin
    b. S-100
    c. CD45
    d. p63
    e. Ebstein-Barr virus (EBV)

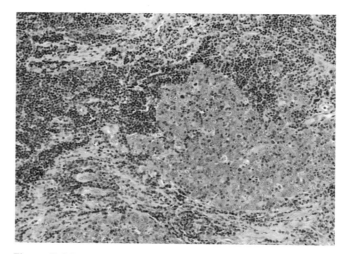

Figure 7.16

25. Which population group in the United States has the LOWEST incidence of nasopharyngeal carcinoma?
    a. Alaskan Eskimos
    b. African Americans
    c. Whites
    d. Third-generation Chinese immigrants

26. The best designation of this nasopharyngeal tumor (Fig. 7.17) is:
    a. Keratinizing nasopharyngeal carcinoma
    b. Nonkeratinizing nasopharyngeal carcinoma
    c. Nasopharyngeal papillary adenocarcinoma
    d. Lymphoma
    e. Olfactory neuroblastoma

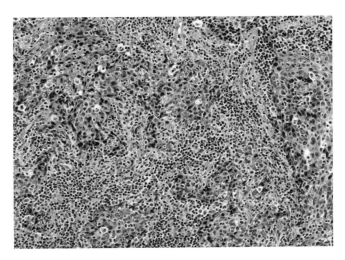

Figure 7.17

27. Which of the following types of nasopharyngeal carcinomas have the LOWEST incidence of EBV positivity?
    a. Keratinizing nasopharyngeal carcinoma
    b. Nonkeratinizing differentiated carcinoma
    c. Undifferentiated nonkeratinizing carcinoma
    d. Lymphoepithelioma

28. The most common neoplasm in the tonsil is:
    a. Squamous papilloma
    b. Lymphangiomatous polyp
    c. Dermoid cyst
    d. Squamous cell carcinoma
    e. Lymphoma

29. The most common islet cell tumor of the pancreas is:
    a. Gastrinoma
    b. Beta-cell tumor
    c. Alpha-cell tumor
    d. Solid pseudopapillary tumor
    e. VIP-producing tumors

30. Risk factors for the development of invasive carcinoma of the larynx include all of the following factors EXCEPT:
    a. EBV infection
    b. Smoking
    c. Heavy alcohol consumption
    d. Male gender

■ Answers

1. **a.** The images show a cellular round cell tumor with rosette formation, and it is consistent with neuroblastoma. Although Wilms tumor is common at this age and may rarely have neuroendocrine differentiation, the absence of WT-1 mutations favors neuroblastoma. **Neuroblastoma** usually stains diffusely with synaptophysin and can be differentiated from Ewing sarcoma, lymphoma, or rhabdomyosarcoma by lack of staining for CD99, CD45, and myogenin, respectively.

2. **a.** The images depict a neuroendocrine tumor with prominent nesting pattern. The clinical presentation, histology, and immunophenotype are characteristics of **paraganglioma**. Hepatocellular carcinoma may have neuroendocrine features; however, the cytologic features and diffuse positivity of chromogranin do not favor hepatocellular carcinoma. Carcinoid tumor may be confused with paraganglioma but is very rare in the retroperitoneal region. S-100 stain will reveal the characteristic sustentacular cells in paraganglioma. Retroperitoneal paragangliomas occur at an earlier age than head and neck paragangliomas do and are most frequently present at 30 to 40 years of age. Functional paragangliomas cause symptoms related to the production of norepinephrine similar to pheochromocytoma.

3. **c.** These S-100 positive cells are called **sustentacular cells.** They are of dendritic origin, but they do not stain with CD21 or CD1a. Their presence is diagnostic of paraganglioma, and their absence correlates with malignant behavior. They may be found in some types of carcinoid tumors of the lungs.

4. **d.** The image shows mature ganglion cells in a background of Schwann cells, thus consistent with **ganglioneuroma.** Ganglion cells are not uniformly seen in the other entities mentioned in the question, except for ganglion cell choristoma, which is a rare skin tumor. Ganglioneuroma usually presents in the retroperitoneum or mediastinum as an encapsulated mass and is a benign tumor.

5. **d.** The image shows the microfollicular pattern of **thyroid adenoma.** The standard therapy of follicular adenoma is lobectomy. The capsule of the tumor has to be histologically examined to rule out the possibility of follicular carcinoma.

6. **c.** The image shows the papillary architecture and the characteristic nuclear morphology of **papillary thyroid carcinoma** (nuclear grooves and clear nuclei). Alteration of the RET oncogene on chromosome 10q11.2 is a characteristic feature of this type of thyroid cancer. Somatic (not germline) rearrangements of RET/PTC genes are found in up to 80% of papillary thyroid carcinoma.

7. **b.** The image shows hyperplastic C cell in interfollicular and intrafollicular locations. Germline RET mutations are found in patients with MEN type 2 and results in **C-cell hyperplasia** and medullary carcinoma. C-cell hyperplasia is the precursor lesion of medullary thyroid carcinoma.

8. **a.** Ectopic **adrenal rests** are found in approximately 5% of herniorrhaphy specimens of male children. The circumscription, small size of the nodule, and cytologic features help to differentiate it from metastatic renal cell carcinoma.

9. **a.** Patients with **MEN type 1** develop adenomas of the anterior pituitary gland, pancreas, and parathyroid gland. Hyperplasia and adenomas involving the adrenal cortex and the thyroid are less commonly found. Soft-tissue lipomas, foregut carcinoids, and multiple leiomyomas are also in the spectrum of the disease. Pheochromocytoma and medullary carcinoma of the thyroid are part of MEN type 2 spectrum.

10. **e.** **Hyalinizing trabecular adenoma** of the thyroid is a type of adenoma with prominent hyaline appearance. The trabecular arrangement resembles paraganglioma, and the tumor may have nuclear grooves and psammoma bodies similar to papillary carcinoma. Some authors consider it a histologic variant of papillary carcinoma rather than a distinct identity.

11. **c.** Cytology shows **small round blue cell tumor.** The differential diagnosis of such type of tumors in the nasal cavity includes olfactory neuroblastoma, lymphoma, melanoma, pituitary adenoma, neuroendocrine carcinoma, and sinonasal undifferentiated carcinoma. Resolving this differential diagnosis often requires immunostaining and electron microscopy. The ultrastructural presence of neuroendocrine secretory granules is seen in olfactory neuroblastoma and pituitary adenoma. Neuroendocrine carcinoma may have rare granules, but they also have cell junctions. In these cases, neuroendocrine markers will be positive. Absence of neurosecretory granules and presence of cell attachment junctions favor sinonasal carcinoma. Positivity for cytokeratin and epithelial membrane antigen is also present in carcinomas. Electron microscopy is also useful to demonstrate melanosomes in melanoma. Choice *e* is consistent with lymphoma. Regular neuroblastoma is very rarely present in the nasal cavity.

12. **a.** These are **neurosecretory granules,** which are present in pheochromocytoma and tumors with neuroendocrine differentiation. These tumors stain with neuroendocrine markers including synaptophysin, chromogranin, CD56, and NSE.

13. **b.** Favorable prognosis in patients with **neuroblastoma** is seen in patients less than 18 months of age, with stage I or II disease, and having histology showing low mitotic karyorrhectic index, abundant Schwannian stroma, and ganglionic differentiation. Patients with MYCN amplification and diploidy have adverse prognosis. Advance clinical stage is also associated with bad prognosis except for metastasis to skin, liver, and bone marrow in patients less than 1 year, which is associated with better prognosis than to other sites.

14. **d. Black adenoma** refers to adrenal or thyroid adenoma with dark pigment. The pigment represents lipofuscin or melanin.

15. **d.** The image shows tumor cells with abundant, clear cytoplasm and central nuclei. The differential diagnosis is mainly between adrenocortical tumor and renal cell carcinoma invading the adrenal gland. These tumors resemble each other, and additional tests are often required to differentiate between the two. Adrenocortical carcinoma is more likely to express Melan-A, inhibin, and synaptophysin than renal cell carcinoma, while the latter is more likely to express cytokeratin and CD10. Chromogranin-positive adrenal tumors will have a different histologic appearance, and Ki67 proliferative index would not differentiate between these entities.

16. **b. Adrenocortical adenomas** need to be differentiated from carcinomas. Tumor weight of more than 500 gm, presence of necrosis, high mitotic activity, especially atypical mitoses, high Ki-67 proliferative rate, and capsular or vascular invasion correlates with recurrence and metastasis. Aneuploidy, not diploidy, also favors carcinoma. Marked nuclear pleomorphism can be found in both entities.

17. **c. Cushing syndrome** is most commonly adrenocorticotropic hormone (ACTH)-dependent; an example is excess production of ACTH by a pituitary adenoma, which subsequently results in adrenal hyperplasia. The pathology of adrenal gland in these cases is usually diffuse or micronodular hyperplasia. Macronodular hyperplasia is seen in only 10% to 20% of cases.

18. **b.** The histology shows tumor cells in abundant myxohyaline stroma. This appearance can be found in both polymorphous low-grade carcinoma and mixed tumor. **Polymorphous low-grade adenocarcinoma** is a tumor of minor salivary glands and is found in the hard palate, cheeks, and lips. The histology resembles mixed tumor and adenoid cystic carcinoma. Adenoid cystic carcinoma, however, usually has a cribriform pattern in a less myxoid stroma. The absence of sarcomatous pattern is against the diagnosis of carcinosarcoma.

19. **c.** An epithelial tumor with cartilaginous mesenchymal component in the parotid gland is most likely **pleomorphic adenoma**. Pleomorphic adenoma is the most common neoplasm of the salivary glands and presents as painless, slow-growing neoplasm. This tumor is characterized by architectural pleomorphism. Myoepithelial and mesenchymal components frequently stain with S-100. However, it is a benign tumor and does not usually involve the facial nerve. It can recur if treated by enucleation. Partial or total parotidectomy and surgical excision with a margin of normal tissue are the surgical options of choice.

20. **c.** "Schneiderian" epithelium refers to mucosal lining of the nasal cavity and nasal sinuses. Squamous papilloma arising in this epithelium usually has three morphologic variants. Exophytic fungiform papilloma is usually located on the nasal septum, while inverted papilloma is nonseptal. These two variants are associated with HPV infection, while oncocytic **schneiderian papilloma** is not associated with HPV.

21. **b.** Histology shows numerous eosinophils and clumped degenerating basophilic cells in background of eosinophilic mucin, characteristic of allergic sinusitis. Special stains reveal the presence of few fungal forms. Aspergillus and dematiaceous fungi such as *Curvularia*, *Alternaria*, and *Bipolaris* are involved in most cases of **allergic fungal sinusitis**. Mucormycosis results in fulminant invasive disease, which is usually seen in immunosuppressed patients.

22. **d. Chalazion** is a lipogranuloma that characteristically occurs in the meibomian glands. All of the above-mentioned lesions can have granulomas but in different locations.

23. **a.** The presence of atypical squamous elements with few mucous cysts is characteristic of intermediate-grade to high-grade mucoepidermoid carcinoma. **Mucoepidermoid carcinoma** is the most common malignant tumor of the salivary glands and is characteristically more common in women than in men. Histologically, it may be confused with pleomorphic adenoma, but the lack of myoepithelial cells and mesenchymal components is characteristic of mucoepidermoid carcinoma. The tumor can recur and metastasize to lymph nodes and other organs. High-grade tumors are associated with high mortality rate.

24. **c. Squamous cell carcinoma** of the upper aerodigestive tract is the most common origin of lymph node metastasis involving the head and neck. Cytokeratin, p63, and EBV can be used to confirm the diagnosis. Melanomas and thyroid carcinomas are also not common as lymph node metastasis. S-100 is positive in melanomas. Although lymphoma can occur in the head and neck lymph node, the histology does not support that, and CD45 will not be helpful.

25. **c.** The incidence of **nasopharyngeal carcinoma** is highest in Southern Chinese, Chinese in Hong Kong, and Eskimos. The incidence is high in Chinese immigrants and decreases among second- and third-generation immigrants. In non-Asian population, the incidence is high in adolescents of African descent.

26. **b.** The image shows the lymphoepithelioma lesion of nasopharyngeal carcinoma. The poor differentiation and lack of keratinization are consistent with nonkeratinizing nasopharyngeal carcinoma.

27. **a.** Nonkeratinizing carcinoma is the most common type of **nasopharyngeal carcinoma** (NPC) in endemic areas and is closely related to EBV infection. Keratinizing squamous cell carcinoma is a rare subtype of NPC and is not as strongly associated with EBV infection. Signs of EBV infection were identified in primary tumors as well as distant metastasis. Lymphoepithelioma is a histologic appearance of

nonkeratinizing NPC cells intimately associated with lymphocytes in and around the tumor cells.

28. **a. Squamous papilloma** represents 75% of the all benign tonsillar tumors and is not usually associated HPV. Lymphangiomatous tonsillar polyp is a rare lesion found incidentally in patients who have sensation of foreign body. Squamous cell carcinoma is the most common malignancy followed by lymphoma.

29. **b. Beta-cell tumors** are the most common islet tumors of the pancreas and, when functioning, are also referred to as insulinomas because they secrete insulin. Alpha-cell tumors secrete glucagon. G-cell tumors or gastrinomas are the most common tumor in patients with MEN type 1.

30. **a. Carcinoma of the larynx** typically occurs in men over the age of 50 who are heavy cigarette smokers and who consume alcohol. HPV may play a role in the pathogenesis, but EBV virus is not associated with it.

■ Recommended Readings

Rosai J. *Rosai and Ackerman's surgical pathology*, 9th ed. Philadelphia: Mosby, 2004.

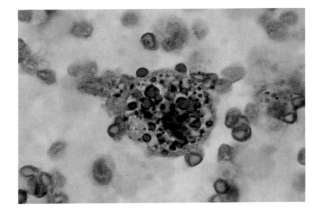

Respiratory System

Ronald M. Przygodzki

■ Questions

1. In the assessment of an open lung biopsy for interstitial lung disease, all of the following should be requested and/or performed EXCEPT:
   a. CT, or high-resolution CT scans of lung
   b. Inflation of specimen(s) with formalin before processing for histology
   c. Biopsy of tips of lobes and lingula
   d. Multiple biopsies from different lung sites
   e. Small samples from the biopsies to be sent to microbiology for analysis

2. Classic features of Erdheim-Chester disease include all of the following EXCEPT:
   a. Involvement of long bones and lung
   b. Infiltration of histiocytes staining with S100 and CD1a
   c. Diffuse infiltration by foamy histocytes along lymphatic routes including septae, pleura, perivascular, and peribronchiolar interstitium
   d. Infiltration by histiocytes lack prominent nuclear grooving
   e. Infiltration by eosinophils

3. You receive a bronchoalveolar lavage from a patient from a local nursing home. You perform routine stains, including the following oil red O stain (Fig. 8.1). Which of the following statements is NOT correct?
   a. A similar picture can occasionally be seen in milk-fed infants.
   b. Inert lipids (e.g., vegetable oil) will cause little inflammatory reaction.
   c. Assessment with this stain does not require special handling during preparation.
   d. This result may also be seen in lung sampling distal to obstruction.
   e. These cytoplasmic droplets are not birefringent.

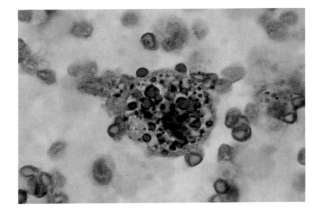

Figure 8.1

4. Cells normally found in the bronchial-bronchiolar epithelium include all of the following EXCEPT:
   a. Clara cells
   b. Kulchitsky cells
   c. Serous cells
   d. Goblet cells
   e. Aschoff cells

5. You are reviewing a wedge biopsy of lung, where you note the presence of giant cells and granulomata within bronchovascular bundles. The differential diagnosis you need to consider includes all of the following EXCEPT:
   a. Intravenous drug abuse
   b. Wegener granulomatosis
   c. Methotrexate lung toxicity
   d. Hypersensitivity pneumonitis
   e. Systemic lupus erythematosus

6. Review of a lung sample from a patient with diffuse lung process reveals alveolar spaces filled with amorphous pink material. All of the following tests should be performed EXCEPT:
   a. Periodic acid-Schiff (PAS) with and without diastase
   b. Acid-fast bacillus (AFB) stain for *Nocardia*
   c. Gomori methenamine-silver (GMS) for *Pneumocystis*
   d. Test for autoantibodies to GM-CSF
   e. Mutation detection tests for surfactant protein B

7. This condition (Fig. 8.2) may be associated with all of the following EXCEPT:
   a. Viral pneumonia
   b. Surfactant deficiency
   c. Ground-glass appearance on radiograph
   d. Hyperlucent emphysematous lungs
   e. Administration of chemotherapeutic agents

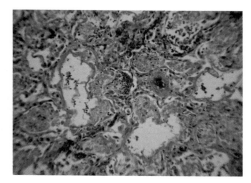

Figure 8.2

8. Wegener granulomatosis (WG) is characterized by:
   a. Necrotizing vasculitis and capillaritis
   b. Necrotizing granulomas involving upper and lower respiratory tract
   c. Glomerulopathy
   d. Response to cytotoxic drugs
   e. All of the above

9. The presence of eosinophilic infiltrates in a lung sample is found in all of the listed disease entities EXCEPT:
   a. Drug reactions
   b. Hodgkin disease
   c. Whipple disease
   d. Collagen vascular disease
   e. Churg-Strauss syndrome

10. Features characteristic of the acute phase of bronchopulmonary dysplasia include:
    a. Submucosal fibrosis
    b. Mucous gland atrophy
    c. Medial hyperplasia of the pulmonary arteries
    d. Squamous metaplasia
    e. Bronchiolitis obliterans

11. All of the following statements regarding small cell carcinoma of the lung are correct EXCEPT:
    a. It expresses CD56 and synaptophysin.
    b. It produces ACTH hormone.
    c. It arises centrally in most cases.
    d. It invades lymphatic vessels.
    e. It commonly presents as an exophytic mass.

12. Idiopathic pulmonary hemosiderosis (IPH) is associated with:
    a. Antiglomerular basement membrane disease
    b. Liver hemosiderosis
    c. Eosinophilia
    d. Wegener granulomatosis
    e. Pulmonary hypertension

13. Which of the following is NOT in keeping with clinicopathologic features of inflammatory myofibroblastic tumor (IMT)?
    a. Foci of gross hemorrhage and/or necrosis
    b. Growth into large airways and blood vessels
    c. Hyperglobulinemia, leukothrombocytosis, and weight loss
    d. Low mitotic activity
    e. Calcifications

14. Neuroendocrine granules may ultrastructurally be seen in the following lung tumors EXCEPT:
    a. Small cell carcinoma
    b. Adenocarcinoma
    c. Squamous cell carcinoma
    d. Mesothelioma
    e. Large cell neuroendocrine tumor

15. Which of the following is correct regarding grade II neuroendocrine carcinomas?
    a. Azzopardi effect is frequently seen.
    b. Most tumors are diploid.
    c. They display a mitotic rate of >5 per 10 high-power fields.
    d. They have a low mortality rate of 5% at 5 years.
    e. The transcription factor p53 is mutated in all cases.

16. The most common malignant tumor of the lung in children is:
    a. Pleuropulmonary blastoma
    b. Carcinoid tumor
    c. Rhabdomyosarcoma
    d. Metastatic tumor
    e. Mucoepidermoid carcinoma

17. Bronchioloalveolar carcinoma:
    a. Of the mucinous type has a worse prognosis than nonmucinous type
    b. Of the nonmucinous type is immunohistochemically negative for TTF-1
    c. Arises centrally in the lung

d. Is less common in children than squamous carcinoma
e. Is associated with myopathic-myasthenic syndrome (Lambert-Eaton syndrome)

18. Sclerosing hemangioma:
    a. Occurs mainly in adult women
    b. Is a fast-growing tumor
    c. Is negative for cytokeratin
    d. Metastasizes to lymph nodes
    e. Is similar in histology to cavernous hemangioma

19. You have a patient with non–small-cell lung carcinoma (NSCLC). Your patient's oncologist requests your assessment of this tumor in light of current EGFR receptor inhibitors. Which of the following statements is correct?
    a. EGFR receptor inhibitors can be used on all NSCLC.
    b. Immunohistochemical (IHC) assessment of EGFR receptor is superior to flourescent in situ hybridization (FISH).
    c. Exon 20 mutations are associated with better therapeutic outcome.
    d. EGFR inhibitor-sensitive mutations include exon 19 (delE746-750).
    e. EGFR mutation in exons 18 to 24 lead to inactivation of receptor.

20. A 3-mm nodular proliferation of spindle cells in the lung of a patient with bronchiectasis most likely is:
    a. Minute meningothelioid nodule
    b. Tumor with carcinoid features
    c. IMT
    d. Leiomyoma
    e. Sugar tumor

21. Thymic tumors commonly associated with myasthenia gravis include all of the following EXCEPT:
    a. Cortical thymoma
    b. Medullary type A thymoma
    c. Mixed thymoma
    d. Lymphocyte-rich thymoma
    e. Thymic carcinoma

22. Which of the following statements about this lung tumor (Fig. 8.3) is true?
    a. Tumors located peripherally near the pleura are less common than central tumors.
    b. Unlike other lung tumors, it is not immunoreactive for TTF-1.
    c. The tumor is highly aggressive with low survival rate.
    d. By electron microscopy, it contains rhomboidal crystals.
    e. It arises from Clara cells.

23. These are lung sections (Fig. 8.4) from a patient with:
    a. Kidney transplant
    b. Congestive heart failure
    c. Renal cell carcinoma

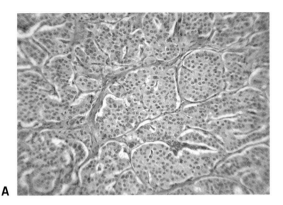

A

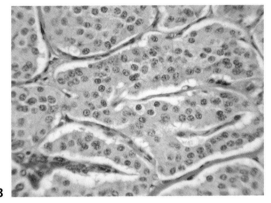

B

Figure 8.3

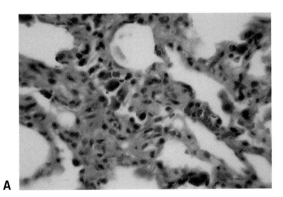

A

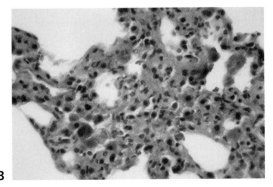

B

Figure 8.4

d. Wegener granulomatosis
e. Interstitial pneumonia

24. Pneumocystis pneumonia commonly occurs in all of the following conditions EXCEPT:
    a. Hyper IgM syndrome
    b. Acquired immunodeficiency
    c. Severe combined immunodeficiency (SCID)
    d. Common variable immunodeficiency
    e. Bare lymphocyte syndrome

25. Which of the following statements regarding "sugar" tumor of the lung is true?
    a. It is commonly located centrally.
    b. Cells show deeply eosinophilic granular cytoplasm.
    c. Cells are positive for HMB-45 and CD117 immunostains.
    d. Mitoses are abundant.
    e. It contains abundant mucin.

26. Creola bodies are found in bronchoalveolar lavage specimens from patients with:
    a. Sarcoidosis
    b. Lipoid pneumonia
    c. Adenovirus infection
    d. Asthma
    e. Mitral heart valve disease

27. Masson bodies are characteristically seen in which of the following types of interstitial lung disease?
    a. Respiratory bronchiolitis-associated interstitial lung disease (RB-ILD)
    b. Lymphoid interstitial pneumonia (LIP)
    c. Cryptogenic organizing pneumonia (COP)
    d. Desquamative interstitial pneumonia (DIP)
    e. Usual interstitial pneumonia (UIP)

28. Squamous cell carcinoma of the lung may show ectopic production of:
    a. ACTH
    b. Calcium
    c. ADH
    d. PTH-like peptide
    e. HCG

29. A tumor involving the lung parenchyma and the pleura and diffusely expressing TTF-1 is LEAST likely to be:
    a. Small cell carcinoma
    b. Adenocarcinoma
    c. Squamous cell carcinoma
    d. Undifferentiated large cell carcinoma
    e. Mesothelioma

30. Bronchial-associated lymphoid tissue (BALT) lymphoma:
    a. Is the most common lymphoma of the lung

b. Is usually high grade with a bad prognosis
c. Is a nodular proliferation of large pleomorphic cells
d. Cells express CD10 and CD56
e. Is associated with EBV infection

31. This pulmonary explant (Fig. 8.5) was from a patient with a long history of asbestos exposure. Which of the following statements is correct regarding this malignancy?
    a. The tumor is usually confined to the lung.
    b. Pleural effusion is rare.
    c. Electron microscopy of the epithelioid variant of this tumor is not helpful.
    d. Calretinin, WT1, and CD141 (thrombomodulin) are used to support the diagnosis of this tumor.
    e. TTF-1 is positive in this tumor.

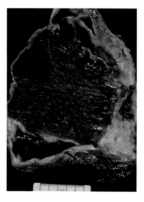

Figure 8.5

32. Which of the following statements is INCORRECT regarding this specimen (Fig. 8.6)?
    a. The patient's symptoms included cough.
    b. Deletion of codon 508 of the CF gene is often present.
    c. Mucus plugging of bronchioles is a secondary phenomenon.
    d. Rare individuals may have Cushing syndrome.
    e. Young to middle-aged individuals are usually affected with this disease.

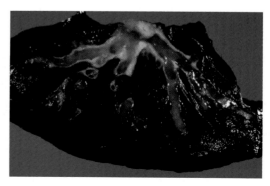

Figure 8.6

33. The diagnosis of the following 1.0-cm tumor (Fig. 8.7) is:
    a. Atypical adenomatous alveolar hyperplasia
    b. Adenoid cystic carcinoma
    c. Fetal adenocarcinoma of lung
    d. Mucinous bronchioloalveolar carcinoma
    e. Metastatic thyroid carcinoma

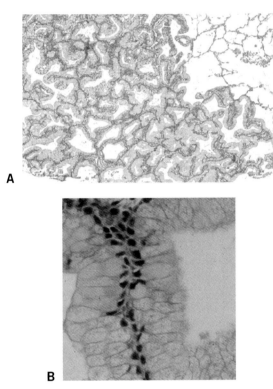

Figure 8.7

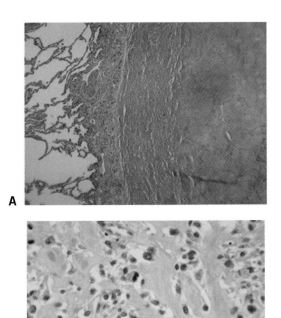

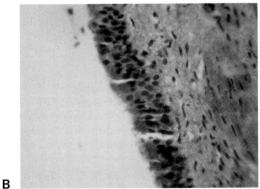

Figure 8.8

34. The best diagnosis for the following lung tumor
    (Fig. 8.8) from a young man is:
    a. Large cell undifferentiated pulmonary carcinoma
    b. Fibroinflammatory reaction
    c. Mesothelioma
    d. Teratoma
    e. Metastatic osteosarcoma

35. You receive this specimen from a young man with an
    anterior unilocular mediastinal mass (Fig. 8.9). Which
    of the following statements is INCORRECT with re-
    spect to this tumor?
    a. The mass may have alveolar tissue.
    b. It may be found in the pericardium as well as below
       the diaphragm.
    c. It occasionally may be lined by metaplastic squa-
       mous epithelium.
    d. Cartilaginous tissue may be present.
    e. Communication with the tracheobronchial tree is
       often present.

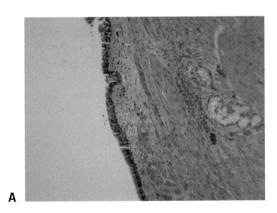

Figure 8.9

■ Answers

1. **c.** In taking biopsies of the lungs, tips of lobes and lingual are to be avoided. Inflation of the surgical specimen with formalin should be performed to avoid specimen atelectasis, which makes assessment of interstitial lesions difficult. All of the remaining items should be performed, as well as sampling for electron microscopy.

2. **b. Erdheim-Chester disease** is a rare disease characterized by infiltration of histiocytes staining variably with S100, but **not staining with CD1a**. In addition to the foamy histiocytes, the disease may also display presence of multinucleated histiocytes, eosinophils, plasma cells, and few lymphocytes. The main differential diagnosis of this disease is Langerhans cell histocytosis.

3. **c.** The oil red O stain reveals lipid droplets within macrophages. This is a feature found in **aspiration pneumonia**. Slides made from BAL material requires that they are not mounted using conventional methods including xylene washes, rather an aqueous mount is needed to retain lipid vacuoles.

4. **e.** Clara cells are columnar nonciliated bronchial cells with a role in surfactant and protease inhibitor production. Kulchitsky cells are basally oriented cells with numerous neuroendocrine granules, with unknown specific function to date. Serous and goblet cells secrete serous and mucinous excretions, respectively. **Aschoff cells are found in rheumatic carditis**.

5. **e.** Patients with systemic lupus erythematosus (SLE) present with pleuritis, siderophages, and capillaritis in the acute phase. A second presentation in SLE consists of a cellular plasmacytic/lymphocytic interstitial pneumonia with variable amounts of fibrosis, categorized as a nonspecific interstitial pneumonia. **Giant cells and granulomas are however not present**. The remaining disease entities contain the features noted in the question.

6. **c.** A diagnosis of **pulmonary alveolar proteinosis (PAP)** requires the exclusion of several possible entities including edema, infection, and the like. The intra-alveolar material present in PAP is PAS-positive, diastase resistant, excluding several other disease entities. *Nocardia* infection is known to be associated with PAP, hence its exclusion needs to be performed. The exudate in *Pneumocystis* pneumonia is foamier as compared with PAP. Autoantibodies to GM-CSF are found among adults with acquired PAP. Mutation on surfactant protein B is in the congenital form, and is lethal.

7. **d.** This H&E picture depicts **hyaline membrane disease**. The membrane may become fragmented and faintly basophilic by the action of bacteria. The lungs are usually firm and atelectatic and **not emphysematous**.

The remaining entities are potential differential disease to be considered; however, each has unique features not depicted in this H&E.

8. **e.** The granulomas in WG are characterized by involvement of bronchovascular regions, including large vessels, inflammatory infiltrate rich in eosinophils, and a less-defined appearance compared with the granulomas in sarcoidosis. Early changes may be as subtle as neutrophilic capillaritis of the alveoli.

9. **c.** Rare pulmonary involvement with **Whipple disease** is known. Sheets of histiocytes with PAS positive granules along bronchovascular bundles are typically noted. Eosinophils are rarely seen.

10. **e.** The most significant injury is at the level of bronchioles and acini with obstructive **necrotizing bronchiolitis**. Late phase of the disease is characterized by fibrosis, metaplasia and atrophy.

11. **e.** Small cell carcinoma **seldom presents as exophytic endobronchial lesions** as would be noted with bronchial carcinoids. It usually presents with circumferential infiltration beneath the bronchial mucosa.

12. **c.** IPH is associated with the presence of large numbers of hemosiderin-laden macrophages in BAL specimens. **Eosinophilia** and iron deficiency anemia are seen, usually with normal renal function and no associated immunological diseases. Wegener granulomatosis should have components of giant cells, granulomata, and presence of ANCA positivity for confirmation.

13. **a.** IMT are biologically borderline tumors that **rarely display necrosis or hemorrhage**. Nearly 50% of patients with IMT show fever, anemia, hyperglobulinemia, leukothrombocytosis, and weight loss. Mitotic activity is readily evident. Calcifications are commonly seen. Surgery is the primary mode of treatment; however, a low rate of recurrence may be present given the nature of the tumors spreading peripherally. The tumor is peripherally located and commonly occurs in children. The tumor shows cytogenetic rearrangements that activate the ALK receptor in chromosome 2p23, but the t(2;5) translocation is not characteristic. This tumor recurs in 25% of cases and may undergo malignant transformation, especially when there is an increased area of necrosis, bizarre giant cells, poor circumscription, and an increased mitotic rate of >3 per 50 high-power fields.

14. **d. Mesotheliomas** reveal elongated plasmalemmal microvilli on the cell surfaces with a length-to-diameter ratio of 10:1 or more. **Neuroendocrine granules are not seen**. All lung tumors to a greater or lesser extent may contain neuroendocrine granules, with small cell carcinoma being best recognized for this characteristic.

15. **c.** Grade II neuroendocrine carcinomas (atypical carcinoids) usually are aneuploid. Mortality for these tumors is rather high and can reach 30% to 50% in

2 years. The Azzopardi effect is represented by the collection and accretion of densely basophilic smudged nucleic acid material adjacent to tumoral blood vessels. This is most commonly associated with small cell neuroendocrine carcinoma. P53 is wild-type in all cases, as compared with small cell neuroendocrine carcinoma where most tumors are.

16. **d.** Although all the tumors noted may occur in children, the most common event is **metastatic tumor** from other sites, especially osteosarcoma.

17. **a.** Squamous cell carcinoma is rarer than the bronchioloalveolar type in children. Mucinous type-bronchioloalveolar carcinoma has a worse prognosis than nonmucinous type. Lambert-Eaton syndrome is a feature of small cell neuroendocrine carcinoma.

18. **a.** Sclerosing hemangiomas are slow-growing tumors. They arise from type 2 pneumocytes and display positivity for cytokeratin and EMA.

19. **d.** EGFR inhibitors are used only in NSLCL that failed initial chemotherapy response. FISH is superior in detection of EGFR receptor than IHC detection. Exon 20 mutations are associated with resistance to inhibitor therapy. EGFR mutation in exons 18 to 24 leads to constitutive activation. EGFR mutations with sensitivity to EGFR inhibitors include exon 19 (delE746-750) and exon 21 (L858R).

20. **b.** **Carcinoid tumorlets** are usually seen in patients with bronchiectasis and intralobar sequestration. They must not exceed 4 mm in maximal radial dimension. They occur within or around bronchovascular sheaths.

21. **e.** **Thymic carcinoma** is the only thymic disease that is not associated with myasthenia gravis.

22. **a.** Carcinoid tumors **arise from Kulchitsky cells** and rarely present with carcinoid syndrome. Central carcinoids are more common than peripheral carcinoids, and are usually located near bronchi/bronchioles. Tumors have a high survival rate. Cells contain neurosecretory granules and react with neuroendocrine markers, TTF-1, Grimelius stain, and may react with S-100.

23. **a.** This is pneumonia caused by **cytomegalovirus** with usual viropathic changes. Situations in which this infection can occur include AIDS and postorgan transplantation.

24. **d.** *Pneumocystis* pneumonia usually occurs with cellular immunodeficiency such as SCID and is rarely seen in antibody deficiency syndromes other than **Hyper IgM syndrome**.

25. **c.** **Epithelioid myomelanocytoma** (pulmonary "sugar tumor") contains abundant glycogen and is typically located in the peripheral lung. The cells are positive for HMB-45 and CD117 and may also be positive with muscle specific actin, S100 and NSE, as well as microphthalmia transcription factor 1.

26. **d.** Creola bodies are found in patients with **asthma**. They are ciliated columnar cells sloughed from the bronchial mucosa. Other common findings in the sputum of asthma patients include Charcot-Leyden crystals, Curschmann spirals, and eosinophils.

27. **c.** Masson bodies are dense eosinophilic fibroblastic plugs in the bronchioles and are characteristically seen in **organizing pneumonia**.

28. **d.** Squamous cell carcinoma can cause hyperparathyroidism.

29. **e.** TTF-1 is expressed in about three quarters of adenocarcinoma and in several other lung carcinoma types. Squamous cell carcinoma rarely stains with TTF-1. Nuclear staining should be used as true positive staining. This stain is very useful in determining whether a pleural-based tumor is or is not a **mesothelioma**; however, it should not be used in exclusion of other stains affirming lung origin (e.g., mucin, etc.).

30. **a.** **BALT lymphoma** is a nodular proliferation of small monotonous B lymphocytes, which do not express CD10 or CD56. It is a low-grade tumor, similar to MALT lymphoma.

31. **d.** The gross picture is that of a **pleural mesothelioma**. The tumor typically begins with studding of the pleural surface, becoming confluent and obliterating the pleural cavity. Invasion of contiguous structures including peripheral lung parenchyma, great vessels, myocardium, and soft tissue of chest may all occur. Pleural effusions are common. Bushy plasmalemmal microvilli are seen in the epithelioid variant, and are diagnostic. TTF-1 is positive in most pulmonary adenocarcinomas and many adenosquamous carcinomas. Mesotheliomas are consistently negative for TTF-1, whereas calretinin, WT1, and CD141 are used as inclusive stains for mesothelioma.

32. **b.** The picture depicts a **grade I neuroendocrine carcinoma** (classical carcinoid) located in the bronchus (tan intrabronchial mass in superior aspect of the picture). Although bronchiectatic changes with mucus plugging are noted, this is secondary to the plugging of the airway by the carcinoid, and is not a result of cystic fibrosis.

33. **d.** The tumor presented is a **mucinous bronchioloalveolar carcinoma**. Lack of sclerosis and inflammation removes this tumor from adenocarcinoma. Distinction between atypical adenomatous alveolar hyperplasia and a small bronchioloalveolar carcinoma is dependent on size, that is, those less than 5 mm are considered to be the former.

34. **e.** This **metastatic osteosarcoma** reveals a rounded mass however highly pleomorphic cytology embedded within an osteoid matrix. Key note in the question is that the patient is young, thereby removing large cell undifferentiated pulmonary carcinoma and mesothelioma. The pleomorphism is too extensive for this to be a reactive process. Other mesodermal leaves are missing to categorize this tumor into a teratoma.

35. **a.** This is a **bronchogenic cyst**, in which alveolar tissue is never present. The main differential diagnosis of this tumor is congenital pulmonary airway malformation (CPAM) and esophageal duplication cyst. Presence of submucosal glands, location of mass, and lack of double muscle layer excludes an esophageal duplication cyst. Interestingly though, both may be lined by ciliated columnar cells. Lack of alveolar tissue excludes CPAM, and is useful in situations when bronchogenic cysts occur within the lung proper.

■ Recommended Readings

Leslie KO, Wick MR. *Practical pulmonary pathology: A diagnostic approach,* 1st ed. Philadelphia: Churchill Livingstone, 2005.

Pfeifer JD. *Molecular genetic testing in surgical pathology,* 1st ed. Philadelphia: Lippincott Williams & Wilkins, 2006.

O'Leary TJ. *Advanced diagnostic methods in pathology,* 1st ed. Philadelphia: Saunders, 2003.

Travis WD, Colby TV, Koss MN, et al. *Non-neoplastic disorders of the lower respiratory tract,* 1st Series, Fascicle 2, Atlas of Nontumor Pathology. Washington, DC: The Armed Forces Institute of Pathology, 2002.

9

Cardiovascular System

Atif Ahmed

■ Questions

1. Which of the following statements is true about the human heart?
   a. It develops from two tubes that later divide into four chambers.
   b. It is first recognizable at 15 days of gestation.
   c. It starts to pump at 8 weeks of gestation.
   d. Tetralogy of Fallot is the most common congenital anomaly.
   e. Congenital heart defects are present in 6 per 100,000 live births.

2. The most common chromosomal abnormality associated with congenital heart disease is:
   a. 46,XY inv (3)(p21q22)
   b. Deletions in chromosomal region 22q11.2
   c. 45XO chromosomal karyotype
   d. Trisomy 21
   e. Trisomy 18

3. The most common valvular abnormality in the United States is:
   a. Mitral valve prolapse
   b. Aortic valve disease
   c. Subaortic stenosis
   d. Pulmonic stenosis
   e. Rheumatic mitral stenosis

4. Congenital heart anomalies LEAST frequently associated with microdeletions in chromosome 22q11 include:
   a. Persistent truncus arteriosus
   b. Tetralogy of Fallot
   c. Interrupted aortic arch
   d. Patent ductus arteriosus
   e. Right-sided aortic arch

5. In complete transposition of the great vessels, there is:
   a. Atrioventricular (AV) discordance with ventriculoarterial concordance
   b. AV discordance associated with ventriculoarterial discordance
   c. AV concordance associated with ventriculoarterial discordance
   d. AV concordance associated with ventriculoarterial concordance

6. What is the most likely cause of this lesion (Fig. 9.1), which is seen in endomyocardial biopsy of a heart transplant recipient patient?
   a. Effect of chemotherapy
   b. Recurrent Chagas disease of the heart
   c. Direct effect from placement of pacemaker wires
   d. Acute transplant rejection
   e. Restrictive cardiomyopathy

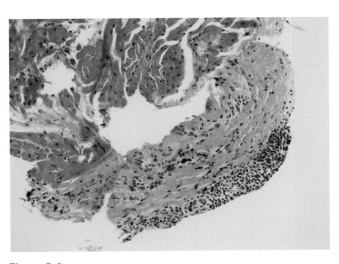

Figure 9.1

7. What is the most common metastatic tumor to the heart?
   a. Prostatic carcinoma
   b. Carcinoma of the lung
   c. Rhabdomyosarcoma
   d. Melanoma
   e. Colon carcinoma

8. What is the most common cardiovascular abnormality seen in patients with congenital rubella syndrome?
   a. Patent ductus arteriosus
   b. Interrupted aortic arch
   c. Coarctation of the aorta
   d. Ventricular septal defect
   e. Transposition of the great vessels

9. Brown-Brenn is a special stain that is used in which of the following conditions?
   a. To delineate loss of elastic tissue in Marfan syndrome patients
   b. To highlight intracellular lipid
   c. To stain Gram-positive bacteria
   d. Is a stain for myxoid degeneration in heart valves
   e. To stain mycobacterial organisms

10. These are histologic sections of a tumor identified in the heart of a 37-year-old woman with signs of mitral valve stenosis (Fig. 9.2). Which of the following statements best describes this lesion?
    a. It is the most common primary heart tumor found in this age group.
    b. It is most commonly located in the right ventricle.
    c. It can regress spontaneously without treatment.
    d. It is an aggressive tumor with potential for metastasis and high mortality.
    e. It is a hamartomatous lesion.

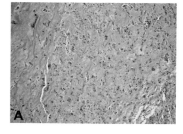

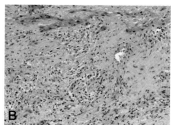

Figure 9.2

11. What is the most common artificial heart valve used in surgical practice?
    a. Bioprosthetic heart valve
    b. Björk-Shiley valve
    c. Medtronic-Hall tilting disk valve
    d. St. Jude valve
    e. Starr-Edwards valve

12. All of the following morphologic cardiomyopathic changes are associated with Adriamycin therapy EXCEPT:
    a. Loss of cross striations in the myocytes
    b. Inflammatory infiltrate of mononuclear cells
    c. Myocytolysis
    d. Loss of cytoplasmic myofilaments
    e. Vacuolization of cardiac myocytes

13. A heart transplant recipient has undergone an endomyocardial biopsy 2 months after the transplant (Fig. 9.3). Additional significant histologic findings to look for in the biopsy that will determine the management of this patient include the identification of:
    a. Nodular subendocardial lymphocytic infiltrate
    b. Interstitial fibrosis
    c. Calcifications
    d. Diffuse myocyte necrosis
    e. Vascular intimal proliferation

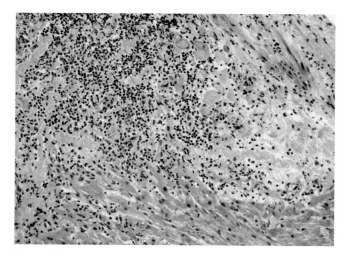

Figure 9.3

14. Which of the following best describes cardiac "MICE"?
    a. They appear as calcified amorphous nodules on imaging studies.
    b. They are attached to the pericardium.
    c. They are identified in cases of infective endocarditis.
    d. They are composed of histiocytes and mesothelial cells.
    e. They are cardiac masses seen in the atrioventricular nodal region.

15. Fibromuscular dysplasia differs from atherosclerotic lesions in that it:
    a. Results in fibroid necrosis of the vessel wall
    b. Causes calcifications of small blood vessels
    c. Is a congenital condition that commonly occurs during the first decade of life
    d. Does not cause arteriosclerosis
    e. Does not cause luminal occlusion

16. Which of the following statements best describes thromboangiitis obliterans?
    a. It is commonly found in mesenteric vessels of elderly people.
    b. It can be identified on radiograph by calcification of arteries.
    c. It is a painless form of arteritis, in contrast to temporal arteritis.
    d. It shows predilection for the aortic arch.
    e. It is associated with smoking.

17. A 74-year-old man presented with recurrent headaches and tenderness on the side of his head. A temporal artery biopsy is performed (Fig. 9.4). Which of the following statements applies to this condition?
    a. The absence of giant cells in this biopsy excludes the diagnosis of temporal arteritis.
    b. The biopsy shows organized thrombus.
    c. The histologic findings are consistent with polymyalgia rheumatica.
    d. This condition results as a complication of a bacterial infection.
    e. The diagnosis of polyarteritis nodosa with thrombosis can be made from this biopsy.

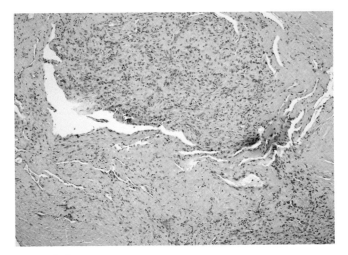

Figure 9.4

18. Aschoff bodies are defined as:
    a. Thickened endocardial ridges in the left atrium
    b. Collections of large histiocytes with vesicular nuclei

c. Interstitial or perivascular areas of fibrinoid necrosis surrounded by inflammatory infiltrate
    d. Valvular excrescences seen in cases of rheumatic endocarditis
    e. Nodular foci of valvular myxoid change

19. A 25-year-old woman presented with fever, arrhythmias, and deteriorating cardiac function. An endocardial biopsy was performed (Fig. 9.5). The most likely cause of this lesion is:
    a. Ischemic myofibrillar necrosis
    b. Human immunodeficiency virus
    c. Picornavirus infection
    d. Hypersensitivity reaction to antibiotics
    e. Kawasaki disease

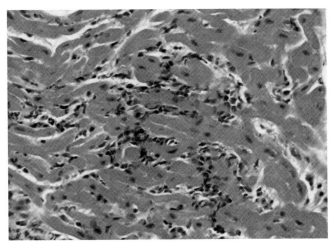

Figure 9.5

20. A suspected case of infective endocarditis repeatedly yielded negative bacterial blood culture tests. The most likely cause of this "culture negative" endocarditis is:
    a. HACEK group
    b. Clostridium
    c. Brucella
    d. Legionella
    e. All of the above

21. Cardiomyopathy can result from accumulation of all of the following substances EXCEPT:
    a. Hemosiderin
    b. Glycogen
    c. Amyloid material
    d. Carnitine
    e. Mucopolysaccharides

22. Radiation damage to the heart most commonly results in the development of:
    a. Mesothelioma of the pericardium
    b. Chronic constrictive pericarditis

    c. Ventricular rhabdomyoma
    d. Sarcoidosis
    e. Valvular calcifications

23. Which of the following cardiac tumors commonly undergoes spontaneous regression?
    a. Fibroma
    b. Rhabdomyoma
    c. Myxoma
    d. Rhabdomyosarcoma
    e. Teratoma

24. Which of the following substances helps prevent the development of atherosclerosis?
    a. Homocystine
    b. Fibrinogen
    c. Antioxidants
    d. C-reactive proteins
    e. Lipoprotein a

25. All of the following statements about arterial calcification in the elderly are true EXCEPT:
    a. It involves small- and medium-sized vessels.
    b. It most commonly involves the lower extremities.
    c. It can result in ischemic gangrene.
    d. It is associated with varicose veins.
    e. It is a complication of diabetes.

26. Pathologic features of Churg-Strauss disease (CSD) differ from Wegener granulomatosis (WG) in that:
    a. CSD shows a characteristic eosinophilic infiltrate.
    b. CSD does not affect renal vessels.
    c. CSD disease does not show the development of granulomas.
    d. CSD affects only small vessels.
    e. Pulmonary infiltrates are present in WG and not in CSD disease.

27. Pathologic changes in the heart and lungs related to pulmonary hypertension include all of the following conditions EXCEPT:
    a. Plexiform arteriopathy
    b. Increased right ventricular load
    c. Atheromatous narrowing of the right coronary artery
    d. Subendocardial ischemic myocardial necrosis
    e. Tricuspid valve insufficiency

28. This myocardial condition (Fig. 9.6) may be caused by all of the following agents EXCEPT:
    a. Antihypertensive medications
    b. Coxsackie B virus
    c. Chagas disease
    d. Hypereosinophilic syndrome
    e. Hypersensitivity to penicillin

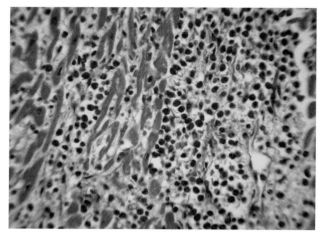

Figure 9.6

29. This picture (Fig. 9.7) represents a section of the left coronary artery. The diagnosis is:
    a. Microscopic polyarteritis
    b. Polyarteritis nodosa
    c. Churg-Strauss Disease (CSD)
    d. Leukocytoclastic vasculitis
    e. Henoch-Schönlein purpura (HSP)

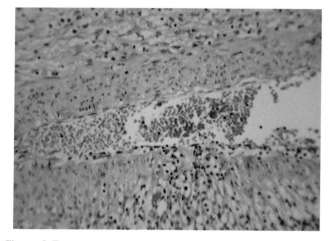

Figure 9.7

30. This section (Fig. 9.8) represents an area of infarction in the heart. The age of this infarct is most likely:
    a. 6 to 8 hours
    b. 24 hours
    c. 1 to 3 hours
    d. 3 days
    e. 10 days

31. Changes in the liver resulting from right-sided heart failure include:
    a. Nutmeg appearance
    b. Lobular fibrosis
    c. Fatty changes in periportal hepatocytes
    d. Centrilobular hepatocyte necrosis
    e. All of the above

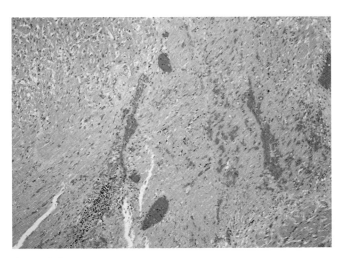

Figure 9.8

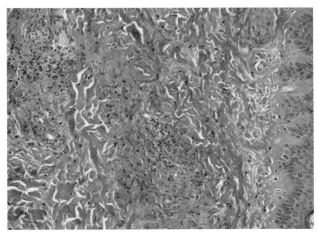

Figure 9.9

32. What is the most common cause of cystic medial degeneration of the aorta in patients older than 50 years?
   a. Marfan syndrome
   b. Hypertension
   c. Turner syndrome
   d. Idiopathic
   e. Syphilis

33. All of the following conditions can cause aneurysm of the ascending aorta EXCEPT:
   a. Mönckeberg medial calcification
   b. Syphilitic aortitis
   c. Takayasu disease
   d. Marfan syndrome
   e. Giant cell aortitis

34. Which of the following types of vasculitis is mediated by immune complex deposition?
   a. Wegener granulomatosis
   b. Churg-Strauss angiitis
   c. Microscopic polyangiitis
   d. Henoch-Schönlein purpura
   e. Polyarteritis nodosa

35. A 40-year-old man developed red-purple plaques that are subsequently biopsied (Fig. 9.9). The most likely diagnosis is:
   a. Leukocytoclastic vasculitis
   b. Churg-Strauss angiitis
   c. Microscopic polyangiitis
   d. Henoch-Schönlein purpura
   e. Polyarteritis nodosa

■ Answers

1. **b.** The heart develops from a single tube and is first recognizable at 15 days of gestation. Congenital heart diseases have an incidence of 6 per 1,000 live births. Chamber septal defects are the most common congenital heart anomaly.

2. **d.** Trisomy 21 is the most common cytogenetic abnormality and is specifically associated with complete atrioventricular canal defect and left ventricular outflow obstruction. Turner syndrome (45XO) is commonly associated with bicuspid aortic valve and coarctation of the aorta and DiGeorge syndrome (deletions in chromosomal region 22q11.2) is associated with persistent truncus arteriosus.

3. **a.** Mitral valve prolapse occurs in 1% to 3% of the population and is most commonly seen in Marfan syndrome. Other common valvular disease includes congenital aortic valve disease, which commonly presents at 50 to 70 years of age and manifests as stenosis in most cases.

4. **d.** Conotruncal malformations, commonly associated with velocardiofacial syndrome (deletions in 22q11), include persistent truncus arteriosus, absent ductus arteriosus, interrupted aortic arch, tetralogy of Fallot, and right-sided aortic arch. Coarctation of the aorta is less common. Patent ductus arteriosus, on the other hand, is commonly associated with trisomy 21 and congenital rubella infection.

5. **c.** This is the typical scenario of complete transposition: the aorta ascends parallel and to the right of the pulmonary artery. There is AV concordance because the right atrium communicates with the right ventricle from which the aorta arises and the left atrium is in continuity with the left ventricle from which the pulmonary artery arises.

6. **d.** The image shows "Quilty lesion," which is a dense endocardial collection of lymphocytes. This phenomenon is seen in heart-transplant patients receiving cyclosporine therapy and is not related to rejection.

7. **b.** Carcinoma of the lung is the most frequent metastatic tumor to heart, followed by lymphoma, breast carcinoma, and other tumors.

8. **a.** Congenital heart defects result from rubella infection in the first 3 months of gestation. The most common anatomic defects include patent ductus arteriosus, pulmonary artery stenosis, and systemic arterial hypoplasia.

9. **c.** Brown-Brenn stain is a modified Gram stain for bacteria. This stain is indicated in cases of infective endocarditis endocardial vegetations.

10. **a.** Cardiac myxoma is the most common primary tumor of the heart and constitutes 50% to 80% of primary heart tumors. It is most commonly located in the atrium and characteristically presents as a heart murmur that changes with time and position.

11. **a.** The most common artificial heart valves are bioprosthetic valves. The remaining choices are examples of mechanical valves.

12. **b.** Cardiomyopathy related to Adriamycin is characterized by myofibrillar loss and vacuolar degeneration of heart myocytes. Electron microscopy reveals distension and swelling of the endoplasmic reticulum. Inflammation is notably minimal to absent.

13. **d.** The image shows a focus of perivascular lymphocytic infiltrate consistent with acute rejection. The management of the patient depends on the rejection grade as determined by additional histologic findings. The degree and distribution of lymphocytic infiltrate, the presence of neutrophils, and myocyte necrosis are all factors pointing toward advanced grading of acute rejection.

14. **d.** Cardiac "MICE" are benign "mesothelial incidental cardiac excrescences" identified as endocardial collections of histiocytes and mesothelial cells and are mostly found incidentally at autopsy. These can be mistaken for carcinoma; otherwise they have no clinical significance.

15. **d.** Fibromuscular dysplasia is a nonarteriosclerotic lesion that affects large and medium vessels and occurs in the third and fourth decades of life. It results in disorganization of the vessel muscular wall, arterial narrowing, and aneurysm formation. On the other hand, atherosclerotic lesions are characterized by proliferated spindle and lipid cells in the intima with fragmentation of the internal elastic lamina and hyaline degeneration of the smooth muscle layer. Both lesions can result in arterial stenosis and ischemia.

16. **e.** It is a rare disease that affects men in 20 to 30 years of age and is associated with smoking. It affects the blood vessels of the extremities and can result in gangrene.

17. **b.** Temporal artery biopsy is indicated in suspected cases of temporal arteritis, which is characterized by destruction of the vessel wall with inflammatory infiltrate containing giant cells. The arteritis results in fragmentation and degeneration of the internal elastic lamina. The histologic changes are segmental. Although the presence of giant cells is a significant finding, a negative biopsy does not rule out the diagnosis. The image shows a medium-sized artery with partial occlusion by organized thrombus. The inflammation that is characteristic of temporal arteritis is absent. However, this diagnosis cannot be completely excluded.

18. **c.** Aschoff bodies are found in 80% to 90% of cases of fatal myocarditis. Central areas of fibrinoid necrosis are surrounded by mixed inflammatory or granulomatous infiltrate and are present in the perivascular or subendocardial interstitium of the interventricular septum. Other histologic finding in rheumatic fever include MacCallum patches, which are thickened subendocardial ridges in the left atrial endocardium immediately above and perpendicular to the posterior leaflet of the mitral valve; they represent evidence of

diffuse valvitis. Anitschkow cells are enlarged histiocytes with basophilic cytoplasm and vesicular nuclei with a dense central bar of chromatin. These cells are found in cases of acute rheumatic endocarditis.

19. **c.** The image shows an interstitial infiltrate of lymphocytes with myocyte necrosis, findings that are consistent with a diagnosis of myocarditis. Myocarditis is defined as the presence of inflammatory infiltrate associated with myocyte injury and necrosis in the absence of ischemic changes such as contraction band necrosis. Picornaviruses, especially coxsackie type B, are the most common causes of myocarditis.

20. **e.** Partly treated streptococci can also cause negative cultures.

21. **d.** Infiltration of the myocardium by various substances can lead to cardiomyopathy. This occurs in amyloidosis, hemosiderosis, hemochromatosis, and glycogenosis. On the other hand, systemic deficiency of muscle carnitine leads to cardiomyopathy.

22. **b.** Chronic pericarditis and pericardial constriction are the most common manifestations of radiation damage to the heart. Histology in these cases will show dense fibrosis with calcification and scant inflammatory infiltrate.

23. **b.** Rhabdomyomas are usually multiple, located in the ventricles, and can present from infancy through childhood. They are associated with tuberous sclerosis, and they may spontaneously regress.

24. **c.** Accumulation of homocystine, lipoprotein a, and C-reactive proteins predispose to atherosclerosis. Food rich in antioxidants helps prevent atherosclerosis. Antioxidants help remove oxygen radicals which play a role in the development of atherosclerosis.

25. **d.** Arteriosclerotic changes in the elderly lead to calcifications and thrombosis that may occur in the distal aorta, aortic bifurcation, and distal arteries leading to intermittent claudication and ischemia of the extremities. Varicose veins affect the superficial veins of the legs and are not commonly associated with calcifications.

26. **a.** CSD is a form of allergic granulomatosis with vasculitis and is typically associated with eosinophilia and history of asthma. Histologically, CSD is characterized by eosinophilic infiltrate, which is not usually seen in Wegner granulomatosis. Both diseases involve the medium and small vessels. Renal disease, granulomas, and pulmonary infiltrate can occur in both diseases with varying severity.

27. **c.** Pulmonary hypertension affects the right side of the heart with resultant increase in right ventricular preload and afterload. Right ventricular ischemia subsequently results from decreased coronary perfusion and not by atheromatous narrowing of the supplying coronary artery.

28. **b.** Eosinophilic myocarditis is usually caused by hypersensitivity reactions to drugs and parasites. Viral myocarditis is usually lymphocytic myocarditis.

29. **b.** Kawasaki disease is a form of polyarteritis nodosa-like vasculitis involving the coronary vessels and manifests with fever and complete heart block. Microscopic arteritis and HSP affects small blood vessels.

30. **d.** The image shows coagulative necrosis and the presence of infiltrating lymphocytes. Neutrophils usually infiltrate the necrotic muscle at 2 to 3 days, followed by lymphocytes and then macrophages, which become most noticeable at 5 to 10 days. Fibroblasts invade the area of infarction at 10 to 14 days.

31. **e.** Chronic venous outflow obstruction as in heart failure results in centrolobular pallor, necrosis, and eventually fibrosis with central-central bridging fibrosis. In advanced cases, it can result in cirrhosis "cardiac sclerosis."

32. **b.** Cystic medial degeneration of the aorta can occur in both hypertension and Marfan syndrome. The histology includes cystic medial change with loss of elastic tissue and accumulation of ground substance. Marfan syndrome is the most common cause in patients younger than 30 years. Both conditions can result in aortic dissection.

33. **a.** Aneurysm of the ascending aorta can be caused by aortitis, Takayasu disease, and Marfan syndrome. Mönckeberg medial calcification is a common finding in elderly people and usually involves small- and medium-sized arteries such as in the lower legs, breast, thyroid, and temporal arteries.

34. **d.** Henoch-Schönlein purpura is a systemic vasculitis syndrome affecting small vessels and is seen in the skin, kidneys, and other organs. The vasculitis is caused by deposition of immune complexes containing IgA. The remaining choices are not mediated by immune complex deposition.

35. **a.** Leukocytoclastic vasculitis is an inflammatory process with destruction of small dermal blood vessels. The inflammatory infiltrate is composed of neutrophils and karyorrhectic debris is usually prominent. Eosinophils may also be seen, especially in drug-induced cases. The etiology is unknown in most cases but can be secondary to drug eruption, collagen vascular diseases, Henoch-Schönlein purpura, and neoplasia.

■ Recommended Readings

Rosai J. *Rosai and Ackerman's surgical pathology*, 9th ed. Philadelphia: Mosby, 2004.

Stocker JT, Dehner LP. *Pediatric pathology*, 2nd ed. Philadelphia: Lippincott Williams & Wilkins, 2002.

Urinary System

Bungo Furusato and Isabell A. Sesterhenn

Questions

1. Hereditary papillary renal cell carcinoma is a syndrome characterized by predisposition to develop multiple, bilateral papillary renal tumors. Linkage analysis mapped the gene to chromosome:
   a. 7q31
   b. 3p25
   c. 10q11
   d. 11q13
   e. None of the above

Questions 2–4 pertain to the following patient:

A 5.5-cm cortical mass in the right kidney was incidentally found in a 61-year-old African American man. He had a history of heavy smoking. Macroscopically, the tumor was organ confined and had a multinodular predominantly yellow cut surface (Fig. 10.1).

2. Which histologic type would you expect from this picture?

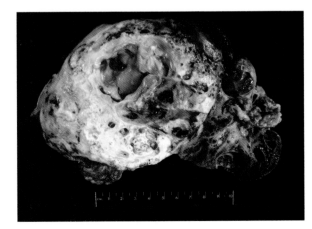

Figure 10.1

a. Conventional (clear cell) renal cell carcinoma
b. Chromophobe carcinoma
c. Papillary carcinoma
d. Renal medullary carcinoma
e. Renal cortical adenoma

3. The patient was found to have sickle cell anemia. Based on the pathologic findings, the prognosis (overall 5-year survival) for this type of tumor is:
   a. Fairly good (approximately 60%)
   b. Extremely good (approximately 95%)
   c. Good (approximately 80%)
   d. Virtually 100% survival
   e. Virtually 0% survival

4. This type of tumor possibly can contain granular/eosinophilic cells. This feature can also be found in:
   a. Chromophobe carcinoma
   b. Papillary carcinoma
   c. Oncocytoma
   d. All of the above
   e. None of the above

5. Simple cysts are the most common cystic lesion of the kidneys. Their incidence rate increases with:
   a. Age
   b. Cholesterol level
   c. Blood pressure
   d. Hormone level
   e. None of the above

6. Several classifications of renal cystic diseases have been proposed based on microscopic findings, clinical presentation, or radiologic appearance.

The primary distinctions are genetic and nongenetic. Which of the following is NOT a genetic cystic disease?
a. Adult polycystic kidney disease
b. Infantile polycystic kidney disease
c. Juvenile nephronophthisis
d. Medullary sponge kidney
e. None of the above

7. What is the correct association between polycystic kidney disease and liver pathology?
a. Autosomal dominant polycystic kidney – hepatic cysts
b. Autosomal recessive polycystic kidney – hepatic cysts
c. Autosomal dominant polycystic kidney – congenital hepatic fibrosis
d. Medullary sponge kidney – congenital hepatic fibrosis
e. None of the above

8. Which are the most common sites of metastases from renal cell carcinoma?
a. Lung, bone, and liver
b. Bladder, colon, and prostate
c. Esophagus, stomach, and duodenum
d. Anal canal, liver, and esophagus
e. None of the above

9. A 33-year-old man with intermittent gross hematuria shows bloody efflux from the right ureteral orifice. The patient has Klippel-Trenaunay syndrome. What type of renal tumor is most likely?
a. Multilocular cystic renal cell carcinoma
b. Angiomyolipoma
c. Hemangioma
d. Cystic nephroma
e. None of the above

10. What syndrome is commonly associated with angiomyolipomas?
a. Klippel-Trenaunay syndrome
b. Sturge-Weber syndrome
c. Klinefelter syndrome
d. Stauffer syndrome
e. Tuberous sclerosis

11. Which cytoplasmic organelle is characteristically increased in oncocytomas on electron microscopy?
a. Centrioles
b. Lysosomes
c. Rough endoplasmic reticulum (RER)
d. Golgi apparatus
e. Mitochondria

12. Does renal cell carcinoma ever occur concurrently with renal oncocytomas? The best answer is:

a. No. It never happens.
b. Yes. It occurs concurrently with 60% of oncocytomas.
c. No. It occurs concurrently with soft tissue tumor.
d. Yes. It occurs concurrently in approximately 10% of oncocytomas.
e. Unknown

13. Nephroblastoma accounts for up to 80% of urologic cancers in patients under age 15. In North America, what is the incidence of nephroblastoma in children less than age 15?
a. 1 per 1,000,000
b. 7 per 1,000,000
c. 21 per 1,000,000
d. 49 per 1,000,000
e. 98 per 1,000,000

14. Most children with WAGR syndrome (Wilms tumor, aniridia, genitourinary malformation, and mental retardation) have a chromosomal deletion on what chromosome?
a. 11p
b. 3p
c. 7q
d. 8p
e. 17q

15. Nephroblastoma is very uncommon in the newborn but has been described in approximately 1% of patients with a positive family history. This is thought to be inherited in an autosomal dominant manner. What is the approximate incidence of bilateral sporadic nephroblastomas?
a. 5%
b. 25%
c. 50%
d. 75%
e. 100%

16. A 58-year-old mother of four had repeated attacks of renal colic and showed an enlarged kidney. The kidney appeared as a dense, fibrotic, distorted mass with four or five calculi in the pelvis, 2 to 4 cm each. The parenchyma exhibited ovoid, soft, bright yellow areas of necrosis. There appeared to be extensive cortical fibrosis. What is the most likely diagnosis shown in Figures 10.2A and 10.2B?
a. Xanthogranulomatous pyelonephritis
b. Tuberculosis of the kidney
c. renal cell carcinoma - clear cell type
d. Intrarenal adrenal cortex
e. None of the above

17. A 2-year-old complained of abdominal pain. The mother felt a tumor in the upper abdomen. Imaging studies revealed a large mass in the left

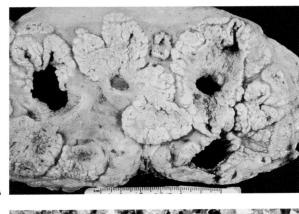

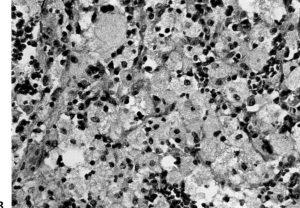

Figure 10.2

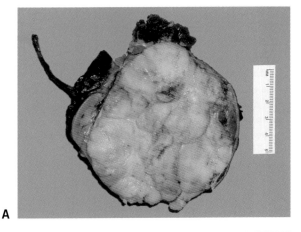

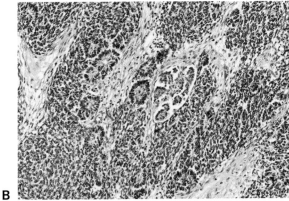

Figure 10.3

kidney. The kidney measured 10 × 8 × 7 cm and contained a partially encapsulated gray to tan tumor with focal areas of hemorrhage. What is the most likely diagnosis as shown in Figures 10.3A and 10.3B?

a. Nephroblastoma (Wilms tumor)
b. Dysgenesis of kidney
c. Multilocular cystic nephroma
d. Mesoblastic nephroma
e. Neuroblastoma

18. A 56-year-old man presented with hematuria and costovertebral pain. Imaging studies indicated a tumor in the upper pole of the right kidney. In the upper pole of the nephrectomy specimen was a soft, spherical tumor with yellow, hemorrhagic, and gray areas. It was 8 cm in diameter, encapsulated, focally calcified, and apparently confined within the kidney. What is the most likely diagnosis as shown in Figures 10.4A and 10.4B?

a. Malakoplakia of kidney
b. Xanthogranulomatous pyelonephritis
c. Renal abscess
d. Oncocytoma
e. Renal cell carcinoma - clear cell type

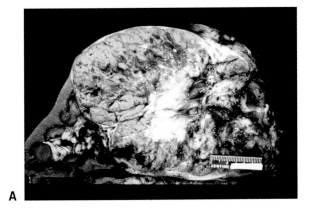

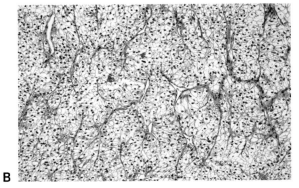

Figure 10.4

19. A 45-year-old man was discovered to have a large asymptomatic renal tumor during a routine examination. At surgery, a circumscribed, soft, tan, hemorrhagic tumor was identified measuring 2.3 cm × 1.7 cm that bulged but did not appear to invade the capsule. The remaining renal parenchyma was grossly unremarkable. Representative cross-sections were submitted. Hale colloidal iron stain was negative. What is the most likely diagnosis as shown in Figures 10.5A and 10.5B?
   a. Renal cell carcinoma – chromophobe cell type
   b. Xanthogranulomatous pyelonephritis
   c. Renal oncocytoma
   d. Malakoplakia of kidney
   e. Carcinoid

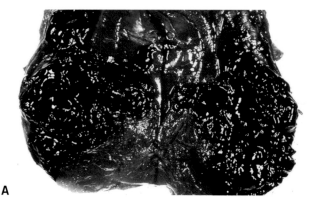

A

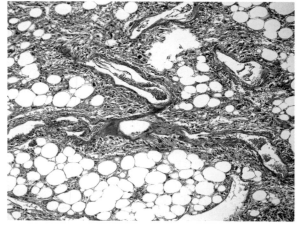

B

Figure 10.6

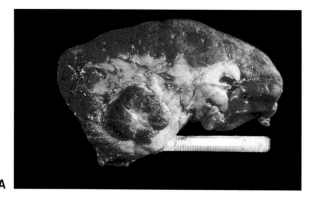

A

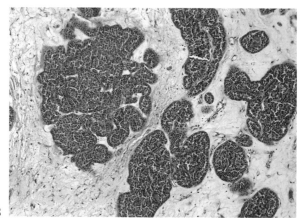

B

Figure 10.5

20. A 35-year-old woman was admitted in shock. Tenderness and a mass in the upper abdomen were found. Nephrectomy was performed. The most likely diagnosis as shown in Figures 10.6A and 10.6B is:
   a. Renal cell carcinoma, pleomorphic
   b. Leiomyosarcoma
   c. Angiomyolipoma
   d. Wilms tumor (nephroblastoma)
   e. Carcinosarcoma

21. What is the most common risk factor contributing to the development of urothelial carcinoma?
   a. HPV infection
   b. Cyclophosphamide treatment
   c. Cigarette smoking
   d. *Schistosoma hematobium*
   e. None of the above

22. Radical cystectomy is the recommended treatment for bladder adenocarcinoma. What is its approximate incidence in relation to all bladder cancers?
   a. 50%
   b. 25%
   c. 10%
   d. 75%
   e. <2%

23. Fluorescence in situ hybridization (FISH) is primarily used for assessing the response to intravesical therapy such as BCG in patients with superficial bladder cancer. Which chromosome is NOT included in this FISH method?
   a. Chromosome 3
   b. Chromosome 7
   c. Chromosome 9
   d. Chromosome 10
   e. Chromosome 17

24. Urothelial carcinoma in situ (CIS) frequently has alterations of what molecular markers?
   a. P53
   b. VHL
   c. P63
   d. TMPRSS2-ERG gene fusion
   e. None of the above

25. A 39-year-old woman with history of labile hypertension was found to have a large mass arising from the posterior bladder wall on cystoscopic examination (Figs. 10.7A, 10.7B). Which diagnosis would you expect?
   a. Paraganglioma
   b. Nested variant of urothelial carcinoma
   c. Granular cell tumor
   d. Metastatic carcinoma
   e. Malignant melanoma

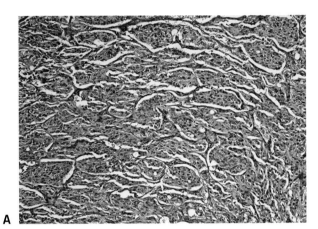

A

B

Figure 10.7

26. This 61-year-old man, over a period of several months, developed urinary frequency, hesitancy, and minimal hematuria. This progressed to macroscopic hematuria. The most likely diagnosis as shown in Figure 10.8 is:
   a. Bullous cystitis
   b. Chronic cystitis

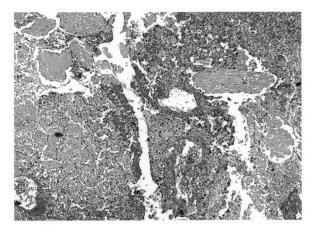

Figure 10.8

   c. Localized amyloidosis
   d. Malakoplakia
   e. Necrotizing cystitis

27. A 45-year-old man presented with a large tumor filling the bladder. Total cystectomy was done. What is the most likely diagnosis shown in Figures 10.9A and 10.9B?
   a. Urothelial carcinoma
   b. Rhabdomyosarcoma

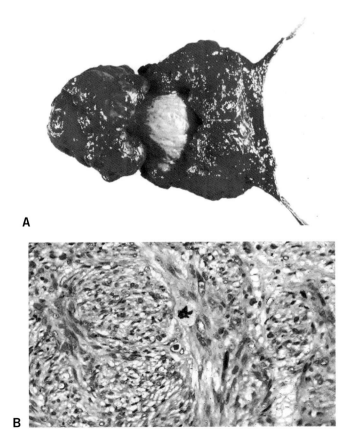

A

B

Figure 10.9

c. Carcinosarcoma

d. Leiomyosarcoma

e. Spindle cell carcinoma

28. Five years before the onset of recurrent dysuria, a patient had a rupture of the bladder, which was surgically repaired. What is the most likely diagnosis shown in Figures 10.10A and 10.10B?

a. Clear cell adenocarcinoma

b. Glandular metaplasia

c. Endometriosis

d. Prostatic carcinoma

e. Nephrogenic adenoma

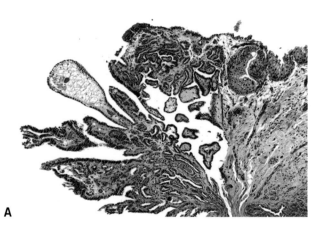

A

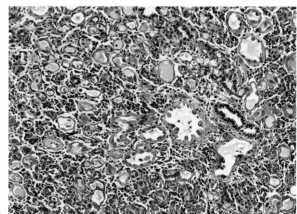

B

Figure 10.10

29. A 42-year-old woman presented with hematuria. A mass was palpable in the bladder and adjacent anterior abdominal wall. Cystoscopy revealed ulceration in the dome. A 1.5-cm tumor nodule in the wall of the dome partially protruded into the ulcerated mucosa. It was mucinous and cystic. A strip of tissue from the bladder to umbilicus was also excised and contained similar nodules of

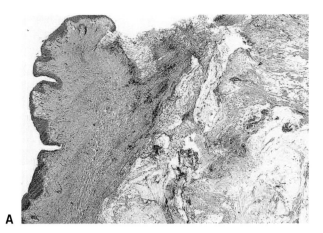

A

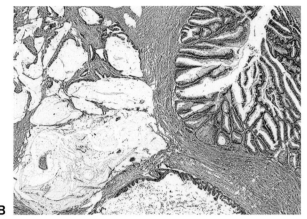

B

Figure 10.11

cystic and mucinous tumor. What is the most likely diagnosis shown in Figures 10.11A and 10.11B?

a. Urothelial carcinoma

b. Urachal rest

c. Urachal adenocarcinoma

d. Glandular cystitis

e. Urothelial carcinoma with glandular differentiation

30. A 45-year-old man had one episode of gross, painless hematuria. Cystoscopy revealed a papillary tumor in the dome and another on the left lateral wall. A 6.5 × 5.0 cm lesion was excised from the dome (Fig. 10.12). The most likely diagnosis is:

a. Papillary urothelial carcinoma - Grade II (High grade)

b. Papillary cystitis

c. Infiltrating urothelial carcinoma - Grade III (High grade)

d. Papilloma

e. Inverted papilloma

31. Hematuria and cloudy urine in a 63-year-old man led to cystoscopy, which showed an ulcerated lesion of the

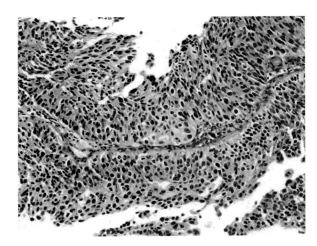

Figure 10.12

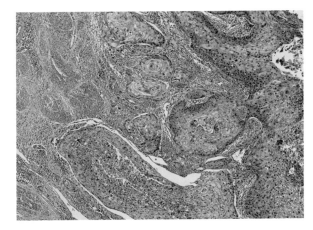

Figure 10.13

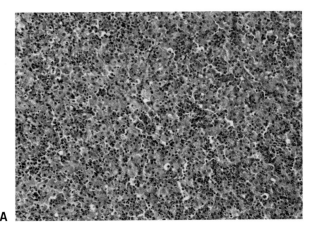

A

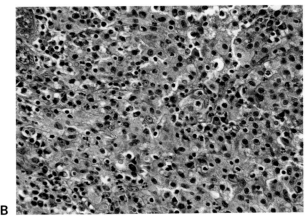

B

Figure 10.14

bladder. The anterior wall of the bladder was replaced by a neoplasm that measured about 10 × 5 cm (Fig. 10.13). The most likely diagnosis is:

a. Leukoplakia
b. Squamous cell carcinoma
c. Urothelial carcinoma
d. Schistosomiasis
e. Normal bladder

32. This 23-year-old woman had symptoms of cystitis and increasing difficulty voiding. Cystoscopy revealed a firm, elevated brown lesion at the bladder neck partially occluding the urethra. What is the most likely diagnosis as shown in Figures 10.14A and 10.14B?

a. Radiation cystitis
b. Infiltrating urothelial carcinoma
c. Malakoplakia
d. Acute cystitis
e. Signet ring carcinoma of bladder

33. A 4-year-old boy presented with painful urination, obstructive symptoms, and severe urgency and straining. What is the most likely diagnosis shown in Figure 10.15A–C?

a. Lymphoma of bladder
b. Rhabdomyosarcoma
c. Undifferentiated carcinoma of bladder
d. Paraganglioma
e. Pseudotumor of bladder neck

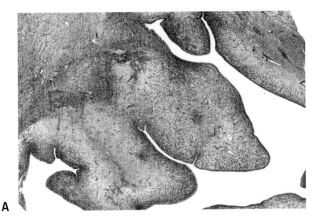

A

Figure 10.15 (continues)

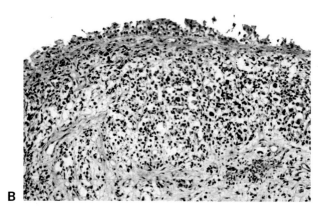

B

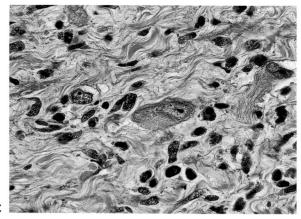

C

Figure 10.15 *(continued)*

34. A 45-year-old man had dysuria and hematuria. A hemorrhagic area in the left lateral wall of the bladder was found (Fig. 10.16). The most likely diagnosis is:
   a. Normal bladder
   b. Thiotepa effect on normal bladder
   c. Carcinoma in situ
   d. BCG effect
   e. Reactive hyperplasia

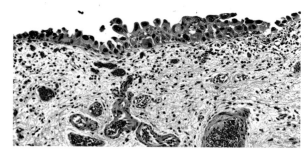

Figure 10.16

35. A 65-year-old woman presented with dysuria and hematuria. The prior history is unremarkable except for hysterectomy 25 years ago. This lesion was identified on cytoscopic examination (Fig. 10.17). The most likely diagnosis is:
   a. Squamous cell carcinoma
   b. BCG effect

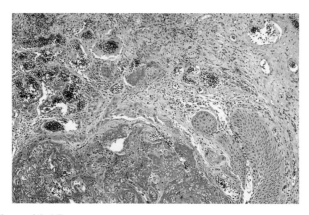

Figure 10.17

   c. Radiation cystitis
   d. Amyloidosis
   e. None of the above

36. Loss of WT1 gene function may occur in any of the following conditions EXCEPT:
   a. Juvenile granulosa cell tumor
   b. Desmoplastic small round blue cell tumor
   c. Nephrogenic rests
   d. Glomerulonephritis
   e. Cystic nephroma

37. The most frequent congenital renal neoplasm is:
   a. Mesoblastic nephroma
   b. Wilms tumor
   c. VHL–associated clear cell carcinoma
   d. Familial papillary renal call carcinoma
   e. Neuroblastoma

38. Histologic changes in the kidneys of patients with minimal change disease include:
   a. Segmental increase in mesangial matrix and cellularity
   b. Cortical and medullary interstitial fibrosis
   c. Proliferation of visceral epithelial cells
   d. Thickened capillary walls
   e. Infiltration by neutrophils

39. The risk of developing acute glomerulonephritis after streptococcal infection by a nephritogenic strain is:
   a. 100%
   b. 70%
   c. 15%
   d. 1%
   e. 50%

40. Glomerular diseases, which are most likely to recur in transplant kidneys, include all of the following EXCEPT:
   a. Membranoproliferative glomerulonephritis
   b. Diabetes mellitus

c. IgA nephropathy
d. Antiglomerular basement membrane disease (anti-GBM)
e. Fibrillary glomerulopathy

41. Characteristic pathologic features of lupus nephritis include which of the following?
   a. "Full house" immunofluorescent profile
   b. Wire loop lesions
   c. Tubuloreticular bodies
   d. Electron-dense deposits with fingerprint-like pattern
   e. All of the above

42. The term "sclerosis" refers to:
   a. Accumulation of eosinophilic PAS-positive, silver-negative structureless material that stains red with trichrome stain
   b. Accumulation of eosinophilic PAS-positive, silver-positive structureless material that stains blue-green with trichrome stain
   c. Accumulation of eosinophilic PAS-negative, silver-negative fibrillar material that stains blue-green with trichrome stain
   d. Accumulation of fibrillar material with characteristic configuration in x-ray diffraction analysis
   e. None of the above

43. Negative renal biopsy findings by light microscopy and immunofluorescence may be seen in:
   a. Minimal change disease
   b. Thin glomerular basement membrane disease
   c. Alport syndrome
   d. Lupus nephritis
   e. All of the above

44. The most common glomerulopathy worldwide is:
   a. IgA nephropathy
   b. Postinfectious glomerulonephritis
   c. Membranous glomerulonephritis
   d. Membranoproliferative glomerulonephritis
   e. Crescentic glomerulonephritis

45. Glomerulonephritis developing a few days after upper respiratory tract infection is most likely:
   a. Henoch-Schönlein purpura
   b. IgA nephropathy
   c. Minimal change disease
   d. Membranoproliferative glomerulonephritis
   e. Membranous glomerulonephritis

46. The most common lesion in diabetic nephropathy is:
   a. Nodular Kimmelstiel-Wilson lesion
   b. Diffuse glomerulosclerosis
   c. Fibrin caps
   d. Capsular drops
   e. Epithelial crescents

47. Interstitial nephritis is commonly associated with:
   a. The chronic use of nonsteroidal anti-inflammatory drugs
   b. Hemolytic uremic syndrome
   c. Renal artery stenosis
   d. Graft-versus-host disease in the kidney
   e. Diabetic nephropathy

48. Glomerular tip lesions are characteristically associated with:
   a. Diabetic glomerulopathy
   b. Focal segmental glomerulosclerosis
   c. Lupus nephritis
   d. Light chain disease
   e. Hemolytic uremic syndrome

49. A renal biopsy that is considered adequate for Banff classification should have a minimum of:
   a. 7 to 10 glomeruli and 1 artery
   b. 10 glomeruli and 2 arteries
   c. 5 to 7 glomeruli
   d. 5 glomeruli and 2 arteries
   e. 7 glomeruli, 10 tubules, and 2 arteries

50. A kidney transplant patient suspected of having transplant rejection had undergone a renal biopsy, which was subsequently stained with C4d (Fig. 10.18). Which of the following statements about this immunofluorescence result can be regarded as correct?
   a. The patient is considered to have mild cellular rejection.
   b. The staining is diffusely positive in tubular basement membranes.
   c. This result excludes the presence of rejection.
   d. C4d will give better results if performed with immunohistochemistry on paraffin-embedded tissue.
   e. This result indicates in situ activation of complement.

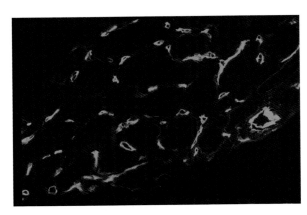

Figure 10.18

■ Answers

1. **a. Hereditary papillary renal cell carcinoma** is a cancer syndrome mapped to chromosome 7q31.1–q34, a region containing the MET oncogene, which is mutated in hereditary papillary renal cell carcinoma families. Although trisomy 7 is commonly associated with sporadic papillary renal cell carcinomas, only 13% of sporadic papillary tumors have MET mutations, suggesting that sporadic and hereditary disease may develop by different mechanisms. Cytogenetic features of most common renal neoplasm are as follows: WT1 gene on chromosome 11p13 in nephroblastoma, p57/kip2 gene on chromosome 11p15 in nephroblastoma associated with Beckwith-Wiedemann syndrome, VHL gene on chromosome 3p25 in clear cell renal cell carcinoma associated with von Hippel-Lindau syndrome, MET gene on chromosome 7q31 in papillary renal cell carcinoma associated with hereditary papillary renal cell carcinoma.

2. **a.** See comment in Answer 4.

3. **a.** See comment in Answer 4.

4. **d. Renal cell carcinoma** clear cell type (conventional type), is characterized by a multinodular/multicolored tumor mass with a predominantly yellow-colored cut surface. In general, the yellow color corresponds to the lipid-rich tumor cells. The growth pattern is usually solid but occasionally a cystic growth pattern composed of multiple cysts varying in size up to 2 to 3 cm in diameter occurs. On light microscopy, the clear cell areas are the result of extensive, intracytoplasmic accumulation of glycogen, phospholipids, and neutral lipids because of characteristic disturbances of increased glucose 6-phosphate levels, activated glycosis, and reduced gluconeogenesis. As the malignancy becomes more anaplastic (grade 1–3), the amount of cholesterol decreases. Conventional renal cell carcinoma are composed of a mixture of clear cells and granular cells. This granular cell pattern can be found in chromophobe renal cell carcinoma, oncocytoma, and papillary renal cell carcinoma.

5. **a.** The incidence rate of **simple renal cysts** increases with age. In general, they are asymptomatic. They can be solitary to multiple and are usually located in the cortex. The size varies but is usually <5 cm.

6. **d.** Genetic **renal cystic diseases** include adult (autosomal dominant) polycystic kidney disease, infantile (autosomal recessive) polycystic kidney disease, juvenile nephronophthisis (autosomal recessive), medullary cystic disease (autosomal dominant), and autosomal recessive and rare multicystic disorders (von Hippel Lindau, tuberous sclerosis, etc.). Nongenetic renal cystic diseases include multicystic dysplastic kidney, benign multilocular cyst, simple cyst, medullary sponge kidney, sporadic glomerulocystic kidney disease, acquired renal cystic disease, and calyceal diverticulum.

7. **a.** Autosomal dominant polycystic kidney disease is associated with hepatic cysts that become evident with increased age. Autosomal recessive polycystic kidney disease is associated with congenital hepatic fibrosis in all affected surviving individuals.

8. **a.** The common sites are lung, liver, bone, lymph nodes, adrenal, brain, opposite kidney, heart, spleen, and skin. Liver metastasis is associated with an ominous prognosis. Adrenal metastasis occurs in <19% in ipsilateral and 10% to 11% in contralateral adrenal. Adrenal metastasis is more common with large upper pole tumors in patients with metastatic disease. The most common sites and approximate frequency of **metastasis of renal cell carcinoma** are lung in 50% to 60%, lymph nodes, liver, and bone in 30% to 40% each, opposite kidney in 10% to 25%, and brain in 5%.

9. **c.** Ninety-five percent of **hemangiomas** present with intermittent gross hematuria. There is no gender or side predilection. Twelve percent are multifocal and a few bilateral. Sometimes the lesions are seen in the renal pelvis. The tumor diameter ranges from 1 to 2 cm. Treatment can be embolization, laser ablation, or partial nephrectomy. However, this depends on location and size.

10. **e.** This is an autosomal dominant inherited disease associated typically with multiple and bilateral **angiomyolipomas**, mental retardation, and adenoma sebaceum. Angiomyolipoma in these patients frequently develops in late childhood. Although this tumor occurs in 80% of patients with tuberous sclerosis, <40% of patients with angiomyolipoma have features of tuberous sclerosis.

11. **e.** The abundant mitochondria are responsible for the eosinophilic cytoplasm seen in the polygonal, uniform cells of **oncocytomas**. Mitotic figures are rare.

12. **d.** Approximately 10% of oncocytomas occur concurrently with renal cell carcinoma in either the ipsilateral or contralateral kidney. The renal cell carcinoma can be a separate tumor or can be embedded in the oncocytoma.

13. **b.** The estimated incidence approaches 7 per 1,000,000. **Wilms tumor** is the most common renal malignancy in childhood. Fifteen percent of nephroblastomas are associated with congenital anomalies. Nephroblastoma is approximately 2 to 8 times more common in patients with horseshoe or fused kidneys. Several other genitourinary abnormalities such as renal hypoplasia, ectopia, duplications, hypospadias, and cryptorchidism have been reported in association with Wilms tumor.

14. **a.** Most children with **WAGR syndrome** have a chromosomal deletion on chromosome 11p13, the chromosomal abnormalities most commonly reported associated with nephroblastoma. The gene at this locus has been cloned and designated the WT1 tumor suppressor gene. A second Wilms tumor locus,

WT2, has been identified on chromosome 11p15.5. Approximately 20% of patients with Wilms tumor have loss of heterozygosity (LOH) on chromosome 16q, and 11% of Wilms tumor patients have LOH on chromosome 1p.

15. **a.** The incidence of bilateral sporadic **nephroblastomas** is 5% (4% synchronous, 1% metachronous). Most of these are found in kidneys with the perilobar type of nephrogenic rests. Forty percent of cases with nephrogenic rests have unilateral Wilms tumors. Nephrogenic rests are found in 90% of patients with bilateral Wilms tumors.

16. **a. Xanthogranulomatous pyelonephritis** is commonly seen in patients with staghorn calculi. Characteristic band of golden yellow tissue outlines the dilated calyces and renal pelvis. The mucosa is ulcerated. Histologically, the lesion shows a zonal change involving all areas of the kidney. There is hyalinization or fibrosis of the cortex with only a few glomeruli remaining. A middle zone shows inflammation, many foam cells (vacuolated macrophages), proliferating small vessels, and a deep zone contains necrotic debris, blood, and fibrin in the area of destroyed medulla and calyces.

17. **a. Nephroblastoma**, a favorable histology. Grossly, the tumor has an encephaloid appearance. The typical nephroblastoma consists of three elements, all seen on this slide: epithelial, stromal, and blastemal. The darkly staining, intensely cellular areas are the undifferentiated nephrogenic component. In places, these appear to differentiate into tubules, occasionally glomeruloid structures—all lined by neoplastic cells. The above structures are contained in a poorly differentiated spindled mesenchymal stroma. This has a myxoid or fibroblastic appearance. Occasionally, this stromal component may show differentiation to skeletal muscle or cartilage. The presence of nuclear anaplasia is defined as hyperchromasia, nuclear enlargement to three times that of the nonanaplastic cells and multipolar aneuploid mitoses. Recognition of diffuse unfavorable histology is important because it is associated with poor response to treatment.

18. **e.** This is renal cell carcinoma, clear cell type, grade 1. The macroscopic appearance is typical of a **clear cell renal cell carcinoma**. Histologically, the tumor cells are clear, show a definite organoid arrangement supported by a rich "sinusoidal" vascular network. Clear cell carcinomas can be solid, tubular, cystic or papillary. Nuclear anaplasia is generally more marked in tumor cells with granular/eosinophilic cytoplasm. In contrast, the foamy histiocytes of xanthogranulomatous pyelonephritis occur in sheets and there is almost invariably a considerable number of inflammatory cells.

19. **c. Renal oncocytomas** are usually large, 6 to 7 cm in diameter. Macroscopically, the tumor is well circumscribed, red brown, or mahogany colored with a central scar. Microscopically, the small cells are arranged in nests, tubules, and sometimes in microcysts or macrocysts associated with an acellular stroma. The cells are often discohesive. The cytoplasm is intensely eosinophilic because of the large number of mitochondria, and the nuclei are mainly round with conspicuous nucleoli. Commonly, clusters of bizarre nuclei can be seen. Irrespective of the size, the tumor is benign. The differential diagnosis includes chromophobe renal cell carcinoma.

20. **c.** The presence of blood clots should raise the suspicion of **angiomyolipoma**. The tumor consists of the typical triad of fat, smooth muscle, and thick-walled blood vessels. The most characteristic feature is the relationship of the smooth muscle component to the adventitia of the vessels. The smooth muscle cells may show considerable pleomorphism, but mitoses are quite rare. The fat cells vary markedly in size. Angiomyolipomas may be predominantly myogenous or lipomatous, which is reflected in the gross appearance. Not infrequently, because of variation in size and shape of the cells and hemorrhage and necrosis, these tumors are misdiagnosed as malignant. Only rare malignant angiomyolipomas have been reported. The rare epithelioid variant consists of cells with eosinophilic cytoplasm and prominent nucleoli. The cells are often clustered around blood vessels. This variant of angiomyolipoma may be malignant, particularly if it contains cells with marked nuclear anaplasia. Angiomyolipomas are positive for smooth muscle and melanoma markers to variable degree.

21. **c. Cigarette smoking** is probably the most important risk factor associated with urothelial carcinoma of the bladder and upper urinary tracts in industrialized countries. The risk increases two- to sixfold in a patient with a history of significant tobacco abuse when compared to the nonsmoking population. *Schistosoma hematobium* is an important risk factor for squamous cell carcinoma (less frequent in urothelial carcinoma) of the urinary bladder in regions where this infection is endemic. Cyclophosphamide causes hemorrhagic cystitis and increased risk for urinary bladder cancer following long-term administration.

22. **e.** The incidence of primary **adenocarcinoma of the bladder** is <2% of all bladder cancers. The urothelial carcinoma accounts for approximately 90% of all bladder cancers. Adenocarcinoma is a frequent complication of exstrophy and urachal remnants. There are several types of adenocarcinoma: not otherwise specified, mucinous, enteric, signet-ring cell, clear cell, and mixed pattern. Signet-ring carcinoma can present as diffuse thickening of the bladder wall mimicking linitis plastica. The coexistence of cystitis glandularis (enteric metaplasia, mucinous metaplasia) is in favor of primary adenocarcinoma. It is always necessary to exclude metastasis from another primary and direct extension from the GI tract.

23. **d.** FISH detects the aneuploidy of chromosomes 3, 7, and 17 loci as well as the loss of 9p21 locus.

24. a. **P53 and RB genes** are the most frequent molecular markers implicated in urothelial carcinoma.

25. a. The histologic features of **paraganglioma**, including the zellballen, are characteristic. The tumor cells are negative for cytokeratin AE1/3, CK7, and CK20. They are strongly immunoreactive for chromogranin and synaptophysin. Sustentacular cells are highlighted on immunostaining for S-100. The combination of labile hypertension, the presence of a bladder mass, and the histologic features are diagnostic features of paraganglioma. Most of these tumors are well circumscribed. Dissection of the muscularis propria should raise the question of malignancy.

26. c. Suprapubic cystostomy and urethrostomy revealed an irregular, thick, hard bladder wall and mucosa involving the trigone and proximal urethra. The impression was gained that this represented a tumor. There are numerous deposits of pink staining, homogeneous, acellular masses in the lamina propria typical of **amyloid**, and the special stains such as Congo red and immunohistochemistry were confirmatory.

27. d. **Leiomyosarcoma** of the bladder is indistinguishable from leiomyosarcoma in any location. These tumors are the most common malignant mesenchymal tumor of the bladder. They account for <1% of all bladder malignancies.

28. e. **Nephrogenic adenoma** consists of delicate papillations of the surface with associated tubules and microcysts in the adjacent stroma. These are lined by cuboidal epithelium, occasionally columnar or flat. The cytoplasm is usually pink, sometimes clear. At times, the cells present a hobnail appearance, and tubules often have prominent basement membranes. The tubules resemble renal tubules, hence the designation of these as nephrogenic adenoma. Inflammatory cells and vascular congestion are also present.

29. c. At one margin of the slide, the tumor approaches the bladder surface. The bladder epithelium is normal and there is chronic inflammation of the lamina propria. The muscularis propria contains large lakes of mucin and columnar cells consistent with **urachal** adenocarcinoma. On the right side of Figure 10.11B, a villous adenoma is seen. The section was taken from the junction of urachal tract and bladder dome.

30. a. This is **papillary urothelial carcinoma**, grade II (high grade). The thin fibrovascular core is lined by urothelium with focal loss of cell polarity. Some areas are similar to the cellular changes to grade I carcinoma. For the most part, however, the nuclei are hyperchromatic and variable in size and shape indicative of a high grade carcinoma. Therefore, it is diagnosed as grade II. The complete loss of cell polarity resulting in complete disorganization and the marked nuclear anaplasia of grade III carcinoma are not present.

31. b. This is **squamous cell carcinoma**. Squamous epithelium infiltrates the muscularis propria in irregularly outlined nests. There are nuclear anaplasia and easily identifiable keratinization.

32. c. This is **malakoplakia**. In the lamina propria, a dense aggregation of histiocytes is seen. These are identified by abundance of pink-granular cytoplasm and round vesicular nuclei. Many intracellular inclusions (Michaelis-Gutmann bodies) are present. The latter take several forms: small, blue spherules with a clear halo or similar bodies having a bull's eye appearance, that is, spherule with a central blue dot. There is also acute and chronic inflammation.

33. b. This is **embryonal rhabdomyosarcoma**, botryoid type. The polypoid masses are typical of the botryoid variant of embryonal rhabdomyosarcoma. Underneath the urothelial surface is a dense band of small clusters of round cells with scattered rhabdomyoblasts referred to as cambium layer. By immunohistochemistry, the tumors are positive for myogenin, Myo D1, Desmin, and Actin. The prognosis is favorable compared with the deeply invasive variants of embryonal rhabdomyosarcoma.

34. c. This is carcinoma in-situ (CIS). The epithelium shows marked cellular anaplasia: variation in the size, shape, and staining intensity of nuclei involving the entire epithelial thickness. There is loss of cellular cohesion with shedding of tumor cells. The term includes mucosal changes corresponding to grade II and grade III urothelial carcinoma. The abnormality does not have to involve the entire thickness of the mucosa but it can be pagetoid, involve cystitis cystica or von Brunn nests. The loss of cellular cohesion can be so severe that the mucosa is completely denuded or only individual tumor cells cling to the surface (clinging variant of CIS).

35. c. The histology is typical of **acute radiation cystitis**. The combination of fibrin deposits associated with hemorrhage and reactive epithelial proliferation into the lamina propria should raise the question of radiation injury, particularly when the cell nests have squamoid appearance and show nuclear pleomorphism. These features are often misinterpreted as squamous cell carcinoma. Acute radiation cystitis can develop decades following radiation treatment. On inquiry, it was revealed that this patient had hysterectomy for uterine carcinoma followed by radiation therapy.

36. e. Loss of **WT1 gene** function characteristically occurs in Wilms tumor, WAGR syndrome, and Denys-Drash syndrome, and desmoplastic small round cell tumor. It has also been described in nephrogenic rests and mesoblastic nephroma but not in cystic nephroma.

37. a. **Congenital mesoblastic nephroma** usually occurs in the first 3 months of age.

38. a. **Minimal change disease** is usually negative on histology. Few histologic changes are described and

are compatible with the diagnosis of minimal change disease. These include a slight increase in mesangial matrix and cellularity and focal interstitial fibrosis.

39. c.

40. d. Anti-GBM disease, lupus, and postinfectious glomerulonephritis are rare to recur in transplanted kidneys.

41. e. Hyaline thrombi are also seen.

42. b. Glomerular **sclerosis** stains with PAS, silver and trichrome stains. Option "a" refers to hyalinosis, and option "c" refers to fibrosis. Glomerular sclerosis is seen in focal segmental glomerulosclerosis, idiopathic focal sclerosis, congenital nephrotic syndrome, and diabetes mellitus.

43. e.

44. a. **IgA nephropathy** is the most common glomerular disease and is more common in Japan and Europe than in the North America.

45. b. **IgA nephropathy** usually develops few days after upper respiratory tract infection. In comparison, postinfectious glomerulonephritis usually evolves over several weeks, not days.

46. b. **Diffuse glomerulosclerosis** is the most common glomerular manifestation of diabetes mellitus, and is characterized by increase in mesangial matrix and basement membrane (GBM) thickening. The most common immunofluorescence pattern is diffuse linear IgG localized along GBM and tubular basement membrane.

47. a. Many commonly used therapeutic agents, particularly NSAIDs and β-lactam antibiotics, can cause interstitial nephritis.

48. b. These lesions appear at the hilum of the glomerulus at the opening of the proximal tubule, and appear as foam cells within dilated capillaries sometimes accompanied by hyalinosis.

49. b. Specimens containing 7 to 10 glomeruli and 1 artery are considered marginal, <7 glomeruli or no arteries are considered unsatisfactory.

50. e. **C4d** provides evidence of complement activation and supports the diagnosis of humeral rejection. C4d staining can be performed with immunofluorescence or immunohistochemistry. Staining is considered positive if there was widespread strong linear circumferential peritubular capillary staining. Immunohistochemical stains on paraffin-embedded tissue are associated with decreased sensitivity and increased intra- and interobserver variability compared with immunofluorescence.

11

Male Reproductive System

Bungo Furusato and Isabell A. Sesterhenn

■ Questions

1. A 35-year-old man detected a small nodule in his left scrotum (Fig. 11.1). Which is the correct diagnosis?
   a. Adenomatoid tumor
   b. Sertoli cell tumor
   c. Malignant mesothelioma
   d. Metastatic adenocarcinoma
   e. Yolk sac tumor

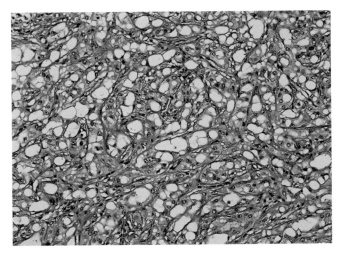

Figure 11.1

2. What is the normal upper limit for alpha-fetoprotein (AFP) in the adult?
   a. 2 μg/mL
   b. Up to 4.5 μg/mL
   c. Up to 9 μg/mL
   d. Less than 1 μg/mL
   e. Not detectable

3. In a patient with mixed germ cell tumor containing 40% or more of embryonal carcinoma, with vascular invasion and with clinical stage I disease, what is the frequency of microscopic metastases to the retroperitoneal lymph nodes at the time of orchiectomy?
   a. Never in clinical stage I
   b. Less than 2%
   c. Approximately 5%
   d. Approximately 13%
   e. Approximately 30%

4. What is the most common germ cell tumor in prepubertal boys?
   a. Seminoma
   b. Yolk sac tumor
   c. Teratoma
   d. Leydig cell tumor
   e. Embryonal carcinoma

5. Which serum level of AFP would you expect in a patient with this germ cell tumor (Fig. 11.2)?
   a. 30 μg/mL
   b. Up to 9 μg/mL

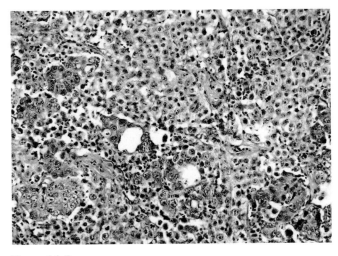

Figure 11.2

c. 520 μg/mL

d. 150 μg/mL

e. 3000 μg/mL

6. A 2-year-old boy has an orchiopexy for an inguinal testis. The pediatrician would like to know what is the risk of developing a germ cell tumor?
   a. Less than 15%
   b. Approximately 30%
   c. Approximately 40%
   d. Approximately 90%
   e. None of the above

7. A 28-year-old patient had a right orchiectomy for stage I nonseminomatous mixed germ cell tumor (NSGCT) confirmed by pathology. What is the chance of having or developing a germ cell tumor in the opposite testis?
   a. Approximately 20%
   b. Approximately 35%
   c. Approximately 4%
   d. Approximately 57%
   e. None of the above

8. What other disease can cause an increased serum level of human chorionic gonadotrophin (HCG)?
   a. Lung cancer
   b. Prostate cancer
   c. Colon cancer
   d. All of the above
   e. None of the above

9. What type of genetic disorder is associated with the large cell calcifying Sertoli cell tumor?
   a. Carney syndrome
   b. Gardner syndrome
   c. Angelman syndrome
   d. Beckwith-Wiedemann syndrome
   e. None of the above

10. A 65-year-old man presented with a testicular mass. Radical orchiectomy was performed. The histology was consistent with spermatocytic seminoma. Which of the following statements correctly describes this entity?
    a. It is regarded as the testicular tumor of older men.
    b. It is not reported in children, cryptorchid testis, or extratesticular sites.
    c. It contains three cell types: abundant intermediate-sized cells, small lymphocyte-like cells, and larger cells.
    d. It does NOT show elevation of AFP or HCG.
    e. All of the above.

11. A 30-year-old man presented with a cystic mass in the head of the right epididymis (Fig. 11.3). The most likely diagnosis is:
    a. Papillary cystadenoma
    b. Simple epididymal cyst
    c. Appendix epididymis
    d. Paradidymis
    e. Benign papillary mesothelioma

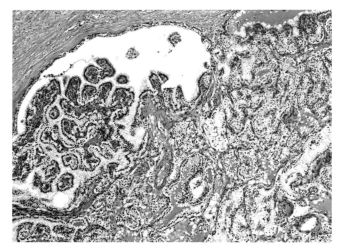

Figure 11.3

12. A 35-year-old man was found to have a left testicular mass. On gross examination, the lesion consisted of a small (around 10 mm) whitish encapsulated nodule located in the testicular parenchyma (Fig. 11.4). The diagnosis is:

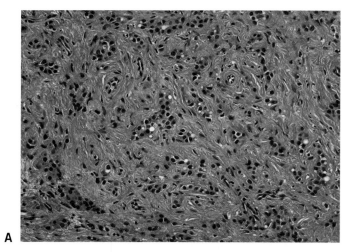

A

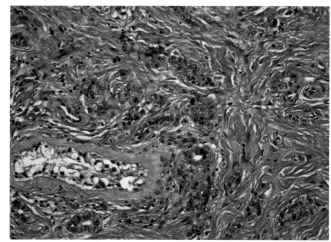

B

Figure 11.4

a. Adenomatoid tumor
b. Metastatic carcinoma of the prostate
c. Sclerosing Sertoli cell tumor
d. Metastatic carcinoma of the lung
e. Benign papillary mesothelioma

13. A 46-year-old man presented with a firm spermatic cord mass of several years' duration. It has increased in size over the past 2 to 3 years. The tumor was excised along with a hydrocele sac (Fig. 11.5). The most likely diagnosis is:
a. Malignant mesothelioma
b. Sclerosing liposarcoma
c. Nodular periorchitis
d. Vasitis nodosa
e. Benign papillary mesothelioma

a. Seminoma with syncytiotrophoblastic cells
b. Seminoma
c. Embryonal carcinoma
d. Choriocarcinoma
e. Spermatocytic seminoma

15. A mother detected an enlarged testis in her 2-year-old boy. The orchiectomy specimen revealed a circumscribed tumor with multiple small cysts replacing most of the testis (Fig. 11.7). Some of the cysts contained mucoid fluid. What is the diagnosis?
a. Yolk sac tumor
b. Embryonal carcinoma
c. Mixed germ cell tumor
d. Teratoma
e. Cystic dysgenesis

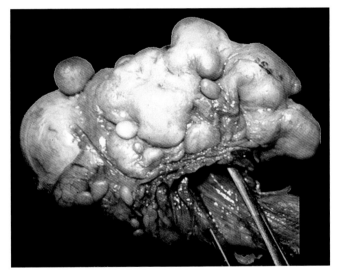

Figure 11.5

14. A 46-year-old man presented with a heavy feeling, pain, and swelling in the scrotum (Fig. 11.6). HCG was slightly elevated. AFP was negative. The diagnosis is:

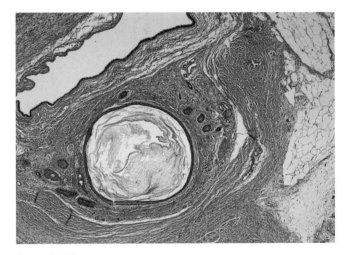

Figure 11.7

16. A 21-year-old man noticed a right testicular mass of 1 month's duration. In the lower pole of the testis was a mass measuring 5 cm in diameter. Grossly, it had a variegated appearance. The histology (Fig. 11.8A and 11.8B) is typical of:

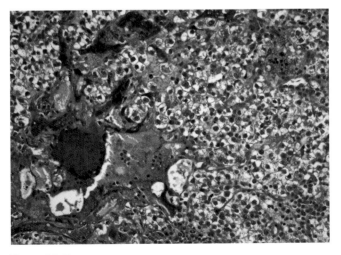

Figure 11.6

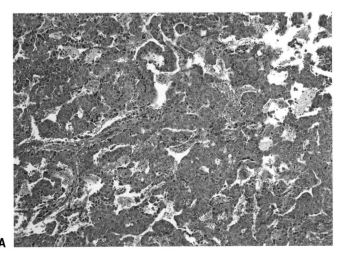

A

Figure 11.8 (continues)

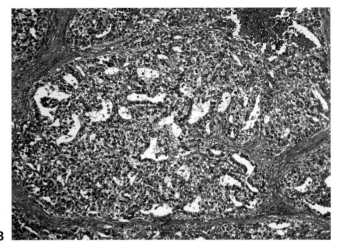

B

Figure 11.8 *(continued)*

a. Embryonal carcinoma and seminoma
b. Embryonal carcinoma and yolk sac tumor
c. Solid yolk sac tumor
d. Embryonal carcinoma
e. Malignant Sertoli cell tumor

17. A 24-year-old man with an infertility problem had a testicular biopsy (Fig. 11.9A and 11.9B). The histology indicates:

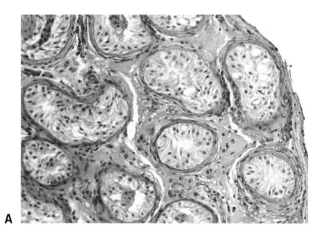

A

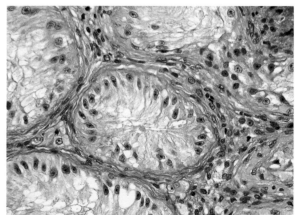

B

Figure 11.9

a. Sertoli-cell-only syndrome
b. Healed mumps orchitis
c. Klinefelter syndrome
d. Intratubular malignant germ cell neoplasia unclassified
e. Maturation arrest

18. A 68-year-old man complained of gradually enlarging testis of 6 months' duration. No tumor markers were performed. The prostate was also hard. The testis measured 6 × 5 × 4 cm and contained a homogeneous yellowish white tumor that had some nodularity, replaced the parenchyma, and extended into the epididymis (Fig. 11.10). What is the correct diagnosis?

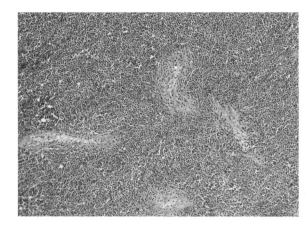

Figure 11.10

a. Seminoma
b. Lymphoma
c. Leydig cell tumor
d. Metastatic lung carcinoma
e. Spermatocytic seminoma

19. A 67-year-old man had swelling of the left scrotum for 3 weeks, which initially was thought to be a

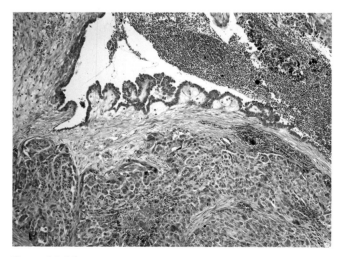

Figure 11.11

hydrocele. When herniorrhaphy was performed, the spermatic cord was found to be enlarged (7–8 cm in diameter). A tumor appeared to arise near the epididymis and extend up the cord. The tunica was studded with numerous granular, nodular lesions. The testicular parenchyma was grossly uninvolved (Fig. 11.11). The diagnosis is:
a. Malignant mesothelioma
b. Adenomatoid tumor
c. Metastatic carcinoma of the prostate
d. Yolk sac tumor
e. Reactive mesothelial proliferation

20. A mother noticed that her child had an enlarged right testis (Fig. 11.12A and 11.12B). What is the diagnosis?
a. Mature teratoma
b. Gonadoblastoma
c. Sertoli cell tumor
d. Yolk sac tumor
e. Adenomatoid tumor

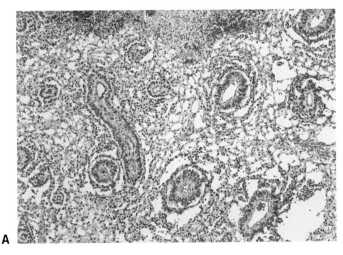

A

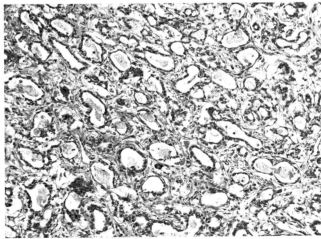

B

Figure 11.12

21. A 27-year-old man presented with a palpable groin mass (Fig. 11.13). He had no detectable testis in the scrotum. What is the diagnosis?
a. Mixed germ cell tumor
b. Seminoma
c. Undescended testis
d. Embryonal carcinoma
e. Intratubular germ cell neoplasia unclassified

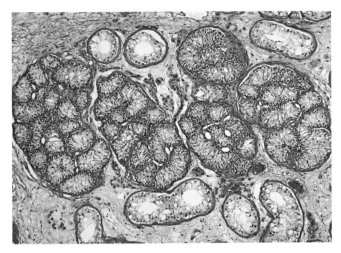

Figure 11.13

22. This 23-year-old man had a testicular biopsy (Fig. 11.14). Which condition does he have?
a. Leydig cell tumor
b. Seminoma
c. Cryptorchid
d. Leydig cell hyperplasia
e. Sertoli cell tumor

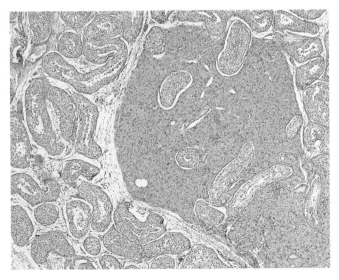

Figure 11.14

23. A 27-year-old man presented with an asymptomatic right scrotal mass discovered during a routine physical

examination. The cut surface of the testis revealed a well demarcated, whitish-gray round cyst. It was 1.7 cm in diameter with a laminated, soft, friable center (Fig. 11.15). The testis was otherwise normal. The diagnosis is:

a. Seminoma
b. Spermatocele
c. Leydig cell tumor
d. Epidermoid cyst
e. Dermoid cyst

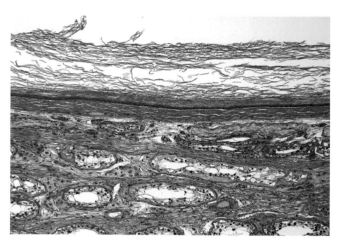

Figure 11.15

24. This 53-year-old white man had swelling of the left testis 2 years previously, which partially subsided. One month before orchiectomy, the swelling recurred and was associated with pain. The testis contained a light yellow, spherical lesion about 1.5 cm in diameter (Fig. 11.16). This was soft and somewhat friable. A similar, smaller lesion was located in the opposite pole. There was considerable fibrosis of the tunica and cord. What is the diagnosis?

a. Seminoma
b. Lymphoma

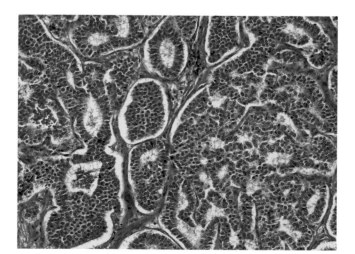

Figure 11.16

c. Leydig cell tumor
d. Carcinoid
e. Sertoli cell tumor

25. A 36-year-old man sustained an injury to his right testis 1 year ago, which was followed by enlargement of the testis. Two months before admission, he experienced hemoptysis and gynecomastia. A right orchiectomy was performed. The cut surface of the testis showed a large area of recent hemorrhage (Fig. 11.17). What is the diagnosis?

a. Seminoma
b. Lymphoma
c. Leydig cell tumor
d. Choriocarcinoma
e. Seminoma with syncytiotrophoblastic cells

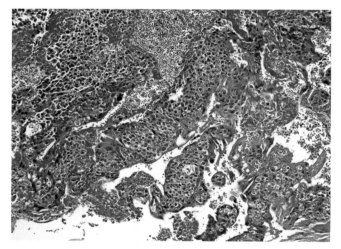

Figure 11.17

26. A 58-year-old man had bilateral orchiectomy as part of treatment for prostatic adenocarcinoma. One testis was slightly enlarged and had a firm, irregular mass replacing approximately one third of the parenchyma (Fig. 11.18A and 11.18B). What is the correct diagnosis?

a. Metastatic prostate carcinoma
b. Carcinoid
c. Leydig cell tumor
d. Lymphoma
e. Sertoli cell tumor

27. A 20-year-old African American man was found to have a testicular tumor. In the orchiectomy specimen, the testicular parenchyma was largely replaced by a yellowish brown tumor mass (Fig. 11.19). What is the diagnosis?

a. Malakoplakia
b. Carcinoid
c. Leydig cell tumor
d. Granulomatous orchitis
e. Leydig cell hyperplasia

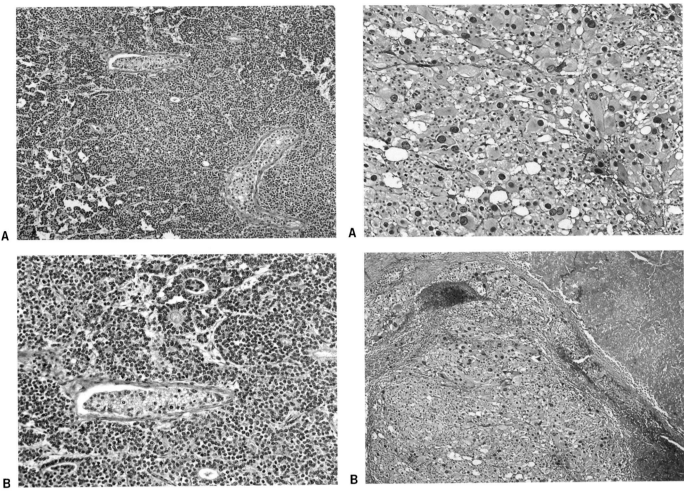

Figure 11.18

Figure 11.20

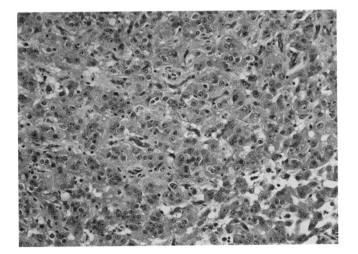

Figure 11.19

a. Malignant Leydig cell tumor
b. Carcinoid
c. Leydig cell tumor
d. Sertoli cell tumor
e. None of the above

28. A 71-year-old man presented with a mass in the right testis. He was otherwise asymptomatic. The testis contained a 3-cm tumor, which was yellowish tan in color and largely necrotic. It was entirely confined within the testis (Fig. 11.20). What is the diagnosis?

29. An 81-year-old man presented with symptoms suggestive of incarcerated hernia. The swelling had evolved over a period of 22 months. The testis was firm and variably yellow, gray to pink in color. Nodular masses of similar tumor tissue extended to the spermatic cord (Fig. 11.21). What is the diagnosis?
a. Malignant Leydig cell tumor
b. Malignant mesothelioma
c. Malignant gonadal stromal tumor with Sertoli cell differentiation
d. Choriocarcinoma
e. Sertoli cell tumor

30. Your patient is 12 years old and phenotypically female with external and internal genitalia of female configuration. Karyotyping revealed a mosaic of XO/XY. An ovoid structure 2.8 × 1.7 × 1.2 cm covered by a

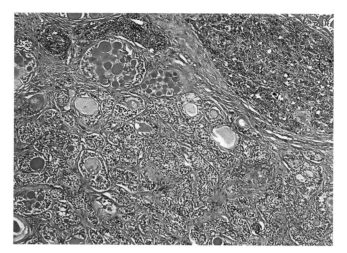

Figure 11.21

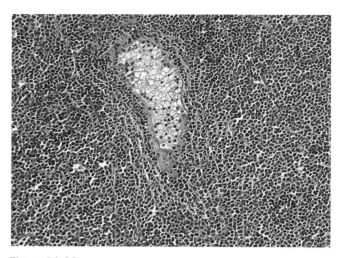

Figure 11.23

glistening membrane was found in the right adnexa and removed. The cut surface was translucent, tan-yellow, and had one small hemorrhagic focus (Fig. 11.22). What is the diagnosis?

a. Seminoma
b. Gonadoblastoma arising in a dysgenetic testis
c. Granulosa cell tumor
d. Ovotestis
e. Prepubertal testis

32. A 45-year-old man presented with an indurated area on the dorsum of his penis. Total penectomy was performed (Fig. 11.24). What is the most likely diagnosis?

a. Melanoma
b. Kaposi sarcoma
c. Bowen disease
d. Chronic inflammation
e. Paget disease

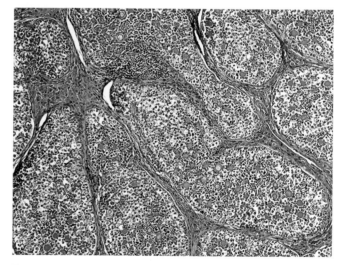

Figure 11.22

31. A 68-year-old patient was admitted for bilateral inguinal hernia and found to have a right testicular tumor. The testis was moderately enlarged and firm. The parenchyma was replaced by a yellowish white neoplasm (Fig. 11.23). What is the diagnosis?

a. Malignant Leydig cell tumor
b. Gonadal stromal tumor
c. Plasmacytoma
d. Sertoli cell tumor
e. Chronic orchitis

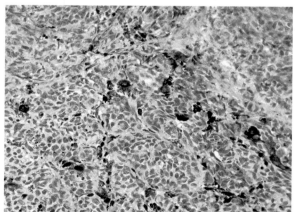

A

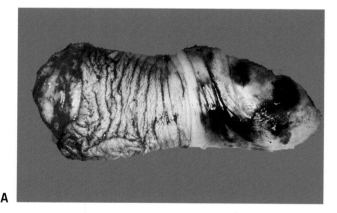

B

Figure 11.24

33. A 30-year-old man had a firm, flat lesion on the fore-skin that was said to be suspicious for carcinoma. The excised foreskin contained a light tan, firm, plaque-like lesion that was 0.5 cm in diameter (Fig. 11.25). What is the most likely diagnosis?
   a. Kaposi sarcoma
   b. Nonspecific acanthosis
   c. Paget disease
   d. Lichen sclerosis (Balanitis xerotica obliterans), prepuce
   e. Bowen disease

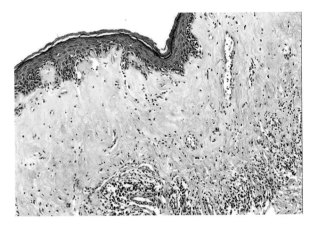

Figure 11.25

34. This 30-year-old man presented with warty lesions of the prepuce that has been present for 1 year. The foreskin contained several linear, papillary areas, each measuring about 2 cm in length (Fig. 11.26). What is the most likely diagnosis?
   a. Pseudoepitheliomatous hyperplasia
   b. Giant condyloma
   c. Bowen disease
   d. Condyloma acuminatum, prepuce
   e. Paget disease

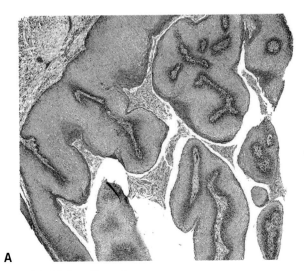

A

Figure 11.26 (continues)

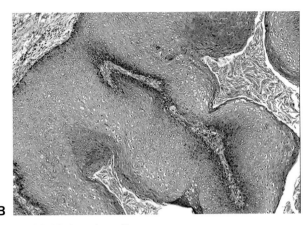

B

Figure 11.26 (continued)

35. This 80-year-old man developed bladder carcinoma and died 2 years later with generalized metastases. Several weeks prior to death, induration of the distal penis was noted. The penis became indurated throughout (Fig. 11.27). What is the most likely diagnosis?
   a. Angiosarcoma
   b. Squamous cell carcinoma, well differentiated
   c. Squamous cell carcinoma, poorly differentiated
   d. Metastatic carcinoma
   e. None of the above

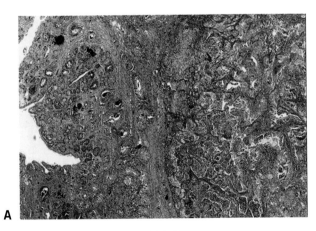

A

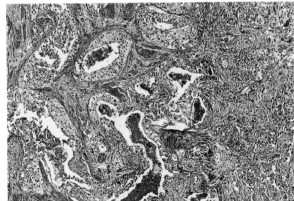

B

Figure 11.27

36. A 48-year-old man gave a history of a small lump on the penis for 8 or 9 years. A crusting, plaque-like lesion measuring 0.6 cm was located on the shaft. It was felt to resemble psoriasis (Fig. 11.28). What is the most likely diagnosis?
    a. Bowenoid papulosis
    b. Kaposi sarcoma
    c. Bowen disease, skin of penis
    d. Chronic inflammation
    e. None of the above

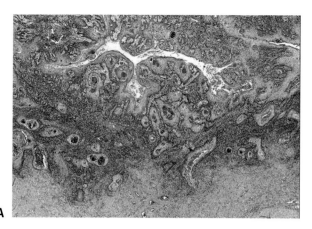

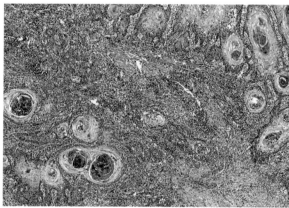

A

B

Figure 11.29

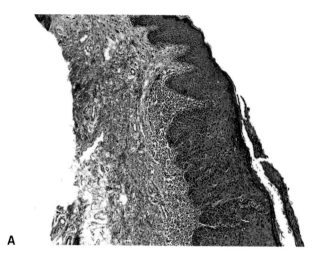

A

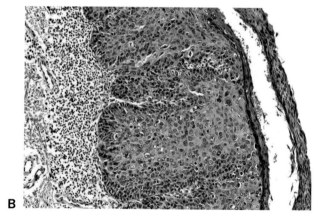

B

Figure 11.28

37. A 46-year-old man developed a lesion on the inner surface of the prepuce 3 weeks prior to circumcision. It remained unchanged after 10 days of antibiotic treatment. An elevated, firm, red-brown lesion measuring 2.8 × 2.8 × 1.5 cm was described (Fig. 11.29). The urologist is asking for preliminary results for patient consultation. What is the most likely diagnosis?
    a. Bowenoid papulosis
    b. Kaposi sarcoma
    c. Bowen disease, skin of penis
    d. Squamous cell carcinoma
    e. Pseudoepitheliomatous hyperplasia

38. The prostate gland develops from dual embryonic derivation, urogenital sinus, and Wolffian duct. Which of the following is of Wolffian duct origin?
    a. Peripheral zone
    b. Transitional zone
    c. Seminal vesicle
    d. Anterior fibromuscular stroma
    e. None of the above

39. Which of the following statements does apply to the basal cells?
    a. Prostatic acini and ducts are lined by basal cells and secretory cells.
    b. Basal cells express high molecular weight cytokeratins, which may be detected by 34betaE12.
    c. In general, basal cells form a thin and continuous layer that separates the secretory epithelium from the basement membrane.
    d. Normal basal cells express PSA.
    e. All of the above are correct.

40. "Normal" PSA levels range from 0 to 4 ng/mL. Age-specific normal reference ranges and acceptable rates of change in the PSA value over time (PSA velocity) have

been delineated and may enhance the identification of individuals at risk for disease. PSA was approved by the FDA in 1986. What percentages of cancers are found in men with "normal" PSA levels?
a. Approximately 15% to 20%
b. Approximately 40%
c. Approximately 60%
d. Approximately 80%
e. All of the above are incorrect.

41. What type of events can adversely affect PSA results?
a. Digital rectal exam
b. Urinary retention
c. Insertion of Foley catheter
d. Recent prostate biopsy
e. All of the above are correct.

42. The half-life of serum PSA is about 2 to 3 days depending on the testing method used. Based on this data, one should wait at least 21 days following manipulation of the prostate to allow for sufficient time before drawing a serum PSA to obtain reliable results. The digital rectal exam (DRE) is another procedure in assessing patients who are at risk for prostate cancer. What is the accuracy of detecting prostate cancer by DRE alone?
a. Approximately 50%
b. Approximately 70%
c. Approximately 40%
d. Less than 40%
e. All of the above are incorrect.

43. What are the potential agents being studied and suggested to prevent prostate cancer?
a. 5-alpha-reductase inhibitors (Dutasteride)
b. Vitamin D
c. COX-2 inhibitor
d. Lycopene
e. All of the above are correct.

44. A 64-year-old man underwent radical retropubic prostatectomy. The pathology report revealed disease involving the entire left side of the gland with no capsular penetration. The lymph nodes were negative for cancer. What is his pathologic stage by American Joint Commission on Cancer (AJCC) staging systems?
a. pT3b, N0, Mx
b. pT3b, N0, M0
c. pT3b, N1, M0
d. pT2b, N0, Mx
e. None of the above.

45. A 65-year-old man presented with lower urinary tract symptoms that were 12/5 attributed to an enlarged prostate. Urologist performed transurethral resection

of the prostate (TURP). The specimen consisted of 21 grams of prostatic tissue. Pathologic findings were consistent with nodular hyperplasia except for several fragments with the histology in these images (Fig. 11.30). What immunohistochemical stain would be most helpful?
a. AMACR
b. CK7
c. S100
d. P53
e. CK20

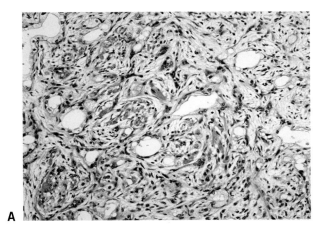

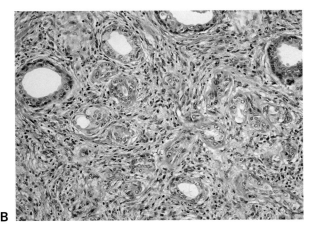

Figure 11.30

46. A 60-year-old man with a serum PSA level of 3.5 ng/mL had lower urinary tract symptoms. A TURP was performed. A total of 13 grams of chips were obtained, and all the tissue was submitted for review (Fig. 11.31). The diagnosis is:
a. High-grade prostatic intraepithelial neoplasia (HGPIN)
b. Ductal adenocarcinoma
c. Urothelial carcinoma involving the prostate
d. Prostatic urethral polyp

47. A 63-year-old man noted gradually increasing fre-
    quency and decreasing size of urinary stream. Rectal
    examination revealed a small area of induration on the
    left side (Fig. 11.32). The diagnosis is:
    a. Prostatic carcinoma – Gleason score 6 (3+3), well
       differentiated
    b. Prostatic carcinoma – Gleason score 7 (3+4), poorly
       differentiated
    c. Hyperplasia
    d. Atrophy of prostate
    e. Normal seminal vesicle

48. A 65-year-old man with symptoms of prostatism had a
    soft prostate on rectal examination. The histology of
    the transurethral resection specimen revealed which of
    the following (Fig. 11.33):
    a. Urothelial carcinoma of bladder invading the prostate
    b. Squamous metaplasia due to estrogen defect
    c. Prostatic carcinoma – Gleason score 8 (4+4), poorly
       differentiated
    d. Hyperplasia of prostate
    e. Irradiation effect on prostate

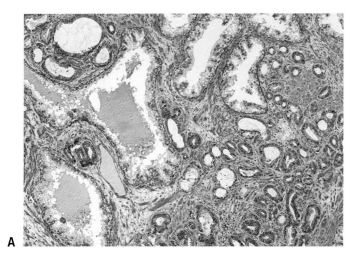

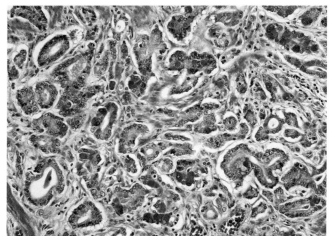

A

B

Figure 11.32

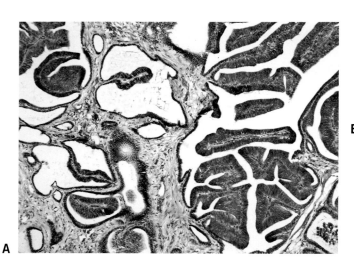

A

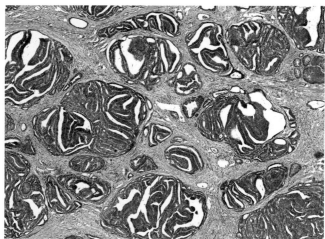

B

Figure 11.31

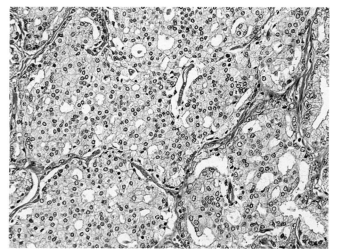

Figure 11.33

49. A 72-year-old man presented with symptoms of prostatism (Fig. 11.34). He has:
   a. Prostatic adenocarcinoma, well differentiated, Gleason score 6 (3+3)
   b. Rectal adenocarcinoma extending to the prostate
   c. Atrophy
   d. Papillary prostatic carcinoma
   e. Glandular hyperplasia of prostate

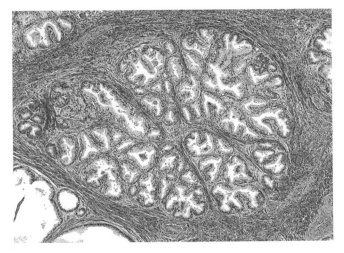

Figure 11.34

50. This 67-year-old man with a long-standing history of prostatism had a transurethral resection (TURP) (Fig. 11.35). The diagnosis is:
   a. Prostatic intraepithelial neoplasia (PIN)
   b. Atrophy
   c. Hyperplasia
   d. Urothelial carcinoma of prostatic ducts
   e. Basal cell hyperplasia

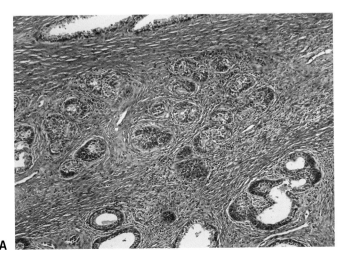

A

Figure 11.35 (continues)

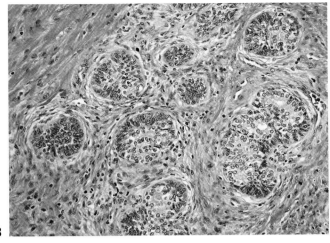

B

Figure 11.35 (continued)

51. This 66-year-old man with symptoms of prostatism had a hard indurated prostate. An indwelling catheter was used for a few days. The diagnosis from this image (Fig. 11.36) is:
   a. Carcinoma
   b. Acute prostatitis
   c. Urothelial carcinoma
   d. Granulomatous prostatitis
   e. Infarct of prostate

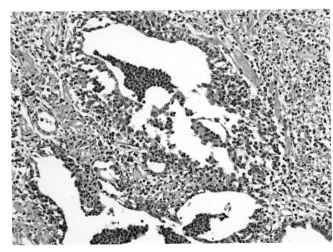

Figure 11.36

52. This 68-year-old man had carcinoma of the prostate which was treated with estrogen. Several months later, another biopsy was obtained (Fig. 11.37). Immunohistochemically, PSA and PAP were positive in these lesions. What is the diagnosis?
   a. Prostatic carcinoma showing estrogen effect
   b. Acute prostatitis
   c. Prostatic carcinoma, poorly differentiated, Gleason score 10 (5+5)
   d. Granulomatous prostatitis
   e. Xanthoma

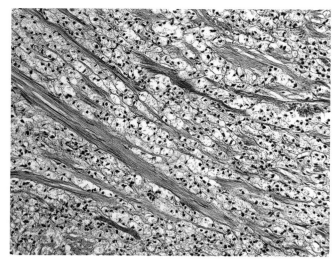

Figure 11.37

53. A 60-year-old man presented with symptoms of urinary obstruction and an enlarged prostate. The clinical impression was benign prostatic hypertrophy (BPH). Which immunohistochemical profile do you expect (Fig. 11.38)?

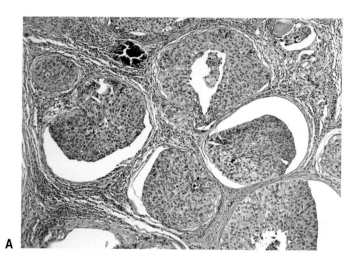

A

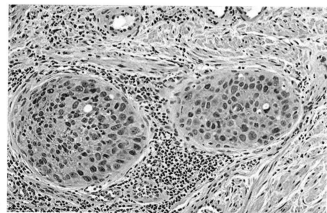

B

Figure 11.38

a. PAP +, PSA −, P63 −
b. PAP −, PSA +, P63 −
c. PAP +, PSA +, P63 −
d. PAP −, PSA −, P63 +

54. A 49-year-old man presented with symptoms of urinary obstruction and elevated PSA levels up to 5.3 ng/mL. A TRUS-guided needle biopsy was performed. The histology showed glands suspicious for prostatic adeno-carcinoma in the H&E section (Fig. 11.39). However, the lesion was negative for PSA and PAP. What is the diagnosis?

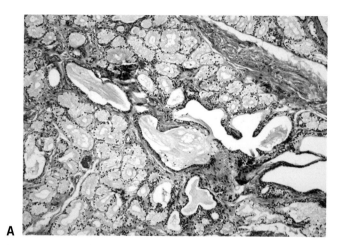

A

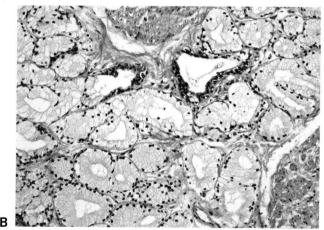

B

Figure 11.39

a. Prostatic carcinoma – Gleason score 6 (3+3), well differentiated
b. Cowper gland
c. Hyperplasia
d. Atrophy of prostate
e. Normal seminal vesicle

55. A 59-year-old man developed urinary retention as a result of what was believed to be prostatic hyperplasia.

The prostate weighed 65 grams and prostatectomy was performed (Fig. 11.40). The diagnosis is:

a. Prostatic carcinoma – Gleason score 10 (5 + 5), poorly differentiated
b. Malignant lymphoma
c. Granulomatous prostatitis
d. Urothelial carcinoma of the prostate
e. Acute prostatitis

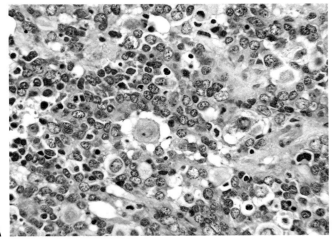

A

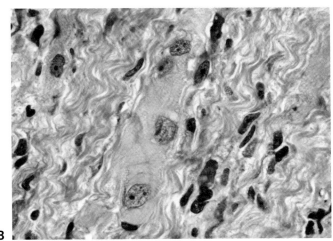

B

Figure 11.41

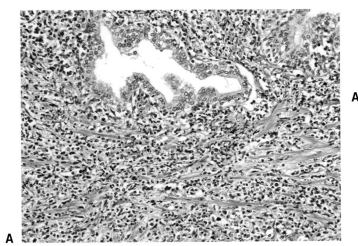

A

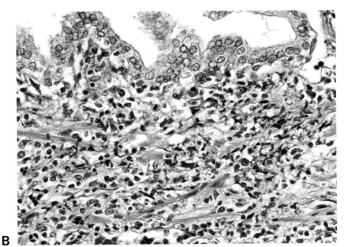

B

Figure 11.40

56. At the age of 17, this patient presented with irritative voiding symptoms and fullness of the bladder. On cystoscopy, polypoid masses protruding from the trigone were seen. The histology (Fig. 11.41) is diagnostic of:

a. Kaposi sarcoma
b. Leukemia
c. Leiomyosarcoma
d. Extrarenal rhabdoid tumor
e. Embryonal rhabdomyosarcoma of the prostate

57. A 48-year-old man came to the urologist because of a history of slight fever and chills. His fever was gradual in onset. He also complained of perineal and back pain,

which is worse toward the sacral area. Rectal examination showed a tender prostate. Otherwise, the patient seems healthy. The laboratory studies showed slightly elevated WBC count and PSA. The urologist is consulting you whether a prostate biopsy or prostatic massage sample can help diagnose this patient. What will you recommend to the urologist?

a. Send post prostatic massage sample for cultures
b. Ask for prostate biopsy to rule out prostate cancer
c. Recommend urethral catheterization
d. First send culture of midstream urine sample
e. None of the above

58. A 65-year-old man with BPH was treated with either Finasteride or an alpha-1 blocker, but this was not specified in the clinical history. After 6 months of treatment, his symptoms improved remarkably, and his prostate decreased in size. Which of the following histologic patterns was most likely present at the time of initiation of treatment?

a. Glandular hyperplasia
b. Stromal hyperplasia consisting predominantly of smooth muscle

c. Stromal hyperplasia consisting predominantly of fibroblasts
d. None of the above

59. This 63-year-old man had an elevated PSA and an indurated prostate on rectal examination. Biopsies were taken (Fig. 11.42). Immunohistochemically, PSA and PAP were positive. What is the diagnosis?
    a. Prostatic carcinoma, Gleason score 6 (3 +3)
    b. Acute prostatitis
    c. Atrophy
    d. Seminal vesicle
    e. Verumontanum gland hyperplasia

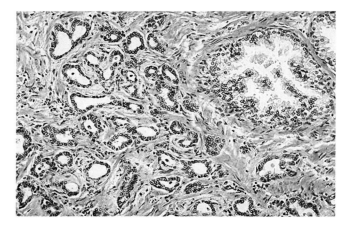

Figure 11.42

60. In which entity do you expect to see these structures (Fig. 11.43)?
    a. Benign prostatic acini
    b. Prostatic adenocarcinoma
    c. Variants of glandular hyperplasia
    d. Infarcts
    e. All of the above

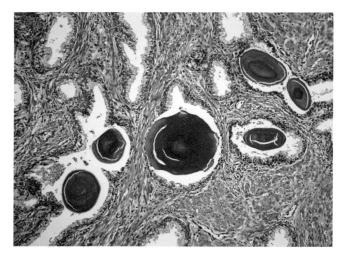

Figure 11.43

61. A 63-year-old man with an elevated serum PSA level underwent extended needle biopsies. One of these had this appearance (Fig. 11.44). What is the diagnosis?
    a. Prostatic adenocarcinoma, well differentiated, Gleason score 3 + 3
    b. Prostatic intraepithelial neoplasia
    c. Benign prostatic glands
    d. Seminal vesicle
    e. Verumontanum gland hyperplasia

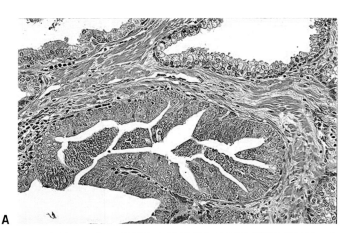

A

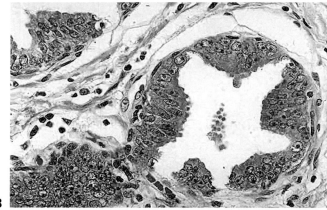

B

Figure 11.44

62. This 63-year-old man was treated with hormone therapy for prostatic carcinoma. Several months later, follow-up biopsies were obtained. Immunohistochemically, PSA and PAP were negative. The image (Fig. 11.45) depicts:
    a. Prostatic carcinoma showing hormone effect
    b. Atrophy
    c. Residual carcinoma with treatment effect
    d. Seminal vesicle
    e. Verumontanum gland hyperplasia

63. A 55-year-old man presented with hematuria. On cystoscopy (Fig. 11.46), no abnormalities of the bladder mucosa were seen. Because the serum PSA was mildly

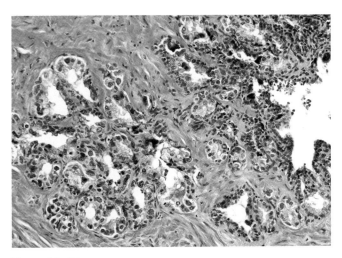

Figure 11.45

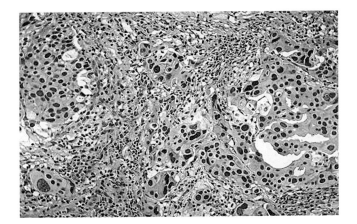

Figure 11.46

elevated, the patient underwent prostate needle biopsies. The diagnosis is:
a. Prostatic adenocarcinoma
b. Nephrogenic metaplasia
c. Urothelial carcinoma involving the prostatic ducts
d. Metastatic clear cell carcinoma
e. None of the above

64. A 63-year-old man with an elevated serum PSA level underwent extended needle biopsies. One of these had this appearance (Fig. 11.47). What is the diagnosis?
a. Prostatic adenocarcinoma, Gleason score 3 + 3
b. Postatrophic hyperplasia
c. Cribriform hyperplasia.
d. Seminal vesicle
e. Verumontanum gland hyperplasia

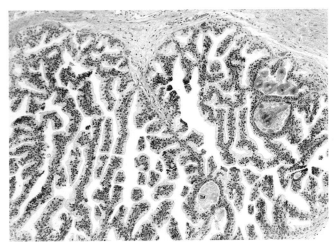

Figure 11.47

■ Answers

1. **a. Adenomatoid tumor** is a common paratesticular tumor involving the epididymis, tunica, and, rarely, the spermatic cord. These tumors can be found in association with the uterus, fallopian tubes, ovaries, and retroperitoneum adjacent to the adrenal. Histologically, the tumor consists of fibrous stroma with varying amounts of smooth muscle and inflammatory infiltrate. The epithelial cells are mesothelial in origin and form solid strands or cords. The cytoplasm contains vacuoles, which often coalesce resulting in cystic spaces with a "spider web" appearance.

2. **c.** The upper limit of serum AFP is up to 9 μg/mL. The half-life is 4 to 5 days.

3. **e.** In this setting, there is a 30% chance of having retroperitoneal metastasis. In a mixed germ cell tumor with more than 40% of embryonal carcinoma and vascular or lymphatic invasion, the likelihood of stage II disease increases.

4. **b.** Yolk sac tumors account for up to 60% of germ cell tumors in infants and children.

5. **b.** Elevated serum levels of AFP are generally due to the presence of yolk sac tumor either in pure form or in association with other germ cell tumor types. AFP production is also seen in glandular or in hepatoid elements of teratoma. About 13% of embryonal carcinomas may show AFP production in isolated or small groups of tumor cells and are not associated with detectable serum level elevations. Seminoma is generally negative for this marker histologically and serologically.

6. **a.** The patient with cryptorchidism has a 3 to 5 times increased risk of developing testicular cancer. Therefore, the lifetime probability of developing a germ cell tumor is approximately 3.5% to 14%.

7. **c.** The patient has a 2% to 5% chance of having a contralateral tumor and has a more than 20-fold increased risk for tumor development compared with the general population. Intratubular germ cell neoplasia can be identified in about 5% to 6% in the contralateral testicular biopsy. It is important to teach patients about testicular tumors to perform regular self-examination of the contralateral testis.

8. **d.** Ectopic HCG production can be seen in any malignancy, particularly carcinomas. Such tumors often have marked nuclear anaplasia. The ectopic HCG production can cause elevated serum levels of HCG. Other placental glycoproteins (e.g., human placental lactogen, PLAP, etc.) can also be identified in nongerm cell tumors.

9. **a. Carney syndrome** is a rare disorder characterized by mucocutaneous pigmentation, atrial myxoma, endocrine tumors (pituitary, adrenals), and large cell-calcifying Sertoli cell tumors. The latter are often bilateral and consist of large eosinophilic cells resembling Leydig cells. The cells form cords or tubules.

The calcifications vary in extent. Some of these tumors are malignant.

10. **e. Spermatocytic seminoma** is a rare neoplasm comprising about 2% to 5% of testicular germ cell tumors. There is no correlation with cryptorchidism. It usually arises in older men around age 50 to 55 and has not been reported in prepubertal children or adolescents. It has not been reported in extratesticular sites, or in association with other germ cell tumors. Clinically, most patients present with painless swelling, which may be present for years. There are cases with bilateral synchronous or metachronous involvement. There are reported cases of spermatocytic seminoma with metastases. However, only one well-documented case is known. Spermatocytic seminoma is rarely associated with sarcoma; these tumors metastasize as sarcomas.

11. **a. Papillary cystadenoma of epididymis** is a benign tumor that accounts for about one third of all primary epididymal tumors. Mean age is 36 years. It often involves the head of the epididymis. About two thirds of papillary cystadenomas of the epididymis occur in patients with von Hippel-Lindau syndrome. In this setting, they are more frequently bilateral. The tumor consists of cuboidal to low columnar clear cells lining dilated ducts and papillae with a single- or a double-layer epithelium. The tumors resemble clear cell renal cell carcinoma.

12. **c. Sertoli cell tumors** account for about 1% of all primary testicular tumors. They can occur at any age but are most common in the fourth to fifth decades (it ranges from 20–80 years old). There are several subtypes: Sertoli cell tumors not otherwise specified, large-cell calcifying Sertoli cell tumor, sclerosing Sertoli cell tumor, lipid-rich Sertoli cell tumor, and the Sertoli cell tumor with heterologous elements. Sclerosing Sertoli cell tumors are not associated with hormonal symptoms. Grossly, the lesion is usually small (0.4–1.5 cm in diameter) and consists of solid, white to yellow-tan nodules. Microscopically, it is composed of cords, solid or hollow tubules, and nests of Sertoli cells set in a densely collagenous stroma. The nuclei vary from large to small, and the cytoplasm is pale and sometimes vacuolated. Immunohistochemically, vimentin and inhibin are present in the neoplastic cells. Pancytokeratin (AE1/3) may be focally positive. All the reported cases had a benign outcome.

13. **c. Nodular periorchitis** (fibrous pseudotumor, fibromatous periorchitis) of the tunica and paratesticular soft tissue typically arise as painless scrotal masses that may be associated with a hydrocele or history of trauma or infection. Typically, these masses are multinodular, but in rare cases they are diffuse, encasing the testis. Microscopically, they consist of collagen with calcifications and focal inflammatory cells.

14. **a.** This is a typical **seminoma** associated with varying numbers of large multinucleated giant cells with abundant pink cytoplasm. Often, the cytoplasm contains

vacuoles, which may contain erythrocytes. The syncy-tiotrophoblastic cells are usually accompanied by hemorrhage. They can cause elevated serum levels of HCG depending on their number. This type of seminoma has the same prognosis as pure seminoma.

15. **d. Teratomas** are often cystic and consist of all three germinal layers (ectoderm, mesoderm and endoderm). The cysts are lined by various types of epithelium. Some are squamous with keratin-filled lumina, others are mucinous and resemble large bowel epithelium, or respiratory in type (pseudostratified and ciliated). Between the cysts are hair follicles, sweat and sebaceous glands, smooth muscle, and fat. All the tissues may be mature, immature, or both. Teratoma in the prepubertal child is diploid and benign. However, in the postpubertal male, teratomas (mature or immature) are commonly aneuploid and present with metastasis in about 30% to 40% at initial presentation. Therefore, teratomas in the adult male are not referred to as benign irrespective of their histologic appearance.

16. **d.** Although some areas consist of solid sheets of cells, much of the tumor is arranged in glandular and papillary structures. The cells are large and the nuclei tend to be irregular and variable in shape or contour. The cells of **embryonal carcinoma** differ from those of seminoma, chiefly in that cell borders are usually ill-defined, nuclei are vacuolated rather than stippled with fine chromatin granules, and the nuclei tend to be more irregular in shape compared with the rounded seminoma cell. The cells are larger than those of seminoma.

17. **a.** In Sertoli cell-only syndrome, seminiferous tubules are devoid of germ cells and are lined by thin pale-staining Sertoli cells only (wind-swept appearance).

18. **b.** The tumor is located mainly in the interstitium. Note that the cells have very little cytoplasm in contrast to seminoma. The nuclei are irregular in shape and smaller than seminoma cells. The prostate biopsy also revealed lymphoma. **Lymphomas** of the testis may be the primary manifestation of this disease and are usually seen in men older than 50 years of age. Generalized lymphoma usually develops within 2 years, and bilateral testicular involvement is seen in about 25% of cases.

19. **a.** Macroscopically, the tumors consist of nodular excrescences studying the tunica with or without diffuse thickening of the tunica vaginalis and/or albuginea. Histologically, the mesothelial lining of the tunica is prominent and multilayered. The cells extend into the adjacent soft tissue as an epithelial-like tumor with solid areas, as well as tubules, acinar, and papillary structures. The cells generally contain abundant pink cytoplasm with nuclear pleomorphism. The lining mesothelial cells of the tunica are hyperchromatic, hyperplastic, and represent the site of origin of the neoplasm. Four months following surgery, tumor nodules recurred in the cord adjacent to the incision. **Malignant mesothelioma** of the tunica is often a manifestation of systemic disease involving peritoneal and/or pleural surfaces.

20. **a.** Microscopically, **yolk sac tumors** are variable and 10 subtypes are recognized. In most instances, several of these coexist. The glandular/alveolar pattern, microcystic, and micropapillary patterns are the most common. The neoplasm forms numerous glandular spaces, some of which are quite large, others minute. Some of the smaller glands resemble fat cells or endothelial-lined spaces, but these, in fact, are lined by flattened or cuboidal cells with clear or pink cytoplasm and irregular vesicular nuclei. There is also a papillary component. Some of these have a prominent central vascular core constituting the so-called glomeruloid structure referred to as the Schiller-Duval body (Fig. 11.12A).

21. **c.** In **cryptorchid testis**, the walls of the tubules have a hyalinized, thickened appearance. The tubules contain only Sertoli cells, recognized by their stringy, vacuolated cytoplasm and the fact that their nuclei have prominent nucleoli. The best evidence of cryptorchidism is the presence of small, tightly packed seminiferous tubules filled with immature Sertoli cells. In contrast to the Sertoli cells in the adjacent atrophic tubules, the immature Sertoli cells appear very dark with elongated hyperchromatic nuclei.

22. **d.** The section shows a large nodule of Leydig cells. It contains seminiferous tubules. The chief difference between **Leydig cell hyperplasia** and Leydig cell tumor is the presence of entrapped tubules seen in hyperplasia. The reason for the Leydig cell hyperplasia is not apparent.

23. **d.** The section shows the wall of a cyst composed of mature squamous epithelium, consistent with **epidermoid cyst**. The cyst contains keratin. The absence of skin appendages distinguishes this cyst from the dermoid cyst. This lesion is benign. The question if this tumor is a monophasic teratoma is still unsettled. Rare epidermoid cysts are associated with intratubular germ cell neoplasia, unclassified.

24. **d.** The tumor consists of numerous clusters and cords of **carcinoid** cells. The cells are uniform and occasionally form glandular lumina. Three years later, there was no evidence of systemic tumor and 5HIAA was negative. The lesion is probably primary in the testis. Carcinoids can be a component of teratoma, metastatic or primary in this site. In association with teratoma, they are included in the category of "teratoma with somatic type malignancy."

25. **d.** Most of the **choriocarcinoma** is hemorrhagic and necrotic. At the margin of the hemorrhage, however, there is some viable tumor. Two distinct cell types are seen: the large cells with large, densely staining nucleus (often multiple) and eosinophilic cytoplasm, which sometimes has large vacuoles, and the smaller cells having a vesicular nucleus, single nucleolus, and finely vacuolated cytoplasm. This tumor usually is detected in the metastases. HCG levels are often high.

26. **a.** The interstitium of the testis contains sheets of cells with scanty, ill-defined cytoplasm and round, hyper-

chromatic nuclei. Some of the nuclei have a prominent nucleolus and some do not. In some places, the cells form small acini, which identify this as an adenocarcinoma. Uninvolved, though atrophic, seminiferous tubules are scattered throughout the tumor. This is a poorly differentiated **prostatic carcinoma** and the interstitial distribution of the tumor, with sparing of the tubules, is characteristic of metastatic lesions to testis.

27. c. In **Leydig cell tumor**, the Leydig cells contain abundant pink cytoplasm with distinct cell borders. The nuclei are round and rather uniform, with finely stippled chromatin and a distinct nucleolus. Numerous, small vascular channels are present throughout the lesion. There is little or no mitotic activity. Gonadal stromal tumors do not show race predilection unlike germ cell tumors. This tumor peaks in the third to sixth decades. The clinical symptoms such as gynecomastia or breast tenderness depend on the hormonal activity of the tumor.

28. a. The cells of this lesion contain abundant pink, sometimes vacuolated, cytoplasm with sharp cell borders. Beyond this, however, the picture differs from the previous Leydig cell tumor in that there is marked anaplasia of the cells, mitotic activity, hemorrhage, and tumor necrosis. **Malignant Leydig cell tumors** are most common in older men.

29. c. The lesion consists of large and small clusters of tumor cells. These are of variable size with scanty cytoplasm and hyperchromatic nuclei. Other fields show numerous mitotic figures and vascular invasion. Thus, it is an anaplastic malignant tumor. In areas, the cells are arranged into a tubular configuration partially encased in a thick, pink basement membrane-like material. These features suggest Sertoli differentiation. Thus, the diagnosis is **malignant gonadal stromal tumor with Sertoli cell differentiation.**

30. b. The gonad is replaced by well-circumscribed masses of germ cells and Sertoli-granulosa cells arranged around pink, round masses resembling Call-Exner bodies. This combination of stromal and germ cells constitutes **gonadoblastoma arising in dysgenetic testis.** There is also marked Leydig cell proliferation. Earlier in life, an immature testis was reportedly removed from the left inguinal area. The most common germ cell tumor arising in gonadoblastoma is seminoma.

31. d. This is **plasmacytoma**. The interstitial distribution of the tumor is typical for hematopoietic and metastatic tumors involving the testis. Plasma cells are somewhat similar to Leydig cells, but differ in these respects: the cytoplasm is purplish red rather than pink, the nucleus contains large chromatin clumps, and the cytoplasm frequently shows a pale cytoplasmic area near the nucleus. As in lymphomas, the testicular involvement may be the initial presentation.

32. a. **Melanoma of the penis** is a rare lesion. Squamous cell carcinoma accounts for more than 95% of penile cancers, while the remaining neoplasms including melanoma, sarcoma, and basal cell carcinoma are rare. The glans and prepuce are the most common sites. The Breslow thickness scale provides important prognostic information. Most of the cases of penile melanoma present with advanced stage and have poor survival. Hematogenous spread pattern seems more common than lymphatic spread due to close proximity to the erectile tissue.

33. d. This is **lichen sclerosis et atrophicus** (Balanitis xerotica obliterans). In the involved areas, the epithelium is thin, and the basal layer of cells shows prominent vacuolization of cytoplasm. Immediately beneath this is a band of relatively acellular, pink-staining, hyalinized stroma. Deep in this band is the inflammatory zone consisting chiefly of lymphocytes. As the process evolves, the acellular band widens and the inflammatory zone is then deeper. There may be detachment of epithelium from stroma to form vesicles or bullae in some cases.

34. d. This is **condyloma acuminatum**. There is growth of the epithelium in two directions: toward the surface to form papillary projections covered with keratin and into the stroma. The latter is particularly characteristic in that each rete peg has a smoothly rounded margin and reaches into the stroma the same distance as adjacent pegs. There may be mitotic activity, but there is no anaplasia and maturation toward the surface is normal and orderly. There is cytoplasmic vacuolization in the middle zone of the epithelium (Fig. 11.26B). When these lesions involve the meatus or urethra, the nuclei are often somewhat larger and irregular, and cells often contain several nuclei. However, these are biologically benign, though often, multicentric and recurrent. HPV types 6/11 are invariably identifiable.

35. d. This shows the typical pattern of **carcinoma metastatic to the penis**. There is extensive filling of vascular lacunae of erectile tissue and adjacent vascular spaces by bladder carcinoma (showing focal squamoid differentiation on the right, Fig. 11.27B). Most such lesions are primary in bladder or prostate and occur as a terminal event.

36. c. This is **Bowen disease**. There is cellular anaplasia involving the full thickness of the epithelium, including loss of polarity and lack of normal maturation toward the surface. Some cells are unusually large, and it is possible to find several cells with bright red cytoplasm: single cell keratinization or dyskeratosis. In situ hybridization usually detects HPV types 16/18. When sweat glands or other adnexal structures do not appear on the slide, one would have to inquire whether it was located on the glans or shaft to distinguish between erythroplasia and Bowen disease. As a rule, Bowen disease will show more bizarre cellularity and dyskeratosis, but in the individual case this is not always reliable. The significance of this distinction lies in the fact that Bowen disease is associated with a high incidence of

visceral or other skin malignancies. The principal differential diagnosis is Bowenoid papulosis, which is usually multifocal with linear distribution of the papules. Histologically, the abnormal cells are less frequent and scattered throughout the otherwise normal epidermis. Also, the patients are usually younger and have a history of venereal diseases.

37. **d.** This is a **well-differentiated squamous cell carcinoma** (SCC). The lesion invading the stroma consists of irregularly outlined finger-like projections of epithelial cells associated with a marked inflammatory infiltrate. In higher power, the tumor shows keratinization. In the left upper corner, the tumor cells are less differentiated and show nuclear anaplasia. The prognosis correlates with the degree of differentiation and stage. The difference between grade 1 (well-differentiated) SCC from grade 3 (poorly differentiated) SCC is that grade 1 SCC shows downward finger-like projections of atypical squamous cells from the papillomatous epidermis. Keratin pearls are present and there is limited cellular atypia and mitotic figures. In contrast, grade 3 SCC shows few or no keratin pearls and marked nuclear pleomorphism, mitosis, necrosis, and deep invasion. The incidence of SCC of the penis in the USA and Europe is approximately 0.5% of all male malignancies. In some African and South American countries, SCC of the penis accounts for around 10% of all diagnosed malignancies in men.

38. **c.** The vas deferens, ejaculatory duct, and seminal vesicle are derived from the Wolffian duct.

39. **d.** The secretory cells (luminal cells) of the prostate only express PSA and PAP. The basal cells are negative. However, in basal cell hyperplasia with secretory differentiation both can be positive, supporting the view that the basal cells are the precursor cells for the secretory cells.

40. **a.** The following list shows the association of PSA levels and risk of cancer:
PSA levels 0 to 2: less than 1%
PSA levels 2 to 4: approximately 15% to 20%
PSA levels 4 to 10: approximately 25%

41. **e.** Several factors are known to affect the serum PSA level. Digital rectal exam, urinary retention, acute prostatitis, recent prostate biopsy, passage of Foley catheter, and any maneuver that manipulates the prostate, will result in temporary elevation of PSA. Following any of these PSA measurements should be delayed to avoid erroneous results.

42. **d.** It has been indicated that digital rectal exam alone detects less than 40% of all diagnosed prostate cancers even when there is a high index of suspicion of glandular abnormalities. However, it is likely that this rate will decrease further with the advent of better detection methods either in serum or urine or in biopsies utilizing molecular markers. The accuracy of clinical staging based on DRE alone in men with palpable lesions is approximately 50%.

43. **e.** Dutasteride (Avodart) inhibits both type 1 and type 2 forms of 5-alpha reductase. Vitamin D induces cell cycle arrest and has an antiproliferative effect on prostate cancer cells. COX 2 inhibitors selectively block prostaglandin production and may reduce expression of several androgen inducible genes. Lycopenes are antioxidants that may inhibit prostate cancer cell growth. Other agents such as green tea-derived polyphenoles induce apoptosis, inhibit cell growth, and dysregulate the cell cycle. Selenium inhibits cell proliferation and induces apoptosis. Vitamin E has shown direct antiandrogen activity.

44. **d.** Using AJCC criteria, organ-confined disease involving more than one half of the lobe but not more than one lobe with negative lymph nodes is classified as pT2b, N0, Mx disease.

45. **c.** **Sclerosing adenosis** consists of relatively circumscribed small acini in a cellular myxoid stroma. Some of the glands can be surrounded by a prominent basement membrane. The glands vary in size, and some appear to consist of only one or two cells. The basal cell layer is positive for 34βE12 and P63. The key feature of sclerosing adenosis is the immunoreactivity for S-100 protein and smooth muscle actin in the basal cells indicating myoepithelial differentiation unlike basal cells in benign or hyperplastic glands. It is not uncommon to see some degree of nuclear pleomorphism.

46. **b.** The tall columnar cells with amphophilic cytoplasm are typical of the **ductal variant of prostatic adenocarcinoma**. They often have a papillary component, particularly in the periurethral region. Several patterns have been described: cribriform, individual glands, and solid. The cells are positive for PAP, PSA, and other secretory cell markers. The presence of basal cells is variable. The prognosis is guarded with a metastatic rate of 25% to 50% at presentation. Often, the ductal component is associated with an acinar carcinoma, which may determine the prognosis. It may be difficult to separate the ductal adenocarcinoma from high-grade prostatic intraepithelial neoplasia and intraductal spread.

47. **a.** This is **well-differentiated prostatic carcinoma** – Gleason Score 6 (3+3). The tumor consists of numerous round or elongated small glands infiltrating between the large benign glands. The carcinoma lacks the complex saw-tooth configuration of hyperplasia, and the glands are closely packed. The glands are generally lined by a single layer of cells, with darker cytoplasm. The nuclei are generally larger than normal. The chromatin is usually coarse with prominent red nucleoli. The nuclei can be vacuolated. Focally, the tumor cells have intensely eosinophilic granular cytoplasm indicating paracrine or endocrine differentiation (Fig. 11.32B). The latter is a common finding in prostatic adenocarcinoma and should not be confused with small cell carcinoma.

48. **c.** This is **poorly differentiated prostatic carcinoma** – Gleason Score 8 (4+4). In poorly differentiated carcinomas, the prostate may be soft on palpation.

PSA levels may be within "normal" range due to functional dedifferentiation of the tumor cells. Sometimes, it is necessary to utilize more than one of the immunohistochemical markers for secretory cells to substantiate the diagnosis of a poorly differentiated prostatic carcinoma.

49. **e.** In **hyperplasia of prostate**, the prostatic nodules consist of fibromuscular stroma surrounding clusters of glands. Some are normal, some may be dilated, and others are closely packed. Hyperplasia is seen best in those glands having a papillary or saw-tooth contour. These papillations may occasionally bridge across the lumen but always maintain a delicate fibrovascular core. In this example, there is no stromal hyperplasia.

50. **e.** This is **basal cell hyperplasia**. There are several small compact acini obliterated by several layers of cells with scant cytoplasm. The nuclei are round or oval, bland, and have occasional small nucleoli. In some of the acini, the cells show more abundant pale cytoplasm, indicating secretory differentiation. The stroma in basal cell hyperplasia is often also hyperplastic.

51. **b.** This is **acute prostatitis**. Many of the glandular lumina are filled with polymorphonuclear leukocytes. In these areas, there is destruction of glandular epithelium. In the involved regions of the prostate, the stroma is extensively infiltrated by the same type of inflammatory cells.

52. **a.** This is **prostatic carcinoma with estrogen effect**. The cytoplasm has a clear or vacuolated appearance, and the nuclei are small and dark (pyknotic). Note that many of the clear or vacuolated spaces contain several of these dark nuclei, indicating that the cell membranes have been destroyed or ruptured.

53. **d.** This is **high-grade urothelial carcinoma** (grade III). The prostatic glands show the typical saw-tooth configuration of hyperplasia. Adjacent glands and ducts are largely filled by sheets of cells with abundant pink cytoplasm and pleomorphic nuclei. There are numerous mitotic figures. Urothelial carcinomas are negative for PAP and PSA but positive for basal cell markers, such as P63 and 34βE12.

54. **c.** This is **Cowper gland**. Note the lobules of acini, each with an associated dilated duct. There is complete uniformity of acini, and the lining cells have small nuclei. The cells have abundant pale to bluish cytoplasm and contain mucin.

55. **b.** There is diffuse infiltration of the prostate by atypical lymphocytes, consistent with **malignant lymphoma**. Lymphomas usually involve the fibromuscular stroma with preservation of the epithelial components. It has no definite affinity for the glands, as is seen in prostatitis, nor it is associated with proliferation, metaplasia, destruction, or other alterations of glandular epithelium where it contacts this epithelium, as in prostatitis. The destruction of the glands is usually a late phenomenon.

56. **e.** In **embryonal rhabdomyosarcoma**, most of the tumor cells are small with hyperchromatic nuclei and scant cytoplasm. Scattered throughout are larger cells with abundant pink or eosinophilic cytoplasm. These are rhabdomyoblasts. A few show cross striations. In other areas, the cells are spindle shaped. This histologic picture associated with the polypoid configuration seen in the trigone constitutes sarcoma botryoides. Postoperative cobalt therapy was given. Seven months after diagnosis, the patient died with generalized metastases. Typically, these patients present with simultaneous obstruction of the rectum and bladder neck.

57. **d.** This patient seems to be suffering from **acute prostatitis**. In younger patients, sexually transmitted organisms such as *Chlamydia* and gonococci are most common. In elderly patients, urinary tract pathogens such as *E. coli* (gram-negative rods) are the usual causes. In both age groups, the etiologic agent is usually identified by Gram stain and culture of a midstream urine sample. Prostatic massage may disseminate infection. The first procedure asks for culture of midstream urine sample.

58. **a.** The drug which was used in this setting suggests **Finasteride**. Medical treatment with Finasteride (5-alpha reductase inhibitor) inhibits the conversion of testosterone to dihydrotestosterone. It acts on the epithelial components of the prostate glands and reduces the size of the prostate. Alpha-1 blockers affect the smooth muscle of the prostate and bladder. Patients with predominantly smooth muscle hyperplasia may best respond to alpha-1 blockers, but this does not result in reduction of size like Finasteride treatment.

59. **c.** In **atrophy**, the glands typically have retained a lobular architecture, are small and lined by cells with scant cytoplasm and hyperchromatic nuclei. Depending on the degree of atrophy, PAP and PSA can be identified in the remaining secretory cells, particularly in evolving or partial atrophy. Several patterns can be recognized: 1) lobular (simple); 2) sclerotic; 3) cystic; and 4) postatrophic hyperplasia. Combined patterns may also present. Atrophy is most commonly misdiagnosed as carcinoma due to the small glandular size, particularly in the evolving stages. Stains for P63 and high molecular weight keratin (34βE12) may be helpful. In some cases, especially when the atrophy is along the edge of a biopsy or when distortion or secondary inflammation is present, the diagnosis may be difficult and again special stains for basal cell makers should be employed. Atrophy is commonly associated with chronic inflammation.

60. **e.** **Corpora amylacea** are commonly seen in benign glands and glandular hyperplasia, but can occasionally be encountered in prostatic carcinoma.

Corpora amylacea may vary in size and shape but are most frequently rounded. They can act as nidus for prostatic calculi. They differ from the needle-shaped crystalloids which are more commonly seen in carcinomas but can also be seen in benign glands.

61. **b.** In **prostatic intraepithelial neoplasia** (PIN), native glands are lined by secretory cells with nuclear enlargement, prominent nucleoli, and dark cytoplasm. Basal cells can be identified even in the H&E-stained section. The cellular features are indistinguishable from those of prostatic adenocarcinoma but invasive features are absent. By immunohistochemistry, PIN can have the same immunohistochemical profile as prostatic carcinoma with exception of the presence of variable numbers of basal cells. At the present the diagnosis of PIN should be restricted to high-grade lesions. PIN is considered to be one of the precursor lesions of prostatic carcinoma.

62. **d. Seminal vesicles** are rarely seen in transurethral resections (TURP) and needle biopsies, unless they are sampled for staging purposes or to monitor treatment response. The seminal vesicle is characterized by a central lumen with complex branches surrounded by smooth muscle. This pattern can present problems, especially when the overall glandular configuration and central lumen are not recognized. Helpful features to recognize seminal vesicle include the presence of cytoplasmic golden-brown lipofuscin pigment and large hyperchromatic and pleomorphic nuclei at the luminal site. These cells are interpreted as involutional change. The cellular variation invariably seen in seminal vesicles is unusual for prostatic carcinoma. Lipofuscin pigment may be present in normal, hyperplastic, preneoplastic (PIN), and carcinomatous glands, and per se is not diagnostic of seminal vesicle. When the epithelial atypia and cellular variation are not present, negative immunohistochemistry for prostatic-specific antigen (PSA) and prostatic acid phosphatase (PAP) is helpful. Additionally, the 34βE12 stain shows basal cells in seminal vesicles, which of course are generally absent in prostatic adenocarcinoma. Ejaculatory duct epithelium has a similar morphology to that of the seminal vesicle. Ejaculatory ducts, however, are surrounded by a band of loose fibrovascular connective tissue and lack the well-formed muscular wall of seminal vesicle.

63. **d.** This is **urothelial carcinoma involving prostatic ducts and infiltrating prostatic stroma**. Recognition of stromal invasion is important for staging and treatment. The ducts are obliterated by cells with marked nuclear pleomorphism and anaplasia. The cell borders are distinct. The cells suggest urothelial carcinoma, which can be substantiated by immunohistochemistry: the cells are negative for PAP, PSA, prostein, and PSMA. AMACR is also negative. The expression of CK 7 and CK20 supports the diagnosis of urothelial carcinoma. In most urothelial carcinomas involving the prostate, random bladder biopsies including the bladder neck/prostatic urethra will show urothelial carcinoma in situ, in the bladder neck often as a pagetoid variant.

64. **e. Verumontanum gland hyperplasia** is often identified as an incidental finding in radical prostatectomy specimens rather than in needle biopsies due to its central location. The lesion is characterized by closely packed, round glands with bland secretory cells and characteristic golden or brownish proteinaceous secretions and/or corpora amylacea. Basal cells are usually identified, and there is a lack of nuclear anaplasia. Prostatic urethral tissue is often seen nearby, and islands of transitional cell epithelium may be present in or adjacent to the proliferating verumontanum glands.

■ Recommended Readings

Cheng L, Bostwick DG (Eds). *Essentials of anatomic pathology,* 2nd ed. New York: Springer-Humana Press, 2006.

Eble JN, Sauter G, Epstein JI, Sesterhenn IA (Eds). *World Health Organization classification of tumours. Pathology and genetics of tumours of the urinary system and male genital organs.* Lyon, France: IARC Press, 2004.

Petersen RO, Sesterhenn IA, Davis CJ. *Urologic pathology,* 3rd ed. Philadelphia: Lippincott Williams & Wilkins, Wolters Kluwer Health, 2009.

Rosai J, Ackerman LV. *Ackerman's surgical pathology,* 9th ed. St. Louis, MO: Mosby-Year Book, Inc., 2004.

Zhou M, Magi-Galluzzi C (Eds). *Genitourinary pathology.* New York: Elsevier, 2006.

12

Breast and Female Reproductive System

Valerie A. Fitzhugh, Joann Habermann, and Debra S. Heller

■ Questions

1. A 54-year-old multiparous woman presents with a painless, poorly defined subareolar mass, accompanied by thick, white nipple secretions. The histology of the lesion is shown (Fig. 12.1). Which of the following is TRUE of the lesion?
   a. It is associated with cigarette smoking.
   b. The lesion is characterized by a dilatation of ducts, inspissation of breast secretions, and a marked periductal and interstitial chronic granulomatous inflammatory reaction.
   c. The periductal and interductal inflammation is manifested by heavy infiltrates of neutrophils.
   d. The mass is an intraductal papilloma.
   e. This lesion is not usually mistaken as carcinoma clinically.

2. All of the following findings are associated with fibrocystic changes of the breast EXCEPT:
   a. Cysts
   b. Apocrine metaplasia
   c. Fibrosis
   d. Atypical ductal hyperplasia
   e. Adenosis

3. Which set of findings is most commonly seen in proliferative breast disease without atypia?
   a. Moderate to florid epithelial hyperplasia, apocrine metaplasia, sclerosing adenosis, papilloma
   b. Atypical lobular hyperplasia, apocrine metaplasia, radial scar, fibroadenoma with complex features
   c. Moderate or florid hyperplasia, sclerosing adenosis, papilloma, radial scar
   d. Duct ectasia, cysts, radial scar, sclerosing adenosis
   e. Fibroadenoma without complex features, radial scar, papilloma, atypical lobular hyperplasia

4. The most common risk factors for breast cancer include all of the following EXCEPT:
   a. Age
   b. Age at menarche
   c. Race
   d. Age at first live birth
   e. Second-degree relatives with breast cancer

5. Which of the following is true regarding to the hereditary breast cancer gene *BRCA1*?
   a. The gene is located on chromosome 13q12.3.
   b. It functions as an anti-apoptotic factor.
   c. Patients have late onset of breast carcinoma.
   d. Other locations where carcinoma can occur include ovary, colon, and pancreas.

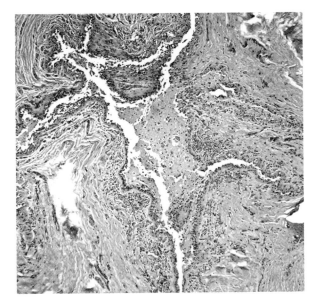

Figure 12.1

e. There is a lower incidence of medullary carcinoma, poorly differentiated carcinomas, ER and PR negativity, and HER-2/*neu* negativity.

6. A 66-year-old woman has a mammographic density and presents with the lesion shown (Fig. 12.2). Which of the following is true of this lesion?
   a. It is characterized by solid sheets of low-grade nuclei and central necrosis.
   b. The necrotic cell membranes commonly calcify and are detected on mammography as clusters or linear and branching microcalcifications.
   c. Periductal concentric fibrosis and chronic inflammation are uncommon.
   d. Extensive lesions are never palpable as an area of vague nodularity.
   e. It is one of the subtypes of invasive carcinoma.

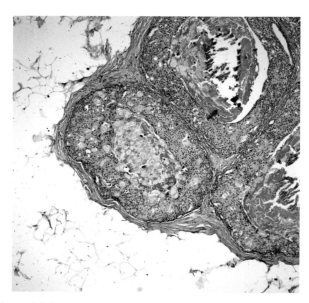

Figure 12.2

7. Which of the following is true regarding the molecular characteristics of lobular carcinoma?
   a. Most show a loss of chromosome 16q22.1 that includes a cluster of at least eight genes responsible for cell-cell adhesion, including e-cadherin and β-catenin.
   b. HER-2/*neu* overexpression is extremely common in well to moderately differentiated types.
   c. Poorly differentiated tumors have a tendency to overexpress hormone receptors.
   d. Tumors with better differentiation tend to show aneuploidy on DNA ploidy analysis.
   e. The E-cadherin on the opposite chromosome (i.e., the one that does not show loss) is upregulated by mutations.

8. Which of the following statements is true regarding fibroadenomas?

a. The lesion is generally benign and occurs in patients between 45 and 60 years of age.
b. The lesion "giant fibroadenoma" is most common in white women in the adolescent years.
c. The stroma of fibroadenoma is usually made up of CD34 positive fibroblasts and scattered factor XIIIa positive dendrophages.
d. The lesions tend to increase in size both during pregnancy and as the patient ages.
e. In cases with apocrine metaplasia, the metaplastic cells are negative for GCDFP-15.

9. All of the following statements regarding the evolution of ductal carcinoma in situ (DCIS) into invasive ductal carcinoma are true EXCEPT:
   a. The transformation to an invasive phenotype does not occur in all cases.
   b. If the transformation from DCIS to invasive ductal carcinoma does occur, it can take years to decades.
   c. The risk of transformation is lower in cases of comedocarcinoma than in noncomedo types of DCIS.
   d. The microscopic type of DCIS correlates closely to the invasive type seen later.
   e. Some invasive ductal carcinomas go through a very short in situ stage before becoming invasive, leading to difficulty in detecting them clinically before invasion.

10. The lesion shown was excised from the breast of a 58-year-old woman (Fig. 12.3). Which of the following immunohistochemical markers will be most helpful in establishing the diagnosis?
   a. Cytokeratin AE1/AE3
   b. Epithelial membrane antigen (EMA)
   c. Gross cystic disease fluid protein-15 (GCDFP-15)
   d. E-cadherin
   e. Lactalbumin

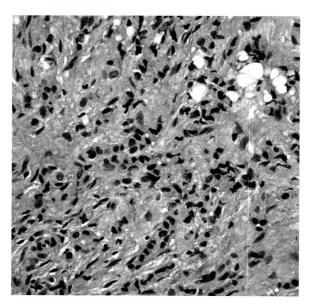

Figure 12.3

11. Which of the following characteristics is necessary for the pathologic diagnosis of inflammatory carcinoma of the breast?
    a. There must be clinical inflammation and edema of the skin of the breast.
    b. Dermal lymphatic invasion must be seen histologically.
    c. Calcifications must be identified radiographically.
    d. Large clear cells must be seen in the epithelial layers of the breast.
    e. The lesion of the nipple of the breast must be differentiated from eczema.

12. Which of the following immunohistochemical stains is most useful in the differential diagnosis of Paget disease of the breast and melanoma?
    a. Carcinoembryonic antigen (CEA)
    b. Cytokeratin 7
    c. HMB-45
    d. Epithelial membrane antigen (EMA)
    e. Cytokeratin AE1/AE3

13. Which of the following is true in the comparison of phyllodes tumor and fibroadenoma?
    a. Phyllodes tumors and fibroadenomas do not fall within the same age group.
    b. Fibroadenomas and phyllodes tumors are always easily distinguishable.
    c. Phyllodes tumors tend to show a dense stromal hypercellularity.
    d. The mitotic count is unimportant when attempting to determine whether the neoplasm is a fibroadenoma or a phyllodes tumor.
    e. Unlike fibroadenomas, phyllodes tumors are not diagnosed at small size.

14. A 58-year-old woman presents with a well-circumscribed breast mass. The histology is demonstrated (Fig. 12.4). Which of the following is true of this lesion?
    a. Grossly, foci of hemorrhage are infrequent.
    b. This tumor has weak immunoreactivity for MUC2 and increased immunoreactivity for MUC1 when compared with ductal carcinoma not otherwise specified.
    c. The mucin in this lesion is extracellular and may be of acid or neutral type.
    d. Of these lesions, 75% show features consistent with endocrine differentiation.
    e. Grossly, these lesions are poorly defined.

15. A 51-year-old woman presents with a 1-cm breast mass. The lesion was excised and the histology is shown. (Fig. 12.5) Which of the following is the *best* answer?
    a. The lesion can be easily differentiated from radial scar and microglandular adenosis on microscopic examination.

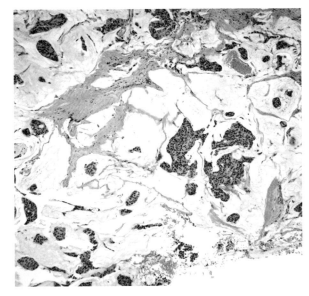

Figure 12.4

    b. These lesions can be characterized by angulated glands, apical blebbing, and luminal calcifications.
    c. It is unusual for these tumors to be underdiagnosed as a benign process on fine needle aspiration biopsy.
    d. Metastases to axillary lymph nodes occur in 50% of cases and the prognosis is poor.
    e. This diagnosis is common, accounting for 35% to 40% of breast carcinoma diagnoses.

16. Which of the following statements about HER-2/*neu* is true?
    a. HER-2/*neu* is an oncogene that encodes a transmembrane glycoprotein with tyrosine kinase activity known as p185, which belongs to the family of epidermal growth factor receptors.

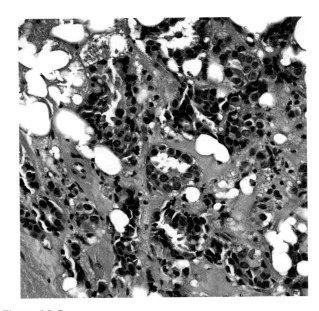

Figure 12.5

b. Its overexpression can be measured by immunohistochemistry but not by fluorescence in situ hybridization (FISH).

c. HER-2/*neu* negativity is an indication to treat a patient with trastuzumab.

d. Overexpression of HER-2/*neu* is a very good predictor of response to chemotherapy and overall survival.

e. There is no improvement in patient response when treatment for HER-2/*neu* therapy is combined with conventional chemotherapy.

17. All of the following lesions can present as a breast mass EXCEPT:
   a. Sarcoidosis
   b. Coccidiomycosis
   c. Silicone reaction
   d. Blunt duct adenosis
   e. Breast abscess

18. A 46-year-old woman has a lesion in association with an intraductal papilloma. The histology is shown (Fig. 12.6). Which of the following is true of this lesion?
   a. This lesion is only seen in association with intraductal papilloma.
   b. This lesion may also be seen in salivary gland tumors.
   c. Carcinoma is not seen in association with these lesions in the breast.
   d. Ultrastructurally, collagen is not seen.
   e. These lesions are positive for Alcian blue.

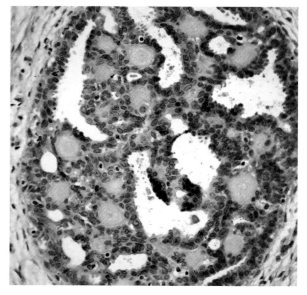

Figure 12.6

19. Which of the following pairs of information correctly stratifies the risk of carcinoma associated with breast hyperplasia?
   a. No or mild hyperplasia: 3 to 4 times the risk for subsequent invasive carcinoma.

b. Moderate or florid hyperplasia: 1.5 to 2 times the risk for subsequent invasive carcinoma.

c. Atypical ductal or lobular hyperplasia: 7 times the risk for subsequent invasive carcinoma.

d. Ductal or lobular carcinoma in situ: 13 to 15 times the risk for subsequent invasive carcinoma.

20. Each of the following tumors is a subtype of ductal carcinoma EXCEPT:
   a. Tubular carcinoma
   b. Mucinous carcinoma
   c. Histiocytoid carcinoma
   d. Cribriform carcinoma
   e. Metaplastic carcinoma

21. A 66-year-old woman is diagnosed with the lesion shown in the photomicrograph (Fig. 12.7). Which of the following is true about this disease?
   a. This invasive tumor does not exhibit the pattern of growth of a classical breast carcinoma.
   b. This lesion frequently shows apocrine differentiation, signet ring morphology and nuclear pleomorphism.
   c. E-cadherin immunostaining is frequently positive.
   d. Expression of p53 and HER-2/*neu* is low.

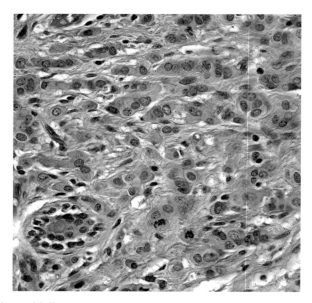

Figure 12.7

22. Which of the following is true regarding angiosarcoma of the breast?
   a. It is not seen following an axillary dissection.
   b. Freely anastomosing vascular channels with malignant endothelial cells are rarely seen.
   c. The tumor is thought to be derived from lymph vessels rather than blood vessels.
   d. The differential diagnosis includes metaplastic carcinoma, acantholytic variant of squamous cell carcinoma, and pseudoangiomatous stromal hyperplasia (PASH).

e. Postradiation angiosarcoma is less common than angiosarcoma de novo.

23. A 27-year-old woman presents with a breast mass that is excised. The histology is demonstrated (Fig. 12.8). Which of the following statements about this lesion is most correct?
    a. It grossly simulates the appearance of invasive carcinoma.
    b. Tumors are on average 10 cm or more in greatest dimension.
    c. The tumor is aggressive and excision should be wide.
    d. The cytoplasm is negative for periodic acid Schiff (PAS) stain.
    e. The overwhelming majority of these cases are malignant.

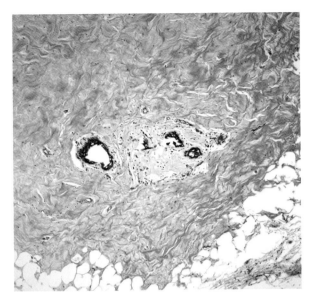

Figure 12.9

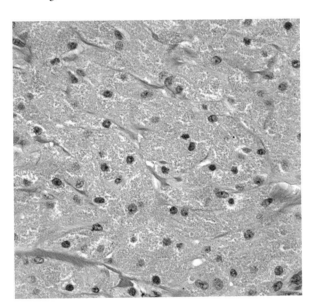

Figure 12.8

24. A breast biopsy is diagnosed as having pseudoangiomatous stromal hyperplasia (PASH). Which of the following statements about PASH is correct?
    a. The spindle cells are immunoreactive for factor VIII-related antigen *Ulex europaeus*, and CD31.
    b. The spindle cells are immunoreactive for CD34 and vimentin.
    c. Breast carcinoma cells are incapable of growing along the pseudoangiomatous spaces.
    d. The pseudoangiomatous pattern is present regardless of the amount of cellularity in the lesion.
    e. There is no relationship between the stromal cells of PASH and the stromal cells of fibroadenoma.

25. A 14-year-old boy developed a nodule below the left nipple. The lesion is excised. The histology is demonstrated (Fig. 12.9). Which of the following statements about the lesion is correct?

a. The lesion can be the result of the hormonal changes of puberty or hormone-secreting tumors.
b. Breast carcinoma is not in the differential diagnosis of this lesion.
c. Epithelial hyperplasia and stromal edema are absent.
d. Histologically similar changes are not seen in the female breast.
e. Hypertrophy of the stromal elements, but not the glandular elements, are seen in this lesion.

26. A perimenopausal woman discovered a large breast mass that was excised. The histology is shown in the figure (Fig. 12.10). Which of the following statements about this lesion is correct?
    a. These lesions acquire vimentin immunohistochemical reactivity but lose reactivity with epithelial markers.

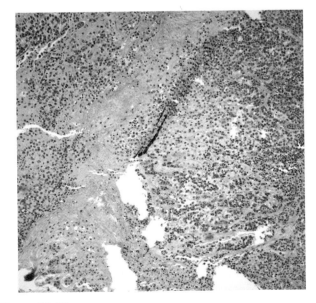

Figure 12.10

b. Subtypes include spindle cell carcinoma, carcinoma with osteoclast-like giant cells, and carcinomas with neuroendocrine features.

c. The behavior of this lesion seems to be more aggressive than that of ordinary invasive ductal carcinoma.

d. The size of the neoplasm at excision is a poor predictor of survival.

e. The sarcomatoid variant of this neoplasm is poorly circumscribed.

27. Which of the following statements is most consistent with inflammatory carcinoma?
    a. Clinically, the breast has a weeping, eczematous lesion that is centered in the nipple.
    b. The lesion is an undifferentiated carcinoma with wide extension into the dermal lymphatic vessels.
    c. Dermal lymphatic invasion is always seen when clinical findings suggest the diagnosis.
    d. Dermal lymphatic invasion has little bearing on the patient's prognosis.
    e. Inflammatory carcinoma rarely simulates the appearance of mastitis.

28. Which of the following statements is true regarding the location of breast carcinomas?
    a. Ten percent of breast carcinomas are multifocal in location.
    b. Breast carcinoma is slightly more frequent in the right breast than in the left.
    c. Five percent of breast carcinomas occur centrally (within 1 cm of the areola).
    d. Approximately 50% of breast carcinomas occur in the upper outer quadrant.
    e. The amount of breast parenchyma in each quadrant has no relation to carcinoma frequency.

29. Which of the following statements about menstrual and reproductive history regarding breast carcinoma is true?
    a. Decreased risk is correlated with early menarche, nulliparity, and late age at first birth.
    b. Oophorectomy before the age of 35 reduces the risk to half that of the general population.
    c. An increase in the risk of breast carcinoma among premenopausal women who have lactated has been documented.
    d. Breast carcinoma risk is increased in postmenopausal women with a hyperandrogenic plasma hormone profile.
    e. Early versus late menopause has no bearing on the risk of developing breast carcinoma.

30. Which of the following statements about the incidence of breast carcinoma in women is true?
    a. Breast carcinoma is the second most common malignant tumor and the leading cause of carcinoma death in women.

b. The incidence of disease is high in North America and northern Europe, intermediate in southern Europe and Latin America, and low in most Asian and African countries.

c. Despite advances in mammography, most breast carcinomas diagnosed in the United States are still larger than 2 cm on initial diagnosis.

d. Mortality continues to steadily fall in countries such as Japan, Costa Rica, and Singapore.

e. Approximately 10,000 women in the United States die of breast carcinoma each year.

31. A 31-year-old woman in her first pregnancy experienced discharge from a mass in the vulva. The lesion was excised and the histology is shown (Fig. 12.11). Which of the following is most consistent with this lesion?
    a. This lesion is a localized focus of hyperplasia in ectopic breast tissue.
    b. The cut surface of the lesion is white without necrotic changes.
    c. This lesion may be seen during pregnancy but not during the puerperium.
    d. Similar changes are not seen in preexisting fibroadenomas.
    e. These lesions are usually poorly delineated at the time of excision.

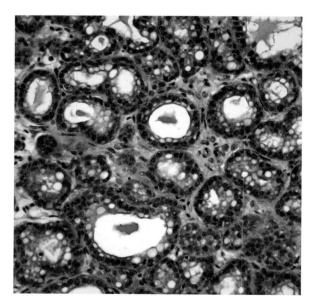

Figure 12.11

32. A 7-year-old girl presents with a white, keyhole-shaped lesion involving the vulva. A biopsy is performed and the histology of the lesion is shown (Fig. 12.12). Which of the following statements is most consistent with this lesion?
    a. The vulvar region presents the least common location of this lesion in children.
    b. Microscopically, the overlying epidermis of this lesion can be hyperplastic.

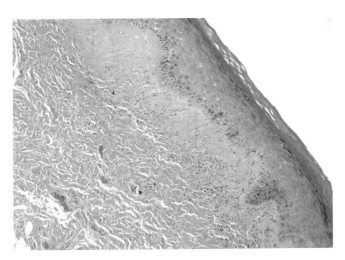

Figure 12.12

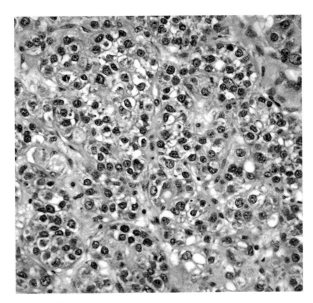

Figure 12.13

c. The minimal histologic criteria for the microscopic diagnosis of this lesion are the presence of a vacuolar interface reaction pattern in conjunction with dermal sclerosis of any thickness.
d. Rare cases of carcinoma associated with this lesion show an underexpression of p53.
e. These lesions are never seen in association with squamous cell carcinoma of the vulva.

33. A woman is diagnosed with Paget disease of the vulva. All of the following statements regarding this disease are true EXCEPT:
a. Clinically, it presents as a crusted, elevated scaling erythematosus rash of the labia majora, labia minora, and/or perianal skin.
b. Immunohistochemically, the tumor cells are positive for MUC1, MUC5AC, EMA, B72.3, and HMB-45.
c. The usual keratin profile of Paget disease of the vulva is CK7+/CK20-.
d. Paget disease of the breast is almost always associated with an underlying carcinoma, while Paget disease of the vulva is not associated with an underlying invasive carcinoma in most cases.
e. Microscopically, large hyperchromatic tumor cells involve the epidermis.

34. A 17-year-old girl presents with vaginal bleeding distinct from her menses. On gynecologic examination, a mass is identified along the lateral wall of the upper vagina and is biopsied (Fig. 12.13). All of the following are true of this lesion EXCEPT:
a. This diagnosis is extremely rare before the age of 12 and after the age of 30; however, a small number of cases occur at the age of 70.
b. All cases are linked to perinatal exposure of diethylstilbestrol (DES).
c. Microscopically, there are tubules and cysts lined by clear cells alternating with more solid areas and

papillary formations as well as hobnail-shaped cells protruding into glandular lumens.
d. The immunohistochemical profile of these tumors is characterized by consistent positivity for CK7, Cam 5.2, 34βE12, CEA, and CA-125.
e. These tumors have ultrastructural characteristics much like lesions of similar type that occur in the endometrium and ovary of older women.

35. The mother of a 2-year-old girl brought her daughter to the pediatrician after noticing a mass protruding from the infant's vagina. She stated that it had the appearance of a bunch of grapes. The lesion was excised. All of the following are true of this lesion EXCEPT:
a. Ninety percent of cases occur in girls under 5 years of age with approximately 66% appearing within the first 2 years of life.
b. The microscopic picture consists of a myxoid stroma, which contains undifferentiated round or spindle cells.
c. The tumor cells tend to crowd around blood vessels and beneath the squamous epithelium.
d. Invasion of the overlying vaginal epithelium may be seen.
e. Foci of neoplastic cartilage may be seen in younger patients with disease lower in the vagina, which is a marker of poor prognosis.

36. Which of the following statements regarding transitional metaplasia of the cervix is true?
a. Tends to be seen in the exocervix of younger women and is rarely associated with atrophy.
b. While it resembles urothelium, it only involves a partial thickness of the mucosa.
c. Immunohistochemical positivity is seen with cytokeratins 13, 17, and 18.

d. The long axes of the urothelial cells are arranged parallel to the surface.

e. Cytokeratin 20 is positive in this condition.

37. All of the following statements regarding cervical tunnel clusters are true EXCEPT:
   a. Tunnel clusters are the result of localized proliferation of exocervix with side channels growing out from it.
   b. Inspissated, deeply eosinophilic secretions may be seen in the glands of the endocervix.
   c. Tunnel clusters have been divided into type A (noncystic) and type B (cystic).
   d. Type A tunnel clusters may be accompanied by a florid glandular proliferation with a certain degree of atypia.
   e. Mitotic activity is practically nonexistent in these lesions.

38. All of the following types of human papilloma virus (HPV) are considered high-risk types EXCEPT:
   a. HPV 16
   b. HPV 33
   c. HPV 35
   d. HPV 18
   e. HPV 11

39. Human papilloma virus is involved in all of the following lesions EXCEPT:
   a. Condyloma acuminatum
   b. Differentiated vulvar intraepithelial neoplasia
   c. Warty vulvar intraepithelial neoplasia
   d. Basaloid vulvar intraepithelial neoplasia
   e. Squamous cell carcinoma of the cervix

40. An 18-year-old sexually active woman had a Pap smear. Based on the results of the Pap smear, a biopsy was performed and the histology is shown (Fig. 12.14). Which of the following is true about her lesion?

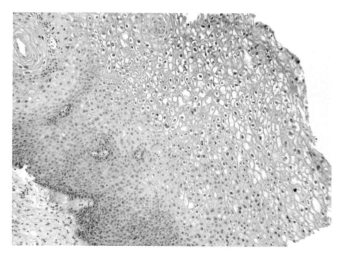

Figure 12.14

a. Her lesion should be described as low-grade squamous intraepithelial dysplasia or cervical intraepithelial neoplasia I.
   b. Her lesion should be described as high-grade squamous intraepithelial lesion or cervical intraepithelial lesion II.
   c. HPV types 6 and 11 are usually responsible for her lesion.
   d. Koilocytic atypia is not a feature of this diagnosis.
   e. A radical hysterectomy will be needed to resolve this lesion as it will not resolve on its own.

41. Squamous cell carcinoma of the cervix consistently expresses all of the following immunohistochemical markers EXCEPT:
   a. AE1/AE3
   b. CEA
   c. P63
   d. Vimentin
   e. Cam 5.2

42. All of the following are poor prognostic factors of cervical squamous cell carcinoma EXCEPT:
   a. Increased size of the primary tumor
   b. Small cell variant of squamous cell carcinoma
   c. The presence of HPV 18
   d. Increased cell proliferation index
   e. The presence of tumor-associated tissue eosinophilia

43. All of the following statements regarding adenocarcinoma of the cervix are true EXCEPT:
   a. Primary adenocarcinomas comprise 40% of carcinomas of the cervix.
   b. The percentage is higher in Jewish women.
   c. The percentage is on the rise in young women.
   d. Cytokeratins, EMA, and CEA are consistently expressed while vimentin is not.
   e. Human papillomavirus infection, particularly types 16 and 18, is seen in most cases of cervical adenocarcinoma.

44. A 35-year-old woman was diagnosed on Pap smear as having atypical glandular cells of undetermined significance. As part of the evaluation, she underwent endometrial biopsy and the histology is shown (Fig. 12.15). Which of the following is the best diagnosis?
   a. Simple hyperplasia
   b. Arias-Stella reaction
   c. Secretory endometrium day 17 to 18
   d. Complex atypical hyperplasia
   e. Endometrial adenocarcinoma

45. A 36-year-old woman has a 3-year history of intrauterine device (IUD) use. She begins experiencing vaginal bleeding, so the IUD is removed and the endometrium

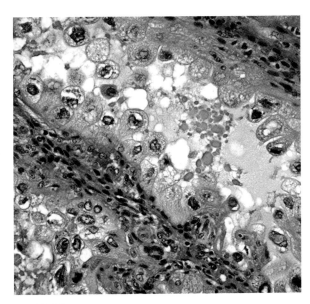

Figure 12.15

is biopsied. The biopsy reveals an extensive lymphocytic infiltrate with occasional plasma cells. The diagnosis is:
a. Acute endometritis
b. Pyometra
c. Secretory endometrium day 23
d. Chronic endometritis
e. Histiocytic endometritis

46. Which day of the menstrual cycle is highlighted by the changes illustrated in the figure (Fig. 12.16)?
a. Secretory endometrium day 26
b. Secretory endometrium day 24
c. Secretory endometrium day 22
d. Secretory endometrium day 19
e. Secretory endometrium day 17

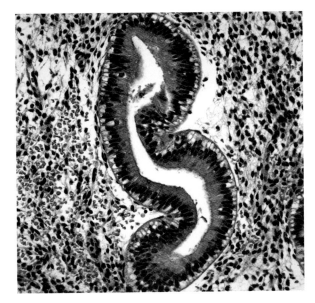

Figure 12.16

47. A 67-year-old woman presents with bleeding. Biopsy confirms the diagnosis of endometrial adenocarcinoma. After hysterectomy, the specimen is seen to have a solid component comprising 45%, a squamous component comprising 10%, and the rest is glandular. Nuclear atypia is minimal. Which of the following is the best grade for this patient's lesion?
a. FIGO grade 1
b. FIGO grade 2, taking into account the solid and squamous portions
c. FIGO grade 2, taking into account the solid portion only
d. FIGO grade 3, taking into account the solid and squamous portions
e. FIGO grade 3, taking into account the solid portion only

48. All of the following are molecular features of endometrial carcinomas EXCEPT:
a. Microsatellite instability
b. p53 mutations
c. DNA aneuploidy in half of cases
d. Mutations in k-ras and PTEN
e. Decreased expression of p21

49. All of the following have been cited as prognostic factors in endometrial carcinomas EXCEPT:
a. Microscopic type
b. p53 underexpression
c. Lymph vessel invasion
d. Angiogenesis
e. Epidermal growth factor receptor (EGFR)

50. Each of the following immunohistochemical markers is present in endometrial stromal sarcomas EXCEPT:
a. CD10
b. H-caldesmon
c. Vimentin
d. Actin
e. Ki-67

51. A 61-year-old woman presented with the lesion shown in the image (Fig. 12.17). Which of the following statements is true of this lesion?
a. Microscopically, this tumor is characterized by an admixture of sarcomatous and carcinomatous areas, resulting in a biphasic appearance.
b. This is a low-grade neoplasm that is well differentiated.
c. Heterologous mesenchymal elements such as fat, cartilage, or skeletal muscle are not commonly seen.
d. These tumors are practically always seen in pre-menopausal women.
e. Cytokeratins are positive in the carcinomatous areas, but never in the sarcomatous elements.

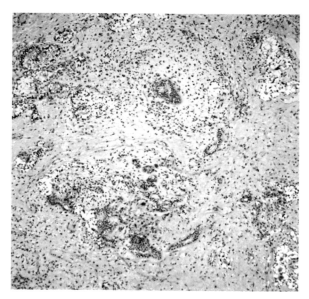

Figure 12.17

52. All of the following immunohistochemical markers are positive in the myometrial lesion seen in the image (Fig. 12.18) EXCEPT:
    a. Smooth muscle actin
    b. H-caldesmon
    c. Vimentin
    d. CD-10
    e. Cam 5.2

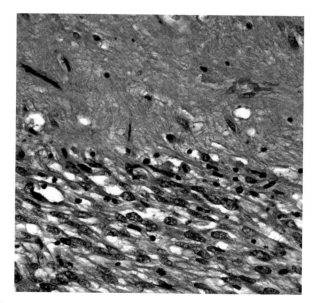

Figure 12.18

53. What are the diagnostic criteria of leiomyosarcoma, listed from most to least important?
    a. High mitotic activity, coagulative necrosis, pleomorphism, cellularity
    b. Cellularity, high mitotic activity, coagulative necrosis, pleomorphism

    c. Pleomorphism, cellularity, coagulative necrosis, high mitotic rate
    d. Coagulative necrosis, high mitotic rate, pleomorphism, cellularity
    e. Coagulative necrosis, pleomorphism, high mitotic rate, cellularity

54. All of the following characteristics of corpus luteum cysts are true EXCEPT:
    a. They are most commonly single.
    b. They are 6 cm or less in greatest dimension.
    c. They typically develop at the end of the menstrual cycle but not during pregnancy.
    d. The cyst wall is composed of luteinized granulosa and theca cell layers.
    e. The fluid contents of the cyst are often bloody.

55. What is the most important criterion for the diagnosis of the lesion in the image (Fig. 12.19)?
    a. Nuclear atypia
    b. High mitotic activity
    c. Lack of stromal invasion
    d. Branching papillary fronds
    e. Exophytic growth pattern

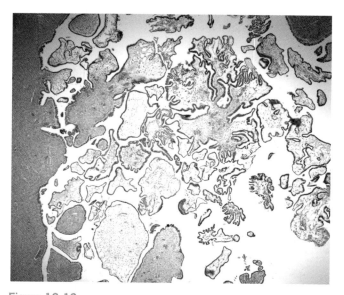

Figure 12.19

56. All of the following immunohistochemical stains are positive in ovarian serous carcinomas EXCEPT:
    a. CK20
    b. CK7
    c. EMA
    d. B72.3
    e. WT1

57. What is the most common ovarian carcinoma?
    a. Mucinous carcinoma
    b. Serous carcinoma
    c. Endometrioid carcinoma

d. Clear cell adenocarcinoma

e. Urothelial carcinoma

58. A postmenopausal woman was noted to have an ovarian mass on ultrasound. The mass was resected and a representative image is shown (Fig. 12.20). This tumor is expected to be negative for which of the following cytokeratins?

a. CK20

b. CK7

c. CK5/6

d. Cam 5.2

e. 34βE12

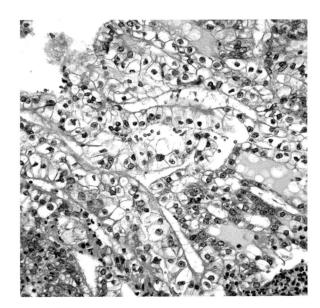

Figure 12.20

59. Which of the following is most commonly seen in immature teratomas?

a. Esophageal tissue

b. Liver tissue

c. Neural tissue

d. Intestinal tissue

e. Cartilaginous tissue

60. Which of the following tumors is LEAST likely seen with struma ovarii?

a. Clear cell adenocarcinoma

b. Mucinous cystadenoma

c. Brenner tumor

d. Carcinoid tumor

e. Papillary carcinoma of thyroid

61. Which chromosome is commonly involved in germ cell and sex cord-stromal tumors of the ovary?

a. 16

b. 13

c. 3

d. 12

e. 21

62. Which special stain is consistently useful in the differential diagnosis between granulosa cell tumors and thecomas?

a. Reticulin

b. Oil Red O

c. PAS

d. Hale colloidal iron

e. Mucicarmine

63. Which of the following endometrial abnormalities can be seen in conjunction with granulosa cell tumors?

a. Endometrial stromal sarcoma

b. Benign stromal nodule

c. Endometrial hyperplasia

d. Endometrial polyp

e. Endometriosis

64. Which pair of immunohistochemical stains is most likely to help differentiate between a granulosa cell tumor and an endometrioid stromal sarcoma of the ovary?

a. CD10 and ER

b. Inhibin and ER

c. CD10 and h-caldesmon

d. CD10 and inhibin

e. Vimentin and ER

65. All of the following are poor prognostic factors of ovarian carcinoma EXCEPT:

a. Tumor spread beyond the ovaries

b. Numerous psammoma bodies

c. Older age

d. Ascites

e. Tumor angiogenesis

66. What is the diagnosis in these abdominal gonads removed from a 10-year-old girl (Fig. 12.21)?

a. Gonadoblastoma

b. Dysgerminoma

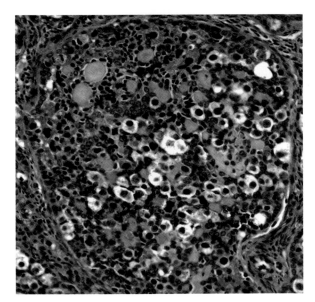

Figure 12.21

c. Sex cord tumor with annular tubules

d. Gynandroblastoma

e. Sertoli cell tumor

67. A 29-year-old pregnant woman presented with vaginal bleeding and absent fetal heart sounds at 25 weeks of gestation. An ultrasound examination was performed followed by hysterectomy because of the bleeding (Fig. 12.22). Tissue from the pregnancy products were sent for chromosomal typing and the results showed:

a. 46,XX

b. 45,XO

c. 69,XXX

d. 92,XXXX

e. 46,XY

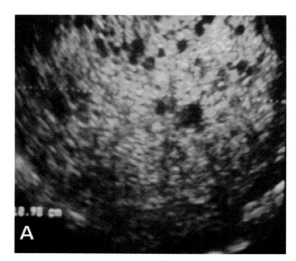

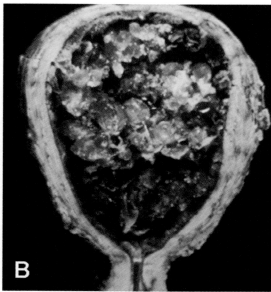

Figure 12.22 (Image provided by Enid Gilbert-Barness, Tampa, FL.)

68. Hysterectomy was performed on a 23-year-old pregnant woman because of severe vaginal bleeding during labor (Fig. 12.23). The diagnosis is most likely:

a. Placenta increta

b. Velamentous insertion of the cord

c. Succenturiate lobe

d. Placenta previa

e. Vasa previa

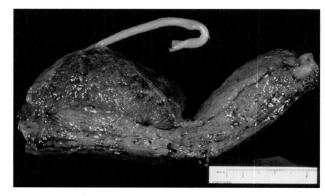

Figure 12.23 (Image provided by Enid Gilbert-Barness, Tampa, FL.)

69. A 36-year old mother with pregnancy-induced hypertension developed abdominal pain and vaginal bleeding and delivered at 36 weeks of gestation. The placenta is shown (Fig. 12.24). The diagnosis is :

a. Fetal thrombotic disease

b. Chorangioma

c. Retroplacental hematoma

d. Hemorrhagic infarction

e. Chorangiosis

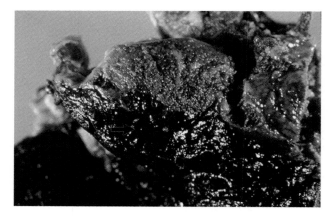

Figure 12.24 (Image provided by Enid Gilbert-Barness, Tampa, FL.)

70. These are cross-sections of an umbilical cord from the
pregnancy of 32-year-old woman with diabetes mellitus
(Fig. 12.25). This lesion is:
  a. Umbilical cord hamartoma
  b. Treated with antifungal therapy
  c. Associated with maternal thrombophilia
  d. Associated with fetal congenital anomalies
  e. Results from excessive cord twisting

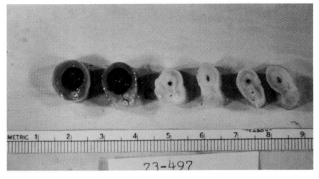

Figure 12.25 (Image provided by Enid Gilbert-Barness,
Tampa, FL.)

■ Answers

1. **b.** The lesion depicted in the image is **mammary duct ectasia**. The history is classic. The lesion is characterized by a dilatation of ducts, inspissation of breast secretions, and a marked periductal and interstitial chronic granulomatous inflammatory reaction. Smoking is associated with periductal mastitis. The infiltrate associated with periductal mastitis consists of lymphocytes and macrophages. Intraductal papillomas do not present with thick secretions. Duct ectasia is of clinical significance because it can be confused with carcinoma by palpation and on mammographic examination.

2. **d.** The histologic findings in **fibrocystic breast** changes are cyst formation, often with apocrine metaplasia, fibrosis, usually secondary to cyst rupture, and adenosis. These are all forms of nonproliferative breast changes. Atypical ductal hyperplasia is a form of proliferative breast disease and is not a component of fibrocystic changes.

3. **c.** Changes of the breast in **proliferative disease without atypia** include moderate to florid hyperplasia, sclerosing adenosis, papilloma, complex sclerosing lesion or radial scar, and fibroadenoma with complex features. **Nonproliferative (fibrocystic) breast** changes include duct ectasia, apocrine metaplasia, cysts, adenosis, and fibroadenoma without complex features, as well as fibroadenomatoid change. Changes of the breast in proliferative disease with atypia include atypical ductal and lobular hyperplasia.

4. **e.** The most common **risk factors** for the development of breast carcinoma as identified by epidemiologic studies include age, age at menarche, age at first live birth, first-degree relatives with breast cancer, history of breast biopsies, and race. A history of second-degree relatives with breast cancer is not identified as a risk factor. Additional recognized risk factors include estrogen exposure, radiation exposure, carcinoma of the contralateral breast or endometrium, geographic influence, diet, obesity, exercise, breastfeeding, and environmental toxins.

5. **d.** The *BRCA1* is located on chromosome 17q21. It is a tumor suppressor gene, not an antiapoptotic factor. Patients tend to have an early onset of breast carcinoma, often in their 40s and 50s. There is a risk of other carcinomas in the ovary, colon, and pancreas. These patients have a greater incidence of medullary carcinoma of the breast, poorly differentiated carcinomas, ER and PR negativity, and Her-2/*neu* negativity.

6. **b.** The lesion depicted here is **comedocarcinoma**. It is characterized by solid sheets of pleomorphic cells with high-grade nuclei and central necrosis. The necrotic cell membranes do indeed calcify and are detected on mammography as clusters or linear and branching microcalcifications. Periductal concentric fibrosis and chronic inflammation are common.

Extensive lesions may be palpable as a vague nodule. It is one of the subtypes of ductal carcinoma in situ (DCIS).

7. **a.** Most invasive **lobular carcinomas** show a loss of chromosome 16q22.1 that includes a cluster of at least eight genes responsible for cell-cell adhesion, including E-cadherin and β-catenin. Well to moderately differentiated tumors are diploid with increased hormone receptor expression and decreased HER-2/*neu* expression. Poorly differentiated tumors tend to be aneuploid with decreased hormone receptor expression and increased HER-2/*neu* expression. The E-cadherin on the opposite chromosome (i.e., the one that does not show loss) is inactivated by mutations, not upregulated.

8. **c.** **Fibroadenomas** are the most common benign breast neoplasm in women from ages 20 to 35. The variant giant fibroadenoma shows a racial predilection for black females in the adolescent years. The stroma of fibroadenomas includes CD34 positive fibroblasts and Factor XIIIa positive dendrophages. While these lesions are seen to increase in size during pregnancy, they decrease in size as the patient ages, leading to increased hyalinization and decreased stromal elements. Fifteen percent of fibroadenomas show apocrine metaplasia, and the metaplastic cells stain positively for GCDFP-15.

9. **c.** While ductal carcinoma in situ **(DCIS)** is accepted as a precursor lesion to invasive ductal carcinoma, progression to an invasive type does not occur in all cases. In most cases, the process of transformation may take years to decades, but in some patients, the interval to transformation is much shorter. There is a definite relation between the microscopic type of DCIS and the invasive component seen later. The risk of transformation in comedocarcinoma is much higher than in cases of noncomedo DCIS.

10. **d.** The lesion depicted in this figure is **invasive lobular carcinoma**, which is highlighted by tumor cells in a single-file pattern and a minimally desmoplastic stroma in many cases. Cytokeratin AE1/AE3, EMA, GCDFP-15, and lactalbumin are common to many lesions of the breast. E-cadherin distinguishes lobular carcinoma from other processes in the breast because of its negative staining pattern. Most cases of lobular carcinoma show a loss of chromosome 16q22.1, resulting in a loss of the E-cadherin gene.

11. **b.** **Inflammatory carcinoma** of the breast was originally a clinical diagnosis (i.e., the entire breast was reddened and warm with edema). Histologic studies of some of the cases revealed an undifferentiated carcinoma invading the dermal lymphatics of the breast. It was found that some cases showed dermal lymphatic invasion without overt clinical symptoms. Calcifications may be seen, but do not contribute to the pathologic diagnosis. Large clear cells in the epidermis are a finding in Paget disease of the breast, as are eczematous type changes of the nipple.

12. c. In **Paget disease of the breast**, one may see intra-cytoplasmic melanin granules in the cytoplasm of the tumor cells. The granules have most likely been transferred from neighboring melanocytes by the process of cytocrinia, in which the tumor cells have imbibed melanin. In this case, and to avoid an erroneous diagnosis of melanoma, the HMB-45 immunostain is most useful, as it will be positive in melanoma and negative in Paget disease of the breast.

13. c. Phyllodes tumors and fibroadenomas are both fibroepithelial lesions of the breast. **Fibroadenomas** are more common before the age of 30, whereas phyllodes occur in the 40s. The stroma is extremely important when trying to decide between a phyllodes tumor and a fibroadenoma. **Phyllodes tumors** are distinguished from fibroadenomas on the basis of cellularity, mitoses, stromal overgrowth, nuclear pleomorphism, and infiltrative borders. Malignant phyllodes tumors show a dense stromal cellularity with mitoses, while it is more common to see a loose connective tissue stroma without mitotic activity in fibroadenomas. phyllodes tumors are often diagnosed at smaller sizes because of increased awareness of breast disease, much like fibroadenomas.

14. c. The lesion in the figure represents **mucinous carcinoma**. It is characterized histologically by small clusters of tumor cells floating in large pools of mucin as seen here. Foci of hemorrhage within these tumors are frequently seen. The tumor has strong cytoplasmic reactivity for MUC2 and decreased reactivity for MUC1 when compared with ductal carcinoma NOS. One quarter to one half of these tumors show endocrine differentiation consisting of argyrophilia, neuron specific enolase positivity, and dense core granules on electron microscopy. The mucin in the tumor is almost entirely extracellular and it may be of acid or neutral type. Grossly, these lesions tend to have sharply defined borders.

15. a. The tumor in this image is an example of **tubular carcinoma**. The angulated shape of the glands and apical snouts are characteristic features of this lesion. Calcifications were noted elsewhere in the lesion. Mitotic figures are absent in these lesions and nuclear pleomorphism is scant. Because of the marked degree of cellular differentiation in these lesions, it is not at all unusual for them to be underdiagnosed as benign. Metastases to the axillary lymph nodes occur in only 10% of cases and the prognosis is excellent. Because of the well-differentiated nature of this lesion, radial scar and microglandular adenosis are important differential diagnostic considerations and are sometimes difficult to differentiate from tubular carcinoma. The diagnosis is relatively uncommon, accounting for a frequency of 1% to 3% in clinical practice.

16. a. HER2/*neu* is an oncogene that encodes a transmembrane glycoprotein with tyrosine kinase activity known as p185, which belongs to the family of epidermal growth factor receptors. Its overexpression can be measured by immunohistochemistry and FISH. The performance of FISH is recommended for immunoreactivity graded 1+ and 2+. Overexpression (or positivity) of HER2/*neu* is seen in more aggressive tumors is an indication to treat patients with trastuzumab (Herceptin), which specifically targets HER2 receptors. Several centers have reported improvement in patient response when HER-2/*neu* therapy is combined with conventional chemotherapy.

17. d. **Blunt duct adenosis** is a histologic diagnosis and a clinically evident mass is not usually associated. Sarcoidosis, coccidiomycosis, breast abscess, and silicone reaction can all cause single or multiple breast masses in patients.

18. b. The histology represented here is that of **collagenous spherulosis**. It is characterized by the presence of intraluminal clusters of generally eosinophilic but sometimes basophilic collagen-rich spherules that seem to arise within the spaces between the epithelial and myoepithelial cells. The lesion can be seen in association with intraductal papilloma and sclerosing adenosis. Exceptionally, foci of lobular carcinoma in situ can involve this lesion. Collagen is seen ultrastructurally in association with basement membrane material and mineral deposition. Collagenous spherulosis can be seen in association with salivary gland tumors. Because this lesion does not contain any type of mucin, it would not be positive for Alcian blue.

19. b. A group convened by the College of American Pathologists recommended grouping patients with fibrocystic **lesions** in the following categories:
   I. No or mild hyperplasia: no increased risk for subsequent invasive carcinoma.
   II. Moderate or florid hyperplasia: 1.5 to 2 times the risk.
   III. Atypical ductal or lobular hyperplasia: 5 times the risk.
   IV. Ductal or lobular carcinoma in situ: 8 to 10 times the risk. (This fourth category, although not fibrocystic breast disease, was added by the group for the sake of completeness.)

20. c. **Histiocytoid carcinoma** is a cytologic variant of invasive lobular carcinoma and therefore does not belong to the invasive ductal carcinoma subgroup. Tubular, mucinous, metaplastic, and cribriform carcinomas are all distinct subtypes of invasive ductal carcinoma.

21. b. This is an example of **pleomorphic lobular carcinoma**. It has the pattern of growth of a classical invasive lobular carcinoma complete with the single cell file pattern of growth but exhibits a marked degree of nuclear pleomorphism and abundant cytoplasm. It frequently shows apocrine metaplasia and focal signet ring morphology. Expression of p53 and HER2/*neu* is very high. Lack of E-cadherin staining is in keeping with the lobular nature of the tumor.

22. d. **Angiosarcoma** can occur secondary to lymphedema following axillary dissection. Microscopically, the diagnostic areas are characterized by freely anastomosing

vascular channels lined with atypical cells. The tumor is thought to arise from blood vessels, not lymph vessels. The differential diagnosis includes metaplastic carcinoma, the acantholytic variant of squamous cell carcinoma, and pseudoangiomatous stromal hyperplasia. Radiation-induced angiosarcomas are actually more common than de novo angiosarcomas and can occur anywhere from 2.5 to 10 years after radiation is given.

23. **a. The histology shown is classic for granular cell tumor.** The cells depicted contain innumerable fine cytoplasmic granules in addition to some larger cytoplasmic granules. The tumors tend to be small and are uncommonly larger than 5 cm. The tumor exhibits benign behavior and local excision is the usual treatment. The large cytoplasmic granules are positive for PAS. It characteristically resembles carcinoma both grossly and clinically, which leads to excision in most cases. Granular cell tumors are benign neoplasms, which carry an excellent prognosis.

24. **b. Pseudoangiomatous stromal hyperplasia** (PASH) is a proliferation of stromal spindle cells of fibroblastic/myofibroblastic origin associated with the formation of artifactual clefts that simulate vascular channels. In the more cellular areas, the pseudoangiomatous pattern may be completely absent. Breast carcinoma cells can grow along the pseudoangiomatous spaces. The spindle cells are negative for FVIII-related antigen, *Ulex europaeus*, and CD31. The spindle cells are immunoreactive for vimentin and CD34. It has been proposed that the stromal cells of PASH are similar to those seen in gynecomastia and fibroadenoma, and that there is a close relationship between these disorders.

25. **a. Gynecomastia** is defined as the enlargement of the male breast which results from hypertrophy and hyperplasia of both the glandular and stromal components. The image shows the characteristic epithelial proliferation surrounded by a hypocellular myxoid halo. It can be a result of the hormonal changes of puberty or of a hormone-secreting tumor. Breast carcinoma is always in the differential diagnosis of this lesion. Histologically similar changes have been reported to occur in the female breast.

26. **c. The lesion shown is an example of metaplastic carcinoma.** It is a ductal carcinoma in which heterologous components are the predominant feature of the lesion (such as the cartilaginous elements seen here). These lesions tend to acquire vimentin positivity in keeping with the mesenchymal elements seen, but occasionally maintain their epithelial staining pattern as well. Subtypes include sarcomatoid carcinoma, spindle cell carcinoma, and carcinoma with osteoclast-like giant cells. The size of the neoplasm at excision is one of the best predictors of survival. These tumors appear to be more aggressive than ordinary invasive ductal carcinomas. The sarcomatoid variant is characteristically well circumscribed.

27. **b. Inflammatory carcinoma** was originally described clinically as a type of breast carcinoma in which the entire breast was red and warm with widespread skin edema, often simulating the appearance of mastitis. Histologic studies revealed that this lesion was indeed an undifferentiated carcinoma with widespread involvement of the dermal lymphatics. Patients have been shown which have the clinical changes of inflammatory carcinoma but lack the dermal lymphatic invasion. This lesion has a poor prognosis.

28. **d. The location of breast carcinoma** is generally indicated by quadrant. Only 3% of breast carcinomas are multifocal in location. Breast carcinomas have been shown to be slightly more frequent in the left breast than the right, with some studies quoting a 13% difference between the two breasts. Seventeen percent of breast carcinomas are located within 1 cm of the areola. Fifty percent of breast carcinomas are located in the upper outer quadrant, a figure related to the high amount of breast tissue in that quadrant. In fact, the marked difference in breast cancer frequency by quadrant is a function of the amount of breast parenchyma per quadrant.

29. **d.** Increased **breast carcinoma risk** is correlated with early menarche, nulliparity, and late age at first birth. Oophorectomy before the age of 35 reduces the risk of acquiring breast carcinoma to one third that of the general population. A decrease in the risk of breast carcinoma among premenopausal women who have lactated has been documented. Breast carcinoma risk is increased in postmenopausal women with a hyperandrogenic plasma hormone profile. Late menopause is also associated with increased breast carcinoma risk.

30. **b.** Breast carcinoma is the most common malignant tumor and the leading cause of carcinoma death in women with more than 1 million new cases diagnosed annually. Approximately 30,000 women die of breast carcinoma in the United States annually. With the advances in mammography in the United States, most cases are <2 cm or are in situ at the time of initial diagnosis. Unfortunately, **mortality** continues to rise in countries such as Japan, Costa Rica, and Singapore. The incidence of breast carcinoma is high in North America and northern Europe, intermediate in southern Europe and Latin America, and low in most Asian and African countries.

31. **a.** The lesion depicted is a **lactating adenoma.** Microscopically, proliferated glands are lined by cuboidal cells which actively secrete milk. This lesion may be seen in the lactating breast as well as in ectopic breast tissue in the axilla, chest wall, or vulva. It is a localized focus of hyperplastic tissue in the lactating breast. It may be seen in pregnancy and in the puerperium. Grossly, these lesions are generally well delineated at the time of excision. The cut surface is gray or tan and necrotic changes are frequent. Lactating adenomas should be distinguished from the proliferative and secretory changes brought on by pregnancy in a preexisting fibroadenoma.

32. c. The lesion depicted here is **lichen sclerosus**. Microscopically, a thick edematous, hypocellular layer (dermis) is seen with a characteristically atrophic epidermis. The vulva is the most common location of affliction in children. In the rare instances where carcinoma has been associated with lichen sclerosus, there is an association with overexpression of p53. The minimal microscopic criteria for this lesion are the presence of a vacuolar interface reaction pattern in conjunction with dermal sclerosis of any thickness. These lesions may be seen in association with differentiated vulvar intraepithelial neoplasia (VIN) and invasive squamous cell carcinoma of the vulva.

33. b. **Paget disease of the vulva** presents clinically as a crusted, elevated scaling erythematosus rash in the labia majora, labia minora, and/or perianal skin. Microscopically large, pale carcinoma cells are identified in the epidermis. The carcinoma cells may form solid nests, glandular spaces, or a continuous layer along the epidermal basement membrane. It shows immunohistochemical positivity for MUC1, MUC5AC, EMA, keratin, CEA, and GCFDP-15. It is negative for HMB-45, an important marker in the differential diagnosis with malignant melanoma. Vulvar Paget disease is usually CK7+/CD20−. Paget disease of the breast is almost always associated with an underlying intraductal or invasive carcinoma, while Paget disease of the vulva is associated with an underlying invasive carcinoma in about 25% to 30% of cases.

34. b. The lesion shown is **clear cell carcinoma of the vagina**. The figure shows prominent clear cell features. The average age of diagnosis is 17 years and is extremely rare before age 12 and after age 30. A small second peak is known to occur at 70 years. Common microscopic features are tubules and cysts lined by clear cells alternating with more solid areas and papillary formations as well as hobnail-shaped cells protruding into glandular lumens. CK7, Cam 5.2, 34βE12, CEA, and CA-125 are consistently positive in these lesions. These lesions share similar ultrastructural characteristics with the clear cell carcinomas of the ovary and endometrium seen in older women. Only two thirds of cases are associated with perinatal exposure to diethylstilbestrol (DES), a nonsteroidal estrogen formerly used to prevent miscarriages and other obstetric complications.

35. e. The lesion described is **botryoid rhabdomyosarcoma**, also known as sarcoma botryoides. Ninety percent of these sarcomas occur in children under five years and approximately 66% occur within the first two years of life. Microscopically, undifferentiated round or stromal cells bathe in a myxoid stroma. Cross striations may or may not be seen in these cells. The tumor cells crowd around blood vessels and beneath the squamous epithelium. The second feature results in a distinctive subepithelial zone known of the "cambium layer of Nicholson." Invasion of the overlying vaginal epithelium may be seen. Foci of neoplastic cartilage may be seen in older patients with disease higher in the vagina; this usually portends a better prognosis.

36. c. **Transitional metaplasia of the cervix** is a condition of older women and is usually seen in conjunction with atrophy. It is resembles the urothelium of the bladder and it involves the entire thickness of the mucosa. The long axes of the urothelial cells are arranged perpendicularly to the surface, and longitudinal grooves may be seen. Immunohistochemical positivity is seen with cytokeratins 13, 17, and 18, as in normal urothelium, but cytokeratin 20 is negative in this condition.

37. a. **Tunnel clusters** are the result of localized proliferation of endocervical glands with side channels growing out through them. Inspissated, deeply eosinophilic secretions may be seen in the involved glands. Tunnel clusters have been divided into type A (noncystic) and type B (cystic). The type A clusters may be accompanied by florid glandular hyperplasia and cytologic atypia. Mitoses are rare.

38. e. The high risk **HPV** types are listed as primarily 16 and 18, but also types 31, 33, 35, 39, 45, 51, 52, 56, 58, 59, 68, 73, and 82. HPV types 26, 53, and 66 have been defined as probably high risk. HPV types 6, 11, 4, 42, 43, 44, 54, 61, 70, 72, and 81 are included in the low risk group.

39. b. **Differentiated vulvar intraepithelial neoplasia** has been described and is not believed to be related to HPV infection. Condyloma acuminatum, warty vulvar intraepithelial neoplasia, basaloid vulvar intraepithelial neoplasia, and squamous cell carcinoma of the cervix are all related to human papilloma virus infection.

40. a. The lesion depicted is **low-grade squamous intraepithelial lesion** or cervical intraepithelial neoplasia I. The figure depicts cells with irregular nuclear membranes, koilocytic atypia, and binucleate cells. Therefore, koilocytic atypia has some bearing in this diagnosis. Squamous intraepithelial lesions are caused by high-risk HPV, not low-risk types like HPV 6 and 11. Low-grade squamous intraepithelial lesions resolve spontaneously in a large number of patients and whether all patients with low-grade lesions need therapy is a controversial issue.

41. d. **Squamous cell carcinomas** consistently express cytokeratins AE1/AE3 and Cam 5.2, CEA (in 90% of cases), and p63. Vimentin is not commonly expressed.

42. e. Increased size of the primary tumor, small cell variant of squamous cell carcinoma, the presence of HPV 18, and increased cell proliferation index are all **poor prognostic factors in squamous cell carcinoma of the cervix**. Tumor-associated tissue eosinophilia has been described as the presence of numerous mature eosinophils in the inflammatory infiltrate of cervical carcinoma. This has been studied in other tissue sites and is regarded as a good prognostic sign.

43. **a.** **Primary adenocarcinoma of the cervix** comprises only 5% to 15% of all carcinomas of the cervix. The percentage is higher in Jewish women and is on the rise on young women. Cytokeratins, EMA, and CEA are consistently present while vimentin is not. HPV infection, particularly types 16 and 18, is seen in most adenocarcinomas of the cervix.

44. **b.** The image is characteristic of the **Arias-Stella reaction**. It is an exaggerated expression of gestational or hypersecretory endometrium in which changes in the endometrial glands are accompanied by prominent nuclear changes manifested by hyperchromasia and nuclear enlargement. Normal and abnormal mitoses may also be present but are uncommon. These changes are almost always focal and are most commonly seen in postabortion curettage specimens, although they occur in both intrauterine and ectopic gestations. The other options would be unusual for a 35-year-old woman.

45. **d.** The description is illustrative of **chronic endometritis**. The histologic picture is dominated by lymphocytes, and more importantly, plasma cells, which are required to make the diagnosis. It may follow pregnancy or abortion, it may be the result of an IUD, or it may be accompanied by pelvic inflammatory disease. Acute endometritis is usually seen in association with abortion, the postpartum state, and instrumentation, and requires the presence of microabscesses. Neutrophilic infiltrates are normally seen in the endometrium on days 26, 27, and 28. Pyometra refers to the accumulation of pus within the endometrial cavity, but no neutrophils are described in the passage. Histiocytic endometritis is a consequence of hematometra where the endometrial mucosa is replaced by lipid laden macrophages. Secretory endometrium on day 23 is marked by prominence of the spiral arterioles.

46. **e.** The figure illustrates the finding of an orderly row of nuclei with homogenous cytoplasm above and vacuoles below, which is seen on day 17. The findings of the other choices are as follows: on day 19 one will see few vacuoles and intraluminal secretions. On day 22, one will see maximum stromal edema. On day 24, one will see collections of predecidual cells appearing around the arterioles. On day 26, one will see solid sheets of predecidual cells with the appearance of a neutrophilic infiltrate.

47. **c.** **FIGO grading** of endometrial carcinoma is performed as follows:
    a. FIGO Grade 1: <5% solid component
    b. FIGO Grade 2: 5% to 50% solid component
    c. FIGO Grade 3: >50% solid component
    Of note, the squamous component has no bearing in the FIGO grading scheme. Also bear in mind that if the degree of nuclear atypia warrants it, the tumor may be upstaged regardless of the architectural grade.

48. **c.** **Microsatellite instability**, overexpression of p53, mutations in k-ras and PTEN, and decreased expression of p21 have all been seen in endometrial carcinomas.

DNA aneuploidy is seen in a quarter of cases, and these cases tend to be of advanced stage. DNA aneuploidy is most commonly seen in serous carcinomas.

49. **b.** p53 overexpression has been described as a **prognostic factor**. Microscopic type is related to prognosis, with serous carcinomas and clear cell carcinomas having poor prognosis. Lymph vessel invasion is a marker of poor prognosis, particularly if present in large quantities. Angiogenesis has been found to be an independent prognostic factor in endometrial carcinomas. Increased expression of EGFR has been suggested to correlate with microscopic grade and a shortened survival time.

50. **b.** **Endometrial stromal sarcomas** are consistently positive for CD-10 and vimentin. Positivity for actin is common. The proliferating cells in the stroma will be positive for Ki-67. H-caldesmon is consistently negative in these tumors but positive in smooth muscle tumors, important in the distinction between ESS and smooth muscle neoplasms.

51. **a.** This image shows the heterologous type of **malignant mixed Müllerian tumor** or MMMT. These are also known as carcinosarcomas. The image shows a carcinomatous component with adjacent cartilage. These are poorly differentiated, high-grade neoplasms that are almost always seen in postmenopausal women. Heterologous elements, such as fat, skeletal muscle, and cartilage are fairly commonly seen in these tumors. They stain positively for cytokeratin not only in the carcinomatous component of the tumor but also in the sarcomatous component in over half of cases. These tumors are characterized microscopically by an admixture of carcinomatous and sarcomatous elements, resulting in a biphasic appearance.

52. **d.** The lesion depicted here is a **leiomyosarcoma**, illustrated here by a smooth muscle background with coagulative necrosis and mitoses. Smooth muscle actin, h-caldesmon, vimentin, and Cam 5.2 are positive in leiomyosarcomas. CD-10, while positive in endometrial stromal sarcomas, is negative in leiomyosarcomas.

53. **d.** The weight of the morphologic factors in **leiomyosarcoma** from most to least important is coagulative necrosis, high mitotic activity, pleomorphism, and cellularity. These factors allow for a fairly accurate prediction of tumor behavior.

54. **c.** **Corpus luteum cysts** are single and usually less than 6 cm in greatest dimension. They may develop at the end of the menstrual cycle or they may occur in pregnancy. The cyst wall is composed of luteinized theca and granulosa cell layers. The contents of the cyst are often bloody, and if the cyst ruptures, hemorrhage into the peritoneal cavity occurs, and the misdiagnosis of ectopic pregnancy can be made.

55. **c.** The lesion depicted in the image is a **borderline serous tumor of the ovary** which as illustrated here has numerous branching papillary fronds in an exophytic growth pattern. These tumors may have nuclear

atypia, high mitotic activity, stratification, and branching papillary fronds. However, it is the lack of stromal invasion that characterizes this lesion as a borderline serous neoplasm.

56. **a.** CK 20 is negative in **ovarian serous carcinomas**. CK7, EMA, WT-1, and B72.3 are all consistently positive in ovarian serous carcinomas. Significantly, WT-1 does not stain uterine corpus serous carcinomas.

57. **b. Serous carcinomas** are the most common carcinomas of the ovary, accounting for 60% to 80% of ovarian carcinomas. Endometrioid carcinomas account for 10% to 25%. Mucinous carcinomas account for 5% to 15%. Clear cell adenocarcinoma and urothelial carcinoma account for far fewer cases.

58. **a.** This is an example of **clear cell adenocarcinoma**. It is characterized histologically by large tumor cells with clear cytoplasm which often contains glycogen, mucin, and fat. Some of the nuclei protrude into the lumina producing the effect called hobnailing. Many different cytokeratins, including CK7, CK5/6, Cam 5.2, and 34βE12, are positive in these lesions. CK20 is consistently negative.

59. **c. Immature teratoma** is a malignant ovarian neoplasm seen most frequently in children and adolescents that is composed of a mixture of embryonal and adult tissues derived from the three germ layers. While any type of tissue may be represented, the most common component is neurally derived. Other structures, such as stomach, esophagus, liver, intestine, and cartilage, may be seen.

60. **a. Struma ovarii** is a teratoma with dominant growth of thyroid tissue. Grossly, the mass tends to have the consistency and color of normal thyroid tissue, and cystic changes may often be seen. This tumor can show any of the changes that occur in the normal thyroid gland, including thyroiditis, hyperplasia, and carcinoma. Struma ovarii can be seen in conjunction with mucinous cystadenoma, Brenner tumor, or carcinoid tumor. A variant of struma ovarii, struma ovarii with clear cells, can mimic clear cell adenocarcinoma, but the two do not usually coexist.

61. **d.** Germ cell and sex cord-stromal tumors consistently show changes in chromosome 12. The germ cell tumors are more likely to have an **isochromosome 12** whereas sex cord stromal tumors are more likely to have a trisomy of chromosome 12. Interestingly, germ cell tumors in the male are also likely to have an isochromosome 12.

62. **a.** Of the special stains listed, reticulin is the most useful in the differential diagnosis between thecoma and granulosa cell tumor. **Reticulin** usually demonstrates reticulin fibers around each individual cell in thecoma as opposed to granulosa cell tumor in which the reticulin highlights groups of cells. Of note, islands of luteinization may be present in thecomas, and these are not reticulin positive.

63. **c.** The endometrium in patients with **granulosa cell tumors** exhibits varying degrees of hyperplasia in about 25% of patients, even when the tumors are extremely small due to the estrogen produced by the tumors. Thecomas has been rarely reported to be associated with endometrial stromal sarcomas. Benign stromal nodules, endometriosis, and endometrial polyps bear no association with granulosa cell tumors.

64. **d. CD10** is positive in endometrioid stromal sarcomas of the ovary. **Inhibin** is positive in granulosa cell tumors. ER can be seen in any estrogen receptor positive tumor. Vimentin is positive in both endometrioid stromal sarcomas and granulosa cell tumors. H-caldesmon is positive in smooth muscle tumors. Therefore, the best pair is CD10 (positive in ESS and negative in granulosa cell tumors) and inhibin (negative in ESS and positive in granulosa cell tumors).

65. **b.** Tumor spread beyond the ovaries, older age, ascites, and tumor angiogenesis are all poor **prognosticators in ovarian carcinoma**. Numerous psammoma bodies have a better prognosis. An extreme example of this is psammocarcinoma, which has a survival much like that of borderline neoplasms.

66. **a.** The tumor shown in the image is a **gonadoblastoma**. It is composed of sharply defined tumor nests with primitive germ cells admixed with Sertoli and granulosa cells. Tumor calcification is usually present. Dysgerminoma is a germ cell tumor of the ovary that is analogous to seminoma in the testis. Sex cord tumor with annular tubules combines the features of a granulosa cell tumor with the growth pattern of Sertoli cells. Morphologically it contains simple and complex annular tubules containing eosinophilic, often calcified, hyaline bodies. Gynandroblastoma is a tumor that contains approximately equal components of granulosa-theca cell and Sertoli-Leydig cell components. Rarely, the sex cord-stromal component can be overgrown by the Sertoli cell component, resulting in a Sertoli cell tumor.

67. **a.** The pictures show the typical ultrasonographic "snow-storm" appearance and the gross vesicular appearance of **complete hydatidiform mole**. No fetus is identified, excluding the possibility of triploidy. The chromosomal karyotype in most cases of complete hydatidiform mole is 46,XX. 46,XY can rarely happen because of dispermy but 46,YY does not occur. Modern therapy of these lesions involves evacuation of the mole followed by monitoring of β-hCG levels. If the β-hCG level rises or plateaus, methotrexate therapy is added.

68. **d.** The image shows a hysterectomy specimen and a **placenta previa** implanted in the lower uterine segment and covering the cervical os. During labor, the placenta tears and vaginal bleeding occurs which may be heavy and require hysterectomy.

69. **c.** The clinical history and the image are consistent with **retroplacental hematoma**, seen on the placental maternal surface. This is the pathologic finding in clinical abruption. It is frequently associated with preeclampsia and may cause decreased placental function and fetal death.

70. d. The image shows a **single umbilical artery (2-vessel cord)** which is associated with maternal diabetes mellitus and fetal congenital anomalies, particularly renal and cardiac malformations. Venous congestion is also present and is often seen in umbilical cords. It does not necessarily indicate thrombophilic disease.

■ Recommended Readings

Crum CP, Lee KR. *Diagnostic gynecologic and obstetric pathology.* Philadelphia: Saunders, 2005.

Kurman R. *Blaustein's pathology of the female genital tract*, 5th ed. New York: Springer, 2002.

Robboy SJ, Mutter GL, Prat J, et al. *Robboy's pathology of the female reproductive tract.* New York: Churchill Livingston, 2008.

Rosen PP. *Rosen's breast pathology*, 3rd ed. Baltimore: Lippincott Williams & Wilkins, 2008.

13

Nervous System, Skeletal Muscle, and Eye

Elisabeth J. Rushing and Mariarita Santi-Vicini

■ Questions

1. This lesion was removed from a 40-year-old man who presented with headaches and ataxia (Fig. 13.1). What is the most likely diagnosis in this case?
   a. Subependymal giant cell astrocytoma
   b. Pilocytic astrocytoma
   c. Arteriovascular malformation
   d. Hemangioblastoma
   e. Angioblastic glioma

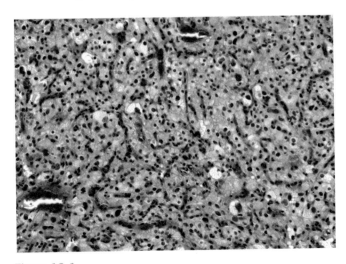

Figure 13.1

2. Microscopic examination of this hippocampus (Fig. 13.2) from a 68-year-old patient who suffered a cardiac arrest during surgery and survived on a respirator for 2 weeks would most likely show the following:
   a. Neurofibrillary tangles in the dentate gyrus
   b. Red, pyknotic neurons (acute neuronal injury) in CA1

   c. Granulovacuolar degeneration
   d. Hirano bodies
   e. Red, pyknotic neurons (acute neuronal injury) in CA2

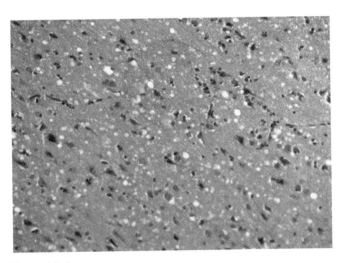

Figure 13.2

3. Which one of the following statements does NOT apply to the abnormality depicted in this gross dissection of the circle of Willis (Fig. 13.3)?
   a. Associated processes include polycystic kidney disease and coarctation of the aorta.
   b. Common at the middle cerebral trifurcation.
   c. A familial inheritance pattern has been noted in fewer than 2% of intracranial aneurysms.
   d. This condition is common in infants and children.
   e. Hemorrhage and secondary infarcts are potential sequelae.

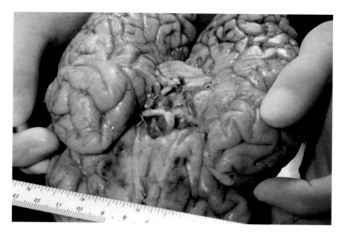

Figure 13.3

4. What is the most likely diagnosis based on this photomicrograph (Fig. 13.4)?
   a. Multisystem atrophy
   b. Unverricht epilepsy
   c. Adult polyglucosan disease
   d. North American blastomycosis
   e. Parkinson disease

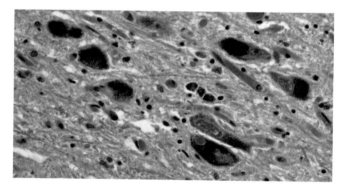

Figure 13.4

5. The differential diagnosis in a 7-year-old child who presented with gait ataxia and this finding (Fig. 13.5) at autopsy should include which of the following entities?

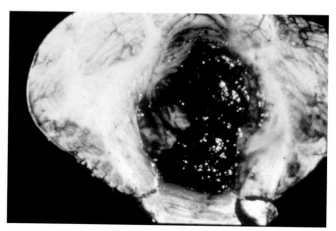

Figure 13.5

a. Glioblastoma multiforme
b. Medulloblastoma
c. Metastasis
d. Hemangioblastoma

6. A 14-year-old boy with this gross finding (Fig. 13.6) most likely presented with the following clinical manifestation:
   a. New-onset seizures
   b. Hemiballismus
   c. Parinaud syndrome
   d. Cortical blindness
   e. Opsoclonus

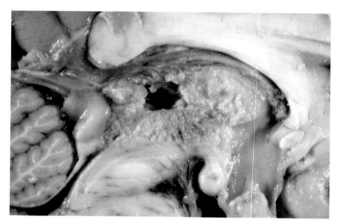

Figure 13.6

7. Which of the following immunohistochemical stains is the most useful for demonstrating axonal spheroids associated with diffuse axonal injury?
   a. Vimentin
   b. Epithelial membrane antigen
   c. Glial fibrillary acidic protein
   d. CD68
   e. β-amyloid precursor protein

8. This is a coronal section from a 52-year-old man (Fig. 13.7). Which statement is FALSE?

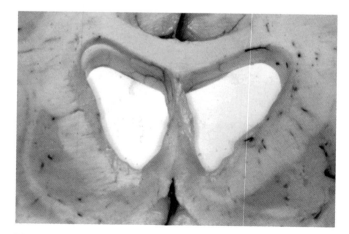

Figure 13.7

a. This disease selectively causes atrophy of the caudate nucleus but spares the putamen.

b. Neuronal loss preferentially affects spiny neurons.

c. CAG trinucleotide repeats characterize this disease.

d. Later generations are affected at an earlier age and often more severely.

e. Clinically, patients usually present with echolalia.

9. Which statement applies to the condition associated with this image (Fig. 13.8)?

a. Filaments within the inclusions contain alpha-synuclein.

b. The nucleus basalis of Meynert is spared.

c. Extensive involvement of the putamen is associated with a type of dementia.

d. Immunohistochemical studies have shown that inclusions in this disease contain significant amounts of gamma amino butyric acid (GABA).

e. Patients typically present with seizures.

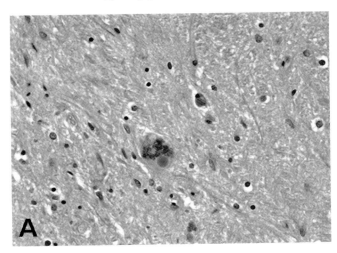

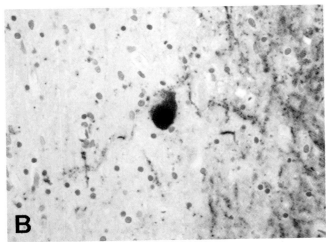

Figure 13.8

10. Which of the following is most likely associated with lobar hemorrhage in the elderly?

a. Metastatic prostate adenocarcinoma

b. Ruptured arteriovenous malformation

c. Cerebral amyloid angiopathy

d. Mycotic aneurysm

e. Capillary telangiectasia bleed

11. A 57-year-old man was found deceased in his lakeside cabin in northern Maine where he was ice fishing. At autopsy, a coronal section of brain showed bilateral hemorrhagic lesions in the globus pallidus (Fig. 13.9). Which of the following is the most likely cause of death?

a. Blunt trauma to the head

b. Anticoagulant overdose

c. Massive ischemic cerebrovascular accident in the distribution of the middle cerebral artery

d. Cerebral aspergillosis

e. Carbon monoxide poisoning

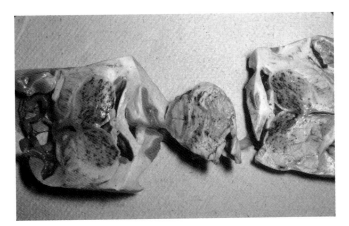

Figure 13.9

12. A 45-year-old missionary returned from Africa suffering from fever and mental confusion. He deteriorated rapidly and died. An autopsy was performed. Which statement does NOT apply to the entity likely diagnosed by the pathologist?

a. These changes are the result of infection with *Plasmodium ovale*.

b. Ring hemorrhages in the brain are a major feature.

c. People with sickle cell trait are less likely to die from infection.

d. Initial infection often causes enlargement of the spleen.

e. Sequestration of infected red blood cells in the blood-brain barrier endothelium is central to the pathologic progression.

13. A 28-year-woman presented with unilateral visual impairment that progressed over the course of several days. Six months later, she developed ataxia and cranial nerve signs. Which one of the following applies to the pathologic findings (Fig. 13.10)?

a. Multiple, circumscribed lesions may be found along the surface of the brainstem.

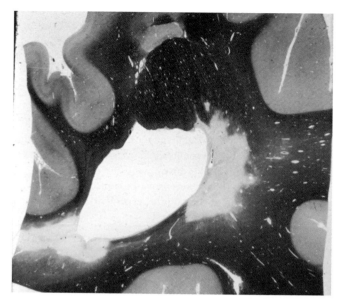

Figure 13.10

b. Lesions are commonly found adjacent to the lateral ventricles.
c. Microscopically, lesions are often macrophage-rich.
d. The Marburg variant is a fulminating form that may be confused with a neoplasm.
e. All of the above

14. Which statement applies to the condition depicted in the photomicrograph (Fig. 13.11)?
    a. The pathologic changes are a result of Heubner arteritis.
    b. The disease is caused by various species of *Ixodes* tick.
    c. Proteinase K-resistant PrP^{sc} can be detected by immunostaining or Western blotting.
    d. It is associated with lactic acidosis and stroke-like episodes.
    e. The disease is caused by deficiency of glutaryl-CoA dehydrogenase.

15. Which of the following genetic alterations is most likely to be associated with this tumor that arose in a 68-year-old man who presented with sudden-onset right hemiparesis (Fig. 13.12)?
    a. Inactivation of p53 and overexpression of PDGF-A
    b. Amplification of epidermal growth factor receptor (EGRF)
    c. Mutation of the copper-zinc superoxide dismutase gene
    d. Mutation in the *Notch-3* gene
    e. The A/ND5 mutation in mtDNA is pathogenic

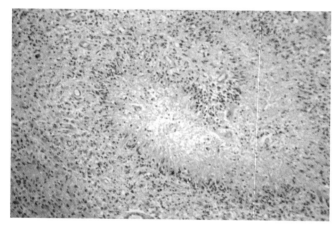

Figure 13.12

16. This 38-year-old woman presented with headaches of increasing severity. Which statement does NOT apply to the entity depicted in this gross photograph (Fig. 13.13)?
    a. It is the most commonly diagnosed primary brain tumor of adults.
    b. Sporadic meningiomas have been linked to chromosome 22 in the region of the NF2 gene.
    c. The tumor expresses estrogen and progesterone receptors.
    d. Clear cell and chordoid are WHO grade 2 variants.
    e. Occasionally present as extracranial tumors.

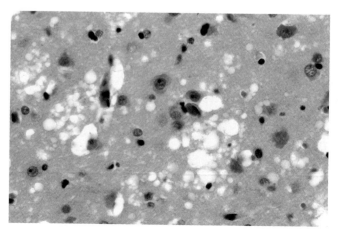

Figure 13.11

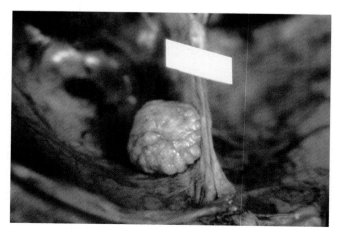

Figure 13.13

17. What is the approximate weight of the brain at the time of birth of a full-term infant?
    a. 120 grams
    b. 240 grams
    c. 800 grams
    d. 1450 grams
    e. 360 grams

18. Which statement is NOT true about lenticular opacities of the eye?
    a. Risk factors include steroids, diabetes, Wilson disease, and aging.
    b. Accumulation of urochrome alters the perception of blue color.
    c. A hypermature form is known as *Morgagnian* opacities.
    d. Typically develop in eyes with shallow anterior chambers.
    e. Congenital cataracts may show autosomal dominant inheritance.

19. Which one of the following entities is linked to high-output cardiac failure?
    a. Telangiectasia
    b. Berry aneurysm
    c. Aneurysm of the great vein of Galen
    d. Arteriovenous malformation
    e. None of the above

20. Which herniation category results in pupillary dilation and impairment of ocular motility on the side of the lesion?
    a. Subfalcine
    b. Transtentorial
    c. Insular
    d. Tonsillar
    e. None of the above

21. Epidural hematoma is most commonly associated with which one of the following lesions?
    a. Rupture of the bridging veins
    b. Trauma to the skull in the region of the temporal bone
    c. Amyloid angiopathy
    d. Bleeding dyscrasias
    e. None of the above

22. What is the most likely diagnosis associated with this image (Fig. 13.14)?
    a. Brainstem glioma
    b. Agenesis of the corpus callosum
    c. Arnold-Chiari malformation (Chiari type II)
    d. Chiari malformation type I
    e. Dandy-Walker malformation

23. What is the etiology for this intraoperative cytologic preparation from a 54-year-old woman with a moderately enhancing right frontal mass (Fig. 13.15)?

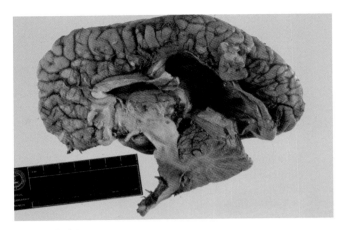

Figure 13.14

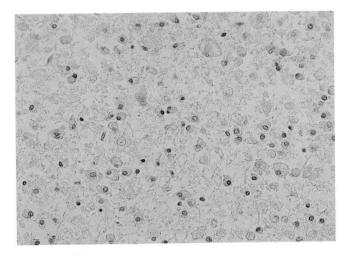

Figure 13.15

    a. Demyelinating lesion
    b. Metastatic carcinoma
    c. Astrocytoma, grade 1
    d. Toxoplasmosis
    e. None of the above

24. Which of the following does NOT apply to malignant peripheral nerve sheath tumors (MPNST)?
    a. Arise from malignant degeneration schwannomas
    b. Associated with neurofibromatosis type I
    c. Follow radiation therapy
    d. Immunoreactive for S100 protein
    e. May arise in a plexiform neurofibroma

25. Other than Niemann-Pick and Tay-Sachs diseases, which one of the following entities may be associated with a cherry red spot?
    a. Central retinal artery occlusion
    b. Age-related macular degeneration
    c. Retinitis pigmentosa
    d. Retinal lymphoma
    e. McArdle disease

26. The pattern of lobar or "knife-edge" atrophy best characterizes which one of the following neurodegenerative diseases?
    a. Corticobasal degeneration
    b. Pick disease
    c. Vascular dementia
    d. Frontotemporal dementia without tau pathology
    e. Diffuse Lewy body disease

27. Which one of the following does NOT apply to contusions?
    a. Wedge-shaped, with the broad base along the surface of the brain.
    b. Microscopically, edema and pericapillary hemorrhage may be present.
    c. Old lesions are most prominent along the base of the sulcus.
    d. Axonal swellings may develop in the vicinity of damaged neurons or remote from the site of impact.
    e. Destruction of the molecular layer of the brain.

28. What is the most likely microscopic finding in this 32-year-old adventure enthusiast who developed encephalitis after spending the summer exploring caves in New Mexico?
    a. Toxoplasma pseudocysts
    b. Negri bodies
    c. Biondi bodies
    d. Hirano bodies
    e. Dürck granulomata

29. This 27-year-old woman presented with rapidly progressive weakness, lethargy, and seizures. Neuroimaging studies showed bilateral hemorrhagic lesions of the temporal lobes. What is the most likely diagnosis?
    a. Methanol toxicity
    b. Hemorrhagic infarct
    c. Neurosyphilis
    d. Herpes encephalitis
    e. Tuberculous encephalitis

30. Which one of these conditions is NOT associated with trinucleotide repeats?
    a. Huntington disease
    b. Lhermitte-Duclos syndrome
    c. Myotonic dystrophy
    d. Fragile X syndrome
    e. Friedreich ataxia

31. An 11-month-old infant presents with an enlarged head circumference. Computed tomography (CT) scans show cystic dilatation of the fourth ventricle, cerebellar vermian dysgenesis, and hydrocephalus. Which of the following is the most likely diagnosis?
    a. Prader-Willi syndrome
    b. Kallmann syndrome
    c. Niemann-Pick disease
    d. Dandy-Walker malformation
    e. Arnold-Chiari syndrome

32. This photomicrograph (Fig. 13.16) is most likely to be associated with which of the following?
    a. Neonate born by vaginal delivery
    b. Follows childhood exanthema
    c. Mosquito bite
    d. Targets the Purkinje cells and hippocampal pyramidal neurons
    e. None of the above

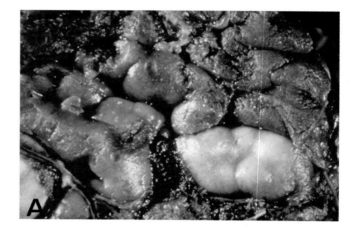

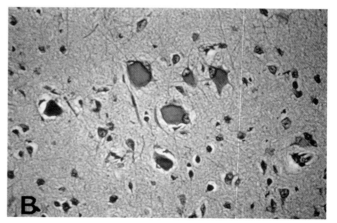

Figure 13.16

33. Which gene mutation is typically associated with the condition depicted in the gross photo (Fig. 13.17)?
    a. Sonic hedgehog
    b. *PTEN*
    c. *LIS*1
    d. *Notch*3
    e. Mutations in the regulatory domain of phenylalanine hydroxylase

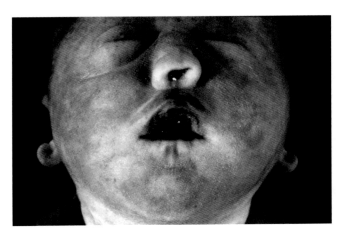

Figure 13.17

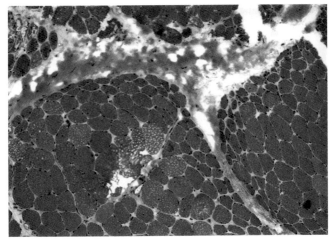

Figure 13.18

34. Which one of the following drug-induced myopathies is characterized by selective atrophy of histochemical type II fibers?
    a. Chloroquine
    b. HMG-CoA reductase inhibitors (or 'statins')
    c. Colchicine
    d. Phenytoin
    e. Methylprednisolone

35. Which one of the following does NOT apply to Duchenne muscular dystrophy?
    a. X-linked inheritance pattern
    b. Becker muscular dystrophy involves the same gene locus.
    c. Panfascicular atrophy is the characteristic histopathologic finding.
    d. Calf pseudohypertrophy
    e. Cardiomyopathy

36. All of the following statements apply to acute inflammatory demyelinating polyneuropathy or Guillain-Barré syndrome EXCEPT:
    a. Clinically, it is characterized by ascending paralysis
    b. Associated with *Campylobacter jejuni* infections
    c. Involves a B cell–mediated immune response
    d. Characterized by inflammation and demyelination

37. Which one of the following does NOT apply to type I myofibers?
    a. High in myoglobin and oxidative enzymes
    b. Stain darkly with adenosine triphosphatase (ATPase) at pH 4.2
    c. Are important for sudden movements
    d. Contain many mitochondria and wide Z–bands
    e. Are rich in mitochondria

38. This type of inflammatory myopathy has the highest risk of developing visceral cancer (Fig. 13.18). The diagnosis is most likely:
    a. Polymyositis
    b. Inclusion body myositis
    c. Juvenile dermatomyositis
    d. Dermatomyositis (adult type)
    e. Overlap syndrome

39. Which one of the following conditions is associated with mutations of the *Notch3* gene?
    a. Cerebral amyloid angiopathy
    b. Cerebral autosomal dominant arteriopathy with subcortical infarcts and leukoencephalopathy (CADASIL)
    c. Frontotemporal dementia with Parkinsonism
    d. Kearns-Sayre syndrome
    e. Holoprosencephaly

40. Which marker is the best for demonstrating the structures in this photomicrograph (Fig. 13.19)?
    a. Alpha-synuclein
    b. Ubiquitin
    c. Glial fibrillary acidic protein
    d. Tau proteins
    e. Transthyretin

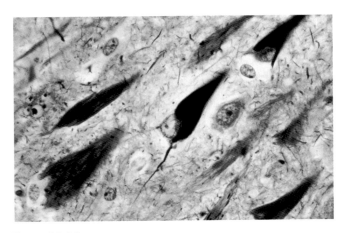

Figure 13.19

41. Which one of the following congenital myopathies is associated with an increased risk of malignant hyperthermia?
    a. Nemaline myopathy
    b. Myotubular myopathy
    c. Mitochondrial myopathy
    d. Central core disease
    e. Inclusion body myositis

42. Which one of the following structures is of similar structure and biochemical composition as corpora amylacea?
    a. Lafora bodies
    b. Negri bodies
    c. Bunina bodies
    d. Biondi bodies
    e. Psammoma bodies

43. Metachromatic leukodystrophy is due to a deficiency of which one of the following enzymes?
    a. β-galactosidase
    b. Arylsulfatase A
    c. Hexosaminidase A
    d. Nonspecific esterase
    e. Hexosaminidase AB

44. Subacute combined degeneration of the spinal cord is caused by which one of the following entities?
    a. Radiation injury
    b. P16 deletion
    c. Vitamin B12 deficiency
    d. Exposure to hexachlorophene in the nursery
    e. Vitamin B6 deficiency

45. In normal corneal architecture, what structure is situated just beneath the epithelial basement membrane?
    a. Descemet membrane
    b. Corneal stroma
    c. Corneal endothelium
    d. Bowman layer
    e. Schlemm canal

46. In which layer of the cornea is copper deposited in Wilson disease (hepatolenticular degeneration)?
    a. Descemet membrane
    b. Corneal stroma
    c. Corneal endothelium
    d. Bowman layer
    e. Retinal pigment epithelium

47. What is the most likely molecular genetic profile of the tumor in this photomicrograph (Fig. 13.20)?
    a. *SOD*1 gene mutation on chromosome 21
    b. 1p19q deletion
    c. 11q22-23 mutation
    d. 4p16.3 mutation
    e. 17q11 mutation

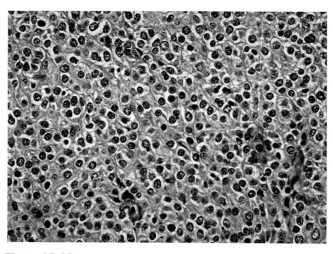

Figure 13.20

48. Which one of the following does NOT apply to HIV meningoencephalitis?
    a. HIV can be detected in CD4-positive mononuclear and multinucleated macrophages and microglia.
    b. Microglial nodules are present.
    c. Multinucleated giant cells are seen.
    d. Multifocal, patchy demyelination.
    e. Micronecrosis is present.

49. In the case of traumatic injury to the brain, diffuse axonal injury is most commonly found in which of the following regions of the brain?
    a. Corpus callosum
    b. Paraventricular and parahippocampal areas
    c. Globus pallidus
    d. Cerebellum

50. Which one of the following is the primary constituent of Z-bands in skeletal muscle?
    a. Myosin
    b. α-actinin
    c. Dystrophin
    d. Sarcoglycan
    e. Myotilin

51. Which one of the following diseases is most likely to be associated with "onion bulbs," indicative of a hypertrophic neuropathy?
    a. Refsum disease
    b. Neuropathic beri-beri
    c. Paraneoplastic neuropathy
    d. Uremic neuropathy
    e. Alcoholic neuropathy

52. Name the most likely diagnosis associated with this coronal section of brain (Fig. 13.21) from a 49-year-old alcoholic man found deceased under a bridge:
    a. Blunt force trauma to the brain
    b. Thiamin deficiency

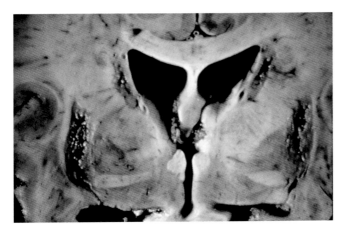

Figure 13.21

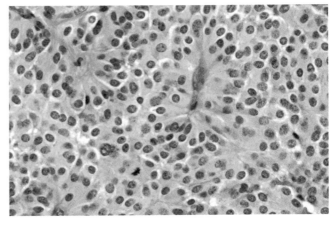

Figure 13.22

c. B12 deficiency
d. Methanol toxicity
e. Vitamin B6 deficiency

53. All of the following entities may be associated with Rosenthal fiber formation EXCEPT:
   a. Craniopharyngioma
   b. Pilocytic astrocytoma
   c. Anaplastic astrocytoma
   d. Alexander disease

54. Which one of the following inclusions is seen in herpetic encephalitis?
   a. Cowdry B
   b. Cowdry A
   c. Renaud body
   d. Biondi body
   e. Bunina body

55. Which of the following conditions may be associated with cerebellar atrophy?
   a. Kernicterus
   b. Chronic alcoholism
   c. Rabies
   d. Reye syndrome

56. A 4-year-old girl presented with nausea and ataxia. A brain biopsy was undertaken; the biopsy photomicrograph (Fig. 13.22) corresponds to which diagnosis?
   a. Medulloblastoma
   b. Pineocytoma
   c. Central neurocytoma
   d. Ependymoma
   e. Oligodendroglioma

57. All the following conditions EXCEPT one are associated with axonal neuropathy?
   a. Thiamine deficiency
   b. Vitamin B₁₂ deficiency

c. Diphtheria toxin
d. Excessive ethanol consumption
e. HMG-CoA reductase inhibitors (or 'statins')

58. The finding in this Gomori-trichrome stained photomicrograph (Fig. 13.23) is suggestive of which one of the following disorders?
   a. Mitochondrial myopathy
   b. Vasculitis
   c. Viral infection
   d. Dysferlinopathy
   e. Tubular aggregate myopathy

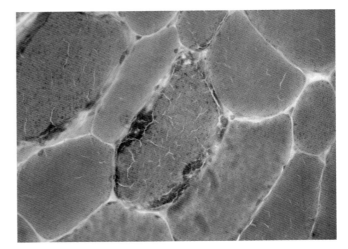

Figure 13.23

59. Microglia are specialized mesoderm-derived cells that typically express which one of the following markers?
   a. GFAP
   b. Neurofilament proteins
   c. CD68
   d. Epithelial membrane antigen (EMA)
   e. CD117 (c-kit)

60. This GFAP-stained section represents a biopsy from a 35-year-old woman who presented with a "mass lesion" noted on MRI scans (Fig. 13.24). What is your diagnosis?
    a. Reactive gliosis
    b. Low-grade astrocytoma
    c. Glioblastoma multiforme
    d. Normal brain
    e. Viral encephalitis

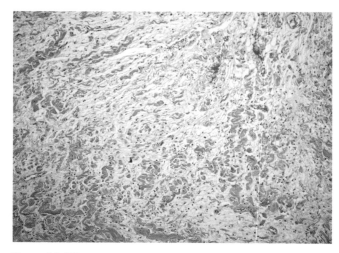

Figure 13.25

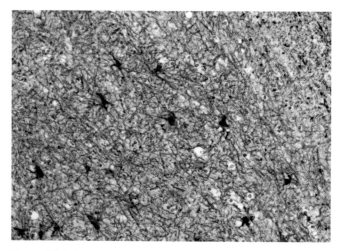

Figure 13.24

61. Alzheimer type II astrocytes are most likely to be encountered in which one of the following conditions?
    a. Lead encephalopathy
    b. Blunt force trauma to the brain
    c. Hepatic encephalopathy
    d. Telencephalic leukoencephalopathy
    e. Carbon monoxide poisoning

62. Subacute sclerosing panencephalitis, a rare disease seen in children and young adults, is thought to be caused by an altered form of which one of the following organisms?
    a. HTLV-1
    b. *Listeria monocytogenes*
    c. Mumps virus
    d. Measles virus
    e. Herpes I

63. Which inherited disease is most likely to be associated with this photomicrograph (Fig. 13.25)?
    a. Tuberous sclerosis
    b. von Hippel-Lindau disease
    c. Neurofibromatosis I (von Recklinghausen disease)
    d. Neurofibromatosis II
    e. Ataxia telangiectasia

64. Which of the following conditions refers to a whitish-yellow, submucosal elevation on the conjunctiva that does NOT invade the cornea?
    a. Staphyloma
    b. Pinguecula
    c. Pterygium
    d. Bullous keratopathy
    e. Coat disease

65. What type of rosette is most commonly seen in this tumor (Fig. 13.26)?
    a. Perivascular pseudorosette
    b. Flexner-Wintersteiner
    c. Pineocytomatous
    d. Homer-Wright
    e. True ependymal rosette

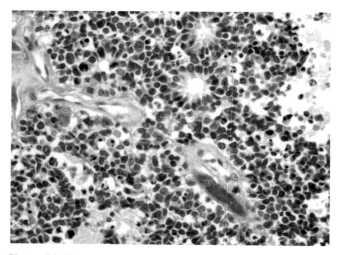

Figure 13.26

66. After swimming in a local freshwater pond, a 15-year-old youth developed altered mental status and drifted into a coma. What is the most likely diagnosis for the biopsy depicted in the photomicrograph (Fig. 13.27)?
   a. Multiple sclerosis
   b. Toxoplasmosis
   c. Necrotizing amebic meningoencephalitis
   d. Cryptococcal meningitis
   e. Granulomatous amebic meningoencephalitis

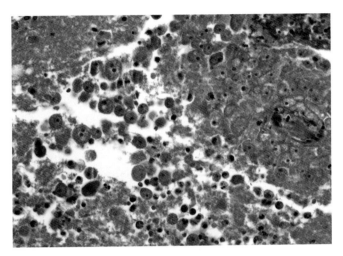

Figure 13.27

67. This 43-year-old diabetic woman presented to the emergency room with a history of headaches for a month. What is the most likely etiology based on this photomicrograph of a Gomori–methenamine silver (GMS)-stained section (Fig. 13.28)?
   a. *Actinomyces* sp.
   b. *Aspergillus* sp.
   c. Zygomycosis (mucormycosis)
   d. Blastomycosis
   e. Coccidioidomycosis

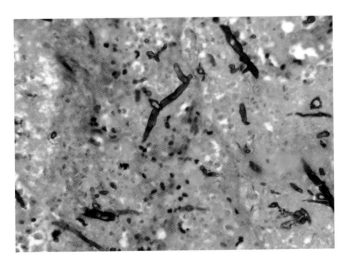

Figure 13.28

68. What is the grade of this tumor (Fig. 13.29) according to the World Health Organization classification of tumors of the nervous system?
   a. Grade 1
   b. Grade 2
   c. Grade 3
   d. Grade 4
   e. None of the above

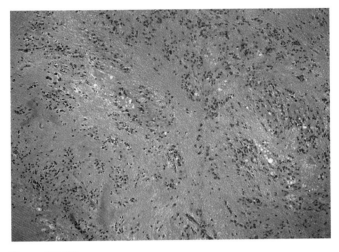

Figure 13.29

69. This 47-year-old man with a past medical history of a renal transplant presented with a 6-month history of dementia, weakness, and visual loss. A brain biopsy was taken (Fig. 13.30). Based on the photomicrograph, what is the most likely diagnosis?
   a. Anaplastic astrocytoma
   b. Acute demyelinating leukoencephalopathy
   c. Pleomorphic xanthoastrocytoma
   d. Progressive multifocal leukoencephalopathy (PML)
   e. Neurosyphilis

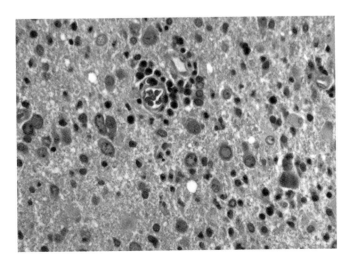

Figure 13.30

70. The tumor shown in the photomicrograph (Fig. 13.31) was removed from the posterior fossa of a 4-year-old child. What molecular genetic abnormality should be evaluated to establish the diagnosis?
    a. Deletion of at least one copy of the *INI1* gene on chromosome 22q
    b. LOH of 1p19q
    c. Translocation 1:14
    d. *PTEN* mutation
    e. Monosomy for chromosome 22

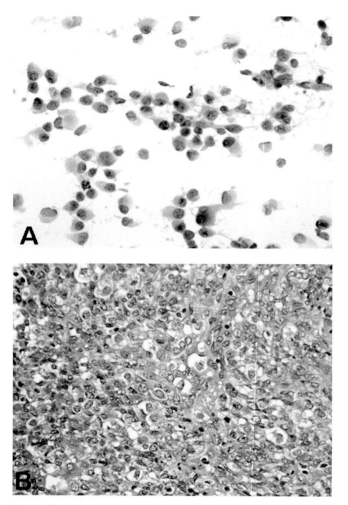

Figure 13.31

■ Answers

1. **d. Hemangioblastoma** is a hypercellular, vascular tumor containing foamy interstitial cells, which represent the actual neoplastic element. Hemangioblastomas occur most commonly in the cerebellum and are often associated with **von Hippel-Lindau syndrome.** Subependymal giant cell astrocytoma is an intraventricular tumor (lateral ventricles) resembling gemistocytic astrocytoma that is usually seen in the context of tuberous sclerosis. Pilocytic astrocytomas are biphasic neoplasms composed of alternating areas of compact spindle cells and more loosely textured zones and often accompanied by Rosenthal fibers.

2. **b.** Acute hypoxic/ischemic injury is associated (if the patient survives at least six hours) with shrunken eosinophilic neurons. Certain populations of neurons are selectively vulnerable, especially large neurons in **CA1 sector of the hippocampus,** the Purkinje cells of the cerebellum, and neurons of layers 3 through 5 of the cerebral cortex. Neurofibrillary tangles, granulovacuolar degeneration, and Hirano bodies are neurodegenerative changes. CA2 is the so-called "resistant zone" of the hippocampus that is less vulnerable to hypoxia/ischemia.

3. **d. Berry aneurysms** involving the circle of Willis are uncommon in children. The photomicrograph shows the basilar aspect of the brain with a berry aneurysm at the trifurcation. The risk of rupture, which produces hemorrhage into the subarachnoid space at the base of the brain, is greatest for females in the fifth decade.

4. **e. Lewy bodies** are inclusion bodies found in **Parkinson disease** and diffuse Lewy body disease. In pure Parkinson disease, Lewy bodies are located predominantly in the pigmented neurons in the substantia nigra (as depicted in the photomicrograph) and locus ceruleus, whereas in diffuse Lewy body disease, they are also found in the cerebral cortex.

5. **b. Medulloblastoma** and **ependymoma** are the second and third most common primary central nervous system (CNS) neoplasms in children. Histopathologically, medulloblastomas are densely cellular "small blue cell" tumors that typically contain frequent mitoses and apoptotic nuclei, and sometimes frank necrosis. Ependymomas are glial neoplasms that are usually recognized by the presence of perivascular pseudorosettes. Overall, low-grade astrocytomas are the most common. In very young children, medulloblastoma is more common than astrocytic neoplasms. Glioblastoma multiforme and metastatic disease are extremely uncommon in children and are much more likely to occur in the over-60 population.

6. **c.** The gross photo shows a midsagittal section of brain with a large mass in the region of the posterior third ventricle. The most common entity in this location in children is a **pineal germinoma. Parinaud syndrome** is associated with dorsal midbrain (pineal region) lesions and is characterized by vertical gaze palsy, convergence-retraction nystagmus, and light-near dissociation. Seizures are typically related to cortical lesions, and hemiballismus occurs with lesions of the subthalamic nucleus. Cortical blindness is seen with bilateral impairment of the posterior occipital lobes, especially those lesions that involve the calcarine fissures bilaterally.

7. **e.** Damage to axons, also termed **diffuse axonal injury (DAI)** or traumatic axonal injury (TAI), is an almost universal finding in cases of mild, moderate, and severe head trauma. Although not specific for trauma, **β-amyloid precursor protein (β-APP)** is a useful stain for highlighting axonal spheroids.

8. **e. Huntington disease** is a rare autosomal dominant inherited disease with a mutation in the IT15 gene, located on **chromosome 4,** which alters the huntingtin protein. There are increased CAG tandem repeat sequences in the gene. The gross photo shows a coronal section of brain with bilateral effacement of the caudate nucleus. Choreiform movement and not echolalia characterize the disease. Echolalia is more common in autism.

9. **a.** In cases of idiopathic **Parkinson disease,** the brain shows pallor of the substantia nigra and locus ceruleus accompanied by neuronal loss, extracellular pigment, and gliosis. The remaining neurons may contain Lewy bodies, which are eosinophilic cytoplasmic structures. Ultrastructurally, Lewy bodies are composed of filaments that form the densely packed core. These filaments are made of **alpha-synuclein,** a lipid-binding protein that can be demonstrated by immunohistochemical methods (image b).

10. **c. Cerebral amyloid angiopathy** is the most common cause of lobar hemorrhage in the elderly. The amyloidogenic proteins, nearly the same as those found in Alzheimer disease, are deposited in meningeal and cerebral vessels, thus weakening their walls and predisposing to hemorrhage.

11. **e. Carbon monoxide poisoning** typically affects both **globus pallidi** and chronic lesions are cavitary.

12. **a. Cerebral malaria** is not caused by *P. ovale,* but by *Plasmodium falciparum,* which infects red blood cells, causing them to clump together (rosetting) and stick to endothelial cells (sequestration). Accordingly, cerebral blood vessels are plugged with parasitized red blood cells containing dots of hemozoin pigment, which leads to stasis and tissue hypoxia. This sets the stage for ring hemorrhages and small collections of inflammatory cells known as **Dürck granulomas.**

13. **e.** All of these statements apply to the diagnosis of **multiple sclerosis.** The photomicrograph shows a sharply demarcated focus of demyelination (myelin pallor) adjacent to the anterior horn of the lateral ventricle in a section stained for myelin.

14. **c. Creutzfeldt-Jacob disease** is a form of spongiform encephalopathy thought to be caused by prions that manifest clinically by rapidly progressive dementia.

The spongiform change is particularly prominent in the cerebral cortex or gray matter of the brain. Accumulation of the abnormal beta-pleated sheet isoform, termed PrP^{sc} for PrP (*p*rotease resistant) and (*sc*rapie) is considered responsible for the pathogenesis of this disease.

15. **b. Glioblastoma multiforme** is an extremely heterogeneous tumor characterized by varying degrees of increased cellularity, pleomorphism, mitoses, endothelial proliferation, and necrosis. **Pseudopalisading necrosis** shown in the photomicrograph is a common feature. Amplification of epidermal growth factor receptor (EGFR) typically indicates a primary (de novo) glioblastoma multiforme, whereas its absence suggests a secondary glioblastoma.

16. **a.** The gross photo shows a dural-based meningioma and not **glioblastoma multiforme,** the most common primary brain tumor in adults.

17. **e.**

18. **d. Cataracts** represent lenticular opacities. Primary closed angle glaucoma develops in eyes with shallow anterior chambers.

19. **c. Vein of Galen aneurysm** is a rare congenital malformation of blood vessels that results in high-output congestive heart failure or may present with developmental delay, hydrocephalus, and seizures. The vein of Galen drains the anterior and central regions of the brain into the sinuses of the posterior cerebral fossa.

20. **b. Transtentorial or mesial temporal herniation** occurs when the medial aspect of the temporal lobe is compressed against the tentorium cerebelli. When this occurs, displacement of the temporal lobe compromises the third cranial nerve, resulting in pupillary dilatation and impaired ocular movements.

21. **b. Epidural hematoma** typically results from trauma, especially fractures, to the skull in the region of the temporal bone that lead to laceration of the middle meningeal artery. This tear results in accumulation of blood under arterial pressure. Patients classically present with a lucid interval followed by rapid decline; immediate neurosurgical intervention is essential to drain the hemorrhage.

22. **c. Arnold Chiari malformation (Chiari type II)** is a condition in which the cerebellar tonsils and medulla oblongata protrude through the foramen, blocking the flow of cerebrospinal fluid. It is usually accompanied by a myelomeningocele.

23. **a.** Acute onset of **demyelinating diseases** can mimic neoplasms clinically and radiographically. This cytologic preparation demonstrates foamy macrophages, which are not typically seen in neoplastic conditions. The young age of the patient would also be unusual in metastatic disease.

24. **a. Malignant peripheral nerve sheath tumors** are malignant sarcomas that arise de novo or from plexiform neurofibromas, but not from schwannomas.

25. **a. Central retinal artery occlusion** is caused by atherosclerosis, which predisposes to thrombosis or embolism from fragments of atheromatous plaques. It may cause a cherry red spot.

26. **b. Pick disease** is a rare form of dementia characterized clinically by early-onset behavioral and personality changes. In addition to lobar atrophy, at the microscopic level, **argyrophilic Pick bodies** are characteristic and can be found in cortical neurons and the dentate gyrus of the hippocampus.

27. **c. Contusions** typically develop along the crest of the gyrus, whereas infarcts are centered at the base.

28. **b. Rabies** is a frequently fatal viral encephalitis that is transmitted to humans by the bite of an infected animal (often raccoons, dogs, or bats). Microscopic examination of the brain reveals neuronal degeneration and inflammation, especially in the rhombencephalon. **Negri bodies,** round eosinophilic cytoplasmic inclusions measuring 1–7 μm, typically found in Purkinje cells of the cerebellum or hippocampal neurons are pathognomonic of rabies.

29. **d. Herpes encephalitis,** caused by herpes simplex virus type 1 (HSV-1), affects infants, children, and adults. Although diffuse, brain involvement is concentrated in the **temporal and frontal lobes** and manifests as hemorrhage and necrosis.

30. **b. Lhermitte-Duclos disease,** also known as dysplastic gangliocytoma of the cerebellum, is thought to represent a hamartomatous growth of the cerebellum. It is one of the recognized manifestations of Cowden syndrome, an autosomal dominant multiple hamartoma syndrome that results most commonly (80%) from a mutation in the *PTEN* gene on arm 10q.

31. **d. Dandy-Walker malformation** occurs more frequently in females than in males and may be associated with a large number of concomitant developmental problems. Of uncertain etiology, the disorder arises during embryogenesis. Predisposing factors include gestational (first trimester) exposure to rubella, cytomegalovirus, toxoplasmosis, warfarin, alcohol, and isotretinoin.

32. **a.** In neonates, brain involvement with **herpes encephalitis** is diffuse, and the usual cause is herpes simplex virus type 2 (HSV-2), which is acquired at the time of delivery.

33. **a. Holoprosencephaly** is the most common developmental anomaly of the human forebrain, and in its most severe form, the cerebral hemispheres fail to completely separate into two distinct halves. Mutations in **sonic hedgehog signaling** are thought to underlie the majority of cases. Affected infants often exhibit severe facial dysmorphism as depicted in the photograph.

34. **e.** Clinically, **steroid myopathy** is associated with proximal weakness and atrophy. Histopathologically, the most common finding is type II myofiber atrophy, a nonspecific alteration, encountered most often in dis-

use atrophy, conditions associated with hypercortisolism, and a variety of collagen-vascular diseases.

35. c. **Panfascicular atrophy** is characteristic of spinal muscular atrophy and not Duchenne or Becker atrophy, which consists of variation in myofiber size, increased endomysial connective tissue, and regenerating fibers.

36. c. **Guillain-Barré syndrome** is an autoimmune-mediated disease involving T cells, is the most common cause of acute motor paralysis in children, and usually follows a febrile and/or viral illness. In epidemics associated with *C. jejuni* infection, many patients are found to have antiglycolipid antibodies. Because these cases involve degeneration of peripheral motor axons without much inflammation, the syndrome has been termed acute motor axonal neuropathy (AMAN).

37. c. **Type 1 myofibers** represent the so-called "red" muscle needed for sustained movements.

38. d. **Dermatomyositis in adults** is associated with a 40% increased risk of visceral cancer. The photomicrograph shows perifascicular atrophy, a common finding in dermatomyositis.

39. b. **Cerebral autosomal dominant arteriopathy with subcortical infarcts and leukoencephalopathy (CADASIL)** is the most common cause of stroke and vascular dementia due to a single mutation. **NOTCH3** encodes a cell surface receptor, which has a role in arterial development and is expressed on vascular smooth muscle cells.

40. d. **Neurofibrillary tangles** are abnormal collections of twisted threads of axonal microtubule-associated protein found inside neurons. They are often basket- or flame-shaped and are highlighted by silver (Bielschowsky) staining (seen in this photomicrograph) or tau immunostaining.

41. d. **Central core disease** is a congenital myopathy that is usually transmitted in an autosomal dominant fashion with variable expression and incomplete penetrance (rare autosomal recessive and sporadic cases) and is almost always due to a mutation in the ryanodine receptor 1 (*RYR1*). **Malignant hyperthermia** susceptibility is associated with this mutation.

42. a. **Lafora bodies** are round, basophilic, PAS-positive inclusions that are seen in neurons and other cells in myoclonic epilepsy of Unverricht. They are identical to corpora amylacea or **polyglucosan bodies**.

43. b. **Metachromatic leukodystrophy (MLD)** is an autosomal recessive lysosomal storage disease that is associated with central and peripheral myelination abnormalities, widespread loss of myelinated oligodendroglia, and the accumulation of metachromatic granules within macrophages. Some patients with clinical MLD have normal **arylsulfatase A** activity but lack an activator protein that is involved in sulfatide degradation. Both defects result in the accumulation of sulfatide compounds in neural and in nonneural tissue, such as the kidneys and gallbladder.

44. c. **Subacute combined degeneration** of the posterior columns of the **spinal cord** is secondary to **vitamin B12 deficiency**.

45. d. The corneal epithelium rests on a collagenous membrane (Bowman membrane). Beneath this layer is the corneal structure, which lies on the Descemet membrane. The innermost layer is the endothelium.

46. a. **Wilson disease** is a rare autosomal recessive disorder of copper metabolism. In this condition, excessive deposition of copper occurs in the liver, brain, and other tissues, notably, in the **Descemet membrane** of the corneal limbus. The genetic defect, localized to chromosome arm 13q, has been shown to affect the copper-transporting adenosine triphosphatase (ATPase) gene (*ATP7B*) in the liver.

47. b. **Oligodendrogliomas** have demonstrated recurrent combined **loss of chromosome 1p/19q**, which represents a favorable prognosis marker and probably a predictor of a good chemosensitivity of the tumor.

48. d. **HIV encephalitis** is a subacute encephalitis involving the white matter is seen in up to 30% of patients with AIDS related to direct invasion of neurons by the neurotropic retrovirus, human immunodeficiency virus type I (HIV). The pathologic hallmarks are **microglial nodules and multinucleate giant cells**. Multifocal, patchy demyelination is a feature of progressive multifocal leukoencephalopathy.

49. a–c. Axonal spheroids are round structures that occur when axons have been damaged by mechanical ("**diffuse axonal injury**") or other forces that disrupt axonal integrity.

50. b. Electron microscopy of skeletal muscle demonstrates dark bands called **Z** bands that separate the repeating units of the sarcomere. Immunolabeling with **alpha-actinin** is concentrated at **Z bands**. Actin, tropomyosin, and troponin were detected along the thin filaments, whereas myosin and paramyosin were localized along the thick filaments.

51. a. **Refsum disease** is an autosomal recessive neurologic disease that results in the malformation of myelin sheaths around nerve cells. Repeated episodes of demyelination and remyelination result in the formation of large onion bulbs in HMSN types IB and III (Dejerine-Sottas), CIDP, and Refsum disease.

52. d. The ingestion of **methanol**, also known as wood alcohol, results in metabolic acidosis, neurologic sequelae, and even death. Methanol is transformed to formaldehyde via the enzyme alcohol dehydrogenase (ADH), then to formic acid, which damages the retrolaminar optic nerve with intra-axonal swelling and organelle destruction. With severe intoxication, common problems are hemorrhagic and nonhemorrhagic damage of the **putamen**. The pathogenesis is unknown.

53. c. **Rosenthal fibers** are irregular, brightly eosinophilic structures that contain heat shock proteins and ubiquitin and can be found in a number of both neoplastic and

nonneoplastic conditions. The most familiar setting is pilocytic astrocytoma, but the nonneoplastic tissue surrounding craniopharyngioma may exhibit dense, "piloid gliosis" with Rosenthal fibers. **Alexander disease** is a rare, sporadic dysmyelinating disease linked to missense mutations in the coding region of the GFAP gene. Rosenthal fibers are found in abundance in periventricular, perivascular, and subpial locations.

54. **b. Cowdry A inclusions** are eosinophilic intranuclear inclusions that may be surrounded by a halo. They are seen in herpes simplex virus (HSV), cytomegalovirus (CMV), and measles infections. Cowdry B inclusions are nonspecific, often multiple, small, and do not exhibit a halo. Poliomyelitis is an example.

55. **b. Ethanol** and certain anticonvulsant medications (such as **phenytoin** and carbamazepine) are cerebellar toxins.

56. **d. Ependymomas** are glial neoplasms characterized by the presence of **perivascular pseudorosettes**. They represent the third most common brain tumor in children, with up to 70% occurring in the posterior fossa. In general, ependymomas arise within, or adjacent to, the ependymal lining of the ventricular system or the central canal of the spinal cord.

57. **c.** The exotoxin produced by *Corynebacterium diphtheriae* is associated with a **demyelinating neuropathy** that typically begins in the paranodal regions of the nerve.

58. **a.** In **mitochondrial** myopathies, Gomori trichrome-stained sections reveal "ragged-red fibers" on light microscopy; these structure represent large, irregularly shaped mitochondria that may contain the so-called "parking lot inclusions" on electron microscopy.

59. **c.** Microglia serve as fixed macrophages within the central nervous and therefore are expected to stain with a variety of macrophage markers such as CD68.

60. **a.** The astrocytes seen in **reactive** conditions have small, regular nuclei and radially arranged slender processes. The cells are evenly distributed and maintain their distance from adjacent cells. In contrast, the constituent cellular elements in astrocytomas are crowded, show tortuous processes, and contain irregularly contoured, hyperchromatic nuclei.

61. **c. Alzheimer type II gliosis** is typically seen in **hyperammonemic states**, such as those seen in hepatic disease. These cells typically lack cytoplasm and exhibit a large clear nucleus, a prominent nucleolus, and margination of chromatin.

62. **d. Subacute sclerosing panencephalitis (SSPE)** is a form of chronic encephalitis of childhood and young adolescence due to **persistent measles virus** infection of the central nervous system. The disease generally occurs 5–10 years after measles infection. In the early stages of the disease, behavioral and personality changes is followed by myoclonic jerks and convul-

sions. The most commonly involved areas in SSPE are periventricular and subcortical white matter.

63. **c.** The photomicrograph is from a **plexiform neurofibroma**, an entity that arises in individuals who lose the wild-type copy of the NF-1 gene on chromosome 17. Neurofibromas are composed of spindle-shaped fibroblasts and Schwann embedded in a collagen-rich, loose myxoid stroma.

64. **b.** A **pterygium** is a fleshy growth that invades the cornea, whereas a pinguecula does not. Both entities are related to solar injury.

65. **b. Retinoblastoma** is the most common primary ocular malignancy of childhood that has been linked to a mutation in the long arm of chromosome 13 (band 13q14). Over 90% of cases occur before 5 years of age. The presence of **Flexner-Wintersteiner** rosettes is a characteristic histopathologic feature of this type of primitive neuroectodermal tumor. These rosettes consist of embryonal cells with high nuclear to cytoplasmic ratios surrounding a membrane-lined lumen.

66. **c. Necrotizing amebic meningoencephalitis** is a fulminating illness caused by *Naegleria* species. Most cases present in children and young adults in summer or fall. The infection is acquired by swimming in warm pools or lakes.

67. **c.** Diabetes mellitus is the predisposing condition in the majority of patients with cerebral form of **zygomycosis**. Pathologic examination often reveals necrotic/infarcted tissue with neutrophilic infiltration with broad nonseptate hyphae (**Mucor**) showing irregular branching. The outcome is usually poor despite surgical excision and antifungal therapy.

68. **a. Subependymoma** is a WHO grade I tumor variant of ependymoma that is most commonly an incidental finding at autopsy. When symptomatic, it usually presents with signs and symptoms of increased intracranial pressure. The most common location is within the posterior fossa, or less frequently, more anteriorly in the ventricular system. Microscopically, these tumors are characterized by small collections of bland, oval cells against a highly fibrillated background.

69. **d. Progressive multifocal leukoencephalopathy (PML)** is characterized by multifocal demyelination caused by the **JC virus**, a member of the papova group. The infection is acquired early in life and reactivated after immunosuppression, such as immunosuppressive medication form transplantation, leukemia/lymphoma, and HIV. Microscopically, the viral inclusions are seen within oligodendrocytes and result in enlarged cells with marginated chromatin. Bizarre-appearing, reactive astrocytes are a common feature.

70. **a. Atypical teratoid rhabdoid (AT/RT)** tumor is a highly malignant neoplasm related histologically and molecularly to rhabdoid tumor of the kidney and other extra-renal, non-CNS counterparts. Almost all

patients are below the age of 2 years. The tumor occurs throughout the CNS with the most frequent location the posterior fossa. The typical lesion is composed of cells with abundant pink cytoplasm (rhabdoid cells), round or reniform, eccentric nuclei, and prominent nucleoli ("a" panel). Many tumors show foci of cells with cytoplasmic clearing (as depicted in the "b" photomicrograph). The tumor cells are diffusely positive for vimentin and focally positive for epithelial membrane antigen (EMA). **Mutation or loss of the *INI1* locus at 22q11.2 is the genetic hallmark of AT/RT.**

■ Recommended Readings

Ellison D, Leila Chimelli L, Harding B, et al. *Neuropathology: a reference text of CNS pathology*. Philadelphia: Mosby, 2003.

Kumar V, Fausto N, Abbas A. *Robbins and Cotran pathologic basis of disease*, 7th ed. Philadelphia: Elsevier, 2004.

Love S, Louis DN, Ellison DW. *Greenfield's neuropathology*, 8th ed. Oxford, England: Oxford University Press, 2008.

PART
II

Clinical Pathology

14

Medical Microbiology and Immunology

Steven D. Mahlen, Elmer W. Koneman, Christopher J. Papasian, and Rangaraj Selvarangan

■ Questions

1. A 2-week-old neonate was brought to the emergency department with probable meningitis. A lumbar puncture was performed, with the following cerebrospinal fluid (CSF) labs: normal glucose, high protein, and pleocytosis with neutrophilic predominance. No organisms were observed on a Gram stain of the CSF. On culture the following day, however, there were many regular, short, non–spore-forming Gram-positive rods on both sheep blood agar and chocolate agar. The organisms were softly beta-hemolytic on blood agar and catalase positive. A Gram stain of the organism from a colony is shown in Figure 14.1. What is the likely identification of this isolate?

   a. *Streptococcus agalactiae*
   b. *Erysipelothrix rhusiopathiae*
   c. *Listeria monocytogenes*
   d. *Corynebacterium jeikeium*
   e. *Bacillus cereus*

2. An uninoculated triple sugar iron (TSI) agar slant is shown in Figure 14.2A. What is the most appropriate description of the inoculated TSI agar slant shown in Figure 14.2B?

   a. Sugar(s) utilized: glucose only; H_2S production: negative; gas production: positive
   b. Sugar(s) utilized: glucose, lactose, and/or sucrose; H_2S production: negative; gas production: positive
   c. Sugar(s) utilized: glucose, lactose, and/or sucrose; H_2S production: positive; gas production: positive
   d. Sugar(s) utilized: glucose and lactose only; H_2S production: negative; gas production: positive
   e. Sugar(s) utilized: glucose and sucrose only; H_2S production: negative; gas production: positive

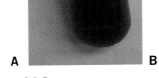

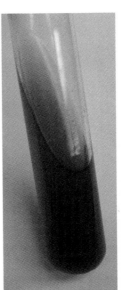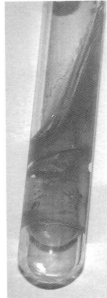

Figure 14.1

Figure 14.2

3. A male patient from southeast India presents with large, painless ulcerative genital lesions and a beefy red penile lesion that has not healed in 6 months. A Wrights stain of a biopsy specimen reveals bipolar-staining rods in macrophages. Bacterial cultures of the biopsy specimen are negative. What is the likely causative agent of these lesions?
   a. *Haemophilus ducreyi*
   b. *Chlamydia trachomatis*
   c. *Treponema pallidum*
   d. *Klebsiella granulomatis*
   e. *Neisseria gonorrhoeae*

4. Which of the following rapid tests best differentiates members of the genus *Staphylococcus* from members of the genus *Streptococcus*?
   a. Catalase
   b. Oxidase
   c. Indole
   d. Coagulase
   e. Pyrase

5. Methicillin resistance in staphylococci:
   a. is encoded by *mecA*
   b. is best detected by disc diffusion by using a cefoxitin disc
   c. means that all β-lactam antibiotics cannot be used for therapy
   d. is enabled by an alteration in the target of β-lactam antibiotics
   e. all of the above

6. How is *Chlamydia trachomatis* typically cultivated?
   a. On standard bacteriologic culture media, such as sheep blood agar
   b. In MRC-5 cells
   c. Coculture of infected peripheral blood mononuclear cells (PBMCs) with activated, allogeneic, noninfected PBMCs
   d. In McCoy cells
   e. In LLC-MK$_2$ cells

7. An oxidase-positive, curved gram–negative rod is isolated on thiosulfate citrate bile salts sucrose (TCBS) agar from a patient with gastroenteritis. The patient had eaten improperly cooked seafood. The isolate is shown in Figure 14.3B on TCBS agar, and an uninoculated TCBS agar plate is shown in Figure 14.3A. A Gram stain of the organism from a colony is shown in Figure 14.3C. What is the most likely identification of the isolate?
   a. *Campylobacter jejuni*
   b. *Plesiomonas shigelloides*
   c. *Vibrio cholerae*
   d. *Vibrio parahaemolyticus*
   e. *Shigella dysenteriae*

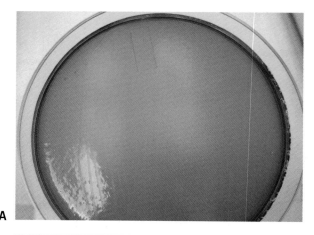

A

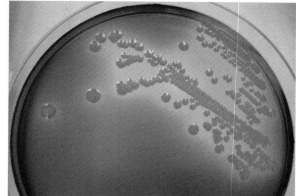

B

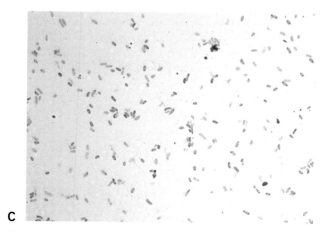

C

Figure 14.3

8. A patient is seen in the emergency department with a wound infection on his right hand. He had been in a fight a few days ago and suffered a clenched fist injury on the same hand when he struck someone else in the face. A wound culture is submitted to the laboratory, and small, Gram-negative coccobacilli are observed on both sheep blood agar and chocolate agar after 48 hours. The colonies are small, pit the agar, and smell like bleach; colonies are shown on sheep blood agar in Figure 14.4. The isolate is oxidase positive, indole negative, and did not grow on

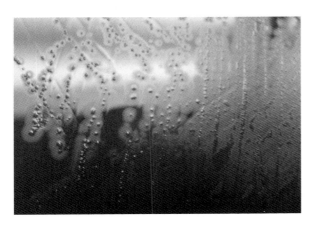

Figure 14.4

MacConkey agar. What is the likely identity of the isolate?
a. *Eikenella corrodens*
b. *Cardiobacterium hominis*
c. *Pasteurella multocida*
d. *Pseudomonas aeruginosa*
e. *Haemophilus influenzae*

9. Based on the sputum Gram stain from a patient with pneumonia shown in Figure 14.5, which of the following genera most likely would NOT be in the differential?
a. *Mycobacterium*
b. *Gordonia*
c. *Nocardia*
d. *Arcanobacterium*
e. *Tsukamurella*

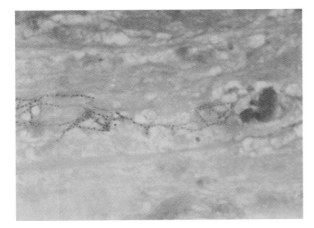

Figure 14.5

10. Mutations in which of the following gene products may be responsible for fluoroquinolone resistance in bacteria?
a. Penicillin–binding protein 2
b. DNA gyrase
c. Dihydrofolate reductase
d. DNA polymerase
e. RNA polymerase

11. An anaerobic, pale-staining, pleomorphic Gram-negative rod is isolated from a patient with an intra-abdominal abscess. Growth of the isolate in the presence of kanamycin (K disk), colistin (Cl disk), and vancomycin (Va disk), and 20% bile (no marking) is shown in Figure 14.6. What is the most likely identity of the isolate?
a. *Fusobacterium nucleatum* subsp. *nucleatum*
b. *Bacteroides fragilis*
c. *Prevotella bivia*
d. *Fusobacterium necrophorum* subsp. *necrophorum*
e. *Bilophila wadsworthia*

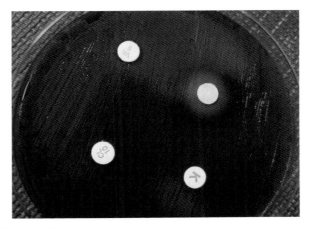

Figure 14.6

12. A faintly staining Gram-negative rod was isolated on buffered charcoal yeast extract (BCYE) agar from a patient with community-acquired pneumonia. The colonies were white in color, as shown in Figure 14.7, and took 4 days to grow. The isolate was biochemically inert. A direct Gram stain of sputum from the patient revealed 3+ white blood cells and no bacteria.

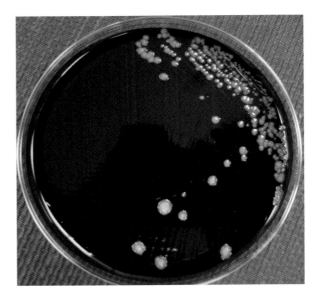

Figure 14.7

Based on this information, what is the likely identity of this isolate?

a. *Pseudomonas aeruginosa*
b. *Bordetella pertussis*
c. *Legionella pneumophila*
d. *Stenotrophomonas maltophilia*
e. *Burkholderia pseudomallei*

13. A catalase-positive, coagulase-negative Gram-positive coccus is isolated from a clean catch urine sample from a female with symptoms of a urinary tract infection. The isolate is PYR test negative and resistant to novobiocin. The organism is shown on sheep blood agar in Figure 14.8. What is the most likely identity of the isolate given the list below?

a. *Enterococcus faecalis*
b. *Staphylococcus aureus*
c. *Staphylococcus epidermidis*
d. *Staphylococcus saprophyticus*
e. *Streptococcus agalactiae*

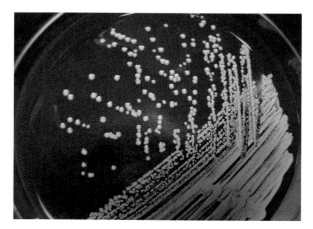

Figure 14.8

14. Which of the following statements about the Venereal Disease Research Laboratory (VDRL) test is correct?

a. It is a serologic assay designed to detect treponemal antibodies.
b. It is the confirmatory assay for a positive rapid plasma reagin (RPR) test.
c. It has the highest sensitivity for primary syphilis.
d. It is a nontreponemal assay that requires microscopic examination.
e. All of the above are correct statements.

15. An acid-fast bacillus is observed in a tissue specimen from a patient with a postoperative leg wound infection. The organism grows in 4 days on a Lowenstein-Jensen agar slant and colonies are buff colored in both light and dark conditions (Fig. 14.9). This growth pattern is most typical of which of the following organisms?

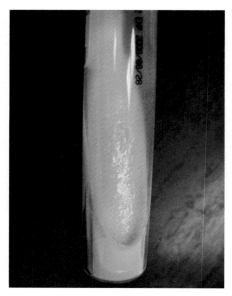

Figure 14.9

a. *Mycobacterium marinum*
b. *Mycobacterium chelonae*
c. *Mycobacterium gordonae*
d. *Mycobacterium ulcerans*
e. *Mycobacterium kansasii*

16. A young man develops a macular skin rash on his abdomen and chest a few days after sitting in a hot tub. A culture of one of the lesions reveals thin gram-negative rods. The isolate grows readily on standard bacteriologic media, is oxidase positive, motile, nonfermentative, and grows at 42°C. Figure 14.10A shows the isolate on MacConkey agar and Figure 14.10B shows the isolate on Mueller-Hinton agar. What is the likely identity of the isolate?

a. *Stenotrophomonas maltophilia*
b. *Acinetobacter baumanii*
c. *Pseudomonas aeruginosa*
d. *Escherichia coli*
e. *Pseudomonas fluorescens*

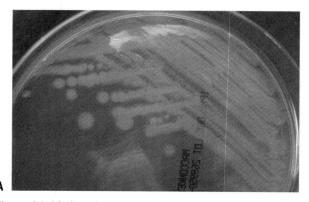

A

Figure 14.10 *(continues)*

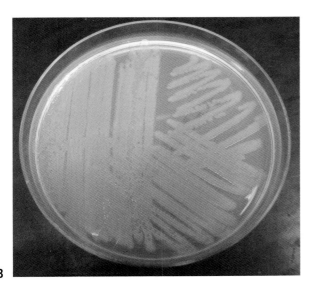

B

Figure 14.10 *(continued)*

17. On which of the following media does *Gardnerella vaginalis* produce β-hemolytic colonies?
    a. Human blood bilayer Tween (HBT) agar
    b. Trypticase soy agar with 5% sheep blood
    c. Cystine-tellurite blood agar
    d. Columbia colistin-nalidixic acid (CNA) agar with 5% sheep blood
    e. All of the above

18. Figure 14.11 shows an organism isolated on sheep blood agar from a clean catch urine specimen from a young woman with a suspected urinary tract infection. A portion of the organism is scraped off of the agar plate to illustrate the growth of the organism. A Gram stain of the organism reveals short Gram-negative rods that stain thicker on both ends of the cells. The isolate is oxidase negative and indole positive. What is the likely identification of the isolate?
    a. *Escherichia coli*
    b. *Proteus mirabilis*
    c. *Klebsiella oxytoca*

    d. *Proteus vulgaris*
    e. *Klebsiella pneumoniae*

19. Which of the following is NOT a characteristic of *Bacillus anthracis*?
    a. Nonmotile
    b. Nonhemolytic on sheep blood agar
    c. Catalase positive
    d. Spores are present.
    e. Motile

20. A young boy is bitten by his pet rat and within a few days develops fever, chills, vomiting, and severe joint pains. A rash soon develops on his palms and soles. Gram-negative rods are isolated from the blood in broth media without the supplement sodium polyanethol sulfonate (SPS). The rods are extremely pleomorphic and filamentous, and are oxidase- and catalase negative. What is the likely identity of the isolate?
    a. *Pasteurella multocida*
    b. *Leptospira interrogans*
    c. *Eikenella corrodens*
    d. *Streptobacillus moniliformis*
    e. *Cardiobacterium hominis*

21. A week after he removed an embedded tick, a 38-year-old male hunter from Arkansas presents with a fever, chills, myalgia, malaise, an intense headache, nausea, and vomiting. No rash is present. The patient is thrombocytopenic (18,000 platelets/μL), has mildly elevated liver function tests, and is mildly leukopenic (neutropenia). Intracellular inclusions are observed in monocytes in a buffy coat preparation from a peripheral blood smear. What is the likely identity of this organism?
    a. *Ehrlichia chaffeensis*
    b. *Anaplasma phagocytophilum*
    c. *Rickettsia rickettsii*
    d. *Orientia tsutsugamushi*
    e. *Rickettsia typhi*

22. The isolate shown on the sheep blood agar plate in Figure 14.12 grew only in an anaerobic atmosphere and

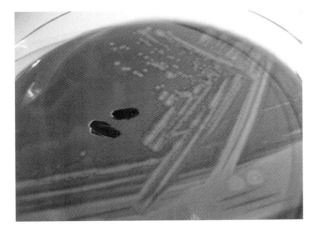

Figure 14.11

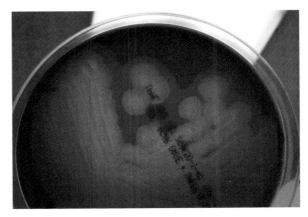

Figure 14.12

stained as large, boxcar-shaped Gram-positive rods. No spores were present on the Gram stain. The isolate is from a case of myonecrosis. What is the most likely identification of this isolate?
 a. *Clostridium tetani*
 b. *Clostridium botulinum*
 c. *Bacillus cereus*
 d. *Clostridium perfringens*
 e. *Bacillus anthracis*

23. A patient has an oral abscess drained. A yellow, grainy substance resembling sulfur granules is expressed from the abscess. A Gram stain of the material reveals pleomorphic Gram-positive rods that have rudimentary branches, as shown in Figure 14.13. The organisms were modified acid-fast stain negative, grew better in an anaerobic atmosphere than in aerobic conditions, and were catalase negative. What is the likely identification of the isolate?
 a. *Corynebacterium jeikeium*
 b. *Actinomyces israelii*
 c. *Nocardia farcinica*
 d. *Nocardia asteroides*
 e. *Corynebacterium xerosis*

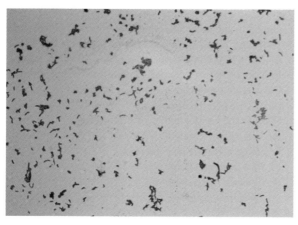

Figure 14.13

24. A 37-year-old woman presents to her physician with fever, chills, headache, and a nonproductive cough. Pharyngeal erythema is noted on examination. A chest x-ray reveals consolidation in her left lower lobe. Her history is significant in that she keeps budgerigars and parrots at home. Sputum is obtained, but no organisms are observed from a direct Gram stain and no growth occurs on artificial culture media. Given these results and the patient's history, what is the most probable causative agent?
 a. *Legionella pneumophila*
 b. *Streptococcus pneumoniae*
 c. *Chlamydophila pneumoniae*
 d. *Mycobacterium tuberculosis*
 e. *Chlamydophila psittaci*

25. A 3-year-old child is brought to the emergency department by his parents. The child has a fever, rash, and nuchal rigidity. A lumbar puncture is performed. The following results are obtained from the CSF: glucose <20, protein 244, slightly cloudy, and 98% polymorphonuclear cells. A gram stain reveals many white blood cells and many Gram-negative diplococci as shown in Figure 14.14. The following day, there were many colorless colonies on chocolate agar. The isolate was oxidase positive and catalase positive. In addition, it produced acid from glucose and maltose. What is the identity of the isolate?
 a. *Moraxella catarrhalis*
 b. *Streptococcus pneumoniae*
 c. *Haemophilus influenzae*
 d. *Neisseria meningitidis*
 e. *Neisseria gonorrhoeae*

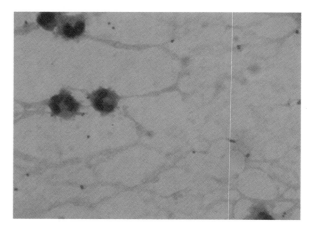

Figure 14.14

26. MacConkey-sorbitol agar is used to isolate:
 a. *Shigella* species
 b. *Escherichia coli* O157:H7
 c. Non-O157:H7 *Escherichia coli* strains
 d. *Salmonella* serotypes
 e. *Yersinia enterocolitica*

27. A Gram-negative coccobacillus is isolated on Bordet-Gengou agar (Fig. 14.15) from a 3-year-old child with a 1-week history of a mild cough and a runny nose. The child has received no immunizations. The isolate is oxidase positive, nonmotile, nitrate-reduction negative, and urease negative. In addition, it did not grow on either sheep blood agar or MacConkey agar. What is the likely identification of the isolate?
 a. *Bordetella bronchiseptica*
 b. *Legionella pneumophila*
 c. *Bordetella pertussis*
 d. *Bordetella parapertussis*
 e. *Brucella melitensis*

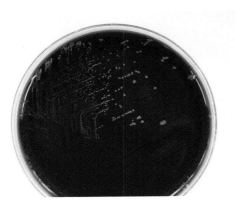

Figure 14.15

28. An individual eats fried rice from an Asian restaurant and within two hours is ill with vomiting and nausea. What is the most likely explanation for this individual's illness?
   a. The individual ingested food contaminated with enterohemorrhagic *Escherichia coli*.
   b. The individual ingested food contaminated with *Campylobacter jejuni*.
   c. The individual ingested food contaminated with preformed *Bacillus cereus* emetic toxin.
   d. The individual ingested food contaminated with *Salmonella* species.
   e. The individual ingested food contaminated with preformed *Clostridium perfringens* enterotoxin.

29. The organism shown in Figure 14.16 was isolated from the blood from a patient hospitalized with pneumonia. The organism is a lancet-shaped Gram-positive coccus in pairs and short chains, is catalase negative, and is bile sensitive. An optochin disk (P disk) was placed on the first quadrant of the sheep blood agar plate in Figure 14.16. Based on these results and the patient's illness, what is the most likely identity of the isolate?
   a. Viridans streptococci
   b. *Streptococcus pneumoniae*
   c. *Streptococcus pyogenes*
   d. *Streptococcus agalactiae*
   e. *Enterococcus faecalis*

30. An *Enterococcus faecium* isolate is cultured from the blood of a patient with endocarditis. The isolate is vancomycin resistant. Which of the following is NOT true regarding this isolate?
   a. Vancomycin resistance is due to an alteration of the target in enterococci.
   b. *E. faecium* is naturally resistant to vancomycin.
   c. *E. faecium* is part of the normal gastrointestinal flora of most humans.
   d. *E. faecium* isolates are nearly always resistant to ampicillin and penicillin.
   e. Vancomycin resistance is acquired by *E. faecium* isolates.

31. A 47-year-old man from California presents to the Emergency Department with fever, headache, back pain, malaise, and hepatosplenomegaly. The patient revealed that he had consumed unpasteurized goat milk that had been imported from Mexico. In 3 days, Gram-negative coccobacilli are isolated from blood culture specimens. The isolate is urease positive in about 2 hours. Given the patient's history and illness, what is the most likely identification of the isolate?
   a. *Brucella canis*
   b. *Brucella abortus*
   c. *Francisella tularensis*
   d. *Brucella suis*
   e. *Brucella melitensis*

32. A 23-year-old man presents to the Emergency Department with vomiting, diarrhea, abdominal cramps, and fever. The patient says that about a day ago he ate chicken cooked on a grill at a barbecue. A sample of the patient's diarrhea is submitted for stool culture, and the organism observed on the xylose lysine deoxycholate (XLD) agar plate shown in Figure 14.17 is isolated in aerobic conditions. What is the most likely identification of the isolate?
   a. *Shigella sonnei*
   b. *Shigella dysenteriae*
   c. *Campylobacter jejuni*
   d. *Salmonella* subspecies Enteritidis
   e. *Escherichia coli* O157:H7

33. An individual who handles fish presents with a well-defined, violaceous lesion on his right index finger. The lesion is painful, and the finger has swelled.

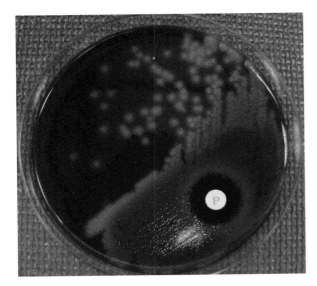

Figure 14.16

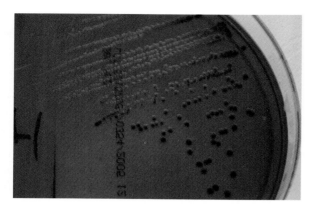

Figure 14.17

A biopsy specimen is sent for culture and in 24 hours nonhemolytic, pleomorphic Gram-positive rods are isolated on sheep blood agar and chocolate agar. The isolate is catalase negative. It was inoculated into a triple sugar iron (TSI) agar slant, and the result is shown in Figure 14.18 (left slant shows an uninoculated control, right slant is the isolate). What is the identity of the isolate?

a. *Listeria monocytogenes*
b. *Erysipelothrix rhusiopathiae*
c. *Arcanobacterium haemolyticum*
d. *Corynebacterium ulcerans*
e. *Bacillus anthracis*

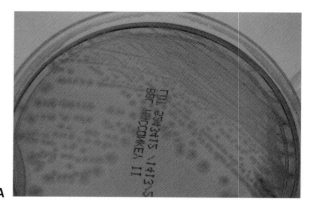

A

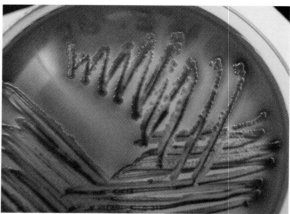

B

Figure 14.19

35. An acid-fast bacillus is cultured from a patient with chronic pulmonary disease. The isolate took about 30 days to grow, and Figure 14.20 shows the organism grown in the dark (left slant) and when exposed to light (right slant). What is the most likely identity of the isolate?

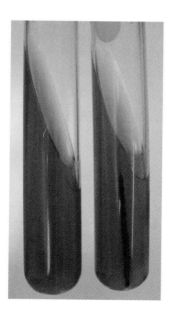

Figure 14.18

34. Which statement concerning the MacConkey agar plate shown in Figure 14.19A is incorrect?
a. The organism is a nonlactose fermenter.
b. The organism is a lactose fermenter.
c. The organism may be a *Salmonella* species.
d. The organism may be a *Shigella* species.
e. The organism may be a *Proteus* species.

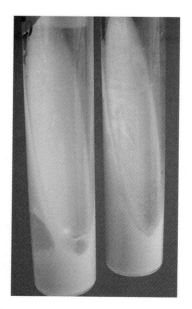

Figure 14.20

a. *Mycobacterium kansasii*
b. *Mycobacterium avium-intracellulare*
c. *Mycobacterium tuberculosis*
d. *Mycobacterium gordonae*
e. *Mycobacterium abscessus*

36. A 5-year-old boy is bitten on the arm by a 6-month-old kitten and develops cellulitis. An oxidase-positive, catalase-positive, Gram-negative coccobacillus is isolated from purulence from the wound. The isolate, shown in Figure 14.21, grows well in aerobic conditions on sheep blood and chocolate agars in 24 hours, does not grow on MacConkey agar, and is indole positive. What is the most likely identity of the isolate?
    a. *Eikenella corrodens*
    b. *Haemophilus influenzae*
    c. *Pasteurella multocida*
    d. *Bartonella henselae*
    e. *Pseudomonas aeruginosa*

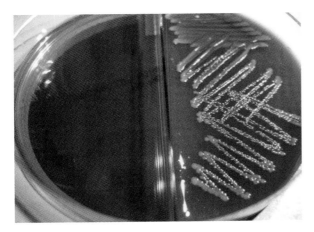

Figure 14.21

37. A 26-year-old man from rural Massachusetts is seen by his physician with symptoms of fatigue, chills, fever, headache, and malaise. The patient has a small red lesion with an annular rash at the site of a previous tick bite on his trunk. The patient reports that he pulled a small tick from the site of the lesion a few weeks ago. What is the most likely agent of the patient's disease?
    a. *Rickettsia rickettsii*
    b. *Borrelia burgdorferi*
    c. *Borrelia recurrentis*
    d. *Leptospira interrogans*
    e. *Francisella tularensis*

38. A 28-year-old woman presents to the Emergency Department with fever, vomiting, bloody diarrhea, and abdominal pain. She says that she may have eaten undercooked chicken a few days ago at a party. A curved, faintly staining Gram-negative rod (Fig. 14.22) was isolated on specialized blood agar from a stool sample submitted to the lab. The isolate is oxidase positive and grew in a microaerophilic atmosphere at 42°C. The isolate did not grow on either MacConkey agar or Hektoen enteric agar in an aerobic atmosphere. In addition, leukocytes were observed in a methylene blue stain of the stool. Based on this evidence, what is the likely identity of this food poisoning agent?
    a. *Vibrio cholerae*
    b. *Escherichia coli* O157:H7
    c. *Salmonella* serotype Typhi
    d. *Campylobacter jejuni*
    e. *Shigella sonnei*

Figure 14.22

39. Figure 14.23 depicts a disk diffusion test with a *Klebsiella pneumoniae* isolate. The isolate is resistant to ceftazidime (zone size 12 mm); the zone size for ceftazidime-clavulanic acid is 22 mm. Which of the following is true for this scenario?
    a. The isolate is confirmed to be an extended spectrum β-lactamase (ESBL) producer.
    b. The disk diffusion test shown in Figure 14.23 is an ESBL screening test, not a confirmatory test.
    c. This is a typical pattern of antibiotic resistance for *Escherichia coli.*
    d. The disk diffusion test shown in Figure 14.23 is invalid because the zone size for ceftazidime-clavulanic acid should be less than the ceftazidime zone size to confirm an ESBL.
    e. The isolate is confirmed to be an AmpC hyperproducer.

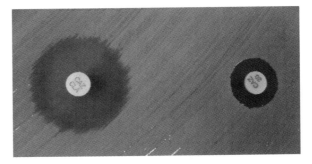

Figure 14.23

40. A 35-year-old man from Virginia is brought to the Emergency Department by his wife with a rash, fever, nausea, vomiting, diarrhea, and abdominal pain. His illness began 3 days ago with a fever, headache, and myalgias. The rash started on the trunk but has since spread to the patient's palms and soles. A week ago he went hunting and pulled a deeply embedded tick off of his trunk after he got home. Given the patient's history and symptoms, what is the most likely etiologic agent?
    a. *Coxiella burnetii*
    b. *Rickettsia prowazekii*
    c. *Anaplasma phagocytophilum*
    d. *Borrelia burgdorferi*
    e. *Rickettsia rickettsii*

41. A 45-year-old woman injection-drug user presents to the Emergency Department with fever, chills, and malaise. A physical examination of the patient reveals swelling, pain, and erythema at a drug injection site on her left arm. Purulent material is submitted to the lab from the injection site. A Gram stain of the pus reveals many Gram-positive cocci in chains and many white blood cells. In 18 hours, a β-hemolytic, catalase-negative, Gram-positive coccus is isolated. A subculture of the organism on a sheep blood agar plate with a bacitracin disk (A disk) is shown in Figure 14.24. What is the most likely identification of the isolate?

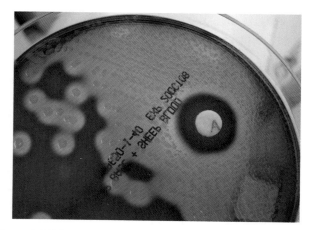

Figure 14.24

    a. *Streptococcus agalactiae*
    b. *Staphylococcus aureus*
    c. *Streptococcus pyogenes*
    d. *Enterococcus faecium*
    e. *Streptococcus milleri* group

42. A 4-year-old Native American boy is brought to a clinic with a fever, malaise, and a sore throat. A white membrane is observed on the child's tonsils. The child has not had all of his immunizations. A throat culture is submitted, and black colonies are observed on cystine-tellurite blood agar after 48 hours of growth. On

Tinsdale agar, the colonies are black with dark brown halos. A Gram stain of the isolate shows pleomorphic Gram-positive rods. The organism is catalase positive and does not produce urease. What is the probable identity of the isolate?
    a. *Streptococcus pyogenes*
    b. *Corynebacterium pseudotuberculosis*
    c. *Arcanobacterium haemolyticum*
    d. *Corynebacterium ulcerans*
    e. *Corynebacterium diphtheriae*

43. A 57-year-old man is hospitalized with sepsis and two sets of blood cultures are drawn. Gram-positive cocci in chains are observed in all four bottles in one day. Subcultures of the bottles reveal catalase-negative, nonhemolytic Gram-positive cocci. The organism grows on a bile esculin agar slant (Fig. 14.25B; Fig. 14.25A is a negative control) and types with the group D Lancefield antigen. In addition, the isolate does not grow in the presence of 6.5% salt. Further testing is performed on the patient, and it is found that he has colon cancer. Based on this information, what is the most likely identity of the blood culture isolate?
    a. *Streptococcus bovis*
    b. *Enterococcus faecalis*
    c. *Enterococcus faecium*
    d. *Streptococcus agalactiae*
    e. *Streptococcus dysgalactiae* subsp. *equisimilis*

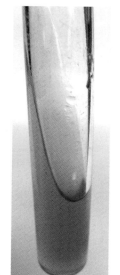 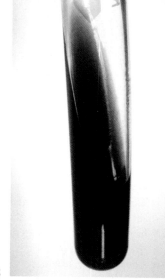

A   B

Figure 14.25

44. Which of the following is often used to isolate *Mycoplasma pneumoniae*?
    a. A8 agar
    b. SP-4 medium
    c. McCoy cells
    d. Middlebrook 7H10 agar
    e. BACTEC 12B medium

45. A 70-year-old woman with chronic obstructive pulmonary disorder (COPD) developed fever, cough, and purulent sputum. Patchy infiltrates were observed on a chest x-ray, and a sample of her expectorated sputum was sent to the lab for analysis. A Gram stain of the sputum revealed many small, Gram-negative coccobacilli and many white blood cells. On culture, a Gram-negative coccobacillus grows only on chocolate agar after 24 hours in increased CO_2 (Fig. 14.26A); the isolate does not grow on either sheep blood agar or MacConkey agar. X and V factor requirements were determined as shown in Figure 14.26B. Furthermore, the isolate was found to be nonhemolytic on rabbit blood agar. Based on these data, what is the most likely identity of the isolate?

   a. *H. influenzae*
   b. *Haemophilus parainfluenzae*
   c. *Haemophilus haemolyticus*
   d. *Haemophilus paraphrophilus*
   e. *Haemophilus parahaemolyticus*

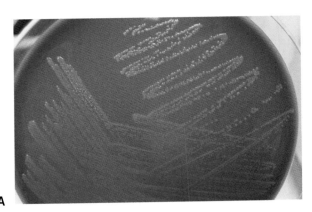

A

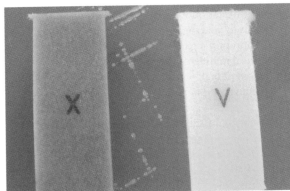

B

Figure 14.26

46. A 5-year-old girl returns from a trip to India with her family and a week later develops diarrhea that lasts for 4 days. Then, she gradually develops fever, abdominal pain, sore throat, and chills. A physical exam of the girl reveals hepatosplenomegaly. Blood cultures are drawn, and Gram-negative rods are observed in all bottles in 24 hours. The isolate is subcultured to solid media. The organism is oxidase negative, indole negative,

urease negative, ornithine decarboxylase negative, and a nonlactose fermenter on MacConkey agar. The isolate was inoculated into a TSI agar slant and is shown in Figure 14.27A. Based on this information and the patient's history, what is the likely identity of the isolate?

   a. *Shigella dysenteriae*
   b. *Edwardsiella tarda*
   c. *Salmonella* serotype Paratyphi A
   d. *Salmonella* serotype Typhi
   e. *Shigella sonnei*

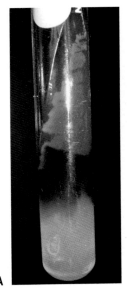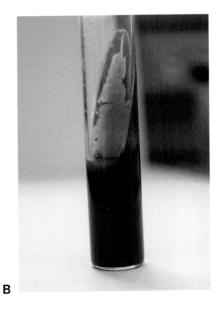

A   B

Figure 14.27

47. A 60-year-old woman inpatient is recovering from surgery and develops diarrhea, fever, and abdominal pain. She had surgery 5 days ago and has been on antimicrobial therapy since then. A stool sample is submitted to the lab, and an anaerobic Gram-positive, spore-forming rod is isolated on cycloserine-cefoxitin-fructose agar (CCFA). The colonies fluoresce chartreuse under UV light. A rapid toxin assay is positive as well. What is the most probable identity of the isolate?

   a. *Clostridium botulinum*
   b. *Clostridium difficile*
   c. *Bacillus cereus*
   d. *Clostridium perfringens*
   e. *Clostridium septicum*

48. A 28-year-old woman presents to her physician with a 3-day history of arthritis in her knees, fever, and dermatitis. The dermatitis consists of several pustular lesions on her extremities. The patient admits that she has had multiple sexual encounters over the past year and that none of her partners used protection. A sample of her knee joint fluid is sent to the lab along with two sets of blood cultures. A Gram stain of the joint fluid reveals moderate white blood cells and few Gram-negative diplococci. The following day, a pure culture

of the organism shown in Figure 14.28 is obtained only on a chocolate agar plate. The isolate is an oxidase positive, catalase positive, Gram-negative diplococcus. In addition, the organism produces acid from glucose but not from maltose, sucrose, lactose, or fructose. What is the identity of the isolate?

a. *Neisseria gonorrhoeae*
b. *Moraxella catarrhalis*
c. *Neisseria meningitidis*
d. *Neisseria lactamica*
e. *Neisseria sicca*

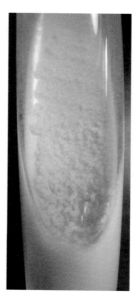

Figure 14.29

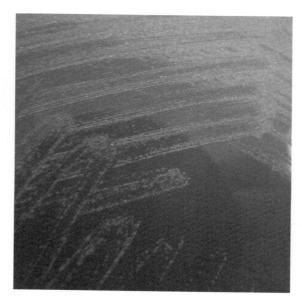

Figure 14.28

49. A 46-year-old HIV-positive man presents to his physician with a recent history of weight loss, fever, night sweats, and a chronic, productive cough. Acid-fast bacilli are observed on a smear of his expectorated sputum. Growth of an acid-fast bacillus is obtained in liquid medium in about 7 days; on solid media, the organism takes about 2 months to grow. The isolate is not pigmented in either light or dark conditions, is pyrazinamidase positive, nitrate reduction positive, niacin positive, and has rough colonies (Fig. 14.29). The identity of the isolate was determined by a DNA hybridization probe. What is the most likely identity of the isolate?

a. *Mycobacterium bovis*
b. *Mycobacterium kansasii*
c. *Mycobacterium tuberculosis*
d. *Mycobacterium avium-intracellulare*
e. *Mycobacterium fortuitum*

50. Which of the following characteristics is often exploited to determine *Helicobacter pylori* colonization?

a. Rapid catalase production
b. Rapid oxidase production
c. Rapid H_2S production
d. Rapid indole production
e. Rapid urease production

51. Of the following observations, which is most specific for indicating a parasite infestation?

a. Bloody diarrhea
b. Hepatosplenomegaly
c. $\geq 15\%$ peripheral blood eosinophilia
d. Chronic cough
e. Cramping abdominal pain

52. Each of the following symptoms may complicate a parasitic infestation EXCEPT:

a. Bloody diarrhea
b. Suprapubic pain
c. Focal itching of the skin
d. Loss of hair
e. Transient pneumonia

53. Which stool fixative has the disadvantage that trichrome-stained smears CANNOT be prepared in it?

a. Merthiolate-iodine-formaldehyde (MIF)
b. Schaudinn fixative
c. Zinc-based Schaudinn fixative (EcoFix)
d. Polyvinyl alcohol (PVA)
e. Sodium acetate, acetic acid, formalin (SAF)

54. Which parasite forms will not be recovered in stool concentrates prepared by the zinc sulfate flotation technique?

a. Hookworm eggs
b. *Giardia lamblia* cysts
c. *Trichuris trichiura* eggs
d. *Diphyllobothrium latum* eggs
e. *Entamoeba histolytica* cysts

55. Why are thick peripheral blood smears in addition to thin smears prepared to help establish the diagnosis of malaria?
    a. Malarial parasitic forms will be detected in light infections.
    b. Visualization of the parasitic forms is improved.
    c. The staining quality of the malarial forms is improved.
    d. There is less interference of staining by the anticoagulant.
    e. The potential exflagellation of gametocytes is reduced.

56. The parasitic form illustrated in the photomicrograph (Fig. 14.30) was observed in a stool specimen concentrate. It can be identified as:
    a. *Entamoeba coli*
    b. *Entamoeba histolytica*
    c. *Dientamoeba fragilis*
    d. *Iodamoeba butschlii*
    e. *Endolimax nana*

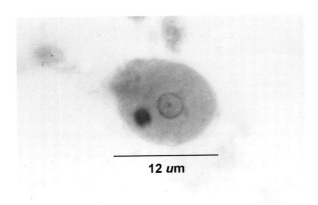

12 um

Figure 14.30

57. Each of the following amoeba when observed in human stool specimens is considered to be a harmless commensal EXCEPT:
    a. *Entamoeba coli*
    b. *Iodamoeba bütschlii*
    c. *Entamoeba dispar*
    d. *Endolimax nana*
    e. *Dientamoeba fragilis*

58. The intestinal protozoan trophozoite illustrated in the photomicrograph (Fig. 14.31) can be identified as the trophozoite of:
    a. *Entamoeba coli*
    b. *Iodamoeba bütschlii*
    c. *Isospora belli*
    d. *Balantidium coli*
    e. *Sarcocystis hominis*

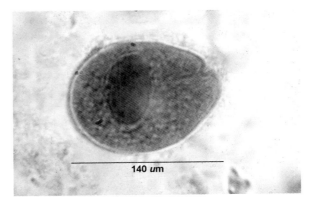

140 um

Figure 14.31

59. Which of the following diagnostic tests is the least sensitive in establishing the identification of the organism illustrated in the photomicrograph (Fig. 14.32)?
    a. Duodenal aspirates or biopsies
    b. The string test, "Enterotest"
    c. "Triple fecal test" (stool exams on 3 consecutive days)
    d. Detection of cysts using direct immunofluorescence
    e. Antigen detection in stool specimens (ELISA)

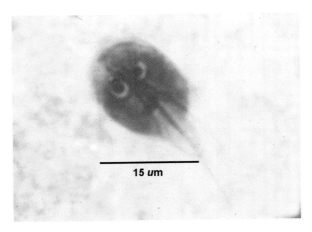

15 um

Figure 14.32

60. The parasitic form illustrated in the photomicrograph (Fig. 14.33) can be identified as the trophozoite of:
    a. *Giardia lamblia*
    b. *Dientamoeba fragilis*
    c. *Chilomastix mesneli*
    d. *Balantidium coli*
    e. *Trichomonas hominis*

61. The group of people most commonly exposed to and infested with the ciliate *Balantidium coli* is:
    a. Cattle ranchers
    b. Pig and swine farmers
    c. Poultry farmers
    d. Wild game hunters
    e. Equestrians

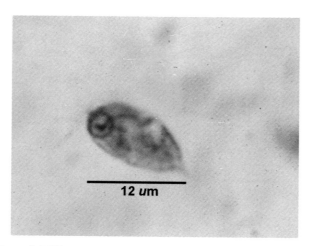

Figure 14.33

62. Each of the following coccidian protozoa has evolved as AIDS-identifying microbes, indicating the need to test for HIV infection when observed in stool specimens, EXCEPT:
    a. *Cryptosporidium parvum*
    b. *Cyclospora cayetanensis*
    c. *Isospora belli*
    d. *Sarcocystis hominis*
    e. *Microsporidium* species

63. The ovum illustrated in the photograph (Fig. 14.34) is estimated to occur in stool specimens of approximately 25% of the world population. What nematode does it represent?
    a. *Ascaris lumbricoides*
    b. *Strongyloides stercoralis*
    c. *Enterobius vermicularis*
    d. *Ancylostoma duodenale*
    e. *Necator americanus*

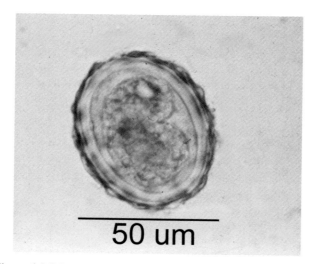

Figure 14.34

64. The ovum illustrated in the photomicrograph (Fig. 14.35), with its barrel-shape and distinctive hyaline bipolar plugs is easy to recognize as *Trichuris trichiura*. Although distinctive, what other nematode produces similar-appearing ova and must also be ruled out?
    a. *Enterobius vermicularis*
    b. *Necator americanus* (hookworm)
    c. *Ancylostoma duodenale*
    d. *Capillaria phillipensis*
    e. *Strongyloides stercoralis*

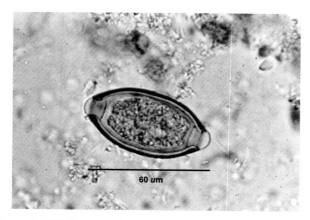

Figure 14.35 (Image taken from Centers for Disease Control and Prevention website at http://phil.cdc.gov/phil/home.asp.)

65. What practice is most effective in making the diagnosis of this appendiceal worm infection (Fig.14.36), particularly in children?
    a. Microscopic examination of stool specimen concentrates
    b. Deep rectal swab
    c. The transparency tape procedure
    d. Stool examination after a saline purge
    e. Visual examination of the perianal buttocks

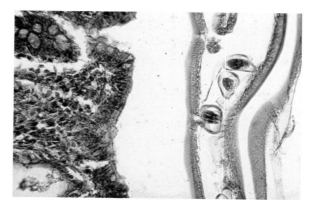

Figure 14.36 (Image taken from Centers for Disease Control and Prevention website at http://phil.cdc.gov/phil/home.asp.)

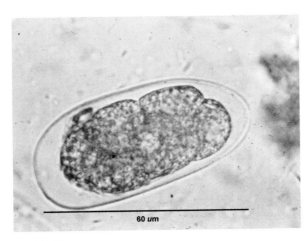

Figure 14.37

66. The ovum illustrated in the photomicrograph (Fig. 14.37), with its thin smooth shell and retraction of the internal cleavage leaving a clear space, is characteristic of which of the following nematodes?
    a. *Necator americanus*
    b. *Ascaris lumbricoides*
    c. *Capillaria philippinensis*
    d. *Trichuris trichiura*
    e. *Enterobius vermicularis*

67. How is the diagnosis of *Strongyloides stercoralis* established in stool specimens?
    a. Observing a low quantitative ova count
    b. Observing rhabditiform lavae
    c. Observing filariform larvae
    d. Detecting an increase in polymorphonuclear inflammatory cells
    e. Identifying ova in stool concentrates using the flotation technique

68. The laboratory identification of *S. stercoralis* rhabditiform larvae can also be made using the agar technique. In this procedure, a small portion of stool concentrate is placed in the center of a blood agar plate. Within 24 to 48 hours, streak lines from the central area of bacterial growth extending to the periphery of the plate may be observed, indicating the migration of larvae. When should this procedure be used?
    a. For all routine stool specimens submitted for "O & P"
    b. Only when strongyloidiasis is clinically suspected
    c. On stools that appear bloody
    d. On stools where an increase in inflammatory cells are seen in direct mounts
    e. When a stool specimen is received with an order of "O & P"

69. What is the primary reason for performing quantitative egg counts when ova suspicious of hookworm are identified in a stool specimen?

    a. To rule out *Strongyloides* infection
    b. To distinguish *Necator americanus* from *Ancylostoma duodenale*
    c. To indicate the severity of infection that may require aggressive therapy
    d. To help predict if invasive filariform infection has occurred
    e. To alert to strictly enforce infection control practices

70. What symptom is specifically related to the filariform larval stage in the hookworm life cycle?
    a. Episodes of acute abdominal pain
    b. Transient pneumonia including a Loeffler-like syndrome
    c. Severe recurrent diarrhea
    d. Development of iron deficiency anemia
    e. Lack of mental development in infested children

71. What is the identification of the ova illustrated in the photomicrograph (Fig. 14.38)?
    a. *Taenia* species
    b. *Diphyllobothrium latum*
    c. *Hymenolepis nana*
    d. *Hymenolepis diminuta*
    e. *Diphyllidium caninum*

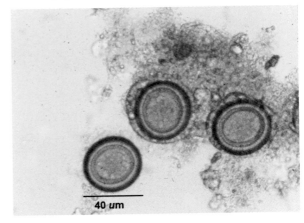

Figure 14.38

72. *Taenia solium* can be separated from *Taenia saginata* only by examination of the adult worm or parts thereof. The scolex of *T. solium* is fitted with a raised rostellum fitted with a ring of hooklets; the scolex of *T. saginata* is smooth. The proglittids of *T. solium* have less than 13 lateral branches; those of *T. saginata* have more than 13. Why is it important to establish this differential identification?
    a. To administer species-specific therapy
    b. *Taenia saginata* is more likely to produce intestinal complications
    c. *Taenia solium* adults are more difficult to eliminate from the intestine
    d. The ova of *Taenia solium* are infective for humans
    e. There is no medical reason to distinguish between these two species

73. Illustrated in the photomicrograph (Fig. 14.39) is a relatively large ovum with a smooth outer surface, a thin shell with a nonshouldered operculum, an abopercular knob at the opposite end, and an internal cleavage that extends to the inner lining of the shell. The identification is:
   a. *Paragonimus westermanii*
   b. *Hymenolepis nana*
   c. *Clonorchis sinensis*
   d. *Diphyllobothrium latum*
   e. *Dipyllidium caninum*

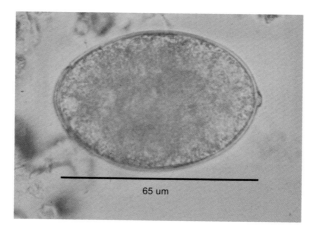

Figure 14.39

74. What is a common complication of an infestation with the fish tapeworm, *Diphyllobothrium latum*?
   a. Prolonged intermittent diarrhea
   b. Iron deficiency anemia
   c. Megaloblastic anemia
   d. Subcutaneous infection (sparganosis)
   e. Seizures and neurologic deficiencies

75. The ovum illustrated in the photomicrograph (Fig. 14.40) can be identified as:

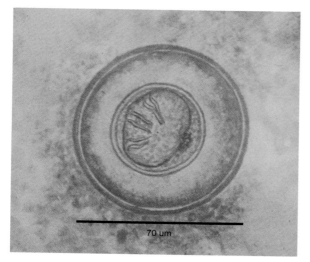

Figure 14.40

   a. *Taenia solium*
   b. *Hymenolepis nana*
   c. *Hymenolepis diminuta*
   d. *Necator americanus*
   e. *Diphyllobothrium latum*

76. The large ovum in the photomicrograph (Fig. 14.41) was observed in a stool specimen. At what anatomic site in the human body does the adult worm most commonly reside?
   a. Cystic cavity in the lung
   b. Portal tract of the liver
   c. Portal veins of the large intestine
   d. Skeletal muscle
   e. Portal veins of the urinary bladder

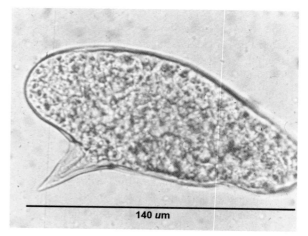

Figure 14.41

77. Illustrated in the photomicrograph (Fig. 14.42) is an H&E-stained section of urinary bladder epithelium and underlying mucosa obtained from a 40-year-old man with intermittent hematuria, lower abdominal pain, and frequency of urination. Parasite eggs are observed in the submucosa. The most likely diagnosis is chronic cystitis secondary to:
   a. *Onchocerca volvulus*
   b. *Trichinella spiralis*

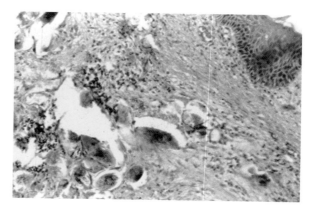

Figure 14.42

c. *Schistosoma mansoni*
d. *Schistosoma haematobium*
e. *Fasciolopsis buskii*

78. How do humans most commonly acquire schistosomiasis?
    a. Ingestion of the meat of uncooked freshwater fish
    b. Ingestion of contaminated drinking water
    c. Direct contact with parasite infested water fowl or fish
    d. Skin penetration while swimming or wading in cer-caria-infested water
    e. Ingestion of metacercaria attached to water plants

79. The large ovum illustrated in this photomicrograph (Fig. 14.43) can be identified as:
    a. *Diphyllobothrium latum*
    b. *Fasciolopsis buski*
    c. *Schistosoma mansoni*
    d. *Paragonimus westermanii*
    e. *Clonorchis sinensis*

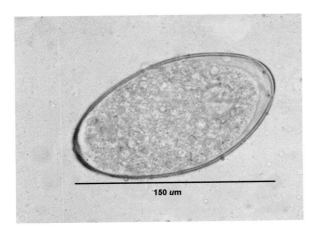

Figure 14.43

80. By which of the following means do humans acquire fascioliasis?
    a. Ingestion of the meat of uncooked freshwater fish
    b. Ingestion of contaminated water
    c. Direct contact with parasite infested water fowl or fish
    d. Skin penetration with cercaria while swimming or wading in infested water
    e. Ingestion of metacercaria attached to water plants

81. Each of the following is a manifestation of infestation with the fluke illustrated in the photograph (Fig. 14.44) EXCEPT:
    a. Cirrhosis and jaundice
    b. Persistence of organisms often for decades
    c. Eosinophilia, particularly in early stages of infestation
    d. Abdominal distress and intermittent diarrhea are minimal
    e. The disease tends to remain low-grade.

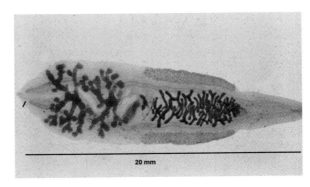

Figure 14.44

82. By which of the following means do humans acquire infestations with *Clonorchis sinensis*?
    a. Ingestion of the meat of uncooked freshwater fish
    b. Ingestion of contaminated water
    c. Direct contact with parasite infested water fowl or fish
    d. Skin penetration with cercaria while swimming or wading in infested water
    e. Ingestion of metacercaria attached to water plants

83. Where in the human body is the adult form of the parasite represented by the ovum illustrated in the photomicrograph (Fig. 14.45) located?
    a. Liver
    b. Large intestine
    c. Brain
    d. Heart
    e. Lung

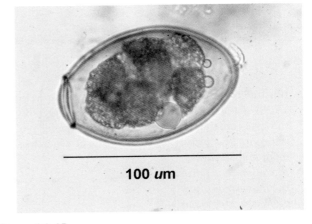

Figure 14.45

84. The intra-erythrocytic parasitic forms observed in the composite photomicrograph (Fig. 14.46) of peripheral blood smears are most consistent with:
    a. *Plasmodium falciparum*
    b. *Plasmodium vivax*
    c. *Plasmodium malariae*
    d. *Plasmodium ovale*
    e. *Babesia microti*

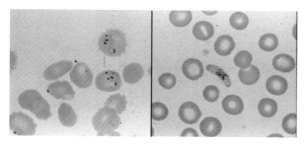

Figure 14.46

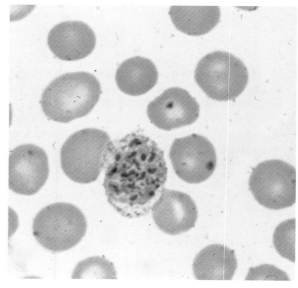

Figure 14.48

85. What species of blood parasite is represented by the peripheral smear illustrated in the photomicrograph (Fig. 14.47)?
   a. *Plasmodium falciparum*
   b. *Plasmodium vivax*
   c. *Plasmodium malariae*
   d. *Plasmodium ovale*
   e. *Babesia microti*

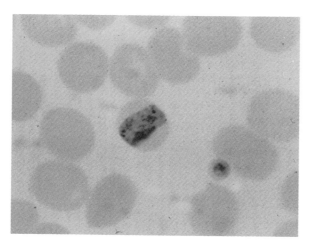

Figure 14.47

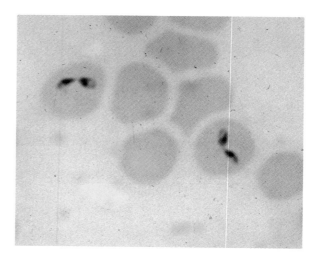

Figure 14.49

86. Illustrated in the center of the photomicrograph (Fig. 14.48) of a peripheral blood smear is an enlarged erythrocyte containing many merozoites, in the form of a schizont. This picture is characteristic of which plasmodium parasites?
   a. *Plasmodium falciparum*
   b. *Plasmodium vivax*
   c. *Plasmodium malariae*
   d. *Plasmodium ovale*
   e. *Babesia microti*

87. Which of the following blood parasites is represented by the intra–erythrocytic forms observed in the peripheral blood smear photomicrograph (Fig. 14.49)?
   a. *Plasmodium falciparum*
   b. *Plasmodium vivax*
   c. *Plasmodium malariae*
   d. *Plasmodium ovale*
   e. *Babesia microti*

88. Which blood parasitic disease is indicated by the peripheral blood picture illustrated in the photomicrograph (Fig. 14.50)?
   a. Onchocerciasis
   b. African trypanosomiasis
   c. Chagas disease
   d. Leishmaniasis
   e. Toxoplasmosis

89. From the bite of which insect do humans become infected with the blood flagellate illustrated in the photomicrograph (Fig. 14.51)?
   a. Reduviid bug
   b. Phlebotomus sandfly
   c. Ixodes tick
   d. Glossina tsetse fly
   e. Anopheles mosquito

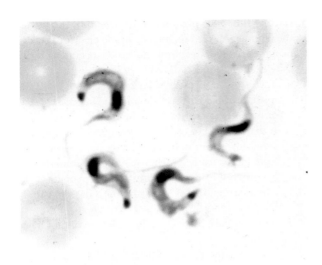

Figure 14.50

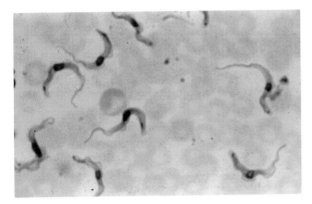

Figure 14.51

90. Illustrated in this photomicrograph (Fig. 14.52) is an intracellular cluster of small histoplasma-like parasitic forms that are called amastigotes. The observation of these forms in tissue sections is characteristic of which hemoflaggelate?

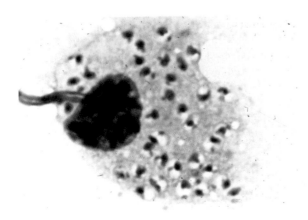

Figure 14.52

a. *Trypanosoma brucei rhodesiense*
b. *Trypanosoma brucei gambiense*
c. *Trypanosoma cruzi*
d. *Leishmania donovani*
e. *Toxoplasma gondii*

91. Each of the following activities predisposes humans to contract toxoplasmosis EXCEPT:
a. Ingestion of raw lamb or pork (steak tartar)
b. Cleaning out cat litter boxes
c. Ingestion of unwashed fruits and vegetables
d. Hiking without applying insect repellant
e. Intravenous injection of illicit drugs

92. Illustrated in the photomicrograph (Fig. 14.53) is the tail section of a microfilaria observed in a peripheral blood smear in which two nuclei are observed extending into the sheathed tail section. To what species of filarial does this belong?
a. *Onchocerca volvulus*
b. *Loa loa*
c. *Wuchereria bancrofti*
d. *Mansonella perstans*
e. *Brugia malayi*

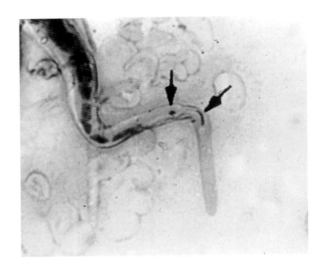

Figure 14.53

93. How is the diagnosis of onchocerciasis most commonly made?
a. By identifying microfilaria in the peripheral blood
b. By demonstrating microfilaria in teased snips of skin
c. Isolating the Simulium black fly at the site of the bite
d. Detecting microfilaria in conjunctival secretions in cases of night blindness
e. Biopsy of subcutaneous nodules to demonstrate the adult worms

94. Illustrated in the photomicrograph (Fig. 14.54) is an H&E-stained section of dissected pieces of skeletal

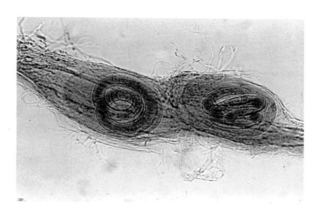

Figure 14.54

muscle containing a pair of larvae. What is the presumptive diagnosis?
a. Visceral larva migrans (*Toxicara canis*)
b. Hydatid disease (*Echinococcus* species)
c. Trichinosis (*Trichinella spiralis*)
d. Sparganum (*Spirometra mansonoides*)
e. Coenurosis (*Multiceps* species)

95. Echinococcosus, or hydatid disease, is a parasitic disease in which humans serve as accidental hosts, in whom cysts develop in the viscera after ingestion of the larval forms. What are the two animal species that serve as definitive and intermediate hosts?
a. Horses and dogs
b. Swine and cattle
c. Dogs and sheep
d. Cats and a variety of birds
e. Foxes and wild rabbits

96. It may be wise to inform physicians in addendum comments to reports that serologic assays are available to establish a definitive diagnosis of each of the following clinically suspected deep-seated parasitic diseases EXCEPT:
a. Toxoplasmosis
b. Trichinosis
c. Cysticercosis
d. Extraintestinal amebiasis
e. Sparganosis

97. Which of the following diagnostic parasitology procedures should the physician be advised that the laboratory will not perform even if specifically included in an "O & P" order?
a. Direct wet mounts for detection of motility in preserved specimens
b. Concentration procedures
c. Acid-fast stains when cryptosporidium is suspected
d. Both concentration and permanent-stained smears on stool specimens
e. Fecal immunoassays on formalin-preserved specimens

98. Each of the following guidelines should be included in the laboratory ward manual or in the electronic order program relative to submitting stool specimens for parasite examination EXCEPT:
a. Two fresh or preserved specimens should be submitted for parasite examination on successive days or on an every-other day schedule.
b. If diarrhea is not one of the symptoms, a single stool should be submitted followed by a specimen collected after using a cathartic on the second day.
c. Stools should not be submitted for parasitic examination on any patient after 3 days in the hospital.
d. The third successive stool specimen will not be accepted.
e. Two specimens should be submitted on successive days for direct EIA assays.

99. Each of the following reports should include an addendum comment relative to the conditions indicated as a guide to appropriate patient care EXCEPT:
a. *Entamoeba histolytica/dispar*: Indicate that not all *Entamoeba histolytica* strains are pathogenic and a clinical correlation is needed before therapy is instituted. EIA procedures are available if it is necessary to specifically identify true *E. histolytica* strains.
b. *Blastocystis hominis*: Indicate whether the concentration of parasitic forms are few, moderate, many, or packed.
c. *Giardia lamblia*: EIA assays should always be performed even if both stool concentrates and stained smear preparations are positive for cysts.
d. *Dientamoeba fragilis*: Indicate that this parasite can be pathogenic, particularly in children, and that therapy should be considered.
e. *Endolimax nana*: Indicate that this amoeba is a common commensal and that therapy should not be instituted.

100. A stool specimen submitted on a patient with recurrent low-grade diarrhea revealed no organisms on direct examination of a stool concentrate or on the stained smear. On the next day, a second stool specimen was submitted with the same results. In the spirit of providing the physician with "how to order" guidelines, what should be the laboratory recommendation?
a. Submit a third stool specimen for O & P exam on the following day.
b. That an order for special acid-fast stains be performed
c. Order O & P plus fecal immunoassays on a stool concentrate
d. Order O & P on stool concentrates and immunoassays for *Cryptosporidium, Cyclospora, and Microspora*
e. Order an agar plate culture for *Strongyloides stercoralis*

101. A 36-year-old woman with elevated AST and ALT levels has serum collected for viral serologic tests. The results of these tests are as follows:
Hepatitis B surface antigen: positive
Hepatitis B surface antibody: negative
Hepatitis C antibody: positive
IgM antibody to hepatitis B core antigen: negative
Total antibody to hepatitis B core antigen: positive
IgM antibody to hepatitis A: negative
IgG antibody to hepatitis A: positive

Which of the following conclusions can you draw from these test results?
a. The patient has acute hepatitis C.
b. The patient has chronic hepatitis C.
c. The patient has acute hepatitis B.
d. The patient has chronic hepatitis B.
e. The patient has chronic hepatitis A.

102. A 37-year-old man with slightly elevated AST and ALT levels has serum collected for serologic tests for viral hepatitis. The results of these tests are as follows:
Hepatitis B surface antigen: negative
Hepatitis B surface antibody: positive
IgM antibody to hepatitis B core antigen: negative
Total antibody to hepatitis B core antigen: positive
IgG antibody to hepatitis A: positive

Which of the following conclusions can you draw from these test results?
a. The patient has acute hepatitis B.
b. The patient has chronic hepatitis B.
c. The patient is immune to hepatitis B by means of vaccination.
d. The patient is immune to hepatitis B through natural infection.
e. The patient has chronic hepatitis A.

103. A 56-year-old man with markedly elevated AST and ALT levels has serum collected for serologic tests for viral hepatitis. The results of these tests are as follows:
Hepatitis B surface antigen: negative
Hepatitis B surface antibody: positive
IgM antibody to hepatitis B core antigen: negative
Total antibody to hepatitis B core antigen: negative
IgG antibody to hepatitis A: positive

Which of the following conclusions can you draw from these test results?
a. The patient has acute hepatitis B.
b. The patient has chronic hepatitis B.
c. The patient is immune to hepatitis B by means of vaccination.
d. The patient is immune to hepatitis B through natural infection.
e. The patient has chronic hepatitis A.

104. A 36-year-old woman with elevated AST and ALT levels has serum collected for viral serologic tests. The results of these tests are as follows:
Hepatitis B surface antigen: negative
Hepatitis B surface antibody: negative
Hepatitis C antibody: positive
IgM antibody to hepatitis B core antigen: negative
Total antibody to hepatitis B core antigen: negative
IgM antibody to hepatitis A: negative

Which of the following conclusions can you draw from these test results?
a. The patient has acute hepatitis C.
b. The patient has chronic hepatitis C.
c. The patient is immune to hepatitis C.
d. The patient has probably been infected with hepatitis C at some point in their life.

105. A 36-year-old woman with elevated AST and ALT levels has serum collected for viral serologic tests. The results of these tests are as follows:
Hepatitis B surface antigen: negative
Hepatitis B surface antibody: negative
IgM antibody to hepatitis B core antigen: negative
Total antibody to hepatitis B core antige: positive

Which of the following conclusions can you draw from these test results?
a. The patient has acute hepatitis B.
b. The patient has chronic hepatitis B.
c. The patient has active hepatitis B infection.
d. The patient is immune to hepatitis B.
e. None of the above

106. An 8-month-old boy is being evaluated because he has had chronic sinusitis, one case of staphylococcal bacteremia, and a case of pneumococcal pneumonia in the past 3 months. Physical examination is normal and a chest x-ray is also normal. Laboratory tests reveal the following:

Serum IgG:	very low
Serum IgM:	very low
Serum IgA:	very low
IgM+ cells:	Within normal limits (WNL)
CD21+ cells:	WNL
CD3+ cells:	WNL
CD4+ cells:	WNL
CD8+ cells:	WNL

Which of the following diseases is consistent with these findings?
a. Bruton disease
b. Transient hypogammaglobulinemia
c. DiGeorge syndrome
d. Severe combined immunodeficiency

107. A 6-month-old girl is evaluated for an immunodeficiency after she is diagnosed with *Pneumocystis* pneumonia. A thymic shadow is not evident on chest

x-ray and physical examination reveals an absence of tonsils. Laboratory studies reveal markedly reduced serum Ig levels, and an almost complete absence of circulating lymphocytes. Which of the following is UNLIKELY to explain these findings?
a. IL-2 receptor deficiency
b. Recombinase activating gene deficiency
c. Deficient expression of MHC class I molecules
d. Adenosine deaminase deficiency
e. JAK-3 tyrosine kinase deficiency

108. A 4-week-old boy is evaluated for a possible immunodeficiency. He had been hospitalized with a bacterial infection of the umbilical stump that was responding to antimicrobial therapy. During this infection, his neutrophil count was markedly elevated to levels that were very abnormal for this type of infection. A Rebuck skin window was performed to evaluate his potential immunodeficiency. In this procedure, the skin of the forearm is gently abraded with a scalpel blade and a cover slip is placed on the abrasion. Every 2 hours, for 8 hours, the cover slip is removed, replaced by a new cover slip, and examined under the microscope. In this way, migration of neutrophils to the damaged skin can be monitored. No neutrophils accumulated on any of the cover slips examined, despite very high neutrophil counts in peripheral blood. Which of the following is likely to account for a mutation in the gene encoding findings?
a. LFA-1
b. B7
c. CD28
d. CD40
e. C-reactive protein

109. A 2-year-old boy with a history of multiple bacterial infections is evaluated for an immunodeficiency. His serum IgM levels are slightly elevated, but his serum IgG, IgA, and IgE levels are markedly reduced. Circulating lymphocytes, B lymphocytes, and T lymphocytes are all within normal limits. This patient most likely has a mutation in the gene encoding in which of the following molecules?
a. LFA-1
b. B7
c. CD28
d. CD154 (CD40 Ligand)
e. C reactive Protein

110. Sera from patients with systemic lupus erythematosus (SLE) are most likely to yield a false-positive result in which of the following tests?
a. Rapid plasma reagin (RPR) test
b. Microhemagglutination-treponema pallidum (MHA-TP)
c. Cold agglutinins
d. Proteus OX 19 antibodies
e. Lyme serology

111. A 36-year-old woman is hospitalized with pneumonia. Her history includes chronic sinusitis of 5 weeks' duration, and urinalysis reveals proteinuria and hematuria. A diagnosis of Wegener granulomatosis is considered. A positive result in which of the following serologic tests would provide the strongest support for this diagnosis?
a. Rheumatoid factor
b. Antinuclear antibody
c. Anti–double-stranded DNA
d. Antineutrophil cytoplasmic antibody
e. Anti-Ro

112. A 33-year-old woman comes to her physician complaining of extremely dry eyes. On questioning, she also indicates that she has had difficulty eating because her mouth has felt very dry recently. Which of the following serologic tests should be ordered to support the diagnosis suggested by these clinical symptoms?
a. Rheumatoid factor
b. Antinuclear antibody
c. Antismooth muscle antibodies
d. Antineutrophil cytoplasmic antibody
e. Anti-Ro and anti-La

113. A 49-year-old woman visits her physician for a physical examination. She does not have any specific complaints, but laboratory tests reveal elevated AST and ALT levels, and subsequent analysis reveals elevated IgG levels. A diagnosis of type 1 autoimmune hepatitis would be most strongly supported by a positive result for which of the following tests?
a. Antimitochondrial antibodies
b. Antinuclear antibody
c. Antismooth muscle antibodies
d. Antineutrophil cytoplasmic antibody
e. Anti-Ro and anti-La

114. A 63-year-old woman who visits her physician for her annual physical examination indicates that she has been unusually tired over the past several months and also complains that her skin has been itching lately. Laboratory data reveals elevated liver function tests, but viral serologic tests do not support a diagnosis of viral hepatitis and there is no history of alcohol abuse. An autoimmune disorder is considered, with primary consideration given to primary biliary cirrhosis. A positive test in which of the following tests would provide the strongest support for this diagnosis?
a. AMA
b. Antinuclear antibody and anti–double-stranded DNA
c. Antismooth muscle antibodies
d. Antineutrophil cytoplasmic antibody
e. Anti-Ro and anti-La

115. A 5-week-old infant whose mother was HIV infected during pregnancy is brought to her pediatrician. Which

of the following tests should be used to determine whether or not the baby is HIV infected?

a. ELISA for serum antibodies
b. Western Blot for serum antibodies
c. RT-PCR for viral RNA
d. ELISA for salivary antibodies
e. PCR for HIV proviral DNA

116. A newborn infant, with various clinical problems is evaluated for the possibility of an in-utero infection. Serologic results are as follows:

IgM anti-toxoplasma antibody: negative
IgG anti-toxoplasma antibody: negative
IgM anti-rubella antibody: negative
IgG anti-rubella antibody: positive
IgM anti-CMV antibody: positive
IgG anti-CMV antibody: negative
RPR: positive
MHA-TP: negative

These serologic tests implicate which of the following organisms in this infection?

a. Toxoplasma
b. Rubella
c. CMV
d. *T. pallidum*
e. None of the above

117. A 67-year-old man with confusion and difficulty maintaining his balance is evaluated for neurosyphilis. A negative result in which of the following tests would provide the strongest evidence against this patient having neurosyphilis?

a. Serum RPR
b. Serum VDRL
c. CSF VDRL
d. Serum MHA-TP
e. CSF MHA-TP

118. A 37-year-old man comes to his physician because of a chronic infection on his right wrist. Due to his history of owning his own pet shop and spending a large amount of time cleaning aquaria, the possibility of *Mycbacterium marinum* infection is considered. In addition to inoculating and incubating media under standard conditions for recovery of *Mycobacterium tuberculosis*, what additional media/incubation conditions should be utilized to maximize recovery of *M. marinum*?

a. Chocolate agar slant at 30°C
b. Chocolate agar slant at 42°C
c. Middlebrook 7H11 slant at 30°C
d. Middlebrook 7H11 at 42°C
e. BCYE agar at 25°C

119. A 46-year-old man with AIDS is seen by his physician because of a chronic infection on his left forearm. A specimen from the lesion had been previously collected and acid-fast bacilli were observed but no organisms were recovered in culture after 3 weeks, and consideration is given to the possibility that he is infected with *Mycobacterium haemophilum*. In addition to inoculating and incubating media under standard conditions for recovery of *M. tuberculosis*, what additional media/incubation conditions should be utilized to maximize recovery of *M. haemophilum*?

a. Chocolate agar slant at 30°C
b. Chocolate agar slant at 42°C
c. Middlebrook 7H11 slant at 30°C
d. Middlebrook 7H11 at 42°C
e. BCYE agar at 25°C

120. Under normal clinical circumstances, a treponemal test is routinely performed after a positive RPR test result is obtained. A positive treponemal test result generally confirms that the patient has syphilis, whereas a negative treponemal test result usually indicates that the RPR test was falsely positive. Which of the following clinical conditions compromises the use of treponemal tests as described and interpreted above?

a. Primary syphilis
b. Pregnancy
c. Systemic lupus erythmatosus
d. Previously diagnosed and treated syphilis
e. Co-infection with *Haemophilus ducreyi*

121. A bronchoalveolar lavage is performed on a 33-year-old man with pneumonia of several weeks duration that has not responded to antimicrobial therapy. Silver stain of a cytology specimen is shown (Fig. 14.55); individual cells are approximately 12 μm in diameter. After 13 days, gray-white fungal hyphae are

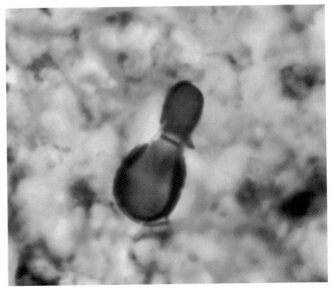

Figure 14.55 (Image taken from Centers for Disease Control and Prevention website at http://phil.cdc.gov/phil/home.asp.)

detected on a variety of fungal culture media incubated at room temperature. This most likely diagnosis in this patient is:

a. Blastomycosis
b. Coccidioidomycosis
c. Candidiasis
d. Sporotrichosis
e. Histoplasmosis

122. A fungal blood culture is collected on a patient with AIDS, high fever, and a pulmonary infiltrate. After 12 days, a whitish mycelial mass is detected on a variety of fungal culture media. After an additional week, the following structures (Fig. 14.56) are detected in the fungal culture; each of these large structures is approximately 12 μm in diameter. The most likely diagnosis in this patient is:

a. Blastomycosis
b. Coccidioidomycosis
c. Candidiasis
d. Sporotrichosis
e. Histoplasmosis

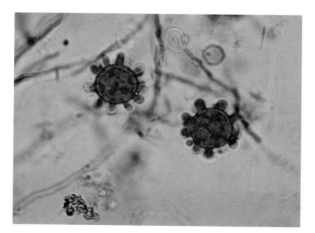

Figure 14.56 (Image taken from Centers for Disease Control and Prevention website at http://phil.cdc.gov/phil/home.asp.)

123. A 37-year-old man is hospitalized with fever and chills. Blood cultures are collected on the day of admission turn positive within 24 hours, yeasts are detected on Gram stain, and the blood cultures are subcultured to blood and chocolate agar plates. The following day, the following structures (Fig. 14.57) are detected with India ink; each individual cell is approximately 5 to 17 μm in diameter. The identity of this isolate is likely to be which of the following?

a. *Candida albicans*
b. *Cryptococcus neoformans*
c. *Malassezia furfur*
d. *Trichosporon beigelii*
e. *Geotrichium candidum*

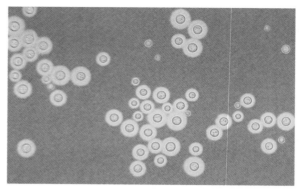

Figure 14.57 (Image taken from Centers for Disease Control and Prevention website at http://phil.cdc.gov/phil/home.asp.)

124. A 57-year-old woman with leukemia is hospitalized due to a rapidly progressive sinusitis. The nasal area has a thick, dark, blood-tinged discharge, and this material is submitted for bacterial and fungal culture. A calcofluor white stain reveals structures with the following morphology (Fig. 14.58); the hyphae range from approximately 10–20 μm in diameter. The following day, several colonies of fungi are detected on chocolate and blood agars, submitted for bacterial culture. The most likely identity of this organism is:

a. *Aspergillus*
b. *Rhizopus*
c. *Penicillium*
d. *Paecilomyces*
e. *Candida*

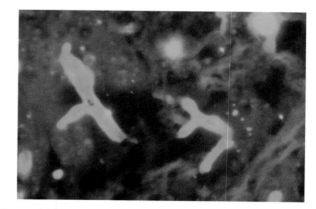

Figure 14.58 (Image taken from Centers for Disease Control and Prevention website at http://phil.cdc.gov/phil/home.asp.)

125. A 57-year-old woman comes to her physician because of three lesions on her right forearm. The first lesion initially appeared approximately 4 weeks earlier, as a small, hard nodule. The second and third lesions each appeared at weekly intervals. The initial lesion has ulcerated, and is now necrotic. The patient had been treated previously with cefazolin, but there did not appear to be any clinical response. A skin biopsy is collected and submitted for KOH examination and fungal culture. Rare elongated yeasts are detected on direct

examination, and growth is detected on fungal media within 48 hours. A lactophenol cotton blue preparation of a scotch tape preparation from 4-day-old cultures is shown (Fig. 14.59). The most likely identity of this organism is:

a. *Candida albicans*
b. *Geotrichium* species
c. *Sporothrix schenkii*
d. *Blastomyces dermatitidis*
e. *Histoplasma capsulatum*

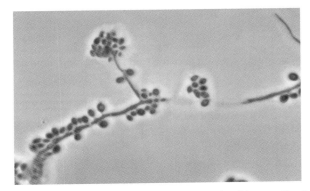

Figure 14.59 (Image taken from Centers for Disease Control and Prevention website at http://phil.cdc.gov/phil/home.asp.)

126. A 23-year-old woman who lives in Thailand comes to the hospital because of skin lesions that have developed on her face and trunk. She is known to be HIV infected and has had several previous opportunistic infections. On examination, her temperature is 100.4°F, her liver appears enlarged, she has generalized lymphadenopathy, and she has many umbilicated papules on her face and trunk. Histologic examination of a skin biopsy from one of the lesions reveals numerous tiny yeasts, and fungal culture of this material reveals a grayish mold that produces a diffusible red pigment after 5 days of incubation at room temperature; a lactophenol cotton blue preparation of this mold is shown in the accompanying figure (Fig. 14.60). On subculture at 37°C,

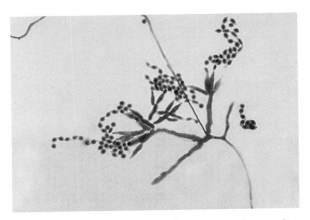

Figure 14.60 (Image taken from Centers for Disease Control and Prevention website at http://phil.cdc.gov/phil/home.asp.)

the mold is readily converted to a yeast. The most likely cause of this infection is:

a. *Candida albicans*
b. *Penicillium marneffei*
c. *Trichosporon beigelii*
d. *Blastomyces dermatitidis*
e. *Coccidioides immits*

127. A skin scraping is collected from the scalp of a 13-year-old boy with three slowly growing bumps on his head. A KOH/calcofluor white examination of this material was negative, but a white filamentous fungus with the microscopic characteristics shown (Fig. 14.61) was recovered after 4 days incubation at room temperature. The large structures shown (Fig. 14.61) are approximately 20 × 70 μm. The most likely genus of this fungus is:

a. *Trichosporon*
b. *Trichophyton*
c. *Microsporum*
d. *Epidermophyton*
e. *Malassezia*

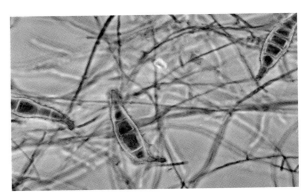

Figure 14.61 (Image taken from Centers for Disease Control and Prevention website at http://phil.cdc.gov/phil/home.asp.)

128. Supplementation of media with which of the following is critical for recovering *Malassezia furfur* in culture?
a. Hemin
b. NAD
c. Cysteine
d. Charcoal
e. Lipids

129. Microscopic examination of a biopsy specimen with KOH/calcofluor white reveals an organism with the morphology shown in the accompanying figure (Fig. 14.62); the structures shown have a diameter of 3–5 μm. This morphology is characteristic of:
a. *Candida*
b. *Rhizopus*
c. *Aspergillus*
d. *Nocardia*
e. *Malassezia*

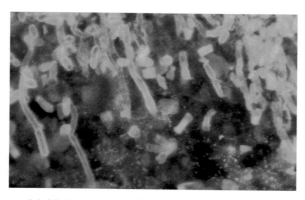

Figure 14.62 (Image taken from Centers for Disease Control and Prevention website at http://phil.cdc.gov/phil/home.asp.)

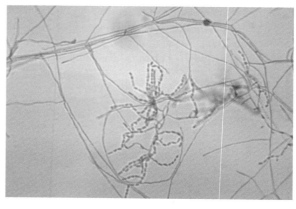

Figure 14.63 (Image taken from Centers for Disease Control and Prevention website at http://phil.cdc.gov/phil/home.asp.)

130. Which of the following *Candida* organisms does not produce pseudohyphae?
    a. *Candida albicans*
    b. *Candida tropicalis*
    c. *Candida krusei*
    d. *Candida glabrata*
    e. *Candida parapsilosis*

131. Which of the following *Candida* spp. is most likely to be resistant to fluconazole?
    a. *Candida albicans*
    b. *Candida tropicalis*
    c. *Candida krusei*
    d. *Candida glabrata*
    e. *Candida parapsilosis*

132. Person-to-person transmission is most likely to occur with which of the following fungal species?
    a. *Blastomyces dermatitidis*
    b. *Coccidiodes immitis*
    c. *Trichophyton rubrum*
    d. *Histoplasma capsulatum*
    e. *Sporthrix schenkii*

133. A bronchoalveolar lavage specimen is submitted for fungal culture. Several yellowish colonies are recovered on brain heart infusion (BHI) agar, but not on BHI with chloramphenicol and cyclohexamide, incubated in ambient air at room temperature for 4 days. Microscopic examination reveals organisms with the morphology shown in the accompanying figure (Fig. 14.63). The diameter of these filaments is approximately 1 µm. The organism grows in the presence of lysozyme. This organism is most likely to be a member of which of the following genera:
    a. *Aspergillus*
    b. *Nocardia*
    c. *Actinomyces*
    d. *Rhodococcus*
    e. *Streptomyces*

134. Which of the following organisms will not stain acid fast with a modified acid-fast stain?
    a. *Cryptosporidium parvum*
    b. *Rhodococcus equi*
    c. *Nocardia asteroides*
    d. *Isosopora belli*
    e. *Streptomyces somaliensis*

135. Several colonies of cream colored cottony fungus are recovered after 4 days' incubation at room temperature from an "eye" specimen. The morphology is as shown in the accompanying figure (Fig. 14.64). The most likely identification of this fungus is:
    a. *Acanthamoeba*
    b. *Fusarium*
    c. *Paecilomyces*
    d. *Aspergillus*
    e. *Penicillium*

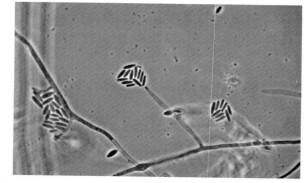

Figure 14.64 (Image taken from Centers for Disease Control and Prevention website at http://phil.cdc.gov/phil/home.asp.)

136. Several colonies of a velvety, dark gray fungus are detected after 2 weeks of incubation at room temperature. The specimen source is a biopsy from the foot of a Haitian immigrant whose foot has been swollen and disfigured for many months. The

microscopic morphology is as shown in the accompanying figure (Fig. 14.65). The most likely identity of this fungus is:

a. *Phialophora*
b. *Cladosporium*
c. *Paecilomyces*
d. *Blastomyces*
e. *Paracoccidioides*

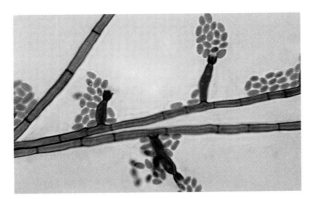

Figure 14.65 (Image taken from Centers for Disease Control and Prevention website at http://phil.cdc.gov/phil/home.asp.)

137. Direct or indirect person-to-person transmission is UNLIKELY to occur with which of the following organisms/infections?
a. Pharyngitis due to *Streptococcus pyogenes*
b. Pneumonia due to *Legionella pneumophila*
c. Diarrhea due to *Shigella sonnei*
d. Hepatitis due to hepatitis A virus
e. Pinworm infection due to *Enterobius vermicularis*

138. A specimen collected from a surgical site infection is submitted for bacterial culture. After 24 hours of incubation, several colonies of beaded Gram-positive bacilli are recovered on blood and chocolate agar plates. These organisms are found to be acid fast with a routine Kinyoun stain. The most likely identity of this isolate is:
a. *Mycobacterium kansasii*
b. *Mycobacterium avium* complex
c. *Mycobacterium gordonii*
d. *Mycobacterium fortuitum* complex
e. *Mycobacterium tuberculosis*

139. Over a 3-week period, the mycobacteriology laboratory experiences an unusually large number of cultures that are positive for acid-fast bacilli. The organisms are recovered on both Middlebrook 7H11 and Lowenstein Jenson solid media, and are typically first detected after approximately 2 weeks of incubation at 37°C. The colonies have a deep yellow-orange pigment when initially recovered, and subcultures in the dark are similarly pigmented. Epidemiologic investigation reveals that the majority of patients from whom these organisms were recovered do not appear to have symptoms compatible with a mycobacterial infection. The most likely identity of these isolates is:
a. *Mycobacterium tuberculosis*
b. *Mycobacterium kansasii*
c. *Mycobacterium avium* complex
d. *Mycobacterium gordonae*
e. *Mycobacterium fortuitum* complex

140. Which of the following conditions is insufficient to qualify an HIV-infected individual as having AIDS?
a. Disseminated tuberculosis
b. CD4 T-cell count $<200/\mu L$
c. Pulmonary histoplasmosis
d. Pneumocystis pneumonia
e. Chronic intestinal crytosporidiosis

141. A patient with which of the following serologic profiles is NOT currently infected with hepatitis D, and CANNOT become infected with hepatitis D virus in the future (see table below)?
a. A
b. B
c. C
d. D
e. E

	Patient A	Patient B	Patient C	Patient D	Patient E
Hepatitis B surface antigen	Positive	Negative	Negative	Positive	Negative
Hepatitis B surface antibody	Negative	Positive	Negative	Negative	Negative
Hepatitis C antibody	Positive	Negative	Positive	Negative	Negative
IgM antibody to hepatitis B core antigen	Positive	Positive	Negative	Positive	Negative
IgM antibody to hepatitis A	Negative	Negative	Negative	Negative	Positive
IgG antibody to hepatitis A	Positive	Negative	Negative	Negative	Negative

142. In addition to *Candida albicans*, which of the following yeasts will produce positive results with a germ-tube test?
a. *Candida glabrata*
b. *Candida krusei*
c. *Candida dublinensis*
d. *Cryptococcus neoformans*
e. *Candida parapsilosis*

143. A 56-year-old woman with fibrosis and atrophy of the skin on her hands, and fibrosis of the skin on her arms, shoulders, and face, is seen in clinic. She also complains that her hands seem to freeze up in cool weather relatively easily, and that it has recently become difficult for her to swallow. A positive result in which of the

following tests would provide the strongest support for a diagnosis of systemic sclerosis?
a. Anti-DNA topoisomerase I
b. Anti-mitochondrial antibodies
c. Anti-nuclear antibody
d. Anti-smooth muscle antibodies
e. Anti-Ro and anti-La

144. A 4-year-old boy is brought to his pediatrician because his face began swelling the previous day and continued to swell over the next 24 hours. His mother indicates that the swelling appears to have decreased slightly in the past few hours. A screening test indicates that the patient's serum C4 levels are markedly reduced. To further diagnose hereditary angioneurotic edema in this patient, quantitation of which of the following would be most useful?
a. C1
b. C1 inhibitor
c. C3
d. C7
e. Total hemolytic complement

145. A complete deficiency in which of the following complement components is most likely to predispose to recurrent, life-threatening infections in early childhood?
a. C1
b. C2
c. C3
d. C4
e. C6

146. Which of the following fungal culture media is least effective for recovering dimorphic fungi from clinical specimens?
a. Brain-heart infusion agar (BHI)
b. BHI agar with chloramphenicol and cyclohexamide
c. Inhibitory mold agar
d. Sabouraud brain heart infusion (SABHI) agar
e. Sabouraud dextrose agar (SDA)

147. Patients with severe neutropenia are at greatest risk for disseminated infection with which of the following fungi?
a. *Histoplasma capsulatum*
b. *Aspergillus fumigatus*
c. *Pneumocystis jiroveci*
d. *Coccidioides immitis*
e. *Trichophyton rubrum*

148. Hyperacute rejection of kidney allografts depends on which of the following pathogenic mechanisms?
a. Type I hypersensitivity
b. Type II hypersensitivity
c. Type III hypersensitivity
d. Type IV hypersensitivity

149. Damage to the kidney in patients with systemic lupus erythematosus (SLE) is due primarily to which of the following pathogenic mechanisms?
a. Type I hypersensitivity
b. Type II hypersensitivity
c. Type III hypersensitivity
d. Type IV hypersensitivity

150. Hematologic abnormalities (e.g., leukopenia, lymphopenia) observed in patients with systemic lupus erythematosus (SLE) is due primarily to which of the following pathogenic mechanisms?
a. Type I hypersensitivity
b. Type II hypersensitivity
c. Type III hypersensitivity
d. Type IV hypersensitivity

151. In evaluating the capacity of peripheral blood leukocytes to respond to various proliferative stimuli, markedly reduced proliferative responses to conconavalin A indicates deficient function of which of the following?
a. CD 3+ lymphocytes
b. CD19+ lymphocytes
c. Antigen presenting cells
d. Neutrophils
e. NK cells

152. In evaluating the capacity of peripheral blood leukocytes to respond to various proliferative stimuli, markedly reduced proliferative responses to irradiated allogeneic leukocytes indicates deficient function of which of the following?
a. CD4+ lymphocytes
b. CD8+ lymphocytes
c. CD19+ lymphocytes
d. Macrophages
e. CD56 lymphocytes

153. A 50-year-old leukemic patient develops fever and a black necrotic lesion on his upper palate. Rhinocerebral mucormycocis is suspected. All of the following statements regarding this disease and its diagnosis are true EXCEPT:
a. A biopsy specimen from tissue around the necrosed area should be submitted for fungal culture.
b. Tissue biopsy specimens submitted for culture should be homogenized thoroughly before plating.
c. Zygomycetes will not grow on cycloheximide containing media.
d. Isolation of the pathogen is achieved in only a small proportion of cases.
e. Rhizopus is the most common pathogen isolated from patients with rhinocerebral mucormycosis.

154. A mold is growing from biopsy material obtained from the hard palate. A rapidly growing white cottony

colony fills the plate within second day of culture. Microscopically, a single sporangiophore is borne singly or in groups opposite rhizoids. Hyphae are non-septate. What is the identity of the organism?
   a. *Rhizopus* spp.
   b. *Rhizomucor* spp.
   c. *Mucor* spp.
   d. *Cuninghamella* spp.
   e. *Saksena* spp.

155. A 65-year-old man is admitted for viral encephalitis. He had fever, myalgias, progressive weakness, and respiratory insufficiency, with the subsequent development of flaccid paralysis. Performance of which of the following tests is most appropriate for confirming a diagnosis of West Nile encephalitis?
   a. PCR on CSF
   b. Serology on CSF
   c. PCR from serum
   d. Viral isolation from CSF
   e. Viral isolation from blood

156. A mycobacterial infection is suspected in association with multiple skin nodules in the scrotum of an AIDS patient. A tissue biopsy is AFB smear positive and submitted for culture. Which of the following incubation or culture conditions is critical to recovering the potential etiologic agents of this infection?
   a. Inoculate ferric ammonium citrate medium and incubate at 30°C
   b. Incubate at 37°C for up to 6–8 weeks
   c. Inoculate liquid medium for efficient recovery
   d. Inoculate Egg-based solid media
   e. Inoculate selective medium to eliminate skin flora

157. Upper lobe fibrocavitary disease is detected in a 60-year-old heavy smoker with preexisting lung disease. He is hospitalized with a productive cough, fatigue, fever, weight loss, and night sweats. His sputum culture is positive for AFB and grows nonchromogenic smooth, colonies after 2 weeks of incubation, which are Niacin negative. What is the most probable cause of his infection?
   a. *M. avium-intracellularae*
   b. *M. tuberculosis*
   c. *M. hemophilum*
   d. *M. gordonae*
   e. *M. simiae*

158. A lymph node biopsy from the neck of a 5-year-old child is submitted for mycobacterial culture. After 2 weeks of incubation, small buff-colored colonies of acid-fast bacteria are growing on the media. What is the most probable identification of the organism?
   a. *M. avium-intracellularae*
   b. *M. marinum*

   c. *M. hemophilum*
   d. *M. gordonae*
   e. *M. simiae*

159. A 50-year-old man is diagnosed with intestinal lipodystrophy. A biopsy of the small intestine demonstrates "foamy" macrophages infiltrating lamina propria containing periodic acid-schiff positive inclusions resembling bacteria. What is the organism causing this disease?
   a. *H. pylori*
   b. *Lactobacillus*
   c. *Tropheryma* spp.
   d. *Actinomyces*
   e. *Nocardia*

160. A teenager is hospitalized with disseminated intravascular coagulation, fever, and refractory hypotension, 2 days after he was bitten by a dog . His medical history is significant for splenectomy 6 months previous to this incident. After 2 days of incubation on blood agar, cultures collected from infected tissue at the site of the bite reveal 2–3 mm diameter spreading, nonhemolytic colonies. What is the most probable identification of the isolated organism?
   a. *Capnocytophaga canimorsus*
   b. *Pastereulla multocida*
   c. *Streptococcus pyogenes*
   d. *Eikenella corrodens*
   e. *Listeria monocytogenes*

161. A 60-year-old woman develops a necrotic lesion on her palms and several small ulcerating nodules on her forearm with purulent discharge. She remembers having sustained numerous pricks on her hand while planting rose plants around her front porch 2 weeks earlier. A dimorphic fungus is recovered from biopsy specimens from these skin lesions. A silver stain of the biopsy from her palm shows small round, oval or cigar-shaped budding yeast cells. What is the diagnosis?
   a. Balstomycosis
   b. Sporotrichosis
   c. Histoplasmosis
   d. Coccidiomycosis
   e. Aspergillosis

162. A germ-tube positive *Candida* sp. is obtained from a HIV-positive patient on fluconazole prophylaxis. It failed to grow at 42°C and does not express beta-glucosidase activity. What is the most probable identification of the *Candida* species?
   a. *C. parapsilosis*
   b. *C. albicans*
   c. *C. dubliniensis*
   d. *C. tropicalis*
   e. *C.glabrata*

163. A teenager is seen in the ophthalmology clinic for blurring of vision due to fungal infection of the cornea. The patient is a soft contact lens user and reports switching to a new lens cleaning solution in the last month. Which of the following molds is most likely to be recovered from corneal scrapings from this patient?
    a. *Alternaria* spp.
    b. *Fusarium* spp.
    c. *Curvularia* spp.
    d. *Acremonium* spp.
    e. *Cladosporium* spp.

164. A rapid antigen test for influenza has a sensitivity of 95% and a specificity of 96%. What is the positive predictive value of the test when the prevalence of the disease is 1%?
    a. 9%
    b. 19%
    c. 39%
    d. 49%
    e. 59%

165. A rapid antigen test for influenza has a sensitivity of 95% and a specificity of 96%. What is the positive predictive value of the test when the prevalence of the disease is 20%?
    a. 19%
    b. 39%
    c. 59%
    d. 79%
    e. 86%

166. How is the performance of an influenza rapid antigen test influenced by a low prevalence of influenza in the community early and late in the influenza season?
    a. False negatives are common.
    b. False positives are common.
    c. No influence on test results.
    d. PPV for the test is high.
    e. PPV for the test is unchanged.

167. The test result that is legally admissible as evidence for sexual abuse in a child for detection of *Chlamydia trachomatis* and *Neisseria gonorrhoea* is:
    a. Direct fluorescent antibody test
    b. Serology
    c. Culture
    d. Nucleic acid detection test
    e. Nucleic acid amplification test

168. A newborn infant has fever and lethargy in the first week of life. Examination of CSF is significant for CSF pleocytosis and MRI shows temporal lobe involvement. Examination of CSF by which of the following methods is most likely to confirm a diagnosis of herpes simplex virus (HSV) encephalitis?
    a. Viral culture
    b. Serology
    c. Direct fluorescent antibody test
    d. Realtime PCR
    e. Reverse transcriptase PCR

169. A teenage girl is seen in the adolescent clinic for complaints of intense itching in the vulvar area and a yellow-greenish, frothy, foul-smelling vaginal discharge. Which of the following diagnoses is most likely?
    a. *Candida* vulvovaginitis
    b. Allergic vaginitis
    c. Bacterial vaginosis
    d. *Trichomonas* vaginitis
    e. Herpes simplex virus infection

170. A 30-year-old volunteer from the Red Cross is admitted for fever and a swollen, painful left leg with blistering skin lesions. In the previous week, he was working in the Mississippi coast removing debris from a recent hurricane. A Gram-negative, lactose fermenting, oxidase-positive bacteria were isolated in pure culture on MacConkey agar. What is the most likely cause of his illness?
    a. *Vibrio cholerae*
    b. *Aeromonas hydrophila*
    c. *Vibrio vulnificus*
    d. *Chromobacter violaceum*
    e. *Pseudomonas aeruginosa*

171. Congenital rubella is suspected in a 1-month-old baby delivered to an immigrant worker with no medical records. The baby shows signs of hepatosplenomegaly, thrombocytopenia, and jaundice. Diagnosis of congenital rubella can be accomplished by all of the following methods EXCEPT:
    a. Detection of rubella specific IgM in the infants serum
    b. Detection of rubella specific IgG in the infants serum
    c. Detection of rubella specific IgG in the infants serum after 6 month of age
    d. An elevated and consistent titer of rubella antibodies detected by hemagglutination inhibition during the first 6 month of life

172. A 5-year old boy is admitted to the hospital for respiratory distress and fever. Fibroblast cell cultures inoculated with a nasal aspirate collected from the patient show large and small rounded, refractile cells with pyknotic nuclei resembling the cytopathic effect of rhinovirus and enterovirus. Which of the following characteristics of rhinovirus can be used to distinguish it from enterovirus?
    a. Rhinovirus is sensitive to low pH.
    b. Enterovirus is sensitive to low pH.
    c. Rhinovirus prefer 37°C to 33°C for growth.
    d. Rhinovirus is susceptible to lipid solvents.

173. Cell cultures inoculated with a respiratory specimen show early signs of viral cytopathic effect. Guinea pig RBCs are used for the hemadsorption test to identify this virus. Which of the following characteristics can be used to detect influenza virus and to distinguish it from parainfluenza virus?
    a. Ability to hemadsorb at 4°C and 25°C
    b. Ability to hemadsorb only at 4°C
    c. Ability to hemadsorb at 37°C
    d. Inability to hemadsorb guinea pig RBC compared to PIV

174. Gram-positive cocci in clusters are seen in two separate peripheral blood cultures from a neonate. The isolate grows on a blood agar plate and is positive for the following tests: clumping factor by slide coagulase test with rabbit plasma, ornithine decarboxylase, and PYR. What is the identity of this organism?
    a. *S. aureus*
    b. *Staphylococcus lugdunensis*
    c. *Staphylococcus intermedius*
    d. *Staphylococcus hemolyticus*
    e. *Staphylococcus schleiferi*

175. A premature infant with *Enterobacter cloacae* sepsis failed to respond to cephalosporin therapy. Minimum inhibitory concentrations (MICs) of isolates obtained during the first and third day of therapy are as follows:

	DAY 1	DAY 3
cefpodoxime	1	0.5
cefotaxime	0.12	0.24
cefoxitin	8	>128
ceftazidime	0.5	0.5
ceftriaxone	0.12	0.06

    What is the most probable explanation for such an increase in MIC with cefoxitin only?
    a. ESBL production
    b. AmpC-inducible resistance
    c. AmpC- plasmid mediated resistance
    d. AmpC-derepressed mutant.
    e. K1 beta-lactamase

176. Plasmid mediated AmpC resistance has been described in all of the following bacteria EXCEPT?
    a. *Klebsiella* spp.
    b. *E. coli*
    c. *Salmonella* spp.
    d. *Enterobacter* spp.
    e. *P. mirabilis*

177. A 55-year old liver transplant patient with *Enterobacter cloacae* sepsis failed to respond to cephalosporin therapy. The isolate obtained during the first day of therapy was susceptible to all cephalosporins tested, however, an isolate obtained on the fourth day displayed resistance to all cephalosporins tested with high MICs as follows: cefpodoxime >128, cefotaxime 64, ceftazidime 64, cefoxitin >128, ceftriaxone 64. What is the most probable mechanistic explanation for this change in susceptibility to cephalosporins?
    a. ESBL production
    b. AmpC-inducible resistance
    c. AmpC- plasmid mediated resistance
    d. AmpC-derepressed mutant.
    e. K1 betalactamase

178. Aerobic culture from an eye grows Gram-positive rods with colonies that are large, circular with granular texture on a TSA sheep blood agar. By phase contrast microscopy, the cells are broad with ellipsoidal spores that do not swell the sporangia. What is the most possible pathogen?
    a. *B. anthracis*
    b. *B. cereus*
    c. *C. perfringens*
    d. *C. septicum*
    e. *B. megaterium*

179. A 15-year-old patient has received consolidation therapy for AML and is scheduled for an allogeneic bone marrow transplant. After 3 weeks of neutropenia, he develops a new onset fever, pulmonary infiltrate, and a halo and cresentric sign on CT of the chest. Histologic examination of a biopsy from the lung shows septate hyphae with acute angle branching, and culture from this specimen grows a blue-green mold with uniserate conidial heads. What is the most probable identification of this mold?
    a. *A. terreus*
    b. *A. fumigatus*
    c. *A. ustus*
    d. *P. marneffii*
    e. *A. versicolor*

180. Several medical students developed abrupt and frequent vomiting 3 hours after ingestion of a potato salad at a summer party. Nearly one third had diarrheal illness the same day, and symptoms had abated in all patients within 24 hours of onset. Which of the following organisms is the most likely cause of their illness?
    a. *Salmonella enteritidis*
    b. *Shigella dysentriae*
    c. *Clostridium perfringens*
    d. *Staphylococcus aureus*
    e. *Campylobacter jejuni*

181. A commercial PCR for *Chlamydia trachomatis* (CT) and *Neisseria gonorrhoea* (GC) detects both pathogens from a single amplification test. A plasmid containing primer binding sites identical to *C. trachomatis* is used as an internal control to monitor inhibition. Your

laboratory identifies a specimen which has high positive signal for CT and negative signal for GC and internal control. How would you report this result?

a. Report CT positive and GC negative
b. Report CT positive but GC indeterminate because of nonspecific inhibition
c. Report CT positive but GC indeterminate because of competitive inhibition
d. No inhibition occurred

182. A 40-year-old previously healthy man from Arizona is admitted to the hospital for fever, chills, and pneumonia with bilateral interstitial pulmonary infiltrates and respiratory compromise resembling acute respiratory disease syndrome. He recently returned from a 1-month trip to Asia and was involved in cleaning of his garage that was infested with rodents. What is the most probable cause of his disease?

a. CMV
b. *Cryptococcus*
c. Aspergillosis
d. Hantavirus
e. LCMV

183. *S. aureus*, isolated from a wound culture, was found to be resistant to erythromycin and susceptible to clindamycin by disc diffusion. However, the zone around clindamycin adjacent to the erythromycin disc was flattened. What is the resistance mechanism of this *S. aureus* regarding clindamycin?

a. Susceptible to clindamycin
b. Constitutive resistance to clindamycin
c. Inducible resistant to clindamycin by methylation of 23S rRNA
d. Resistance by efflux mechanism
e. Overexpression of clindamycin resistance enzyme

184. A teenage bone marrow transplant patient is in the intensive care unit with suspected septic shock. He had previously sustained a puncture wound to his leg in a nearby pond following his last chemotherapy. Ecthyma gangrenosum is suspected and broad spectrum therapy is initiated. A Gram-negative rod is recovered from blood cultures that grows on MacConkey agar, is oxidase positive, and ferments D-glucose. What is the most probable identity of this organism?

a. *E. coli*
b. *P. aeruginosa*
c. *A. hydrophila*
d. *V. vulnificus*
e. *Serratia marcescens*

185. A veterinarian working with primate colonies for a research project on simian immunodeficiency virus presents to a local hospital with diplopia, ataxia, and seizures. Following admission to the intensive care unit

he develops ascending flaccid paralysis. His CSF exam is significant for CSF pleocytosis and elevated protein levels. What is the most likely infection in this patient?

a. Simian immunodeficiency virus
b. Human immunodeficiency virus
c. Herpes simplex virus
d. Herpes B virus
e. Lymphocytic choriomeningitis virus.

186. A 7-year-old boy is admitted to a hospital in Texas during the month of August for seizures and hallucinations; his condition worsened progressively and the patient died within 5 days of admission. The parents report that the boy was swimming in a local pond for several days in the week prior to the illness. What is the most probable pathogen associated with this condition?

a. *S. pneumoniae*
b. Herpes simplex virus
c. *Naeglaria fowleri*
d. *Neisseria meningitidis*
e. Easter equine encephalitis virus

187. A 2-year-old girl is seen in the clinic for complaints of limping for the last month. MRI reveals osteomyelitis of the knee joint and *Kingella kingae* infection is suspected. What is the best method for optimal detection of *K. kingae*?

a. Serology for Kingella
b. PCR of blood for Kingella
c. Inoculation of joint fluid to blood culture media
d. Inoculation of joint fluid on TSA sheep blood agar
e. Inoculation of joint fluid on chocolate blood agar

188. A 25-year-old computer engineer is admitted to a hospital for symptoms of severe muscle pain, fever, and incapacitating joint pain and arthritis for the last 3 weeks. His symptoms started 3 weeks ago upon his return from a business trip to India. What is the most probable cause of his viral illness?

a. Dengue virus
b. West Nile virus
c. Chickungunya virus
d. Yellow fever virus
e. Easter equine encephalitis virus

189. A 1-year-old boy is seen in a Milwaukee emergency room during February and is subsequently admitted for dehydration following acute gastroenteritis. What is the most probable cause of gastroenteritis in this child?

a. Adenovirus
b. Rotavirus
c. Norovirus
d. Calicivirus
e. Astrovirus

190. A 65-year-old kidney transplant recipient is losing renal function. BK virus nephropathy versus rejection of the renal allograft are considered as potential causes of this altered function. What is the best method to implicate BK virus as the reason for loss of allograft function?
    a. BK virus PCR on urine
    b. BK virus PCR on plasma
    c. BK virus culture from urine
    d. BK virus cultre from plasma
    e. BK virus serology

191. An RSV outbreak is suspected in a nursing home. Which of the following tests is acceptable for rapid testing in this setting?
    a. Lateral flow immunochromatographic assay
    b. Direct fluorescent antibody (DFA) test
    c. Culture
    d. RT-PCR
    e. Serology

192. A teenager is admitted to the hospital for toxic shock syndrome with refractory hypotension, hemoconcentration, and profound leukocytosis; she dies within 10 hours of admission. Her history is significant for medical abortion in the last week preceding this illness. Which of the following anaerobic bacteria is associated with this condition?
    a. C. perfringens
    b. Clostridium sordellii
    c. Clostridium septicum
    d. Clostridium tetani
    e. Clostridium innocuum

193. A previously healthy 8-month-old boy is admitted to a hospital in Omaha during mid-July for clinical suspicion of meningitis. His CSF is remarkable for CSF pleocytosis with predominance of lymphocytes, increase in CSF protein, and normal CSF glucose. Which of the following pathogens is the most probable cause for his illness?
    a. Escherichia coli
    b. Listeria monocytogenes
    c. Enterovirus
    d. Herpes simplex virus
    e. Cytomegalovirus

194. Which of the following agar is used for selective isolation of Burkholderia cepacia from sputum of cystic fibrosis patients?
    a. MacConkey agar
    b. CAN agar (Columbia-colistin-nalidixic acid)
    c. CIN medium (cefsulodin-irgasan-novobiocin)
    d. OFPBL agar (oxidative-fermentative base, polymyxinB, bacitracin, lactose)
    e. CVA medium (cefoperazone-vancomycin-amphotericin B)

195. Which of the following clinical material is NOT acceptable for anaerobic culture?
    a. Sputum, expectorated
    b. Blood
    c. Sinus aspirate
    d. Transtracheal aspirate
    e. Urine, suprapubic aspirate

196. Which of the following statements about susceptibility testing of Streptococcus pneumoniae is FALSE?
    a. Microbroth dilution test requires Cation-adjusted Mueller-Hinton broth (CAMHB) supplemented with lysed horse blood.
    b. Disc diffusion test can be used to reliably predict ceftriaxone susceptibility.
    c. Oxacillin disc diffusion zone of = 20 mm indicates susceptibility to penicillin.
    d. Oxacillin zone diameter of = 19 mm may be penicillin susceptible, intermediate or resistant.
    e. Susceptibility to tetracycline indicates susceptibility to doxycycline and minocycline.

197. A 6-month-old child is admitted to the hospital for dehydration due to bloody diarrhea. The physician ordered C. difficile and bacterial stool cultures. The C. difficile antigen test is positive. How would you advise the physician?
    a. The C. difficile result is a false-positive result because colonization has not been reported in this age group.
    b. C. difficile colonization is common in this age group and does not indicate disease.
    c. Recommend physician to cancel bacterial stool cultures because C. difficle is identified as the pathogen.
    d. Inform C. difficile is forwarded to reference laboratory for susceptibility testing.
    e. Suggest that the physician submit stool for rotaviral testing.

198. Which of the following pathogens do NOT require airborne transmission precautions for infection control?
    a. M. tuberculosis
    b. Rubella
    c. Measles
    d. Varicella-zoster virus

199. A lymph node biopsy from a 10-year-old boy grows Gram-negative coccobacillus that is suspicious for Francisella spp. The organism was subsequently confirmed by the state public health lab as Francisella tularensis. What is the select agent rule recommendation for sentinel laboratories that encounter such organisms capable of being used for bioterrorism purposes?
    a. Destroy the organism within 1 week of confirmatory lab test result.
    b. Destroy the organism within 48 hours of confirmatory lab test result.

c. Destroy the organism soon after forwarding it to state public health laboratory for confirmatory test
d. Use the organism for proficiency testing provided written approval of state public health laboratory director is documented.
e. Destroy the organism within 30 calendar days from receipt of confirmatory lab test result.

200. An acute viral gastroenteritis is suspected in travelers abode a cruise ship. What is the most probable cause of this infection?
a. Adenovirus
b. Rotavirus
c. Norovirus
d. Enterovirus
e. Bocavirus

201. Which of the following emerging respiratory viruses do not belong to the group?
a. SARS
b. OC43
c. NL63
d. 229E
e. Bocavirus

202. Which of the following influenza viruses is NOT an avian influenza strain?
a. H5N1
b. H7N7
c. H7N2
d. H3N2
e. H9N2

Answers

1. **c.** *Listeria monocytogenes* is an important cause of meningitis in neonates. Neonatal infection caused by *L. monocytogenes* is similar to that caused by *Streptococcus agalactiae* (group B streptococcus). Both organisms cause an early-onset sepsis syndrome usually acquired in utero, and late-onset meningitis that occurs a few weeks after birth. *S. agalactiae* is catalase negative and is a Gram-positive coccus. *Erysipelothrix rhusiopathiae* is catalase negative and usually causes cutaneous infections or endocarditis in individuals who have had exposure to animals or animal products. *Corynebacterium jeikeium* is a pleomorphic Gram-positive rod that is nonhemolytic on blood agar and most often causes infections such as septicemia and wound infections in immunocompromised patients. *Bacillus cereus* is a spore-forming Gram-positive rod that can cause a variety of infections, including food poisoning and serious eye infections. *L. monocytogenes* is a catalase positive, beta-hemolytic Gram-positive rod that also exhibits the following characteristics: motile only at 25°C, forms a block-type CAMP test pattern, hippurate hydrolysis positive, and H$_2$S negative.

2. **b.** The TSI agar slant is used to show whether gram-negative bacteria can ferment glucose, lactose, and/or sucrose, form gas, and form H$_2$S. The ingredients of TSI agar include: the carbohydrates glucose, lactose, and sucrose, peptones, the pH indicator phenol red, sodium thiosulfate for H$_2$S production, and ferrous sulfate to detect H$_2$S. The concentration of lactose and sucrose is ten times higher than the concentration of glucose. If glucose is the only sugar fermented, acid is produced throughout the medium and initially the whole agar slant is yellow (phenol red turns yellow in the presence of acid). However, because the glucose concentration is so low, the organism will then utilize the peptones present in the medium and release basic products. Peptone utilization occurs aerobically, so the slant reverts to a red color; the butt of the medium remains yellow. This fermentation pattern is called K/A. If lactose or sucrose is fermented in addition to glucose, acid conditions are maintained throughout the medium because of the high concentrations of lactose and sucrose, so the pattern is A/A. If H$_2$S is produced by the organism in question, the butt will turn black. H$_2$S is only produced in an acid environment S, if the butt is black, it is assumed to be "A" for acid production. If gas is produced, gas bubbles will be observed in the butt of the tube.

3. **d.** *Klebsiella* (formerly *Calymmatobacterium*) *granulomatis* is the causative agent of granuloma inguinale, or Donovanosis. This disease is most likely a sexually transmitted disease, characterized by painless ulcerative genital lesions. The primary lesion often becomes a beefy red granulomatous ulcer. The disease is rare in the United States but is more prevalent in southeast India, Papua New Guinea, the Caribbean, Brazil, parts of Africa, southeast Asia, and among Aboriginals in Australia. The organism does not grow on culture media, and is usually diagnosed by observing Donovan bodies (bipolar-stained rods) in macrophages or mononuclear cells. *Haemophilus ducreyi* causes chancroid, and can be cultured on solid media. *Neisseria gonorrhoeae*, a cause of urethritis, disseminated infections, and several other diseases, can also be cultured on solid media. *Chlamydia trachomatis* causes chlamydia and is usually diagnosed by cell culture in McCoy cells or by probe hybridization assays. *Treponema pallidum* is the causative agent of syphilis and does not grow on solid media. It is a spirochete, and is usually diagnosed by nontreponemal and treponemal tests.

4. **a.** Staphylococci are catalase positive, while streptococci are catalase negative. **Catalase** is a test that can be performed in a few seconds to rapidly differentiate these two genera. The test consists of adding a drop of 3% hydrogen peroxide to colony material. If bubbling is observed, the test is considered positive.

5. **e.** Methicillin resistance in staphylococci is encoded by *mecA*. Methicillin resistant organisms are resistant in vivo to all β-lactam antibiotics. The target of β-lactam antibiotics are the penicillin-binding proteins (PBPs) found in the cell wall of bacteria. The product of *mecA* is an altered PBP called PBP2′ or PBP2a. β-lactam antibiotics do not bind well, so they are ineffective. There are a number of ways to detect methicillin resistance. The polymerase chain reaction can be used to directly detect *mecA* from either colony material or directly from specimens. Many laboratories, though, use disk diffusion to determine susceptibilities, and cefoxitin has been found to be the most sensitive indicator of methicillin resistance by this method.

6. **d.** The most common method to cultivate *Chlamydia trachomatis*, an obligate intracellular pathogen, is cell culture in **McCoy cells**. McCoy cells, which are primarily used only to isolate *C. trachomatis*, are derived from a mouse fibroblast cell line. Other cell lines have also been used to cultivate *C. trachomatis*, including HeLa 229, HEp-2, HL, BGMK, Vero, and L cells. *C. trachomatis* cannot be cultivated on bacteriologic culture media. MRC-5 cells are used to cultivate many different viruses, including herpes simplex virus, CMV, and VZV. Coculture of infected peripheral blood mononuclear cells (PBMCs) with activated, allogeneic, noninfected PBMCs is used for HIV, HTLV-1/2, and other viruses. LLC-MK$_2$ cells are used for several viruses, including mumps, parainfluenza, and several types of enterovirus.

7. **c.** Thiosulfate citrate bile salts sucrose (TCBS) agar is a selective medium that is commonly used for isolating *Vibrio* species. TCBS agar usually inhibits other bacteria besides *Vibrio* species. The medium differentiates sucrose–fermenting species, such as *V. cholerae*, from

non–sucrose-fermenting species. When sucrose is fermented, yellow colonies and a yellow precipitate are observed (Fig. 14.3B; compare to uninoculated TCBS plate, Fig. 14.3A). Besides *V. cholerae*, sucrose-fermenting species include *V. alginolyticus*, *V. metschnikovii*, a few strains of *V. vulnificus*, and other species. Nonsucrose-fermenting species include *V. mimicus*, *V. parahaemolyticus*, most strains of *V. vulnificus*, *V. damsela*, and other species.

8. **a.** *Eikenella corrodens* is an inhabitant of the human oral cavity and the gastrointestinal tract. It is associated with human bite wounds, clenched fist injuries, oral surgery, and cellulitis among drug addicts when they lick needles before injection. It also causes endocarditis, and is part of the "HACEK" group of bacteria. *E. corrodens* isolates are well known for their strong bleach-like odor and the fact that colonies may pit the agar (Fig. 14.4). *Cardiobacterium hominis*, another member of the HACEK group, may also pit the agar, but it is indole positive and does not smell like bleach. *Pasteurella multocida* is usually associated with animal bite wounds. *Haemophilus influenzae* usually does not grow on sheep blood agar, and requires X and V factors. *Pseudomonas aeruginosa* grows well on MacConkey agar, and colonies are readily apparent in 24 hours.

9. **d.** The Gram stain depicts a beaded, branching, Gram-positive rod, which was later found to be a *Nocardia* species. Generally, bacteria with high lipid contents in their cell walls, such as organisms from the genera *Mycobacterium*, *Nocardia*, *Gordonia*, and *Tsukamurella*, do not stain completely with the Gram stain, and often appear beaded. Any time a beaded, branching organism is observed in a direct clinical Gram stain, one of these genera should be suspected (*Mycobacterium* species may appear beaded, but may not show branching). All of these genera could also cause pulmonary disease. *Arcanobacterium* species could also cause pulmonary diseases, but they stain as Gram-positive rods, and do not appear beaded.

10. **b.** Resistance to fluoroquinolones in bacteria can arise from mutations in **DNA gyrase**, an enzyme that relaxes supercoiled DNA during DNA replication. Resistance to fluoroquinolones can also be caused by outer membrane mutations that result in a diminished uptake of the antibiotic, or by activation of an efflux pump that removes the antibiotic from the cytoplasm of the organism.

11. **b.** *Bacteroides fragilis* is the most common anaerobe isolated from infections involving anaerobic bacteria. *B. fragilis* is isolated frequently from many types of infections, including intra-abdominal infections, pleuropulmonary infections, pelvic infections, skin and soft tissue infections, and bacteremia. It grows in the presence of 20% bile, and is usually resistant to kanamycin, colistin, and vancomycin (Fig. 14.6). Most other anaerobic Gram-negative rods will not grow in the presence of 20% bile, except *Bilophia wordsworthia* and

Fusobacterium mortiferum-varium. *B. wordsworthia* and the commonly isolated *Fusobacterium* species can be differentiated from *B. fragilis* by their sensitivity to kanamycin and colistin.

12. **c.** *Legionella pneumophila* is a thin, poorly staining Gram-negative rod that primarily causes pneumonia but may also be involved in extrapulmonary infections. It is frequently not observed on direct Gram stains from patient sputum. The medium of choice to culture *L. pneumophila* and other *Legionella* species is BCYE agar. Colonies are often white to bluish white in color, and isolates are biochemically nonreactive. Many laboratories use 16S rRNA gene sequencing to definitively identify *Legionella* species. *Pseudomonas aeruginosa*, *Stenotrophomonas maltophilia*, and *Burkholderia pseudomallei* all grow well on standard bacteriology media in about 24 hours or less, and react to several biochemicals. *Bordetella pertussis* is usually cultured on Regan-Lowe agar or Bordet-Gengou agar, and colonies resemble mercury drops.

13. **d.** *Staphylococcus saprophyticus* is a relatively infrequent cause of urinary tract infection (UTI), but nearly all women are symptomatic when the organism is cultured from their urine. It is the most frequent coagulase-negative staphylococcus isolated from UTIs. *S. epidermidis*, another coagulase-negative staphylococcus, is isolated from urine infrequently, but about 90% of patients are asymptomatic when the organism is cultured. *S. saprophyticus* is resistant to novobiocin, while *S. epidermidis* is sensitive. *S. aureus* is coagulase positive, while both *Enterococcus faecalis* and *Streptococcus agalactiae* are catalase negative.

14. **d.** The VDRL test is a nontreponemal serologic assay that detects reaginic antibodies that flocculate with cardiolipin for measuring a host response to *Treponema pallidum*, the organism that causes syphilis. The VDRL test is read with a microscope. The RPR test is another example of a nontreponemal assay; this test can be read by eye. The nontreponemal assays are usually used as screening assays. They lack sensitivity for primary and late syphilis, however. Positive nontreponemal tests are confirmed with specific treponemal serologic assays such as the FTA-ABS (fluorescent treponemal antibody absorption) test or the TP-PA (*T. pallidum* particle agglutination) test.

15. **b.** *Mycobacterium chelonae* is one of the rapid-growing mycobacteria, and it is usually nonpigmented. Rapid-growing mycobacteria are those in which colonies appear in less than 7 days on solid media. The slow-growing mycobacteria take longer than 7 days to form colonies on solid media. Both *M. kansasii* and *M. marinum* are slow growers that are further classified as photochromogens—that is, their colonies become pigmented when exposed to light. *M. gordonae* is usually thought of as a nonpathogen, and is a slow grower classified as a scotochromogen. Scotochromogen colonies are pigmented in both light and dark conditions. Last,

M. ulcerans is a nonphotochromogen (is not pigmented in either the light or the dark) that is also a slow grower.

16. c. The patient has *Pseudomonas* dermatitis, which is often acquired from whirlpools, hot tubs, etc. *P. aeruginosa* is readily identified as an oxidase-positive, nonfermentative (Fig. 14.10A), motile gram-negative rod that grows well at 42°C. In addition, it produces the bluish green pigment pyocyanin (Fig. 14.10B), and may form other pigments as well. *P. fluorescens* has rarely been implicated in disease, and, like most *Pseudomonas* species except *P. aeruginosa*, does not grow at 42°C. *Escherichia coli* is a fermenter and is oxidase negative. Both *Stenotrophomonas maltophilia* and *Acinetobacter baumannii* are oxidase negative; *S. maltophilia* is motile while *A. baumannii* is not.

17. a. *Gardnerella vaginalis*, which may be involved in bacterial vaginosis, is a Gram-positive rod that often stains gram variable. Colonies of *G. vaginalis* are non-hemolytic on standard sheep blood agar and on CNA. However, on **human blood bilayer Tween (HBT)** agar, *G. vaginalis* produces softly β–hemolytic colonies, and is usually the medium of choice for this organism.

18. d. The urinary tract isolate is exhibiting swarming on sheep blood agar, a characteristic that is common for *Proteus* species. The two most commonly isolated *Proteus* species, *P. mirabilis* and *P. vulgaris*, can be differentiated by the indole test. *P. vulgaris* is indole positive, while *P. mirabilis* is indole negative. *Escherichia coli* and *Klebsiella oxytoca* are also indole positive but do not swarm. *K. pneumoniae* is indole negative and does not swarm. *Proteus* swarming is best observed on sheep blood agar or on chocolate agar. Swarming is not observed on MacConkey agar, due to a higher percentage of agar in the medium.

19. e. All *Bacillus* species are catalase-positive, spore-forming Gram-positive rods. *B. anthracis*, one of the most important human pathogens and a potential bioterrorism agent, is recognized by its **lack of motility** and hemolysis. Any spore-forming Gram-positive rod that is nonmotile and nonhemolytic should be referred to the appropriate public health agency to rule out *B. anthracis*.

20. d. *Streptobacillus moniliformis* is the agent of rat bite fever. The organism is naturally found in the upper respiratory tract of wild, laboratory, and pet rats. Humans can get infected by *S. moniliformis* by bites, or by ingesting contaminated food, milk, or water. When the organism is acquired by ingestion, the disease is called Haverhill fever. *S. moniliformis* is a Gram-negative rod that is very pleomorphic and often forms long filaments. The organism is inhibited by sodium polyanethol sulfonate (SPS), a supplement that is found in most blood culture media. Thus, if *S. moniliformis* is suspected, media without SPS must be used for isolation. In general, it is a nonreactive bacterium for most commonly used biochemical tests. *Pasteurella multocida*, *Eikenella corrodens*, and *Cardiobacterium*

hominis are all oxidase positive, and will all grow in standard blood culture media. *Leptospira interrogans* is a spirochete. A similar disease to rat-bite fever called *sodoku* is caused by the spirochete *Spirillum minus*. sodoku is also spread by rat bites, but occurs most often in Asia.

21. a. *Ehrlichia chaffeensis* is an obligate intracellular pathogen that tends to infect monocytes and macrophages. It is the causative agent of human mono-cytotropic ehrlichiosis (HME). The organisms can be observed in cytoplasmic inclusions in monocytes and macrophages called morulae, although it is rare to find them. The clinical manifestations are similar to Rocky Mountain spotted fever (RMSF) caused by *Rickettsia rickettsii*; however, approximately 90% of patients with RMSF will have a rash, while a rash is present in <50% of cases of HME. In addition, morulae are not observed in patients with RMSF. *Anaplasma phagocytophilum* is the agent of human granulocytotropic anaplasmosis (HGA), and also causes a similar disease. *A. phagocytophilum* tends to infect neutrophils, not monocytes, and can be observed as morulae as well. The agents of HME, HGA, and RMSF are all transmitted by the bites of ticks. *Orientia tsutsugamushi*, the agent of scrub typhus, is transmitted by chigger bites, and is not endemic in the United States. *Rickettsia typhi* is the agent of murine typhus, and is transmitted by flea bites. It does occur in the United States. Diagnosis of many of these intracellular pathogens is usually made by epidemiology factors, clinical manifestations, and serology.

22. d. *Clostridium perfringens* is the most frequent clostridial species isolated from clinical specimens. It is well known as an agent of food poisoning, gas gangrene (myonecrosis), pulmonary infections, and soft tissue infections. *C. perfringens* characteristically produces a double zone of hemolysis on blood agar, as illustrated in Figure 14.12. A Gram stain of *C. perfringens* typically shows large, boxcar-shaped Gram–positive rods that may stain gram variable. While all clostridia form endospores, they are rarely observed in *C. perfringens* isolates. *Bacillus cereus* and *B. anthracis* will grow in both aerobic and anaerobic atmospheres. *C. tetani* and *C. botulinum* are not beta–hemolytic on sheep blood agar.

23. b. *Actinomyces israelii* has been isolated from various oral infections, wound infections, and intrauterine-device-associated infections from the female genital tract. There are many *Actinomyces* species that have been implicated in human infections. While *Actinomyces* species are usually thought of as anaerobes, most will grow in aerobic conditions, although they tend to grow better anaerobically. The majority of *Actinomyces* species are catalase-negative, pleomorphic Gram-positive rods that may form rudimentary branches. They do not stain with the modified acid-fast stain, unlike *Nocardia* species. *Nocardia* species, which are often roughly classified as "aerobic actinomycetes," grow best in aerobic conditions and are catalase

positive. *Corynebacterium* species are also catalase positive, also tend to be aerobes, and do not stain with the modified acid-fast stain.

24. **e.** Most cases of psittacosis, caused by *Chlamydophila psittaci*, involve individuals who have had contact with birds. People at risk include poultry farmers, pet store employees, abattoir workers, veterinarians, and pet owners. The organism is usually spread to humans via the respiratory route. Psittacosis can take many forms, including a subclinical infection, a typhoidal manifestation, and an atypical pneumonia. Like other organisms in the family Chlamydiaceae, *C. psittaci* is an obligate intracellular pathogen with a unique biphasic life cycle; the organism does not stain with the Gram stain and will not grow on artificial bacteriologic media. The transmissible form of *C. psittaci* and other Chlamydiaceae is the elementary body that attaches to host cells. Elementary bodies are internalized after attachment and transform into reticulate bodies. The reticulate bodies replicate and form a cytoplasmic inclusion. The reticulate bodies then transform back into elementary bodies and are released from the host cell. Identification of *C. psittaci* is often made using serologic methods such as complement fixation or microimmunofluorescence, although cell culture and the polymerase chain reaction are useful also. *Chlamydophila pneumoniae* is a common cause of community-acquired pneumonia, but it is not normally associated with exposure to birds. *Legionella pneumophila*, *Mycobacterium tuberculosis*, and *Streptococcus pneumoniae* can all be cultured on artificial media.

25. **d.** The clinical presentation of the child is fairly typical of meningitis caused by *Neisseria meningitidis*. *N. meningitidis* is carried in the nasopharynx in about 15% to 20% of the population, and can cause bacteremia, meningoencephalitis, urethritis, and pneumonia in addition to meningitis. There are 13 serogroups, but most infections are caused by the A, B, C, Y, and W-135 serogroups. There is a vaccine for *N. meningitidis* that covers serogroups A, C, Y, and W-135. *N. meningitidis* is a Gram-negative diplococcus, like many members of the genus *Neisseria*. All *Neisseria* species are oxidase positive, and most are catalase positive. *Neisseria* species can be differentiated from each other by their ability to produce acid from the carbohydrates glucose, maltose, lactose, sucrose, and fructose. *N. meningitidis* produces acid from both glucose and maltose, while *N. gonorrhoeae* produces acid only from glucose. *Moraxella catarrhalis* is also an oxidase-positive, Gram-negative diplococcus, but it does not produce acid from carbohydrates. Nither *N. gonorrhoeae* nor *M. catarrhalis* would be expected to cause meningitis. *Streptococcus pneumoniae* is an agent of meningitis, but it is a Gram-positive, catalase-negative diplococcus. *Haemophilus influenzae* may also cause meningitis, but it is a Gram-negative coccobacillus or short rod and requires X and V factors for growth.

26. **b.** MacConkey agar with sorbitol (often referred to as SMAC) is both a selective and differential medium for **O157 Shiga toxin-producing *Escherichia coli*** strains. Sorbitol is the only carbohydrate in SMAC, instead of lactose, which is in standard MacConkey agar. There are many Shiga toxin-producing *E. coli* serotypes. All of the Shiga toxin-producing strains are capable of causing illness such as bloody diarrhea and hemolytic uremic syndrome (HUS). O157 strains account for about 80% of all cases of HUS in the United States. The O157 strains are unique among other *E. coli* strains (including non-O157 Shiga toxin-producing strains) in that they do not ferment sorbitol. *E. coli* O157 strains appear as colorless colonies on SMAC since they do not ferment sorbitol, while all other *E. coli* strains appear dark pink, since they ferment sorbitol. *Yersinia enterocolitica* and most *Salmonella* species/serotypes ferment sorbitol. About 30% to 40% of *Shigella* isolates ferment sorbitol, but media such as Hektoen enteric agar or xylose lysine deoxycholate (XLD) agar is usually used to isolate *Salmonella* and *Shigella*.

27. **c.** Bordet-Gengou agar is one example of a medium that is used to isolate the fastidious Gram-negative coccobacillus *Bordetella pertussis*, the agent of pertussis or whooping cough, from clinical specimens. Bordet-Gengou medium has a short shelf-life, so Regan-Lowe medium is used more often for the isolation of *B. pertussis*. *B. parapertussis* also may cause a pertussis-like respiratory syndrome; *B. bronchiseptica* has been associated with a few cases of respiratory diseases as well. Both of these organisms will grow on standard bacteriology media such as sheep blood agar and MacConkey agar, although recovery of *B. parapertussis* is enhanced by using Bordet-Gengou agar or Regan-Lowe agar. Both *B. pertussis* and *B. bronchiseptica* are oxidase positive, but *B. parapertussis* is oxidase negative. In addition, *B. pertussis* does not reduce nitrate, does not produce urease, and is nonmotile. *B. parapertussis* produces urease in 24 hours, and *B. bronchiseptica* usually produces urease in 4 hours or less. *B. bronchiseptica* also reduces nitrate and is motile; *B. parapertussis* is negative for both of these characteristics. *Legionella pneumophila* is an agent of pneumonia, but is usually cultured on buffered charcoal yeast extract (BCYE) agar, and is a very nonreactive organism biochemically. *Brucella melitensis* is one of the *Brucella* species that causes brucellosis, a zoonotic, systemic disease. It is oxidase positive and will usually grow on chocolate agar. In addition, *B. melitensis* reduces nitrate, is nonmotile, and is urease positive.

28. **c.** The most likely explanation for the patient's illness is ingestion of a preformed enterotoxin in the fried rice that he ate. One of the most rapid-acting enterotoxins is the **Bacillus cereus** emetic toxin. This toxin typically acts within 1–6 hours of ingestion and usually causes vomiting, nausea, and abdominal cramps. Some

patients get diarrhea as well. Foods associated with *B. cereus* emetic toxin include fried rice and various meat products. *B. cereus* may also produce a diarrheal toxin that takes 10–16 hours before symptoms of diarrhea, vomiting, and abdominal cramps appear. Another very fast acting bacterial toxin is staphylococcal enterotoxin, produced by *Staphylococcus aureus*; this toxin, like the *B. cereus* emetic toxin, acts about 1–6 hours after ingestion. The *Clostridium perfringens* enterotoxin is also fast-acting, causing symptoms of watery diarrhea, abdominal cramps, nausea, and sometimes vomiting about 8–16 hours after ingestion. *Salmonella* species, *Campylobacter jejuni*, and enterohemorrhagic *Escherichia coli* all may cause gastroenteritis. All three organisms must be ingested to cause disease; disease caused by *Salmonella* and *Campylobacter* is not toxin-related, but is instead associated with invasion. Nontyphoidal *Salmonella* strains usually cause symptoms of diarrhea, abdominal cramps, and nausea in 1–3 days after ingestion. *C. jejuni* and other *Campylobacter* species cause bloody diarrhea, fever, vomiting, and abdominal cramping 2–5 days after ingestion. Enterohemorrhagic *E. coli* strains, such as O157 isolates, produce the Shiga toxin. Symptoms are usually produced 1–8 days after ingestion and include bloody diarrhea, vomiting, and abdominal cramping.

29. **b.** *Streptococcus pneumoniae* is classically alpha-hemolytic on sheep blood agar and sensitive to optochin (P disk) (Fig. 14.16). Streptococci are catalase negative, and *S. pneumoniae* often appears as lancet-shaped Gram-positive cocci in pairs or short chains. The gram stain reaction, alpha-hemolysis and optochin sensitivity are initial clues that an isolate is *S. pneumoniae*; many labs will perform a bile test to confirm the organism. *S. pneumoniae* is bile sensitive. In addition, *S. pneumonia* colonies often have a central depression, and may look "donut shaped," and many isolates are also mucoid. The viridans group streptococci are also alpha-hemolytic, but usually appear as Gram-positive cocci in chains and are resistant to optochin as a group. Both *S. pyogenes* and *S. agalactiae* are beta-hemolytic on sheep blood agar, and both also appear as Gram-positive cocci in chains. Enterococci such as *E. faecalis* may appear similar to *S. pneumoniae* on gram stain—that is, as lancet-shaped Gram-positive cocci in pairs and short chains—but they are usually nonhemolytic. *S. pneumoniae* is well known as an agent of community-acquired pneumonia, meningitis, otitis media, and other infections such as bacteremia, endocarditis, and sinusitis.

30. **b.** Enterococci are catalase-negative Gram-positive cocci that often appear as pairs or short chains. Most of the enterococci hydrolyze esculin and grow in the presence of bile and 6.5% sodium chloride. Members of this genus are widespread in nature. In humans, they are usually found in the gastrointestinal tract. *Enterococcus faecalis* is probably the most prevalent of the enterococci

found in the human gastrointestinal tract, followed by *E. faecium* and other species. Enterococci tend to cause opportunistic infections in immunocompromised patients, the elderly, and patients who have been hospitalized for long periods. Enterococci may cause urinary tract infections, wound infections, bacteremia, and endocarditis. *E. faecalis* is the most common of the enterococci isolated in clinical specimens, followed by *E. faecium*. An important problem now in hospitals is the emergence of vancomycin-resistant enterococci (VRE). *E. faecalis* and *E. faecium* acquire vancomycin-resistance. There are a number of vancomycin-resistance phenotypes, but the most common in *E. faecalis* and *E. faecium* are the VanA and VanB phenotypes, encoded by the *vanA* and *vanB* genes, respectively. Of the VRE strains that are isolated in the United States, most are *E. faecium*. Resistance caused by VanA and VanB is the result of an alteration of the cell wall target of vancomycin. Intrinsically, most enterococci are resistant to several antimicrobial agents, such as trimethoprim-sulfamethoxazole and low levels of aminoglycosides. In particular, most *E. faecium* isolates are intrinsically resistant to ampicillin and penicillin, making *E. faecium* a difficult organism to treat, especially if a given isolate is found to be a VRE.

31. **e.** The clinical manifestations are consistent with brucellosis, a zoonotic disease that occurs worldwide. Brucellosis is not common in the United States, but cases occur in Texas and California due to people consuming unpasteurized goat milk products imported from Mexico. *Brucella melitensis* is associated with goats and sheep; *B. abortus* is found in cattle and buffalo; *B. suis* is found in swine (although *B. suis* biovar 4 is found in reindeer and caribou); and *B. canis* occurs in dogs. *Brucella* species are catalase-positive Gram-negative coccobacilli. Most are oxidase positive, and a key characteristic of *B. melitensis*, *B. abortus*, *B. suis*, and *B. canis* is their ability to hydrolyze urea. Most strains of *B. suis* and *B. canis* are urease positive in less than 5 minutes, while most strains of *B. melitensis* and *B. abortus* take longer than 5 minutes. *Francisella tularensis* is also a zoonotic Gram-negative coccobacillus. Humans often acquire *F. tularensis* through vector bites, such as from ticks and deer flies. Some people also get *F. tularensis* after exposure to infected animals such as rabbits, prairie dogs, and zoo animals. *F. tularensis* strains are weakly catalase positive, are oxidase positive, and do not hydrolyze urea.

32. **d.** Nontyphoidal *Salmonella* species cause gastroenteritis with symptoms of diarrhea, abdominal cramps, and often fever. The incubation period for *Salmonella* species is about 1–3 days after consuming contaminated food or water. People typically acquire *Salmonella* after eating contaminated poultry, raw fruits and vegetables, cheese, eggs, meat products, or drinking contaminated milk or water. In addition, some people acquire *Salmonella* from pet turtles. *Salmonella* are oxidase-negative Gram-negative rods in the family

Enterobacteriaceae. The taxonomy of *Salmonella* is somewhat confusing. At the time of this writing, there are two *Salmonella* species: *S. enterica* and *S. bongori*. *S. enterica* is divided into six subspecies; *S. enterica* subsp. *enterica* is subspecies type I, and is the subspecies most often isolated from humans and other warm-blooded animals. Furthermore, *Salmonella* strains are serotyped at public health laboratories based on the O antigen (the outermost part of the lipopolysaccharide layer of the cell wall), the H antigen (the flagella), and the Vi antigen (a capsular polysaccharide, not found in all serotypes). There are many *Salmonella* serotypes. The most common serotypes isolated from human infections in the United States are *S. enterica* subsp. *enterica* serotype Enteritidis, abbreviated *Salmonella* serotype Enteritidis (or just *S*. Enteritidis) and *Salmonella* serotype Typhimurium. Since *Salmonella* and *Shigella* species are common agents of gastroenteritis, media used for stool cultures are designed to select and differentiate these two genera. There are many media available, and most laboratories use MacConkey agar and either Hektoen enteric (HE) agar or xylose lysine deoxycholate (XLD) agar for *Salmonella* and *Shigella*. XLD agar is a red-colored medium that contains xylose, lactose, and sucrose as carbohydrates, lysine to identify bacteria that have the lysine decarboxylase enzyme, phenol red as the color indicator, and ammonium citrate and sodium thiosulfate to determine whether organisms produce H_2S. *Shigella* does not ferment any of the carbohydrates, so colonies appear colorless. *Salmonella* serotypes do not ferment lactose or sucrose, but most serotypes do ferment xylose, and would ordinarily have yellow colonies based on acid production; however, *Salmonella* serotypes use lysine in the medium with the enzyme lysine decarboxylase which produces an alkaline product. This alkalinity counters the acid production, and so *Salmonella* colonies also appear colorless on XLD agar. *Salmonella* species, though, also produce H_2S, so the colonies will have black centers, and this differentiates them from *Shigella* species which are H_2S negative. *Escherichia coli* strains, including *E. coli* O157:H7, produce yellow colonies since they ferment lactose and are lysine decarboxylase negative. *Campylobacter jejuni* does not grow on stool culture media used to select *Shigella* and *Salmonella*, so it requires specialized media—*Campylobacter* blood agar is used in most laboratories—and microaerophilic growth conditions.

33. **b.** *Erysipelothrix rhusiopathiae* is a zoonotic organism that is associated with a wide variety of animals, including pigs, fish, and birds. The organism causes erysipeloid, a localized cellulitis with a violaceous, painful lesion, and also causes bacteremia with or without endocarditis. Humans typically acquire *E. rhusiopathiae* by handling infected animals or animal products, so disease caused by the organism is usually occupational. The organism gets into breaks in the skin

to cause erysipeloid. *E. rhusiopathiae* is gram-positive rod that may form chains. It may take 1–3 days for colonies to appear on media. On sheep blood agar, colonies are usually nonhemolytic and pinpoint after 24 hours of incubation. After 48 hours of incubation, colonies are larger and may appear alpha-hemolytic. *E. rhusiopathiae* is the only clinically relevant gram-positive rod that produces H_2S in triple sugar iron (TSI) agar (Fig. 14.18). In addition, *E. rhusiopathiae* is catalase negative and does not form spores. *Listeria monocytogenes* is catalase positive, H_2S negative, and beta hemolytic on sheep blood agar. *Corynebacterium* species are catalase positive and H_2S negative. *Bacillus anthracis* is catalase positive, forms spores, and is also H_2S negative. *Arcanobacterium haemolyticum* is catalase negative, is beta hemolytic on sheep blood agar, and is H_2S negative.

34. **b.** MacConkey agar is a pink-colored medium used for most types of cultures in the bacteriology laboratory. It is a selective and differential medium used to isolate Gram-negative bacteria. MacConkey agar contains lactose as the only carbohydrate, peptones, bile and crystal violet to inhibit Gram-positive organisms, and neutral red as the pH indicator. Lactose fermentation results in the production of acid, which drops the pH of the medium. Lactose fermenters appear dark red on MacConkey agar, often with a darkish red precipitate around the colonies as well. The primary lactose fermenters include *Escherichia coli*, *Klebsiella* species, and some *Enterobacter* and *Citrobacter* species; Fig. 14.19B shows a lactose-fermenting *E. coli* isolate on MacConkey agar. Non-lactose fermenters, on the other hand, utilize the peptones in the medium, which produces alkaline by-products. Under alkaline conditions, the medium turns colorless, and colonies appear colorless as well (Fig. 14.19A). *Shigella*, *Salmonella*, and *Yersinia enterocolitica* are the primary stool pathogens that do not ferment lactose. However, many members of the Enterobacteriaceae do not ferment lactose, such as *Proteus* species. Thus, MacConkey agar does not differentiate between non–lactose-fermenters, but does select for non–lactose-fermenting Gram-negative bacteria.

35. **a.** Figure 14.20 shows two Lowenstein-Jensen agar slants inoculated with the same slow-growing acid-fast bacillus. Buff-colored (nonpigmented) bacteria are evident on the left slant that was incubated in dark conditions. Yellow-pigmented bacteria are visible on the right slant that was exposed to light. This is typical of certain mycobacteria called photochromogens. In general, mycobacteria are often divided into two groups, the *Mycobacterium tuberculosis* complex and the nontuberculous mycobacteria (NTMs). The NTMs may be further divided into four groups: the photochromogens (develop pigment after exposure to light), the scotochromogens (develop pigment in both the light and the dark), the nonphotochromogens (nonpigmented regardless of the light conditions) and the rapid growers.

The photochromogens, scotochromogens, and nonphotochromogens are all slow-growing mycobacteria—they take longer than 7 days to grow on solid media. Mycobacteria that grow faster than 7 days on solid media are the rapid growers. *M. kansasii* is a photochromogen that is associated with chronic pulmonary infections and occasional extrapulmonary infections such as cervical lymphadenitis and cutaneous infections. *M. avium-intracellulare* causes chronic pulmonary disease, extrapulmonary infections, and disseminated disease, particularly in immunocompromised patients, and is nearly always nonpigmented. *M. tuberculosis* is a nonpigmented, slow-growing organism, and *M. gordonae* is a scotochromogen and is rarely, if ever, considered a pathogen. *M. abscessus* is a rapid-growing species that causes pulmonary infections, disseminated disease, and skin and soft tissue infections.

36. **c.** *Pasteurella multocida* is a commensal found in the nasopharynx and oral cavity of animals, particularly dogs and cats. Humans usually become infected with *P. multocida* after bites or scratches. Some people get infected when pets lick skin lesions or sores. The organism usually causes cellulitis at the site of infection, but may also cause meningitis, arthritis, endocarditis, osteomyelitis, septicemia, and respiratory infections. *P. multocida* is an oxidase-positive, catalase-positive, Gram-negative coccobacillus. It grows well on solid media, although it does not grow on MacConkey agar, and is indole positive. Thus, a Gram-negative isolate from a bite wound that grows well on blood agar but not on MacConkey agar should be suspicious for *P. multocida*. *Eikenella corrodens* is a member of the human oral flora, and also in some animals. It is associated with human bite wounds, clenched fist injuries, oral infections, and endocarditis. It is oxidase positive, does not grow on MacConkey agar, and is catalase- and indole negative. *Haemophilus influenzae* is more fastidious than *P. multocida*, and does not grow on sheep blood agar or on MacConkey agar. It is not associated with animal bite wounds, but instead causes meningitis, pneumonia, epiglottitis, and many other infections. *Bartonella henselae* is associated with cat-scratch disease, bacillary angiomatosis, and bacillary peliosis, but is a slow-growing, fastidious organism that is difficult to culture. *B. henselae* will grow on blood agar, but requires incubation for 4 weeks. *Pseudomonas aeruginosa* is not fastidious, and will grow well on MacConkey agar. It is oxidase positive, but is indole negative.

37. **b.** The nonspecific symptoms with an annular rash, the tick bite history of the patient, and the geographical area of the patient are characteristic of infection with *Borrelia burgdorferi*, the agent of Lyme borreliosis or Lyme disease. *B. burgdorferi* is a Gram-negative spirochete that is now divided into three species: *B. burgdorferi* sensu stricto, *B. afzelii*, and *B. garinii*. *B. burgdorferi* sensu stricto is the only species of the group that has been isolated from humans in North America,

while all three species have been isolated from humans in Europe. The organisms are transmitted to humans by the bite of *Ixodes* ticks. Lyme borreliosis is characterized by an annular-shaped lesion called erythema migrans (EM). EM is present in 60% to 90% of patients at the bite site of the tick. In many patients, the central portion of the lesion fades so that it has a bull's eye appearance. Other symptoms of Lyme borreliosis include headache, fever, fatigue, malaise, arthralgia, and myalgia. Untreated patients can develop neurologic and cardiac complications. *Borrelia recurrentis* is an agent of relapsing fever, and is spread by the human body louse (*Pediculus humanus humanus*). *Leptospira interrogans* is a zoonotic spirochete that is transmitted to humans after contact with urine from infected animals. It causes disease worldwide, with symptoms of fever, chills, headache, abdominal pain, and conjunctival suffusion. Some patients develop icteric disease (Weil disease) and renal failure. *Rickettsia rickettsii* is an obligate intracellular pathogen that is transmitted to humans by tick bites, and does occur on the eastern seaboard. It is more common in the southeastern part of the United States, such as North Carolina, South Carolina, and Virginia. It is not characterized by an EM-like rash, but instead by a petechial rash that often appears on the palms and soles. *Francisella tularensis* can also be spread to humans via tick bites and deer fly bites. It is a gram-negative coccobacillus, and disease is not characterized by an EM-like rash.

38. **d.** *Campylobacter jejuni* causes gastroenteritis characterized by abdominal cramping, fever, and diarrhea, which is often bloody. Fecal white blood cells may be present in stool specimens of patients with *C. jejuni* gastroenteritis. *C. jejuni* infections most commonly occur in the summer months, and people usually acquire the organism by eating contaminated or improperly cooked food. The organism requires specialized media for isolation. A commonly used medium is *Campylobacter* blood agar, which is brucella agar with sheep blood and antimicrobial agents to inhibit normal stool flora. It does not grow on other media used in stool cultures, such as MacConkey agar, Hektoen enteric agar, or xylose lysine deoxycholate (XLD) agar. Thus, a *Campylobacter* blood agar plate is included in the standard media package used when a stool culture is ordered. In addition, *C. jejuni* requires a microaerophilic atmosphere (5% O_2, 10% CO_2, 85% N_2) and is usually cultured at 42°C. It is a curved or S-shaped Gram-negative rod that tends to stain faintly (Fig. 14.22). *C. jejuni* is oxidase positive, catalase positive, and hippurate hydrolysis positive; these characteristics, along with growth at 42°C, serve to differentiate it from other *Campylobacter* species. *Vibrio cholerae* is also an oxidase positive, curved gram-negative rod that causes gastroenteritis. *V. cholerae* strains usually do not cause bloody diarrhea, and they grow aerobically in culture. Thiosulfate citrate bile salts sucrose (TCBS) agar is the selective medium usually

used for *Vibrio* species. *Escherichia coli* O157:H7 causes gastroenteritis that is sometimes characterized by bloody stools, abdominal cramping, and low-grade fever. Like other *E. coli* strains, *E. coli* O157 isolates are oxidase negative and will grow in aerobic conditions. MacConkey agar with sorbitol is the medium usually used to select for *E. coli* O157. *Salmonella* serotype Typhi causes typhoid fever, a disease that presents with a diarrheal phase followed by a febrile illness. The incubation period for *S.* serotype Typhi is 7–14 days on average. The organism grows well on most media, but is usually isolated best from blood cultures or bone marrow cultures. It does not require a special atmosphere for growth, is oxidase negative, and is not curved on Gram stain. *Shigella sonnei* is one of the four different *Shigella* species. *Shigella* species cause bacillary dysentery, and symptoms may include bloody diarrhea, fever, tenesmus, and abdominal cramping. Fecal white blood cells are often found in stool specimens. *Shigella* species do not require a special atmosphere for isolation, are oxidase negative, and are not curved on Gram stain. MacConkey agar and Hektoen enteric agar or XLD agar would be excellent media choices to select for *Shigella* species such as *S. sonnei*.

39. **a.** There are various methods that can be used to confirm the presence of an **extended spectrum beta-lactamase** (ESBL) in certain Gram-negative bacteria. Currently, according to the Clinical and Laboratory Standards Institute (CLSI), ESBL testing should be performed only for *Klebsiella pneumoniae*, *Klebsiella oxytoca*, *Escherichia coli*, or *Proteus mirabilis* isolates. In these organisms, ESBLs are important acquired enzymes. Organisms with ESBLs cannot be effectively treated with the penicillins, cephalosporins, or aztreonam. In *E. coli*, *K. pneumoniae*, and *K. oxytoca*, the following antibiotics can be used to screen for the presence of an ESBL: ceftazidime, ceftriaxone, cefotaxime, cefpodoxime, or aztreonam. Ceftazidime, cefotaxime, or cefpodoxime can be used to screen for ESBLs in *P. mirabilis*. These organisms are not normally resistant to these antibiotics, thus they are good screening agents. Confirmatory testing can be performed by either disc diffusion or by broth microdilution. Figure 14.23 shows an example of a disk diffusion confirmatory test for an ESBL-producing *K. pneumoniae*. By either disk diffusion or broth microdilution, the following combinations are tested: ceftazidime compared to ceftazidime with the beta-lactamase inhibitor clavulanic acid and cefotaxime compared to cefotaxime with clavulanic acid. If an ESBL is present, the zone size in disk diffusion will be at least 5 mm larger around the antibiotic with clavulanic acid inhibitor compared to the antibiotic alone. This is due to the inhibition effect of the clavulanic acid. For example, if the ceftazidime zone size is 16 mm, the ceftazidime with clavulanic acid zone size must be 21 mm or greater to confirm the presence of an ESBL. An ESBL is confirmed if this zone size difference is

noted for either of the pairs of disks. For the broth microdilution confirmatory method, a ≥ 3 twofold concentration decrease must be noted with one of the tested pairs of antibiotics compared to the antibiotic/clavulanic acid counterpart. For example, if the MIC for ceftazidime is 8 μg/ml, the ceftazidime/clavulanic acid MIC must be 1 μg/ml to confirm the presence of an ESBL. In contrast, potential AmpC hyperproducing organisms include *Serratia marcescens*, *Pseudomonas aeruginosa*, *Providencia* species, *Citrobacter freundii*, *Enterobacter cloacae*, *Enterobacter aerogenes*, and *Morganella morganii* (the so-called "SPiCEM" organisms). The AmpC gene for these organisms is chromosomal, and may be induced by low levels of various β-lactam antibiotics. Mutations in the induction pathway may result in AmpC hyperproduction. In addition, there are also plasmid-mediated AmpCs. AmpC hyperproducers are very resistant to β-lactam antibiotics. A good screening test for AmpC hyperproduction is cefoxitin. The AmpC enzymes are resistant to beta-lactamase inhibitors such as clavulanic acid, so the confirmatory tests used for ESBLs cannot be used to confirm AmpC hyperproduction. Currently, there are no CLSI-recommended tests for AmpC confirmation.

40. **e.** *Rickettsia rickettsii* is an obligate intracellular pathogen. It is transferred to humans by tick bites; the usual vector in the United States is *Dermacentor* species (*D. variabilis* in the east and *D. andersoni* in the west). *R. rickettsii* is the etiologic agent of Rocky Mountain spotted fever (RMSF). The incubation period for RMSF averages about 7 days. The disease is initially characterized most often by fever, headache, and myalgia. Some individuals also present with nausea, abdominal pain, vomiting, and diarrhea. The major clinical manifestation, though, is a petechial rash that usually begins 3–5 days after the onset of fever and is present in 90% of all patients. The rash often begins on the wrists and ankles, but may also occur on the trunk. Eventually, the rash spreads to the palms and soles in most patients. RMSF is most common in the southeastern and south central United States. *Rickettsia prowazekii* is the agent of louse-borne or epidemic typhus. It is spread to humans by the human body louse (*Pediculus humanus corporis*). The symptoms may be similar to RMSF, although the rash caused by *R. prowazekii* infection does not normally include the palms and soles. Epidemic typhus is endemic in Mexico, Central and South America, parts of Africa, and in Asia. In the United States, *R. prowazekii* persists in Southern flying squirrels, and humans may acquire the organism via flying squirrel fleas, although it is not a common disease. *Coxiella burnetii* is the causative agent of Q fever. Q fever is a zoonosis that occurs worldwide. Humans are usually infected by inhaling contaminated aerosols when organisms are shed in urine, feces, milk, and in animal birth products. Q fever is usually an occupational disease, and there are

several different clinical manifestations, including a febrile illness, pneumonia, endocarditis, hepatitis, osteomyelitis, and neurologic manifestations. *Anaplasma phagocytophilum* causes human granulocytotropic anaplasmosis (HGA), a disease that is similar to RMSF and human monocytic ehrlichiosis (HME, caused by *Ehrlichia chaffeensis*). Like *R. rickettsii*, *A. phagocytophilum* is transferred to humans by the bite of ticks. However, patients with HGA rarely present with a rash, and HGA tends to occur in the northeastern and upper Midwestern states. Cases occur in northern California as well. *Borrelia burgdorferi* is a spirochete that is also transmitted by ticks. The disease it causes, Lyme borreliosis, is characterized by an annular rash (erythema migrans) that often looks like a bull's eye. The rash of Lyme borreliosis occurs at the bite site of the tick, and does not appear on the palms or soles unless one of those areas is bitten by a tick.

41. c. *Streptococcus pyogenes* is the primary cause of bacterial pharyngitis, and is responsible for many other types of infections, including impetigo, sepsis, soft tissue infections, erysipelas, cellulitis, necrotizing fasciitis, endocarditis, pneumonia, osteomyelitis, and scarlet fever. It is a Gram-positive coccus that appears in chains, is catalase negative like other streptococci, and is susceptible to bacitracin (A disk). *S. pyogenes* colonies on sheep blood agar are large with large zones of beta hemolysis, as shown in Figure 14.24. The A disk is no longer considered confirmatory for identification of *S. pyogenes*; some strains of other beta-hemolytic streptococci are also susceptible to bacitracin. Instead, most labs use a rapid kit to determine the presence of the Lancefield group A antigen present in the cell wall of *S. pyogenes* strains. *Streptococcus agalactiae* is a softly beta-hemolytic streptococcus, and has the group B Lancefield antigen. It is resistant to bacitracin and CAMP test positive. It is associated with many infections as well, such as early-onset neonatal disease, late-onset neonatal meningitis, urinary tract infections, soft tissue infections, pneumonia, and osteomyelitis. The *Streptococcus milleri* group, also known as the *Streptococcus anginosus* group, consists of the organisms *S. anginosus*, *S. constellatus*, and *S. intermedius*. Strains of these organisms may carry the Lancefield group A, C, F, or G antigens, or may have no Lancefield group antigen. In addition, these organisms are variable in their hemolytic pattern. All are resistant to bacitracin, and their colonies are small in relation to *S. pyogenes* and *S. agalactiae*. Organisms in the *S. anginosus* group cause abscesses in the peritoneal cavity, in the brain, and in the oropharynx. *Enterococcus faecium* and other enterococci are associated with infections in immunocompromised patients, the elderly, or those who have been hospitalized for long periods. *E. faecium* is catalase negative, and usually appears as pairs or small chains of Gram-positive cocci. Strains of *E. faecium* are nonhemolytic or alpha hemolytic on sheep blood agar. *Staphylococcus aureus* is a significant pathogen, and causes many of the same diseases as *S. pyogenes*. *S. aureus*, like other staphylococci, is catalase positive. *S. aureus* colonies are usually larger than those of *S. pyogenes*, and are also beta-hemolytic on sheep blood agar.

42. e. *Corynebacterium diphtheriae* is a catalase-positive, pleomorphic, Gram-positive rod that is the causative agent of diphtheria. While rates of diphtheria in the United States have declined dramatically since the introduction of a vaccine, cases still appear in individuals who have not been vaccinated. In the mid-1990s, there was an epidemic of diphtheria in Russia and surrounding countries. Diphtheria may occur as a respiratory disease or as a cutaneous disease. The respiratory disease is characterized by pharyngitis with an associated nasopharyngeal membrane, low-grade fever, adenopathy, and hoarseness. Most of the virulence of *C. diphtheriae* is the result of diphtheria toxin that is encoded by a bacteriophage that infects the organism. The toxin may cause severe complications, such as kidney damage, myocarditis, and neuritis. Nontoxigenic strains may still cause cutaneous disease or endocarditis. To determine toxin production, the Elek test or the polymerase chain reaction is often performed. If *C. diphtheriae* is suspected, specialized media are usually used for culture isolation. Samples should be plated on sheep blood agar and a selective medium such as cystine-tellurite blood agar (CTBA) or Tinsdale medium. *C. diphtheriae* colonies are black on CTBA and black or brown on Tinsdale medium with a brown halo around the colonies. Unfortunately, *C. pseudotuberculosis* and *C. ulcerans* also produce the same types of colonies on CTBA and Tinsdale medium. Because they can cause similar respiratory diseases to diphtheria, *C. diphtheriae* must be differentiated from these two organisms. *C. diphtheriae* is urease negative, while *C. pseudotuberculosis* and *C. ulcerans* are urease positive. *Streptococcus pyogenes* is the main bacterial cause of pharyngitis, but it is a catalase-negative Gram-positive coccus that appears in chains. *Arcanobacterium haemolyticum* is also an agent of pharyngitis. It is a beta-hemolytic, Gram-positive rod. Unlike *C. diphtheriae*, *A. haemolyticum* is catalase negative.

43. a. *Streptococcus bovis* is an organism that closely resembles enterococci on media and shares similar biochemical characteristics in that it grows in the presence of bile, hydrolyzes esculin, and is catalase negative. The enterococci, though, grow in the presence of 6.5% sodium chloride, while *S. bovis* does not. In addition, enterococci are pyrrolidonyl arylamidase (PYR) positive, while *S. bovis* is negative. *S. bovis* is Lancefield group D antigen positive. *S. bovis* is an inhabitant of the human gastrointestinal tract. It primarily causes bacteremia and endocarditis, and there is a strong association between *S. bovis* bacteremia and colon malignancy. All individuals with *S. bovis* bacteremia should be tested for colon carcinoma. *Streptococcus agalactiae*, or group B streptococcus, is beta-hemolytic, is esculin

hydrolysis negative, and does not grow in the presence of bile. *Streptococcus dysgalactiae* subsp. *equisimilis* usually isolates type with either Lancefield group C or G. Most of these isolates are beta-hemolytic on sheep blood agar. *S. dysgalactiae* subsp. *equisimilis* are associated with many of the same infections as *Streptococcus pyogenes*.

44. **b.** The mycoplasmas are the smallest known free-living bacteria. They do not have a cell wall. Several are significant human pathogens. *Mycoplasma pneumoniae* causes community-acquired pneumonia and upper respiratory tract infections. *Mycoplasma hominis* and *Ureaplasma urealyticum* cause urogenital tract infections, systemic diseases in neonates (such as meningitis and pneumonia), and invasive disease in immunocompromised patients. The mycoplasmas can be cultured on solid and liquid media. **SP-4 medium** is often used to isolate *M. pneumoniae*. Cultures should be held for 4 weeks, and most laboratories examine the agar surface every 1–3 days with a microscope to observe colonies. A8 agar medium is used to isolate *U. urealyticum* and *M. hominis*. McCoy cells are used to isolate *Chlamydia trachomatis*. Middlebrook 7H10 agar and BACTEC 12B medium are used to recover *Mycobacterium* species.

45. **a.** *Haemophilus influenzae* is a fastidious, gram-negative coccobacillus. It is a significant human pathogen, and some strains are encapsulated. Encapsulated strains are usually the most pathogenic. There are six known *H. influenzae* capsule types: a, b, c, d, e, and f. Capsule type b was once the most common type involved in serious infections, but there is an effective type B vaccine now. The encapsulated *H. influenzae* strains are associated with meningitis, epiglottitis, cellulitis, pneumonia, septic arthritis, and bacteremia. Nonencapsulated strains cause otitis media, conjunctivitis, sinusitis, and pneumonia and bacteremia in immunocompromised patients. The *Haemophilus* species, in general, require hemin (X factor) and NAD (V factor) for growth. A given *Haemophilus* isolate can be streaked on a plate with both X and V impregnated filter papers to determine which factors are required. If the isolate grows in between the X and V filter papers, then it requires both X and V for growth. *H. influenzae* requires both X and V factors (Fig. 14.26B). *H. haemolyticus* also requires both X and V factors for growth; however, it is beta-hemolytic on rabbit blood agar, while *H. influenzae* is not. Chocolate agar provides both X and V factors, but sheep blood agar provides only hemin. *Haemophilus* species are usually colorless on chocolate agar (Fig. 14.26A). *H. influenzae* will also grow as tiny colonies around *Staphylococcus aureus* streaked on sheep blood agar. This is known as satelliting and occurs because *S. aureus* produces NAD as a by-product. All of the *Haemophilus* "para" (*H. parahaemolyticus*, *H. parainfluenzae*, *H. paraphrophilus*) species require only V factor for growth.

46. **d.** The case presentation and travel history of the child are characteristic for typhoid fever, or enteric fever, caused by *Salmonella* **serotype Typhi**. Other infectious agents, such as malaria, should be ruled out as well. A similar disease is caused by *Salmonella* serotype Paratyphi A. *S.* Typhi characteristically produces a small amount of H_2S in triple sugar iron (TSI) agar. This usually shows as a sliver near the top of the slant (Fig. 14.27A) as compared to *Salmonella* serotype Enteritidis, which produces H_2S like most *Salmonella* serotypes (Fig. 14.27B). Most isolates of *S.* Paratyphi A do not produce H_2S. In addition, *S.* Typhi is ornithine decarboxylase negative, whereas nearly all other *Salmonella* serotypes, including *S.* Paratyphi A, are positive. *Shigella* species do not produce H_2S and cause bacillary dysentery, usually characterized by fever, abdominal cramping, bloody diarrhea, and tenesmus later in the disease course. *Edwardsiella tarda* is another member of the Enterobacteriaceae that may also be an agent of gastroenteritis. It is H_2S positive, indole positive, and ornithine decarboxylase positive.

47. **b.** *Clostridium difficile* causes antibiotic-associated pseudomembranous colitis. It is a frequent cause of hospital-acquired diarrhea. *C. difficile* becomes established in the gastrointestinal tract of people after the normal gut flora has been reduced by prolonged antibiotic therapy. Only toxigenic strains cause disease, although nontoxigenic strains can be isolated as flora from stool specimens. Toxigenic strains of *C. difficile* elaborate toxins TcdA and/or TcdB; strains can cause disease when they produce both or either of the toxins. Rapid antigen assays are commonly used to determine the presence and toxin-production of *C. difficile* from stool specimens. The organism can also be isolated from stool by culture on cycloserine-cefoxitin-fructose agar (CCFA), although this is not the most sensitive method of identification. On CCFA, *C. difficile* strains fluoresce chartreuse under UV light, and colonies smell like horse manure. *Clostridium botulinum* is the agent of botulism. *Clostridium perfringens* causes myonecrosis, bacteremia and food poisoning; there have been some cases reported, though, of *C. perfringens* causing antibiotic-associated diarrhea. *C. perfringens* does not fluoresce chartreuse under UV light on CCFA. *Clostridium septicum* is associated with myonecrosis and bacteremia and also does not fluoresce chartreuse under UV light when cultured on CCFA. *Bacillus cereus* causes food poisoning and may grow anaerobically, but it is not associated with antibiotic-associated diarrhea.

48. **a.** *Neisseria gonorrhoeae* is an oxidase-positive, catalase positive, Gram-negative diplococcus. It is noteworthy among the genus *Neisseria* in that it produces acid only from glucose. *N. gonorrhoeae* causes urethritis, epididymitis, rectal infections, pelvic inflammatory disease, conjunctivitis, pharyngeal infections, and disseminated infections. Disseminated gonococcal infection (DGI) occurs when the organism becomes bacteremic. Most

patients with DGI have fever, arthralgias in the knees and elbows, and a dermatitis that consists of pustules and papules, usually on the extremities. *N. gonorrhoeae* is fastidious and grows best on chocolate agar or specialized media such as modified Thayer-Martin agar or New York City agar. Specialized media for the isolation of *N. gonorrhoeae* contain antibiotics to select for the organism. Colonies of *N. gonorrhoeae* are colorless on chocolate agar. *Neisseria meningitidis* may also cause urethritis and cervicitis that is indistinguishable from that caused by *N. gonorrhoeae*. However, most *N. meningitidis* isolates produce acid from glucose and maltose. *Neisseria lactamica* may cause invasive infections in humans; it produces acid from glucose, maltose, and lactose. *Neisseria sicca* may also cause invasive infections, and it produces acid from glucose, maltose, sucrose, and fructose. *Moraxella catarrhalis* is also an oxidase-positive, catalase-positive, Gram-negative diplococcus. It colonizes the nasopharynx of approximately 1% to 5% of adults and is commonly found in infants. *M. catarrhalis* is associated with otitis media, pneumonia and other respiratory tract infections, bacteremia, and sinusitis. It does not produce acid from glucose, maltose, or other carbohydrates. *M. catarrhalis* can be rapidly identified by performing a spot test for indoxyl-butyrate hydrolysis.

49. **c.** *Mycobacterium tuberculosis* is associated with pulmonary tuberculosis and extrapulmonary infections such as skin, joint, and bone infections, cervical lymphadenitis, pericarditis, pleuritis, and meningitis. Symptoms of pulmonary tuberculosis include fever, night sweats, weight loss, chest pain, and cough. Like other mycobacteria, *M. tuberculosis* has a lipid-rich cell wall with mycolic acids. Most of the mycobacteria stain better with the acid-fast stain. *M. tuberculosis* grows slowly on solid media and can take up to 2 months for colonies to appear. The colonies are nonpigmented and dry and wrinkled in appearance; most strains exhibit cording. Biochemical tests are not performed in most laboratories anymore for the identification of *M. tuberculosis*. Instead, most isolates are identified with DNA probes, by PCR, by DNA sequencing, and other nucleic acid amplification assays, such as the amplified *M. tuberculosis* direct test (AMTD). Biochemically, *M. tuberculosis* is niacin positive, nitrate reduction positive, and pyrazinamidase positive. *Mycobacterium bovis* is in the *M. tuberculosis* group and causes similar infections as *M. tuberculosis*. In contrast to *M. tuberculosis*, it is niacin, nitrate reduction, and pyrazinamidase negative. *M. bovis* is also a slow-growing organism and is nonpigmented. *Mycobacterium kansasii* also causes pulmonary and extrapulmonary infections. It is a photochromogen, so it is pigmented when exposed to light. *Mycobacterium avium-intracellulare* is also associated with pulmonary and extrapulmonary infections. Most strains are not pigmented, and it is a slow-growing organism. *M. avium-intracellulare* is pyrazinamidase positive but niacin and nitrate reduction negative. *Mycobacterium fortuitum* is a rapid-growing organism.

50. **e.** *Helicobacter pylori* is the primary cause of peptic ulcer disease and is a risk factor for gastric carcinoma and gastric lymphomas. The organism is found worldwide, and apparently, it is spread by the fecal-oral route. *H. pylori* survives gastric conditions by generating ammonium ions with the enzyme urease and because it is very motile. It is a curved Gram-negative rod that requires a microaerophilic atmosphere. Culture may be performed to isolate the organism, although diagnosis takes several days. Biopsy specimens from endoscopy are usually used for culture isolation. Breath tests have also been developed to take advantage of the rapid and strong **urease** activity of *H. pylori*. Patients first drink or eat something with ^{13}C- or ^{14}C-labeled urea, then their breath is tested for $^{13}CO_2$ or $^{14}CO_2$. This test yields results in less than 2 hours but false negatives may occur if patients are treated with suppressive agents that do not completely eliminate the organism. Biopsy specimens can also be incubated on urea-containing media for a few hours to determine urease activity; longer incubation may be required to increase sensitivity of this method. Serology is also used to monitor therapy, and a stool antigen test is also available. While *H. pylori* is oxidase positive and catalase positive, neither test is diagnostic for the organism.

51. **c.** The finding of significant **peripheral blood eosinophilia**, in the range of 15% to 50% or higher, should always point to the high possibility of a parasite disease indicating a diagnostic exploration. Although bloody diarrhea, splenomegaly, chronic cough, and cramping abdominal pain may be caused by one or more parasites, these signs and symptoms are less specific and occur with a variety of other conditions.

52. **d. Alopecia** is not a symptom that has been attributed to any parasite disease. The other possible answers to this question are associated with the infestation of one or more parasites. Bloody diarrhea can be caused by invasion of the intestinal mucosa by various parasites, notably *Entamoeba histolytica* and the larval forms of *Strongylodes stercoralis*. Suprapubic pain along with hematuria is one of the hallmarks of *Schistosoma hematobium* infestation. Focal itching of the skin occurs at the sites of penetration of the cercariae of all *Schistosoma* species and may also occur during the subcutaneous migration of larval forms of hookworms and of cutaneous larva migrans and the microfilaria of *Onchocerca volvulus*. Transient pneumonia is caused during the transpulmonary migration stages of the larval forms of ascaris and the hookworms or may take the form of hypersensitivity pneumonitis induced by the lytic products of dying forms of infested parasites.

53. **a.** Any fixative containing formalin, **merthiolate-iodine-formaldehyde** (MIF) for example, is not suitable for the preparation of trichrome-stained smears. The formaldehyde fixes the outer cell

membranes of protozoan trophozoites in such a way that the stain does not penetrate. Although smears prepared after sodium acetate, acetic acid, formalin (SAF) are also inferior to those following other fixatives, the parasitic forms are still microscopically visible. Schaudinn fixative, including the zinc-based version (EcoFix), and Polyvinal alcohol both preserve the trophozoites in fixed specimens without interfering with the preparation of high quality stained smears.

54. **d.** The operculated eggs of *D. latum* and other parasites may not be detected in the clear liquid surface layer of stools processed by zinc sulfate flotation because they tend to pop open in the high specific gravity of the mixture, fill with fluid, and sink to the bottom. The other parasitic forms included as responses to the questions have specific gravities that are lower than the 1.018 of the zinc sulfate, causing them to float to the surface where they will be visualized in mounts or stained smears prepared from the clear surface fluid layer.

55. **a.** Malarial parasitic forms will be **detected in light infections** using thick peripheral smears. The concentration of erythrocytes in a thick smear has a 30X concentration of malarial forms compared to thin films, providing the microscopic visualization of the few parasitic forms that may be present in light infections. However, the staining qualities of the parasitic forms may be compromised, often obscuring the details necessary to make a species identification. Thus, a thin smear must also be prepared whenever parasitic forms are detected in the thick smear preparation to make a species identification. The anticoagulant has no effect on staining, and gametocytes are not stimulated to exflagellate early.

56. **b.** Illustrated in the photograph is a trophozoite of *Entamoeba histolytica*, characterized by the presence of a small central karyosome and the even distribution of chromation along the nuclear membrane. Other key identifying characteristics include a finely granular cytoplasm and the ingestion of an erythrocyte. An additional characteristic of *E. histolytica* observed in direct mounts is the unidirectional motility of this trophozoite. *Entamoeba coli* can be identified by its large and eccentric karyosome, the irregular and clumped distribution if chromatin, and a "junky"cytoplasm, containing undigested debris and liquid vacuoles. The trophozoites of *D. fragilis* possess two nuclei. Neither *Iodamoeba butschlii* nor *Endolimax nana* possess an "entamoeba type" nucleus; that is, there is an absence of chromatin distributed along the nuclear membrane.

57. **e.** *D. fragilis* is known to cause a syndrome of persistent diarrhea, abdominal pain with decrease in appetite, and loss of weight. Carriers are often symptomatic. Each of the other amoeba listed are considered to be harmless commensals. *Entamoeba dispar* is morphologically similar to *E. histolytica*. A report of *Entamoeba histolytica / dispar* is often issued, relying on a clinical correlation to determine if the nonpathogenic *E. dispar*

strain has been recovered. Also, it must be recognized that *D. fragilis* is no longer classified as an "amoeba;" rather is a flagellate, even though flagella are not observed with the light microscope. It is important to recognize, however, that when this protozoan is observed in stool specimens, therapy is in order when clinically indicated.

58. **d.** The large size of this trophozoite as indicated by the micrometer scale immediately points to the ciliate, *Balantidium coli*. The cytostome and prominent macronucleus are additional helpful identifying features. The outer membrane is typically covered with delicate cilia, not well demonstrated in this photomicrograph. The trophozoites of *Entamoeba coli* may be as large as 50 μm in diameter, still only one third the size of *B. coli*. Each of the other protozoan parasites listed as possible responses are small in size, with the oocysts of *Isospora belli* and *Sarcocystis hominis* measuring no more than 30 μm.

59. **a.** Illustrated in the photomicrograph is a trophozoite of *Giardia lamblia*. Of the procedures listed, only direct **aspiration or biopsy of duodenal material** has proven to be insensitive in the laboratory diagnosis of this intestinal flagellate. The string test is more sensitive than duodenal aspiration because the "string" is left in place for a period of 5 hours, sufficient time for *Giardia* trophozoites to adhere. In cases of a single negative stool, repeat samples on successive days may be effective. The detection of *Giardia* cysts in stool specimens using immunofluorescence is more sensitive than examination of unstained mounts, and detection of *Giardia* antigen in stool is commonly used when a diagnosis in suspicious clinical cases has not been established.

60. **c.** Characteristic of the trophozoite of *Chilomaxtix mesneli* is the pear shape, the placement of the nucleus tight against the anterior cell membrane, and the presence of a para- nuclear cytostome ("shepherd's hook"). The characteristic "monkey face" appearance of *G. lamblia* would not be confused with the more mundane features of *C. mesneli*. The trophozoites of *Dientamoeba fragilis* possess a pair of nuclei, and *Balantidium coli* is considerably larger, recognized by its outer membrane covered throughout the circumference by short, delicate cilia, and a prominent kidney-shaped macronucleus. The one characteristic that distinguishes *Trichomonas hominis* is an open space between the anterior nucleus and the cell membrane and the presence of a flagella-carrying undulating membrane along the full length of the body.

61. **b.** Human balantidiosis is most prevalent **where pigs are raised and slaughtered**. Reports of infections in the United States are uncommon. Most human cases have been reported from Latin America, the Far East, and New Guinea.

62. **d.** The incidence of human infestations with each of the coccidian parasites listed as responses to this question,

except *Sarcocystis hominis*, has increased significantly with the advent of AIDS requiring prompt HIV testing when identified in stool specimens.

63. **a.** The brown-colored (bile stained), spherical to slightly oval-shaped ovum with a wart-like, thick shell covered by an albuminous coat is characteristic of *Ascaris lumbricoides*. The ova of each of the other nematode species listed as possible answers to this exercise have a smooth, thin wall. The adult worms of *A. lumbricoides* inhabit the small intestine and have the predilection to migrate, entering such orifices as the common bile duct and pancreatic duct, where complications of obstruction may arise. The female worm may excrete as many as 200,000 ova per day making quantitative counts useless as a predictor of the worm load.

64. **d.** In contrast to *Trichuris trichiura*, the ova of *C. phillippinensis* have flattened, less conspicuous polar plugs and, of more significance, possess a thick shell with radial striations. The ova of each of the other nematodes listed have a thin, smooth wall. Geographic location of the patient, of course, would come in to play as *C. phillipensis*, as the name would suggest, is almost exclusively endemic in the Philippines, Thailand, and other countries in the South China Sea area. Much of the high prevalence in this part of the world relates to dietary habits where ingestion of raw animal meat and organs, uncooked crabs, and small freshwater fish is considered a delicacy. None of the other ova included in the list of responses have a barrel shape nor possess polar plugs.

65. **c.** Although isolated ova of *Enterobius vermicularis* may be microscopically observed in the examination of stool specimens or with a rectal swab, the sensitivity is far less than with **a transparency tape preparation**. It may also be possible to visually detect the small adult female worms, that reach about 10–12 mm (1/2 inch) in length, by visual examination of the perianal area of skin, but microscopic examination would be necessary for confirmation. The most sensitive method is to apply the sticky side of transparency tape on the perianal folds and perineal skin before then sticking it face down to the surface of a glass slide for microscopic examination. Both the characteristic ova, smooth-walled and flattened on one side, often containing a mature larva, and adult worms with their characteristic alar "wings" and the pin-point tail, may be detected. It is best to perform this transparency tape procedure on children early in the morning when female worms most commonly exit the anus to discharge eggs on the surrounding skin.

66. **a.** The smooth, thin-shelled ovum with a clear space under the shell where the internal cleavage has retracted as illustrated in the photomicrograph is characteristic of *Necator americanus*. It should be mentioned that the old-world hookworm, *Ancylostoma duodenale*, and *Strongyloides stercoralis* produce ova that are morphologically indistinguishable. The ovum of *Ascaris*

lumbricoides has a thick shell covered with an albuminous coat. The ova of *Capillaria philippinensis* and *Trichuris trichuria* are barrel-shaped, possess a thick shell with, and display hyaline plugs at either end. The ovum of *Enterobius vermicularis* appears somewhat similar to the hookworms, however, its shell is thicker and flattened along one side, appearing much as a deflated football. A well-developed embryo is usually contained within.

67. **b.** The ova of *Strongyloides stercoralis* are rarely found in stool specimens. Therefore, attempts to make the identification of their ova in stool specimens will most commonly fail by whatever method that microscopic mounts are prepared. Rather, the laboratory diagnosis is made by **observing rhabditiform larvae in the stool specimen**. These larvae average between 250 μm and 300 μm long and have a long buccal cavity and a prominent genital primordium approximately one third of the distance from the tail. *Strongylodies* filariform larvae may also develop while in the intestinal tract, but typically invade the mucosa and disseminate in tissues throughout the body and are rarely seen in stool specimens. Polymorphonuclear leukocytes will not be observed in stool specimens, and the rhabditiform larvae do not appear in the top filtrate in the flotation technique.

68. **b.** It is necessary that the laboratory notify the clinical care team that special techniques will be used for the recovery and identification of *Strongyloides* only when there is a consistent history and **strong clinical suspicion** of strongyloidisis. It is a waste of time and money to implement the agar procedure for all stool specimens. *Strongyloides* does not commonly cause bloody smears and does not commonly elicit an inflammatory reaction making these techniques nondiscriminatory.

69. **c.** High ova counts in cases of hookwork infections may be a signal of **severe infection that may require aggressive therapy**. Complications such as iron deficiency anemia may also develop in patients with heavy infestations. Because female hookworms excrete only about 5,000 eggs per day, a quantitative count of the number of ova in a stool specimen can be correlated with the magnitude of the worm load. Female patients who excrete a concentration of 2000 or more ova/ml, and male patients who excrete over 5000 ova/ml are more likely to experience serious infections that require aggressive therapy to prevent a variety of complications. Also, a patient with an intestinal infestation of 500 or more worms will lose about half a liter of blood per week, leading to chronic iron deficiency anemia with complications of osteoporosis and the formation of bone cysts related to erythroid hyperplasia in the bone marrow. The morphology and number of eggs do not distinguish between hookworm species. Although a very low count may suggest *Strongyloides* infection, the presence of characteristic rhabditiform larvae is the key to making that identification. Hookworm ova do not

develop into filariform larvae in the intestine; rather, this is a characteristic of *Strongyloides*. Infection control practices should be in place for stool specimen processing and examination regardless of what microflora is expected, unrelated to the magnitude of the organism load.

70. **b. Transient pneumonia and Loeffler syndrome** is related to that phase early in the hookworm life cycle when the filariform larvae transmigrate through the lungs. The acute abdominal pain and diarrhea that may occur in hookworm infections is secondary to penetration of the bowel mucosa by the adult worms. Filariform larvae do not develop in the intestine in hookworm infections. Similarly, iron deficiency anemia in heavy infestation, which may also lead to mental retardation in children, is secondary to the chronic iron deficiency anemia not from central nervous system circulation of filariform larvae.

71. **a.** The spherical, thick-walled ovum illustrated in the photomicrograph, displaying distinctive radial striations, is characteristic of *Taenia* species. The two commonly encountered species, *T. solium* and *T. saginata* cannot be distinguished by differences in the morphology of the ova. In more mature ova, not seen in this photomicrograph, three pairs of hooklets may be observed within the developing embryo ("hexacanth embryo"). The remaining ova included as possible responses to this question either possess an operculum (*D. latum*), do not have a striated shell (*Hymenolepis* species), or are arranged in clusters (*D. caninum*).

72. **d.** The ova of *Taenia solium*, once ingested, are **directly infective for humans**. The developing onchospheres hatch in the small intestine and penetrate the intestinal wall and enter the circulation. These invasive larval forms (onchospheres) have a specific proclivity to form cysts in the connective tissues, called cysticerci. Development of these cysts in the brain (neurocysticircosis) may lead to a variety of complications including epileptic seizures and cranial nerve palsies, particularly of the fifth and seventh cranial nerves. Ingesting *Taenia saginata* ova does not predispose one to these complications. The intestinal disease and complications of each of these species is similar and do not require any differences in therapeutic approach.

73. **d.** The ovum illustrated in the photomicrograph is characteristic of the fish tapeworm *Diphyllobothrium latum*. The ovum of *Paragonimus westermanni* is a close "look-alike" based on size and overall appearance; however, its operculum has prominent protrusions ("shoulders") and does not possess an abopercular knob. The ovum of *Clonorchis sinensis* also has a shouldered operculum; however, the ovum is only one third the size of *D. latum*. The egg of *Hymenolepis nana* has a thick shell and an inner membrane containing a prominent hexacanth embryo. The ova of *Dipyllidium caninum* are small (20–25 μm in diameter), smooth, and are arranged in clusters.

74. **c.** *Diphyllobothrium latum* is common among people residing in Northern Europe and Scandanavia, particularly in Finland, in whom **megaloblastic anemia** is a common manifestation. *D. latum* worms have a selective proclivity to adsorb this important vitamin from the intestinal contents, depriving the host from this essential element needed for erythrocyte maturation. The intestinal effects of the adult worm on the intestine are minimal, with only occasional bouts of abdominal pain and diarrhea. Bowel obstruction may occur with oversized worms. Sparganosis is a disease caused by the ingestion of the larval forms of diphyllobothroid tapeworms other than *D. latum*, most commonly infesting dogs and cats. Humans acquire these larval forms from the ingestion of copepods or raw or uncooked flesh of infected amphibians and reptiles. The cystic forms of sparganosis are primarily found in the subcutaneous tissue of the skin, and contrary to the larval forms of *Taenia solium*, do not involve the central nervous system.

75. **c.** The spherical egg, with a thick, smooth outer shell and an inner membrane are characteristic of *Hymenolepis* species. The ovum illustrated in the photomicrograph is that of *Hymenolepis diminuta*, a parasite of rats and mice that is uncommonly found in humans. It differs from the ovum of *Hymenolepis nana*, the dwarf tapeworm found in the intestinal tract of infested humans, by the lack of a pair of polar filaments that emerge from thickenings on either side of the inner membrane. The ova of each of these species possess three pairs of prominent hooklets (hexacanth embryo) within the inner membrane, well illustrated in this photomicrograph. None of the other ova included as possible responses to this question have this outer shell and inner membrane, and do not possess a hexacanth embryo within.

76. **c.** Illustrated in the photomicrograph is an ovum of *Schistosoma mansoni*. The adult worms reside in the **portal vein system of the intestine** where the discharge of ova into the surrounding tissue of the bowel serosa and mesentery results in extensive granulomatous inflammation and fibrosis. Portal fibrosis of the liver may occur, however, resulting from invasion of the portal spaces by ova that are discharged into the portal vein system, not by the presence of adult worms. Cystic cavities in the lung are caused by the adults of *Paragonimus westermanii*, skeletal muscle disease is more likely secondary to infestation with *Trichinella spiralis*, while *Schistosoma haemotobium* selectively occupy the portal veins of the urinary bladder.

77. **d.** Chronic cystitis from deposition of the eggs of *Schistosoma haematobium* in the submucosa of the urinary bladder is well documented. Complications include intermittent hematuria and an increase incidence of squamous cell carcinoma. Chronic inflammation secondary to deposition of eggs from *Schistosoma mansoni* is observed primarily in the large bowel and adjacent

mesentery. The inflammatory nodules of *Onchocerca volvulus* are located in the subcutaneous tissues and caused by migration of adult worms, while the larval forms of *Trichinella spiralis* result in focal chronic myositis of the skeletal musculature.

78. **d.** Infective free-swimming cercaria, recently released into water estuaries from the sporocysts of infected snails, penetrate the water-softened skin of the **swimming or wading human host.** "Swimmer itch" is a prickly itching of the skin at the sites where cercaria have penetrated. Minute petechiae progressing to pruritic papular skin eruptions may be observed as the infection becomes more chronic. Ingestion of contaminated drinking water is commonly caused by *Entamoeba histolytica* or *Giardia lamblia*; ingestion of uncooked fish is associated with *Diphyllobothrium latum* and *Clonorchis sinensis*; while *Fasciola hepatica* and *Fasciolopsis buskii* are contracted from the ingestion of metacercaria on contaminated water plants.

79. **b.** The thin, smooth shell, an indistinct nonshouldered operculum at one end, and extension of the cleavage to the inner membrane of the shell is characteristic of *Fasciolopsis buski*. The ovum of *Fasciola hepatica* also appears similar; however, on close examination, the abopercular margin of the shell of the ova of *F. hepatica* is roughened, while that of *F. buski* is smooth. Serologic tests are available to detect *Fasciola hepatica* ES antigen in stool specimens. The ova of *Schistosoma mansoni* have a thicker shell and a prominent lateral spine. The ova of *Diphyllobothrium latum* also appear similar in overall appearance to those of *Fasciola / Fasciolopsis*; however, they are only approximately half the size. The ova of *both Paragonimus westermanii* and *Clonorchis sinensis* can be distinguished by their shouldered rather than flat opercula and the latter also by its considerably smaller size.

80. **e.** The life cycles of both *Fasciola hepatica* and *Fasciolopsis buskii* progress through the release of a free-swimming, ciliated miracidium that penetrate a snail. Within the snail, sporocysts develop and ultimately transform into free-swimming cercaria that are released and attach as metacercaria to a water plant. Humans most commonly become infected after **ingestion of contaminated water plants,** such as fresh watercress added in salads. Ingestion of lake or stream water would only result in human infections in the rare event that metacercaria may be dislodged from infected plants. Humans do not become infected by ingestion of uncooked freshwater fish or contact with water animals. The direct penetration of the skin by free-swimming cercaria is characteristically seen in Schistosomiasis.

81. **a.** Illustrated in the photograph is the adult of the trematode, *Clonorchis sinensis*, the Chinese liver fluke. Interestingly, even with relatively heavy infestations, clinical manifestations tend to remain low grade. Even with infestation of the liver, **cirrhosis and jaundice are uncommon symptoms.** Organisms may persist for decades in chronic cases, resulting only in intermittent mild abdominal distress and low-grade diarrhea. Eosinophilia is a common peripheral blood manifestation. Only in heavy infections might some degree of portal hypertension evolve, and the chance for cholangiocarcinoma is increased.

82. **a.** Infections with the Chinese liver fluke occur following ingestion of raw or undercooked freshwater fish, a warning to sushi lovers. The other sources of infection included in the response to this question have been addressed before and do not apply to the acquisition of *Clonorchis sinensis*.

83. **e.** The relatively large egg with a prominent shouldered operculum is that of the lung fluke (e), *Paragonimus westermanii*. The final destination is the **peripheral lung** tissue where the adult flukes develop within parabronchial pseudocysts. Eggs are discharged into the bronchioles and may be observed either in expectorated sputum specimens or in the stool after being swallowed. This location is a classic example of organotropism; that is, the affinity of a parasite to seek out and reside within a given organ. Humans acquire this parasite from ingestion of raw or poorly cooked crab meat or crayfish. Upon ingestion, the metacercaria of the parasite hatch in the duodenum. The released larvae first penetrate the full thickness of the bowel wall, enter the abdominal cavity, then transmigrate through the diaphragm and into the pleural space.

84. **a.** Illustrated in the left frame of the photomicrograph are the small ring forms of *Plasmodium falciparum*. Note that multiple rings are observed in some erythrocytes; in others, they are plastered against the outer cell membrane, in what is known as the appliqué or accolade position. Illustrated in the right frame is a crescent-shaped gametocyte that is diagnostic.

85. **c.** The infected erythrocyte demonstrates the band-form of the developing trophzoite of *Plasmodium malariae*, that extend to the borders of outer membrane, in contrast to the more ameboid development of trophozoites characteristic of *Plasmodium vivax* and *Plasmodium ovale*. Remember that the trophozoites for *Plasmodium falciparum* do not develop in the peripheral blood. The intra-erythrocytic parasitic forms of *Babesi microti* also do not develop beyond the ring stage.

86. **b.** The enlarged and somewhat pale infected erythrocyte with a schizont comprised of more than 13 merozoite segments is characteristic of *Plasmodium vivax*. Note also that a few tiny granules are observed in the clear cytoplasm in the lower part of the infected erythrocyte. These are Schuffner dots, another identifying characteristic of vivax malaria.

87. **e.** Observed in the two infected erythrocytes are tiny ring forms that superficially resemble those of *Plasmodium falciparum*. Note the distinctive doublet formation, simulating "rabbit ears." When more mature forms are observed, these ring forms arrange in

tetrads, resembling a "Maltese cross," a pattern characteristic of **Babesia microti**. Babesia is a protozoan disease of animals that is transmitted to humans through the bites of *Ixodes dammini* ticks, which are coinfected with this parasite. *Babesia microti* is the agent of Lyme disease, manifest as varying degrees of malaise, anorexia, fatigue, and muscle aches. The disease may last intermittently for several days or weeks but is usually self-limited. Severe disease, including life-threatening hemolytic anemia and disseminated intravascular coagulation may occur in people with prior splenectomy and in the debilitated elderly.

88. **c.** The extraerythrocytic forms observed in the photomicrograph are **trypomastigotes**. Note the deeply-staining, dot-like kinetoplast lying at the tip of the organism posterior to the central nucleus. An anterior flagellum is observed, that runs the full length of the body, supported by an undulating membrane. The distinctive "C" shape of these trypomastigotes are characteristic of *Trypanosoma cruzi*, the agent of Chaga's disease. The trypomastogotes of African trypanosomiasis are linear rather than curved in shape and are usually present in peripheral smear preparations in larger numbers. The microfilaria of *Onchocerca volvulus* do not circulate in the peripheral blood. The parasitic forms of *Leishmania* species are very small, oval in shape, and represent the amastogotic form. The parasitic forms of toxoplasmosis are bow-shaped and the tachyzoites are not commonly seen in the peripheral blood, rather are seen in tissue aspirates or in histological sections.

89. **d.** The hemoflagellate illustrated in the photomicrograph is one of the African trypanosomes, either *Trypanosoma gambiense* or *Trypanosoma rhodesiense*, the vector of which is the tsetse fly. Infections are acquired through the bites of infected **Glossina tsetse** flies, normally a pest of wild game that serve as the main reservoir of trypanosome infestation. The tsetse fly injects the infective trypomastigotes into the skin, where they enter the circulation. The central nervous system is the primary site of infection, resulting in a syndrome of recurrent fever. The lymph nodes in posterior cervical neck region become enlarged ("Winterbottom's sign"). "Sleeping sickness" is the common outcome of chronic infection, beginning with personality changes and ending with fatigue, confusion, somnolence, and finally death from emaciation and terminal coma. The reduviid bug serves as the vector for *Trypanosoma cruzi*, the phlebotomus sandfly for the *Leishmania donovoni* complex, the Ixodes tick for *Borellia bergdorpheri* (Lyme disease), and the anopheles mosquito is a vector for malaria.

90. **d.** Human **leishmaniasis** is acquired from the bites of *Phlebotomus* sand flies. A cutaneous form of leishmaniasis may manifest as ulcers or sores of the skin and mucous membranes extending from the sites of insect bites. Disseminated leishmaniasis, known as Kala Azar,

involves the liver, spleen, and other organs of the reticuloendothelial system. Close observation of the amastigotes illustrated in the photomicrograph will reveal that each has a small bar-like protrusion at right angles to the nucleus. This is the primordial kinetoplast that is observed in the trypomastigotes of *Trypansoma* species, a helpful clue in separating the leishmanial amastigotes from the small yeast cells of the dimorphic fungus, *Histoplasma capsulatum*.

91. **d.** Toxoplasmosis is not transmitted by insect vectors; therefore, **application of repellants** will have no effect. Toxoplasmosis is caused by a bow-shaped protozoan parasite in the form of tachyzoites that have a predilection for invading the central nervous system. The life cycle involves cats that serve as the final host for the sexual reproduction of the parasite. Humans become infected by direct contact with cats or from a variety of fomites contaminated with oocysts present in cat excrement. Therefore, activities such as cleaning out cat litter boxes or ingesting unwashed fruits and vegetables that may have become contaminated can lead to infection. The ingestion of raw meat of animals that had ingested oocysts from contact with infected cats is another common source, particularly in countries where steak tartar is a delicacy. An increase in infection has also been reported related to the intravenous injection of drugs. The most devastating form of toxoplasmosis is direct placental transfer to newborns from of infected mothers.

92. **e.** The filarial parasites are threadlike worms that inhabit the circulatory and lymphatic channels in cases of human infection. **Brugia malayi** has the pattern illustrated in the photograph, with two nuclei extending into the tail separated approximately 10 μm apart. Filariasis is transmitted from an infected human to another via the bite of a mosquito or tabanid flies (*Loa loa*). The female worms produce microfilaria that circulate in the blood. The species are identified primarily on the pattern of nuclei extending into the sheathed tail section. Nuclei do not extend into the tail of *Wuchereria bancrofti* at all and extend all the way to the end of the tail with Loa Loa. *Mansonella perstans* also produce microfilaria that circulate in the blood, but they are unsheathed and are devoid of a tail. Onchocerca microfilaria remain localized to the infection sites and do not circulate in the peripheral blood.

93. **b.** The adult filarial worms are contained within subcutaneous cysts. The females discharge microfilaria that remain confined to the subcutaneous tissue and do not circulate in the peripheral blood, but can be easily **identified in teased snips of skin**. Microfilaria may also migrate to the eye where they can cause "night blindness." They do not cause conjunctivitis and microfilaria and will not appear in conjunctival secretions. The diagnosis can be made by performing a surgical biopsy of one of the subcutaneous nodules; however, this is only done after all other methods have failed.

The simulium black fly obviously does not remain at the site of the bite.

94. c. The beautiful layout of the larval forms illustrated in this photomicrograph, with their 2 ½ spiral turn is characteristic of *Trichinella spiralis*, the cause of trichinosis. This primary skeletal muscle disease in humans is most commonly acquired by ingesting poorly cooked pork or pork products containing encysted larvae. The larvae penetrate the small intestine, enter the lymphatic and finally become encysted within skeletal muscle. More active muscles, such as the gastrocnemius and the deltoid, are most likely infected and serve as sites for biopsy. Damage to muscles may result in a variety of complications—irregularities in chewing and swallowing, difficulty in breathing, and musculoskeletal dysfunction depending on the site and degree of involvement.

95. c. Echinococcus infections in humans are most common among sheepherders, who use dogs as herd control animals. **Dogs or other carnivores** such as foxes, serve as the definitive host, within the intestines of which the adult *Echinococcus* tapeworms reside. They are relatively small, and composed of four segments—a scolex and three proglottids. Eggs are excreted and spread throughout the pasture. **Grazing sheep or other herbivores** as intermediate hosts, ingest these eggs, within which embryos are carried by the blood stream to the liver, lung, and brain where they develop into echinococcal cysts. Within each of these cysts are produced infective protoscolexes, which in turn evaginate in the dog intestine upon ingestion of cyst-laden viscera. Humans are infected from ingestion of the eggs excreted by dogs, often acquired from the skin and hair while petting and handling these pets. Thus, humans also serve as an intermediary hosts in whom larval-induced cysts also develop in various organs, more commonly the liver and brain.

96. e. Various serologic and immunoassays are available for the definitive diagnosis of most parasitic diseases where conventional diagnostic techniques fall short or are inconclusive. Each of the responses to this question has such tests, either commercially available or available through the services of a public health or reference laboratories. The only exception is **sparginosis**, a superficial parasitic skin infection that can be easily diagnosed by a simple surgical biopsy procedure.

97. a. Stool specimens submitted in formalin cannot be examined for parasite motility. Formalin inactivates the motility of the organism and only a fresh sample can be used for this procedure. Each of the other procedures listed as possible answers should be performed when specifically ordered.

98. d. **The third successive stool specimen will not be accepted.** Each of the guidelines indicated as responses to this question should be published in the laboratory ward manual except the directive that three successive stool specimens should not be submitted.

There may be situations where a series of three daily stools may be needed to establish a diagnosis if the clinical presentation is highly suggestive of a parasitic disease in the face of negative results. If a third specimen is to be submitted, it may be well to collect the specimen following administration of a cathartic. The deterrent to submitting three specimens is that studies have indicated that the chances to have a positive test after two successive negative results is very low and may not be cost-effective.

99. c. The only exception to sending the addendum comments indicated in the responses to this question is the need to perform EIA assays for **detection of *Giardia* antigen** when both stool concentrate and smear preparations reveal cyst forms. The diagnosis has been established and performing a follow-up EIA procedure is unnecessary and costly.

100. d. In cases of persistent diarrhea in the face of repeatedly negative routine O & P examinations, the possibility of undetected *Cryptosporidium*, *Cyclospora*, and *Microspora* must be considered; thus, **an order for acid-fast stain should be submitted**. The fecal immunoassays currently available for detection of many of the coccidian parasites are far more sensitive than the routine O & P procedure and/or the preparation of special stains. Yet, in the event that the antigen titers are too low to be detected in the immunoassay procedure, another extensive search for coccidian oocysts via an O & P exam on a concentrated stool specimen, using the recommended centrifugation speed and time of 500 Xg for 10 minutes should be attempted one more time and acid-fast smears prepared. It may also be well to have more than one microbiologist examine the smear and stain preparations. All other guidelines listed as possible responses to this question will fall short.

101. d. The patient has **chronic hepatitis B** because she is surface, antigen positive, negative for IgM antibody to the core antigen, and positive for total antibody to the core antigen. In this circumstance, the presence of surface antigen indicates an active infection. The absence of IgM and presence of total-core antibodies indicates that the antibodies detected are primarily IgG, the hallmark of a chronic infection when surface antigen is present. For all intents and purposes, chronic hepatitis A does not exist, and IgG antibodies to hepatitis A merely indicates an infection at some point in the past. The presence of antibodies to hepatitis C merely indicates exposure to hepatitis C. A positive test does not distinguish between acute, chronic, or resolved infection.

102. d. The presence of hepatitis B surface antibody indicates immunity to hepatitis B. The presence of total antibody to hepatitis B core antigen indicates that this **immunity developed due to natural infection**.

103. c. The presence of hepatitis B surface antibody indicates immunity to hepatitis B. The absence of total antibody to hepatitis B core antigen indicates that

this **immunity was most likely induced via vaccination**.

104. **d.** Detection of antibody to hepatitis C does not distinguish between **active and resolved infection**. Similarly, if the infection is active, it does not distinguish between acute and chronic hepatitis C. Clinically, chronic hepatitis C is a much more likely event than acute hepatitis C. EIA screening tests occasionally produce false-positive results. Western blots provide somewhat greater specificity for antibody testing, but the ambiguities associated with determining the status of the infected patient remain the same. In many instances, patients should be checked for hepatitis C RNA following a positive antibody test.

105. **e.** The serologic pattern presented is occasionally encountered. Unfortunately, it is not entirely clear what stage of infection this pattern represents. This undoubtedly represents an individual who was infected with hepatitis B at some point, and one of their serologic markers, either hepatitis B surface antigen or hepatitis B surface antibody, have dropped below the detection limits of the assay. If distinguishing these two options is important, serum can be collected for quantitative HBV DNA assays; if viral DNA is detected, the patient still has an active infection. Alternatively, if the patient is given vaccine, and they now produce detectable levels of hepatitis B surface antibody, they were most likely immune with antibody levels dropping below the limit of detection with the assay.

106. **b.** In the cases of DiGeorge syndrome and severe combined immunodeficiency (SCID), you would expect an absence of the thymic shadow on chest x ray. Similarly with SCID, physical examination often reveals an absence of lymphoid tissue (e.g., tonsils). With all of these diseases except **transient hypogammaglobulinemia**, you should expect substantially reduced counts of B cells, T cells, or both, whereas this patient's B- and T-cell counts were within normal limits.

107. **c.** This constellation of laboratory, radiology, and physical findings is consistent with severe combined immunodeficiency (SCID). All of the options provided, EXCEPT **deficient expression of MHC class I molecules** are known to predispose to SCID.

108. **a.** This constellation of clinical and laboratory findings is consistent with leukocyte adhesion deficiency, a state in which leukocytes are impaired in binding to ICAM-1 molecules expressed on endothelial cells in inflamed tissue. This deficient binding to ICAM-1 has been demonstrated to be due to mutations in the gene encoding **LFA-1**, the ligand for ICAM-1. Under these circumstances, the patient has difficulty clearing bacterial infections because leukocytes may attain very high levels within the bloodstream, but cannot leave the vasculature and enter the tissues to fight the infection.

109. **d.** This constellation of clinical and laboratory findings is consistent with a diagnosis of hyper-IgM syndrome. This disease is caused by an inability of T-helper cells to induce isotype switching by B lymphocytes. Consequently, IgM is the predominant Ig class made in these patients and very little IgG, IgA, or IgE is made by their B cells. For effective isotype switching to occur, CD40 on B cells must bind to **CD154** on CD4+ T cells. Mutations in the gene encoding CD154 lead to this disorder.

110. **a.** Patients with SLE frequently have false-positive results in nontreponemal syphilis serologic tests, such as the **RPR and VDRL**, due to antiphospholipid antibodies. The MHA-TP is a treponemal test that is specific for antibodies that react with the organism rather than antibodies that react with phospholipids (which are detected with the nontreponemal tests). False-positive nontreponemal tests are sufficiently common in patients with lupus that it is considered one of the diagnostic criteria for this disease.

111. **d.** ANCA antibodies may be positive in a variety of inflammatory vasculitides but are particularly common in patients with Wegener granulomatosis. The cytoplasmic pattern of ANCA (**c-ANCA**) usually caused by antibodies against serine proteinase 3 (PR-3) is highly specific for Wegener granulamatosis. The other autoantibodies are not at all specific for this disease.

112. **e.** This patient history leads you to consider the diagnosis of Sjøgren syndrome. Although rheumatoid factor and ANA's are often positive in patients with Sjøgren syndrome, they are not specific for this disease. **Anti-Ro and anti-La** are relatively specific for this disease, though their absence does not exclude the diagnosis. Anti-Ro and anti-La are also known as anti–SS-A and anti–SS-B, respectively.

113. **c.** Although anti-nuclear antibodies are often present in patients with type 1 autoimmune hepatitis, this test is also positive in a wide variety of other autoimmune disorders. **Antismooth muscle antibodies** are almost invariably positive in patients with type 1 autoimmune hepatitis and relatively specific for this disorder.

114. **a.** A diagnosis of primary biliary cirrhosis is strongly supported by a positive test for AMA. **AMA antibodies** are found in approximately 90% of patients with primary biliary cirrhosis.

115. **c.** If the mother was HIV infected, the transplacental transfer of maternal IgG will almost invariably result in the baby having anti-HIV antibodies at this age, regardless of whether or not the baby is actually HIV infected. It does not matter what methodology you use, or the specimen selected, you will still be testing for maternal antibodies. RT-PCR for HIV viral RNA in the infant's serum is more reliable than looking for maternal antibodies, but this viral RNA may also be potentially transmitted from the mother and may not reflect active infection. **Detection of proviral DNA** in the baby indicates active viral infection and is the test of choice for detecting of congenital HIV infection.

116. **c.** The only Ig class to cross the placenta is IgG. Consequently, the presence of IgG antibodies in the

serum of a newborn infant merely indicates that the mother had these antibodies. In this case, the presence of IgG antibodies to rubella indicates that the mother is immune to rubella infection. In contrast, IgM antibodies are not transplacentally transferred. Therefore the presence of IgM anti-**CMV** antibodies in this baby's serum indicates in-utero synthesis and in-utero infection. RPR tests are often falsely positive in pregnant women, and that appears to be the case in this situation due to the negative MHA-TP confirmatory test. Even if the MHA-TP test had been positive, it would not have distinguished between congenital syphilis and transplacentally transferred antibodies to *Treponema pallidum*. In actuality, there is little reason to test the baby's serum for IgG antibodies.

117. **d.** It is reasonable to perform nontreponemal tests (e.g. RPR or VDRL) on serum as screening tests for primary or secondary syphilis, but over time, the titer of the antibodies detected by these tests may drop to undetectable levels even in patients with tertiary syphilis. Consequently, a negative RPR or VDRL does not exclude a diagnosis of tertiary syphilis. The CSF VDRL is a fairly specific test, so in the appropriate setting a positive result provides very strong support for the diagnosis of neurosyphilis, but the test is fairly insensitive. Consequently, a negative CSF VDRL does not exclude neurosyphilis. Serum treponemal tests generally remain positive in patients with latent and tertiary syphilis. Consequently, a **negative serum MHA-TP** provides strong evidence against neurosyphilis in a nonimmunosuppressed patient. The MHA-TP test is generally not performed on CSF.

118. **c.** *Mycobacterium marinum* grows poorly, or not at all, at temperatures of 35°C or above. Incubation of routine TB medium at temperatures of 30°C is required for the recovery of this organism.

119. **a.** *Mycobacterium haemophilum* grows poorly, or not at all, at temperatures of 35°C or above. Additionally, the organism requires hemoglobin or hemin for growth, so it will not grow on media routinely used to recover *M. tuberculosis* unless it is supplemented with Fildes supplement, 2% ferric ammonium citrate, an X factor strip, or something similar. An alternative approach is to inoculate **chocolate agar slants** and incubate them at 30° C. Growth is further stimulated in an atmosphere containing 10% CO_2.

120. **d.** Antibodies to *Treponema pallidum* typically can be detected for years in the circulation of patients who were successfully treated for syphilis. Consequently, a patient who was diagnosed with **syphilis** many years ago will still have positive treponemal tests even if they no longer have active infection. Under these circumstances, there is no point in repeating the test, and it can no longer be used to confirm a diagnosis of syphilis in patients with positive nontreponemal screening tests.

121. **a.** *Blastomyces dermatitidis* is a thermally dimorphic fungus. The characteristic morphologic feature (broad-based bud) of this organism is detected in the yeast state at body temperatures.

122. **e.** *Histoplasma capsulatum* is a thermally dimorphic fungus. The characteristic morphologic feature (tuberculate macroconidia) of this organism is detected in the mycelial phase of cultures incubated at room temperature.

123. **b.** *Cryptococcus neoformans* is a monomorphic yeast characterized by its heterogeneity in size and its large polysaccharide capsule that repels india ink, which is particulate. It grows quite rapidly on bacterial culture media and can usually be detected after overnight incubation.

124. **b.** **Rhizopus** is one of the agents of zygomycosis. Other agents of zygomycosis include *Mucor*, *Absidia*, and *Cunninghamella*. All of these organisms are molds only, with large, sparcely septate to aseptate, hyphae.

125. **c.** *Sporothrix schenkii* is a thermally dimorphic mold that most commonly causes chronic subcutaneous infections following traumatic implantation. At body temperatures, elongated yeasts are occasionally seen. Room temperature cultures produce the mycelial phase with the characteristic structures shown.

126. **b.** *Penicillium marneffei* is unusual in that it is the only thermally dimorphic fungus of this genus. It is a common opportunistic pathogen in patient with AIDS in southeastern Asia. The infection often disseminates, but the cutaneous lesions described are often most visible. The characteristics in culture are as described in the case.

127. **c.** Dermatophyte infections are caused by members of three different genera: Trichophyton, Microsporum, and Epidermophyton. The macroconidia shown are characteristic of **Microsporum spp**.

128. **e.** *Malassezia furfur* causes tinea versicolor and has also been reported to produce systemic infections in pediatric patients receiving prolonged courses of intravascular **lipids**. The organism will not grow on routine fungal culture media unless it is supplemented with lipids by adding a few drops of virgin olive oil or a similar source of lipids.

129. **a.** The characteristic morphology shown is that of *Candida* pseudophyphae. The classic feature that helps distinguish *Candida* pseudohyphae from the hyphae of most other organisms is the tendency to constrict at the septations.

130. **d.** Production of pseudohypae is characteristic of virtually all *Candida* species except *C. glabrata*. *C. glabrata* is a fairly small yeast, 2–3 × 4–5 μm.

131. **c.** In most clinical settings, *Candida krusei* is encountered relatively rarely. Nevertheless, at some institutions it has become a very important pathogen in high risk patients. One factor that appears to have selected for this organism in those settings is its resistance to fluconazole. *Candida glabrata* also has a tendency to develop resistance to fluconazole, but fluconazole resistance is significantly more common in *C. krusei*.

132. **c.** Most fungal infections are acquired by exposure to environmental sources. Dermatophytes are one of the exceptions to this rule, as they may be transmitted directly, or indirectly, from person to person.

133. **b.** The small size of this organism distinguishes it from *Aspergillus* spp. The branching filamentous morphology is most consistent with either Actinomyces or *Nocardia* spp. Most *Actinomyces* spp. are obligate anaerobes, though occasional isolates can grow aerobically. The capacity to grow in the presence of lysozyme, however, distinguishes **Nocardia** from *Actinomyces* spp.

134. **e.** A modified acid-fast stain is typically used to help identify the organisms listed in options a through d. *Streptomyces* **spp.** will not stain acid fast by this method, which can be used to help distinguish these organisms from the morphologically similar *Nocardia* spp.

135. **b.** *Fusarium* **spp.** are occasional causes of keratitis as are *Acanthamoeba* and *Paecilomyces*. The characteristic morphology, however, is that of Fusarium.

136. **a.** The agents of phaeohyphomycosis or chromoblastomycosis include a wide variety of dematiaceous fungi. Of the genera listed, **Phialophora** and *Cladosporium* are dematiaceous. The characteristic microscopic morphology shown includes phialids of *Phialophora* spp.

137. **b.** All of the infections listed except *Legionella pneumonia* are readily spread from person to person, either directly or indirectly. Legionella is an aquatic organism that is typically transmitted to humans from environmental sources.

138. **d.** All of the organisms listed except *M. fortuitum* are slow-growing species that typically take a minimum of 7 days to grow on solid media. Further, they are unlikely to grow on routine bacteriologic culture media. *M. fortuitum* is a rapidly-growing mycobacteria that occasionally causes cutaneous/subcutateous infections and will grow as described on routine bacteriology culture media.

139. **d.** The organism described is a scotochromogen, and *M. gordonae* is the only scotochromogen listed. Further, *M. gordonae* is a relatively frequent contaminant in TB laboratories as it is commonly recovered from tap water.

140. **c.** In 1993, the case definition of AIDS was expanded to include HIV infected individuals with CD4 counts below $200/\mu L$ as well as those with pulmonary tuberculosis. Chronic cryptosporidiasis and pneumocystis pneumonia are opportunistic infections indicative of significant immunosuppression. Most patients with AIDS who are infected with *Histoplasma capulatum* will develop disseminated infection. Isolated **pulmonary histoplasmosis**, without dissemination, is not necessarily indicative of significant immunosuppression.

141. **b.** The replication of hepatitis D virus depends on the replication of hepatitis B. Consequently, patients with acute or chronic hepatitis B (patients D and A, respectively) can, potentially, also be actively infected with hepatitis D. Similarly, patients who have never been vaccinated against, or infected with hepatitis B (patients C and E) are not immune to hepatitis B, and are therefore susceptible to hepatitis D infection in the future, should they become infected with hepatitis B. Patients who are immune to hepatitis B cannot develop hepatitis D. The status of immunity or infection with hepatitis A or C have no impact on susceptibility to hepatitis D infection.

142. **c.** The germ tube test is often used to distinguish *Candida albicans* from other yeasts, which are typically negative. *Candida dublinensis* also produces germ tubes, so it can potentially be confused with *C. albicans* if this is the only method of identification used. Fortunately, *C. dublinensis* is relatively rarely encountered in clinical settings, so this problem is usually not significant.

143. **a.** Although many patients with systemic sclerosis are positive for antinuclear antibodies, this test is not at all specific for this disease. **Anti-DNA topoisomerase I** antibodies are rarely encountered in patients who do not have systemic sclerosis, but the sensitivity of this test is only approximately 30% to 40%.

144. **b.** Hereditary angioedema is due to a deficiency in circulating levels of **C1 inhibitor**, with a result of decreased disassociation of C1 complexes activated by the classical pathway. Decreased levels of C1, C3, C7 and total hemolytic complement may be observed in a variety of conditions; they are not, in any way, specific for hereditary angioedema.

145. **c.** C3 is central to all three complement activation pathways, and patients with **C3** deficiencies have an immunodeficiency that manifests similarly to hypogammaglobulinemia. Patients with deficiencies in C1 can still activate complement by the alternate and lectin pathways, and patients with C4 and C2 deficiencies can still activate complement by the alternate pathway. Patients with C6 deficiencies are still capable of generating anaphylatoxins and chemotactic factors by all three pathways. Consequently, deficiencies in complement components other than C3 are not as severe as C3 deficiencies, and may not be clinically evident.

146. **e.** The use of **Sabouraud dextrose agar** as a primary recovery medium is discouraged because it is insufficiently rich to reliably grow dimorphic fungi from clinical specimens. All of the other media are fine for this purpose.

147. **b.** Neutropenia is generally considered as a risk factor for bacterial, not fungal, infections. Immunity to most fungi is generally depends on macrophage activation by CD4 cells, resulting in enhanced phagocytosis and killing, or granuloma formation. **Aspergillus** is one of the exceptions to this general rule. Neutropenia is a significant risk factor for disseminated aspergillosis.

148. **b.** Hyperacute rejection of transplants is attributable to preexisting antibodies against antigens on the graft. In the rare clinical circumstances where this occurs, it is due to ABO mismatches or preexisting antibodies

against MHC antigens. Hyperacute rejection can be avoided by following rules for ABO transfusion when transplanting solid tissues and by testing the recipient's serum for antibodies against MHC antigens of the donor (i.e., performing a crossmatch) prior to transplantation.

149. **c.** Autoantibodies, particularly antinuclear antibodies, of patients with SLE typically combine with soluble antigens and precipitate out in various tissues including the kidney. Complement is fixed, attracting neutrophils, and this classic immune complex mediated pathogenesis contributes to tissue damage.

150. **b.** Patients with SLE generally secrete a wide variety of different autoantibodies, not just antinuclear antibodies. Some patients have antibodies directed against cell surface antigens on white blood cells, resulting in their elimination by **classic type II hypersensitivity** reactions.

151. **a.** Conconavalin A is a classic **T-cell** mitogen used to determine the capacity of T cells to proliferate in vitro.

152. **a.** The test described is a classical mixed lymphocyte reaction in which **T-helper cells** are induced to proliferate by foreign MHC class II alloantigens. Irradiated allogeneic macrophages may serve as a source of stimulating alloantigens, but their intact function is not particularly important to this particular reaction. Proliferation of cytotoxic T cells (CD8), B lymphocytes (CD19), macrophages, or NK cells (CD56) is not usually prominent in this reaction.

153. **b.** Rhinocerebral mucormycocis is an infection of the paranasal sinus that spreads to involve the orbit, face, palate, or brain. Diabetic acidosis and hematologic malignancy are predisposing risk factors for craniofacial involvement. *Rhizopus* is the most prevalent agent of mucormycosis. **Tissue material should not be homogenized** as this procedure kills viable hyphal elements. Careful mincing and planting of the tissue on agar media provide optimum recovery.

154. **a.** *Rhizopus* accounts for approximately 60% of all culture proven cases of human mucormycosis and nearly 90% of the rhinocerebral cases. Microscopically, *Rhizopus* is characterized by sporangiphore/s arranged opposite to rhizoids; *Rhizomucor* species have branched sporangiophores that are anchored to the substratum by short rhizoids.
Mucor spp. do not have rhizoids, and in *Cunninghamella* spp, the sporangiophores have long branches that end in swollen vesicles. The sporangiosphore of *Saksenaea* spp bear sporangia that are flask shaped.

155. **b.** Detection of IgM antibody to WNV in serum collected within 8 to 14 days of illness onset using the IgM antibody-capture, enzyme-linked immunosorbent assay (MAC-ELISA) is the most sensitive method for diagnosing this infection. Since IgM antibody typically does not cross the blood-brain barrier, presence of **IgM in CSF** strongly suggests central nervous system infection. Antibodies to WNV cross-react with other closely related flaviviruses (Japanese encephalitis, St. Louis

encephalitis, yellow fever, dengue). Neutralization assays (plaque reduction neutralization tests) are more specific than routine serologic tests and used for confirmation. Serum IgM levels typically persists for 6 months or longer, hence it is not a useful test to detect current disease. Usefulness of PCR is limited because of the transient and low viremias. With PCR, WNV genetic material can be detected in CSF in up to 50% of patients who present with acute West Nile meningoencephalitis. Virus culture is rarely positive except in autopsy material, generally from the brain and other solid organs.

156. **a.** *Mycobacterium haemophilum* is a common pathogen associated with cutaneous skin nodules in AIDS patients and other immunocompromised patients. *M. hemophilum* has special nutritional and incubation temperature requirement. The organism requires hemin or **ferric ammonium citrate** for growth, which can be readily provided by plating specimens on Chocolate agar. Unlike other mycobacteria that prefer 36°C to 38°C for growth, the optimum incubation temperature for *M. hemophilum*, *M. marinum*, *M. ulcerans*, and *M. chelonae* is 25°C to 33°C.

157. **a.** *M. avium-intracellulare* produces a tuberculosis-like disease in middle-aged white men with history of heavy smoking and alcohol abuse. The organism is slow growing (10–21 days) and appears as buff to yellow pigmented smooth or rough colonies. *M. tuberculosis* is a slow grower but is niacin positive. *M. gordonae* and *M. simiae* are yellow-colored colonies and grow in 2 to 3 weeks. *M. hemophilum* is not associated with this clinical disease and prefers low temperature for cultivation.

158. **a.** *M. avium-intracellulare* is the leading cause of cervicofacial lymphadenitis in children. *M. gordonae* is usually nonpathogenic and occurs as a contaminant in the laboratory. *M. simiae* typically produce disease similar to MAC such as chronic pulmonary disease and osteomyelitis. Although *M. haemophiulm* has been isolated from cervicofacial lymphadenitis in children, it is less common when compared with *M. avium-intracellularae*.

159. **c.** *Tropheryma whippelii* is the causative agent for Whipple disease or intestinal lipodystrophy. The disease predominates in middle-aged white men and is characterized by arthralgia, diarrhea, abdominal pain, and weight loss. The inclusions are Gram-positive bacilli that are found extracellularly. The organism is not cultivable and is diagnosed by nucleic acid amplification.

160. **a.** *Capnocytophaga canimorsus* is a Gram-negative fastidious bacteria colonizing the oral cavity of dogs. It is oxidase and catalase positive and exhibits "gliding motility" on agar medium. *C. canimorus* has been associated with septicemia and other severe infections following dog bite. *Pastereulla multocida* is more commonly isolated following cat bites. *E. corrodens* is associated with human bites.

161. **b. Sporotrichosis** also called as the "rose gardener disease" is caused by a thermally dimorphic fungi

Sporothrix schenckii. At 35°C, the colonies are yeast-like, and at 25°C they appear as mold. The disease begins locally on the skin and spread to lymphatics and in severe cases may involve skeletal system. It may cause pulmonary disease in chronic alcoholics or highly immunosuppressed patients.

162. c. *Candida dubliniensis* is a germ-tube positive *Candida* species similar to *C. albicans*. It was originally isolated from an HIV-positive patient in Dublin, Ireland. Unlike *C. albicans*, it fails to grow at 42°C and does not express beta-glucosidase activity. *C. parapsilosis*, *C. tropicalis*, and *C. glabrata* are germ-tube negative candida species.

163. b. *Fusarium* spp is commonly associated with mycotic eye infections. A recent multistate outbreak was reported by CDC to be associated with a brand name lens cleaning solution that was contaminated with *Fusarium* spp. The appearance of "sickle- or canoe-" shaped macroconidia on microscopic morphology are characteristic of this organism.

164. b.

1% Flu	Positive	Negative	
Positive	TP = 19	FP = 80	PPV TP/(TP + FP) 19/99 = 19%
Negative	FN = 1	TN = 1900	NPV TN/(TN + FN) 1900/1901 100%
	Sensitivity TP/ (TP + FN) 19/20 = 95%	Specificity TN/ (FP + TN) 1900/1980 = 96%	

165. e.

20% Flu	Positive	Negative	
Positive	TP = 380	FP = 64	PPV TP/(TP + FP) 380/444 = 86%
Negative	FN = 20	TN = 1536	NPV TN/(TN + FN) 1536/1556 99%
	Sensitivity TP/ (TP + FN) 380/400 = 95%	Specificity TN/ (FP + TN) 1536/1600 = 96%	

166. b. **False-positive test results are common** during the early and late viral season when the prevalence of the disease is low. It is recommended that positive test results from rapid antigen tests be confirmed by other tests such as culture when incidence of the disease is low in the community.

167. c. **Culture** is the accepted test method to provide evidence for sexual abuse in children. *N. gonorrhoea*

detected by culture needs to be confirmed by two different phenotypic tests to be eligible for use as legal evidence. Nucleic acid amplifaction tests may be used for *C. trachomatis* in the absence of culture, however, a positive amplification test needs to be confirmed by culture or an alternate FDA approved amplification test that detects a distinct region on the *C. trachomatis* not overlapped by the previous amplification test.

168. d. The estimate of neonatal HSV infection is 1 in 3,000 to 20,000 live births. Infection occurs during passage through the birth canal or less commonly by ascending infection. Risk of HSV infection is highest (33% to 50%) in infants born vaginally to a mother with primary genital infection and is much lower in reactivation disease (5%). **Nucleic acid amplification** of HSV-DNA in the CSF specimen is the test of choice due to its high sensitivity and specificity. Viral culture is good for recovering HSV from skin vesicles, mouth, eyes, urine, blood, and stool from neonates. Viral specific antibody develops only several weeks after infection and is not useful for diagnosis of HSV encephalitis.

169. d. *Trichomoas vaginalis* is one of the most common sexually transmitted pathogens associated with vaginits. Infection with this parasite leads to vulvar pruritus, and a frothy, foul smelling discharge which is frequently yellowish green in color. Infection with *Candida* spp. does not produce any odor but produces white, cottage cheese-like vaginal discharge. Bacterial vaginosis produces a "fishy" odor and a thin, homogenous milky white or gray vaginal discharge.

170. c. *V. vulnificus* is associated with severe wound and septicemic illness following exposure to seawater during warm weather conditions. Consumption of raw oysters is the main source for systemic infection. Among the choices given *V. cholera* and *V. vulnificus* are the logical possibilities given the seawater exposure, but *V. cholera* infection is restricted to the gastrointestinal tract. *V. vulnificus* is called the "lactose positive" vibrio and is clinically associated with wound infection.

171. b. Maternal IgG crosses the placenta and can be found circulating in the newborn. **IgM does not cross placenta** and denotes fetal infection. Rubella can also be detected by culture in this patient.

172. a. Rhinoviruses are differentiated from enteroviruses by their **sensitivity to low pH**, resistance to lipid solvents (due to lack of a lipid envelope), and preferential growth at 33°C instead of 37°C. Cellular changes from rhinovirus infection occur earlier in fibroblast cell lines than in epithelial cell lines. Among cell lines commonly used in the clinical laboratory, the human embryonic lung fibroblasts, such as MRC-5 and human embryonic kidney cells, support rhinoviral replication.

173. a. Hemadsorbing viruses such as the influenza and parainfluenza are differentiated based on their ability to hemadsorb at different temperatures. Washed guinea

pig erythrocytes are poured over tube cultures and incubated at 4°C for 30 minutes and observed and reincubated at room temperature for 30 minutes; influenza virus hemadsorbs at 4°C and room temperature while parainfluenza hemadsorb only at 4°C. This is an effective way to detect parainfluenza virus before the development of CPE or in the absence of CPE.

174. **b.** The three Staphylococcal species that are positive by slide coagulase tests detecting clumping-factor are *S. aureus*, *S. lugdunensis*, and *S. schleiferi*. Tube coagulase positive species include *S. aureus and S. intermedius*. Among clumping factor positive species, only *S. lugdunensis* is positive by both ornithine decarboxylase and pyrolidonylarylamidase tests, while *S. schleiferi* is negative in the ornithine decarboxylase test and *S. aureus* is negative by both tests.

175. **b.** Development of resistance in *E. cloacae* during therapy is due to inducible resistance mediated by chromosomal **AmpC β-lactamases**. Inducible resistance typically leads to resistance only against inducing agent. Hence it is necessary to test subsequent isolates from the same source within 3 to 4 days especially when a cephalosporin is used for therapy. Chromosomal AmpC genes are common in the following organisms: *Serratia* spp., *Providencia* spp., *Pseudomonas aeruginosa*, *P. mirabilis*, *Acinetobacter* spp., *Citrobacter* spp, *Enterobacter* spp., and *Morganella* spp.

176. **d.** *Enterobacter* spp. has chromosomal AmpC.

177. **d.** Resistance to all cephalosporins and other beta-lactam antibiotics in *Enterobacter* spp arises from point mutations in the regulatory genes for the chromosomal AmpC; as a result, very high levels of AmpC are constitutively produced.

178. **b.** *Bacillus cereus* is a gram-positive rod that grows aerobically with the characteristics mentioned in the question. This organism is a virulent and destructive ocular pathogen. It is associated with post-traumatic keratitis and enopthalmitis after penetrating trauma. *B. cereus* infections of the eye are emergencies and should be reported to the physician immediately.

179. **b.** Invasive aspergillosis is one of the most common mold infections in immunocompromised patients. Pulmonary infiltrate and the CT findings described are characteristics of mold infection. *A. fumigatus* is the most common mold recognized in bone marrow transplant recipients.

180. **d.** Staphylococcal entrotoxin mediated disease characteristically produces symptoms within 1 to 8 hours of ingestion of enterotoxin-tainted food. *S. aureus* replicates efficiently and produces high levels of toxin in a variety of foods that are held at warm temperatures. Shortly after ingestion of these foods, the preformed toxin upon ingestion causes vomiting and diarrhea. Symptoms usually resolve within 24 hours. The incubation period for *Salmonella*, *Shigella*, and *Campylobacter* infections is 1–3 days and it is the bacterium that causes GI disease. *C. perfringens* causes di-

arrhea and abdominal cramps; vomiting and fever are uncommon. It is usually associated with home-canned foods and the incubation period is in the order of 6–24 hrs.

181. **c.** The purpose of these internal controls is to monitor for inhibition, both nonspecific inhibition from extraneous substances and competitive inhibition. In this scenario, the CT amplified at high levels indicating that nonspecific inhibition was not an issue. The failure of the IC to amplify suggests that exhaustion/depletion of amplification reagents due to rapid consumption by CT amplicon, possibly resulted in a false-negative GC result. Hence, the GC result is indeterminate. A separate reaction to test for GC and IC only can provide accurate result for presence of GC in the specimen.

182. **d. Hantavirus** pulmonary syndrome (HPS) is associated with exposure to rodents (natural hosts) excreta. Hantavirus is an RNA virus of the Bunyaviridae family. Within the Hantavirus genus, Sin Nombre virus (SNV) (host: deer mouse) is the major cause of HPS in the four-corner region of the United States. Characteristic laboratory findings include neutrophilic leukocytosis with immature granulocytes, more than 10% immunoblasts (basophilic cytoplasm, prominent nucleoli, and increased nuclear–cytoplasmic ratio), thrombocytopenia and increased hematocrit.

183. **c.** Macrolide resistant isolates of *S. aureus*, may have inducible resistance to clindamycin due to methylation of the 23S rRNA encoded by the *erm* gene also referred to as MLS$_b$ (macrolide,lincosamide, and type B streptogramin resistance). Alternatively, macrolide resistance may be due to an efflux mechanism encoded by *msr*A gene. Clinical laboratories perform a "D test" to detect inducible resistance to clindamycin in erythromycin-resistant isolates of *S. aureus*.

184. **c.** *Aeromonas hydrophila* is associated with severe septic infections in immunocompromised patients. Wound infections with *Aeromonas species* is usually related to freshwater exposure of open wounds.

185. **d. Herpes B virus,** or cercopithecine herpes virus 1, is indigenous to old-world monkeys. It causes subclinical as well as dermal, oral, genital, and eye lesions in monkeys. Virus is transmitted to humans by contact with infected monkeys and results in a life-threatening CNS infection. In almost all untreated cases, fatal ascending myelitis and encephalopathy occurs. Most infected individuals who survive are left with severe brain damage.

186. **c.** Amoebic encephalitis is most frequently acquired during warm summer months and is associated with swimming in stagnant water bodies. Species of amoeba that can cause such a condition are *Naeglaria fowleri*, *Acantahamoeba* species and *Balamuthia mandirallis*.

187. **c.** *K. kingae* is a fastidious gram-negative coccobacillus associated with suppurative arthritis and osteomyelitis in children less than 5 years old. Pyogenic arthritis is usually monoarticular and frequently involving knees

and may also involve the hips and ankles. The organism grows best in anaerobic conditions with enhanced carbon dioxide. In patients with septic arthritis and osteomyelitis, blood culture is often negative. Joint fluid and bone aspirates should be inoculated into automated blood culture systems to maximize recovery.

188. c. **Chikungunya** virus infection can cause a debilitating illness, most often characterized by fever, headache, fatigue, nausea, vomiting, muscle pain, rash, and joint pain. Acute chikungunya fever typically lasts a few days to a few weeks, but as with dengue, West Nile fever, and other arboviral fevers, some patients have prolonged fatigue lasting several weeks. In addition, some patients have reported incapacitating joint pain, or arthritis which may last for weeks to months. The prolonged joint pain associated with chikungunya virus is not typical of dengue.

189. b. **Rotavirus** is the leading cause of viral gastroenteritis in children less than 5 years old during winter months. Recent introduction of vaccine to rotavirus may reduce the burden of the disease in future years.

190. b. BK virus nephropathy is associated with increasing viral loads in plasma. Viral loads in urine are usually very high and are not specific for the disease process. Urine PCR for BK virus may be a sensitive prognostic tool to identify patients at risk for developing future BK viremia.

191. b. Of the options provided, only EIA and DFA can provide rapid results. EIA has poor sensitivity in adults, so **DFA** may be a better alternative. RSV is a labile virus hence culture has less than optimal sensitivity.

192. b. *C. sordellii* is associated with toxic shock syndrome following medical abortion. Blood cultures are rarely positive and the bacterium is usually detected in the endometrium and placental tissues of affected patients.

193. c. Aseptic meningitis during summer months in children is most often associated with **enteroviral** infection. Enteroviral meningitis clinically mimics bacterial meningitis. About 15 different enteroviruses account for nearly 90% of enterovirus serotypes recovered from children with meningitis in the last 30 years. *E. coli*, *Streptococcus agalactiae*, and *L. monocytogenes* cause bacterial meningitis in the neonate, while HSV is associated with encephalitis in the first few weeks of an infant's life.

194. d. **OFBL** is a selective agar used to isolate *B. cepacia* from CF sputum. MacConkey agar is a selective medium for gram negatives. CNA is selective agar for gram-positive organisms from mixed clinical specimens. CIN is a selective medium for isolation of *Yersinia* spp and CVA is a selective and enriched blood agar medium used for isolation of *Campylobacter* species.

195. a. Expectorated **sputum** is a specimen that is not typically cultured anaerobically because of the high number of anerobes colonizing the upper respiratory tract; cultures of expectorated sputum will almost always contain large numbers of anerobes that are unrelated to the infectious process in most circumstances. Anaerobes can be isolated from the other specimens *b* through *e* and isolation of anaerobes from such specimens is clinically significant.

196. b. The susceptibility of *S. pneumoniae* to cephalosporins can not be reliably determined by disc diffusion. Microbroth dilution (MIC) or Etest methodologies are options for determining the susceptibility *S. pneumoniae* to cephalosporins.

197. b. *C. difficile* colonization is **common in children in who are less than 1 year of age**. Testing for *C. difficile* is not advisable in this age group. The intestinal epithelium of infants who are less than 1 year old lacks receptor for *C. difficile* toxin and consequently these infants do not typically develop disease with this potential pathogen.

198. b. Airborne transmission occurs with MTB, measles and VZV. Patients infected with these pathogens should be isolated in negative pressure rooms. **Rubella**-infected patients are kept in contact and droplet isolation.

199. a. Select agent rule dictates that BT agents need to be destroyed within a week following confirmatory testing.

200. c. **Norovirus** is associated with outbreaks of acute viral gastroenteritis on cruise ships. Rotavirus is a pathogen in children. Although Adenovirus, Enterovirus, and Bocavirus can cause diarrheal illness, they do not have associations with any specific environmental exposures.

201. e. All of the viruses *a* through *d* are RNA viruses of the Coronaviridae family. **Bocavirus** is a DNA virus that belongs to the Parvoviridae family.

202. d. **H3N2** is a human influenza A virus that causes seasonal epidemics on a yearly basis. All other viruses such as avian influenza viruses are documented to have infected humans.

■ Recommended Readings

Forbes BA, Sahm DF, Weissfeld AS. *Bailey & Scott's diagnostic microbiology.* 12th ed. St. Louis: Mosby Elsevier, 2007.

Long SS, Pickering LK, Baker CJ, et al. *Red Book: 2006 report of the committee on infectious diseases.* 27th ed. American Academy of Pediatrics, 2006.

Mandell GL, Bennett JE, Dolin R. *Mandell, Douglas, and Bennett's principles and practice of infectious diseases.* 6th ed. Philadelphia: Churchill Livingstone, Elsevier, 2005.

Murray R. Baron EJ, Jorgensen JH, et al. *Manual of clinical microbiology.* 9th ed. Washington: ASM Press, 2007.

Winn W, Allen S, Janda W, et al. G. *Koneman's color atlas and textbook of diagnostic microbiology.* 6th ed. Baltimore: Lippincott Williams & Wilkins, 2006.

15

Transfusion Medicine

Fouad Boctor and Naomi Luban

■ Questions

1. Irradiated blood products are indicated for all of the following conditions EXCEPT:
   a. Low birth weight newborns
   b. In utero exchange transfusion
   c. Congenital immunodeficiency disorders
   d. Acquired immunodeficiency (HIV)
   e. Severe leukopenia patients receiving granulocyte transfusions

2. Select the blood product that does NOT require irradiation for a patient on an irradiation restriction:
   a. Whole blood
   b. Red blood cells
   c. Granulocytes
   d. Fresh plasma
   e. Fresh frozen plasma

3. The Food and Drug Administration (FDA) requires the periphery of a unit of irradiated blood product receive NOT less than:
   a. 50 G
   b. 35 G
   c. 20 G
   d. 15 G
   e. 10 G

4. The time needed for irradiating a unit of blood is:
   a. 60 minutes
   b. 30 minutes
   c. 20 minutes
   d. 5 minutes
   e. Source half-life

5. A pregnant medical technologist is working in the hospital blood bank and an irradiated platelet unit is ordered for a patient with Wiskott Aldrich syndrome. Which one of the following is correct?
   a. The pregnant medical technologist is excused from irradiating the blood products.
   b. The patient with Wiskott Aldrich syndrome does not need an irradiated platelet unit.
   c. The pregnant medical technologist must wear a lead shield during the irradiation process.
   d. There is no risk to a pregnant medical technologist during the irradiation process.
   e. The risk to the pregnant patient varies depending on the irradiation source.

6. Which of the following associations or agencies is involved in the inspection of a radiation source used in the blood bank?
   a. Food and Drug Administration (FDA)
   b. Nuclear Regulatory Commission (NRC)
   c. American Association of Blood Banks (AABB)
   d. FDA and NRC
   e. AABB, FDA, and NRC

7. Which of the following is the correct biochemical moiety that defines blood group A?
   a. L-fucose
   b. N-acetylgalactosamine
   c. D-galactose
   d. D-mannose
   e. N-acetylneuraminic acid

8. The dominant immunoglobulin isotype found in antibodies to the A and B blood group antigens is:
   a. IgG
   b. IgM
   c. IgA
   d. IgE
   e. IgD

9. Hemolytic disease of the newborn due to ABO discrepancy is a milder disorder than Rh (D) incompatibility. The reason is that:
   a. The placenta contains ABO antigen, which absorbs the AB antigen.
   b. The trophoblasts contain a hydrolytic enzyme that destroys the ABO antibody.
   c. The newborn's red cells have not developed ABO antigen.
   d. The newborn's plasma contains a neutralizing factor for ABO.
   e. The ABO antibody cannot cross the placenta/blood barrier.

10. Conversion of group A to group O is dependent on which enzyme?
    a. Galactosidase
    b. N-acetylgalactosidase
    c. Glucosidase
    d. Neuraminidase
    e. Trypsin

11. Which of the following enzyme would convert group B to group O?
    a. Galactosidase
    b. N-acetylgalactosidase
    c. Glucosidase
    d. Neuraminidase
    e. Trypsin

12. Hemolytic transfusion reactions secondary to platelet transfusions are most likely to occur when the donor is:
    a. Type A
    b. Type B
    c. Type O
    d. Type AB

13. A patient with blood type A2, Rh negative needs two units of red cells; O Rh negative inventory is critically low. Select the most appropriate action.
    a. Type all A red cells for A2 phenotype.
    b. Call the blood center to obtain two units of A2 blood.
    c. Titrate the level of anti A in the patient's serum.
    d. Call the patient's physician and explain the possibility of major hemolytic transfusion reaction if patient is receiving A1 red cells.
    e. Crossmatch and release two units of A1 red cells.

Questions 14–20:

A 47-year-old female patient complained of weakness and confusion for four days. Her husband also noticed red spots on her arms. The laboratory data showed: hemoglobin 9 gm/dl, hematocrit 28%, platelets 25×10^9/L, PT 14 seconds (N 12–16), APTT 28 (N 24–36).

14. What other analyte would be expected to be significantly elevated?
    a. Total protein
    b. White cell count
    c. Lactate dehydrogenase (LDH)
    d. Antiplatelet antibodies
    e. Factor VII

15. Additional laboratory data revealed: LD 1400 IU (N 175–225), creatinine 2.7 mg/dl (N 0.8–1.7), BUN 53 mg/dl (N 24–35). The patient's vital signs are also normal. What is your preliminary diagnosis?
    a. Disseminated intravascular coagulopathy (DIC)
    b. Thrombotic thrombocytopenic purpura (TTP)
    c. Valvular obstruction
    d. Idiopathic thrombocytopenic purpura (ITP)
    e. Toxicity with herbal medications

16. The transfusion medicine physician advised her physician to do plasmapheresis. Which of the following statements concerning the use of plasmapheresis is correct?
    a. It removes fragment red cells.
    b. It increases high molecular weight von Willebrand factor.
    c. It removes platelet antibodies.
    d. It removes high molecular weight von Willebrand factor.
    e. Plasmapheresis will stabilize the hypertension.

17. The most appropriate replacement fluid for plasmapheresis in this patient is:
    a. Saline 0.85%
    b. 2% sodium citrate
    c. Lactated Ringer solution
    d. Fresh frozen plasma
    e. 5% human serum albumin

18. During the apheresis procedure, the patient complained of tingling of her lips. What is the possible cause of this symptom?
    a. Fluid overload
    b. Splenic sequestration of platelets
    c. Decreased ionized calcium
    d. Decreased potassium ions
    e. Increased sodium ions

19. How would you treat this symptom?
    a. Terminate the procedure.
    b. Assure patient and do nothing.
    c. Administer KCl.
    d. Administer NaCl.
    e. Administer Ca gluconate.

20. During the plasmapheresis, the patient received 5% albumin. The patient's blood pressure dropped from 130/85

to 70/35, with facial flushing and extreme anxiety. What is the possible cause of this drop in blood pressure?
a. Hypoglycemia
b. Treatment with a beta blocker
c. Hypothyroidism
d. Treatment with an angiotensin-converting enzyme (ACE) inhibitor
e. Internal bleeding

21. During a routine type and screen, a patient typed as A positive. Three screening cell were 3+ positive. The 12-cell panel showed 3+ positivity for all cells tested. The direct antiglobulin test was negative. These findings best describe:
a. Auto antibody
b. Multiple alloantibodies
c. Antibody against high-frequency antigen
d. Antibody against D antigen
e. Nonspecific reaction

22. What is the most common complication of apheresis?
a. Fluid overload
b. Air embolism
c. Citrate toxicity
d. TRALI
e. Elevated blood pressure

23. What is the most common replacement fluid for plasmapheresis performed for thrombotic thrombocytopenic purpura (TTP)?
a. Saline
b. Plasma protein preparation
c. Intravenous immunoglobulin (IVIG)
d. 5% albumin
e. Plasma

24. Red blood cell anticoagulant/preservative solutions contain all of the following EXCEPT:
a. Dextrose
b. Adenine
c. Monobasic sodium phosphate
d. Calcium citrate
e. Mannitol

25. Red blood cell anticoagulant/preservative solution AS (Adsol) permits storage for up to:
a. 21 days
b. 28 days
c. 35 days
d. 42 days
e. 49 days

26. During red cell storage all the following changes occur EXCEPT:
a. Decreased 2,3 diphosphoglycerate
b. Increased plasma hemoglobin
c. Decreased pH
d. Increased ATP
e. Increased serum potassium

27. Which of the following statements correctly describes the hemoglobin-oxygen dissociation curve for red cells refrigeration stored for greater than two weeks?
a. The curve is shifted to the right.
b. The curve is shifted to the left.
c. There is no change in the position of the curve.
d. The shape of the curve is changed from S (sigmoid) shape to Z shape.
e. The shape of the curve is changed from Z shape to S (sigmoid) shape.

28. Cryoprecipitated antihemophilic factor (AHF) is enriched with all of the following coagulant proteins EXCEPT:
a. Fibrinogen
b. Von Willebrand factor
c. Factor VIII
d. Factor VII
e. Factor XIII

29. When recombinant factor VIII is NOT available, what is an alternative blood product to treat a patient with factor VIII deficiency with a small joint hematoma?
a. Fresh whole blood
b. Plasma-derived von Willebrand factor
c. Cryo-depleted plasma
d. Cryoprecipitate
e. Fresh plasma

30. Thawed pooled cryoprecipitated AHF can be stored at room temperature for a maximum of:
a. 2 hours
b. 4 hours
c. 8 hours
d. 12 hours
e. 24 hours

31. All of the following statements about granulocyte product collected by apheresis are true EXCEPT:
a. It should be irradiated.
b. It may be stored for up to 72 hours.
c. It should be kept at room temperature.
d. It should be stored with gentle agitation.
e. It should be crossmatched with the recipient serum.

32. The antibody implicated in hemolytic disease of the newborn that is most likely to suppress fetal erythropoiesis is:
a. Anti-Fya antibodies
b. Anti-Jkb antibodies
c. Anti-D antibodies
d. Anti-Rh 17 antibodies
e. Anti-K_0 antibodies

33. Which of the following red cell antigens serves as a receptor for plasmodium vivax?
   a. Jka and Jkb
   b. Lewis A and Lewis B
   c. P antigen
   d. Fya and Fyb
   e. Glycophorin A and B

34. All of the following are true for the anti-JKa and anti-JKb antibodies EXCEPT:
   a. They may be missed if present in low titer.
   b. They have high affinity and high avidity.
   c. They require the presence of complement to detect.
   d. They may cause delayed hemolytic transfusion reaction.
   e. They are low frequency antigens and rarely cause hemolysis.

35. All of the following are true for Lewis A and B antigen EXCEPT:
   a. Lewis antigens are glycolipid antigens.
   b. Lewis antibodies are IgM isotype.
   c. Lewis antibodies do not cause hemolytic transfusion reactions.
   d. Lewis antigens are located at glycophorin A and B molecules.
   e. Lewis antigens are well developed in neonates.

36. What are the two most reliable laboratory findings to diagnose thrombotic thrombocytopenic purpura (TTP)?
   a. Low neutrophil count - positive neutrophil antibody assay
   b. Low platelet count - positive anti-platelet antibody assay
   c. Anemia - positive direct antiglobulin test
   d. Low platelet count - low ADAMTS13
   e. Low factor VIII activity–prolonged aPTT

37. The pathophysiology of thrombotic thrombocytopenic purpura is best described as resulting from:
   a. Binding of red blood cells to endothelium
   b. Activation of complement system
   c. Activation of extrinsic coagulation pathway
   d. Formation of red cell thrombus
   e. Binding of platelets to HMW von Willebrand factor

38. Which apheresis fluid is LEAST likely to improve the clinical course of TTP?
   a. Only male plasma
   b. 50/50 plasma and 5% human serum albumin
   c. Cryo-poor plasma
   d. 5% human serum albumin
   e. Fresh frozen plasma

39. Transfusion-associated graft-versus-host disease (TAGVHD) has a worse outcome than bone marrow transplant-associated graft host disease (BMTAGVHD) because:
   a. The cell type responsible for TAGVHD is T lymphocyte while in BMTAGVHD is B lymphocytes.
   b. The bone marrow hematopoietic trilineage is the main target in TAGVHD.
   c. The activation of dendritic cells is augmented in TAGVHD.
   d. Bone marrow transplant protects against GVHD.
   e. Bone marrow transplant patients receive intensive immunosuppression.

40. Transfusion-associated graft versus host disease may occur in all of the following disorders EXCEPT?
   a. Hodgkin lymphoma
   b. Wiskott Aldrich syndrome
   c. IgA deficiency
   d. Patients treated with purine nucleoside analogs such as fludarabine and 2-cholrodeoxyadenosine (cladribine)
   e. Intrauterine red cell exchange

41. The most appropriate measure to prevent transfusion-associated graft-versus-host disease from platelet is:
   a. Wash using automated equipment.
   b. Filter using a leukoreduction filter.
   c. Irradiate using 25G.
   d. Use male only platelets.
   e. Use directed donor platelets.

42. The correct cell type responsible for transfusion-associated graft versus host disease in the animal model based on a number per kilogram is:
   a. Lymphocytes
   b. Nucleated RBCs
   c. CD34 cells
   d. Monocytes
   e. Platelets

43. The correct agent or mechanism responsible for transfusion-related acute lung injury (TRALI) includes the following EXCEPT:
   a. Presence of donor anti HLA class I antibodies in the recipient
   b. Presence of donor antigranulocytes antibodies in the recipient
   c. Presence of recipient antilymphocyte antibodies in the donor
   d. Presence of donor anti-HLA Class I and antigranulocyte antibody in the recipient
   e. Presence of recipient anti-HLA class II antibodies in donor.

44. Platelets have all of the following antigens EXCEPT:
   a. HLA class II antigens
   b. HLA class I antigens
   c. ABO antigens

d. GPIIIb/IIa
e. HPA-1

45. What is the best management strategy for a patient diagnosed with immune thrombocytopenic purpura (ITP) without mucosal bleeding?
   a. Monoclonal antibody treatment
   b. Transfusion of leuko-reduced platelets
   c. Transfusion of irradiated platelets
   d. Immunosuppressive medications
   e. Plasmapheresis

46. What is the most common antibody found in a neonate born with thrombocytopenia?
   a. Anti-HPA-1
   b. Anti-HPA-2
   c. Anti-HPA-3
   d. Anti-HLA class I
   e. Anti-HLA class II

47. Each of the following may be used in the treatment of ITP in a D negative (Rh negative) patient EXCEPT:
   a. Corticosteroids
   b. IVIG
   c. Anti-D antibody
   d. Splenectomy
   e. DDAVP

48. The indications for platelet transfusions include each of the following EXCEPT:
   a. A nonbleeding patient with platelets less than 10,000/μl
   b. A nonbleeding, nonsurgical patient with platelet counts between 10,000 and 50,000/μl
   c. A bleeding patient with platelets less than 50,000/μl
   d. A bleeding patient with acute renal failure and platelets more than 50,000/μl
   e. A bleeding patient with Glanzmann thrombathenia with platelets of 200,000/μl

49. The following criteria define a suitable blood donor EXCEPT:
   a. Hemoglobin minimum of 12.5 g/dl
   b. Age more than 70 years
   c. History of jaundice before age of 11
   d. Age of less than 18 years with parent consent
   e. Received a tattoo one month prior

50. Which one of the following is an indication for blood donation deferral?
   a. Return from traveling to a malaria endemic area less than a year ago
   b. Tattoo performed less than three weeks ago
   c. Receiving recombinant growth factor
   d. Receiving rabies vaccine within the last two weeks
   e. Receiving the flu vaccine two days ago

51. A transfusion-dependent patient received two units of packed red cells. Approximately 8 days posttransfusion, the patient developed severe thrombocytopenia. The probable cause of the thrombocytopenia is:
   a. Idiopathic thrombocytopenia purpura
   b. Thrombotic thrombocytopenia purpura
   c. Acute renal failure
   d. Splenomegaly
   e. Posttransfusion purpura

52. Routine infectious disease testing for blood donors includes the following EXCEPT:
   a. HIV by NAT testing
   b. HCV by NAT testing
   c. Cytomegalovirus by PCR
   d. West Nile Virus by PCR
   e. HTLV I/II by enzyme immune assay

53. A single unit of thawed cryoprecipitated AHF if not transfused immediately should be stored under what conditions?
   a. Eight hours at -20°C
   b. One hour at 4°C
   c. Six hours at 20–24°C
   d. Refreeze the unit
   e. Eight hours at 20–24°C

54. Pooled units of thawed pooled cryoprecipitated antihemophilic factor (AHF) stored at 20–24°C should be transfused within:
   a. 24 hours
   b. 6 hours
   c. 4 hours
   d. 3 days
   e. 5 days

55. Which of the following lectins are used to differentiate between A1 and A2 red cells?
   a. Arachis hypogaea
   b. Glycine max (soja)
   c. Dolichos biflorus
   d. Ulex europaeus
   e. Saliva horminium

56. Plant-derived lectins are chemically composed of:
   a. Complex carbohydrates
   b. Proteins
   c. Glycoproteins
   d. Lipoproteins
   e. Small peptides

57. A 62-year-old woman who received multiple blood transfusions due to chemotherapy-associated anemia, presents with petechia and bleeding eight days post red cell transfusion. The CBC shows hemoglobin of 9.5 gm/dl, hematocrit of 38%, white count of 8.5×10^9/l with 70 % segmented neutrophils, 24% lymphocytes,

5% monocytes and 1% eosinophils, and platelet count of $8.500 \times 10^9/l$. What is the diagnosis?
a. Immune thrombocytopenia purpura
b. Chemotherapy associated thrombocytopenia purpura
c. Viral associated thrombocytopenia purpura
d. Posttransfusion purpura
e. Malignancy associated thrombocytopenia purpura

58. A newborn presents with petechia on the trunk. The baby is diagnosed with neonatal associated thrombocytopenia purpura. The mother is found to have antibodies against rare platelet antigens. The maternal aunt's platelets are transfused to the newborn. Ten days later the baby presents with fever, hepatitis, diarrhea, and dermatitis. The cause of these symptoms is:
a. Posttransfusion hepatitis C disease
b. Budd-Chiari syndrome
c. Hemolytic disease of newborn (HDN)
d. Transfusion-associated graft host disease
e. Bacterial infection due to bacterial contamination of platelets

59. Anaphylactic reactions associated with blood transfusions may occur in patients who are IgA deficient. Which of the following statements about IgA deficiency in populations of European descent is correct?
a. IgA deficiency is very rare in this populations.
b. IgA deficiency is the most common congenital immunodeficiency.
c. It affects 1 in 7000–8000 persons.
d. It affects 1 in 70,000–80,000 persons.
e. It affects 1 in 100,000–200,000 persons.

60. A 57-year-old white man with history of myelodysplastic syndrome and multiple red cell transfusion was found to have anti-Jka, E, and S antibodies. What is the probability of finding compatible red cell units? (Incidence of positive red cells for Jka 77%, E 29%, and S 55% in white population.)
a. 12%
b. 9%
c. 50%
d. 7%
e. 29%

61. The *Standards for Blood Banks and Transfusion Services* are issued by:
a. FDA
b. AABB
c. American Red Cross
d. America's Blood Centers
e. FDA, AABB, America's Blood Centers

62. Which of the following statements about the computer crossmatch is true?
a. Serologic crossmatch must be recorded in computer permanent file.

b. All Blood Bank services must use FDA approved software.
c. Patient who has two ABO and Rh typing with negative antibody screen and no transfusion or pregnancy during last 90 days may transfuse blood with no serologic crossmatch.
d. Patient computer data must be accessed by the Blood Bank personnel only.
e. FDA may have an access to the patient's crossmatch in case of acute hemolytic transfusion reaction.

63. The *Standards for Blood Banks and Transfusion Services* require that a patients' sample must be labeled with which of the following?
a. Patient name and date of admission
b. Two independent unique identifications of the patient and the identification of the phlebotomist
c. Two independent identifications of the patient include patient name, time of the sample drawing, and the phlebotomist ID
d. Patient name, location, bed number, and ID of the phlebotomist
e. Patient name and home address

64. Information on severe adverse reactions to transfusion in adults should be retained for a minimum of:
a. 60 years
b. 10 years
c. 5 years
d. 2 years
e. 1 year

65. Records of patient with clinically significant antibodies must be retained for a minimum of:
a. Indefinite
b. 10 years
c. 5 years
d. 2 years
e. 1 year

66. The FDA drafts guidance for industry to provide Look Back policies for donors at risk for transmission of what disease?
a. Malaria
b. Parvovirus infection
c. Creutzfeldt-Jakob disease
d. HCV infection
e. Hepatitis B infection

67. Red blood cell products used for intrauterine exchange transfusions have all the following characteristics EXCEPT:
a. Leukocyte-reduced
b. Irradiated
c. Rh negative
d. CMV safe
e. Washed

68. Justifications for transfusion of red blood cells are derived from:
    a. AABB Standards
    b. FDA CFR
    c. The hospital code of conduct
    d. CAP survey documents
    e. The clinical condition of the patient based on medical record review

69. Plasma transfusion is indicated for each of the following conditions EXCEPT:
    a. Deficiency of vitamin K depending coagulation factors
    b. Liver disease with elevated coagulation screening tests
    c. Warfarin reversal
    d. Plasma albumin low
    e. Fluid replacement for thrombotic thrombocytopenic purpura during apheresis

70. The quality of platelet concentrates derived from whole blood follow which FDA-mandated criterion?
    a. Platelet counts $>5.5 \times 10^{10}$ in 95% of the tested units
    b. Platelet counts $>5.5 \times 10^{10}$ in 100% of the tested units
    c. Platelet counts $>5.5 \times 10^6$ in 75% of the tested units
    d. Platelets count $>5.5 \times 10^6$ in 100% of the tested units

71. The quality of platelets collected by apheresis and labeled as leukocytes-reduced follow which FDA-mandated criterion?
    a. Less than 5×10^6 leukocytes
    b. Less than 5×10^7 leukocytes
    c. Less than 5×10^9 leukocytes
    d. Less than 5×10^2 leukocytes

72. In Fisher and Race CDE terminology, if a patient phenotype is D negative, C negative, and E negative, the haplotype is:
    a. $R^1 r'$
    b. $R^2 r''$
    c. $R^0 r$
    d. $r' r$
    e. rr

73. Rh genes encode nonglycosylated polypeptides on what chromosome?
    a. Chromosome 6 large arm
    b. Chromosome 1 short arm
    c. Chromosome 9 short arm
    d. Chromosome 4 long arm
    e. Chromosome X

74. In Fisher and Race CDE terminology, if a patient's phenotype is D positive, C negative, and e negative the type is:
    a. $R^1 r$
    b. $R^0 r$
    c. Rr
    d. $R^2 R^1$
    e. $R^2 R^2$

75. The genes encoding the glycosyltransferases that produce A and B red cell antigens are located on which chromosome?
    a. Chromosome 6
    b. Chromosome 1
    c. Chromosome 9
    d. Chromosome 4
    e. Chromosome 2

76. The Rh system is complex blood group phenotype controlled by:
    a. One gene
    b. Two genes
    c. Three genes
    d. Four genes
    e. Five genes

77. Antigens of the MNS system are carried on:
    a. Glycophorins A and B
    b. Glycophorin A
    c. Glycophorin B
    d. Rh system
    e. Kell system

78. A person who lacks Ss antigens may lack the U antigen and may develop anti-U following a red blood cell transfusion. The person is a member of which ethnicity?
    a. White
    b. Hispanic
    c. Black
    d. Asian
    e. Arabic

79. The McLeod phenotype lacks which of the following red cell antigen system?
    a. Kidd system
    b. Duffy system
    c. MNS system
    d. Kell system
    e. Rh system

80. In Fisher and Race CDE terminology, if patient phenotype is D positive, c negative and E negative, the haplotype is:
    a. $R^1 r'$
    b. $R^2 r$
    c. $R^z r$
    d. $R^2 R^1$
    e. $R^1 R^1$

81. A white female, blood type A, Rh positive, received two units of compatible red cells postpartum. During

her second pregnancy, the prenatal screening tests for red cell antibodies are positive with all of the screening cells and panels. Her direct antiglobulin test is negative. Her red cell Rh phenotype is D positive and negative for the other Rh antigens. What is her red cell Rh phenotype?

a. R^1r
b. R^zR^y
c. D- -
d. Rr
e. R^1R^2

82. Newborn red blood cells differ from those in the adult. Which antigens are present on newborn red blood cells?

a. Le^a Le^b
b. Le^a only
c. Le^b only
d. Le^a, Le^b, and I
e. None of the above

83. A patient with sickle cell disease is found to have an anti-G antibody. What other antibody might this patient have?

a. Anti-M and N
b. Anti-S and S
c. Anti-Jka and Jkb
d. Anti-D and C
e. Anti-c and e

84. The majority of transfusion associated acute lung injury (TRALI) cases are caused by:

a. Clerical or managerial error
b. Platelets specific antibody HPA-1
c. Undetected anti red cell antigen in donor plasma
d. Anti HLA/granulocytes antibody in donor plasma
e. Fluid overload

85. What is the fluid permitted by FDA and AABB to be administered simultaneously with blood or blood components within the same IV line?

a. Lactated Ringer solution
b. 0.45% sodium chloride
c. 0.9% sodium chloride
d. Any medication
e. IVIG

86. A woman who is Rh (D) negative delivered a Rh (D) positive newborn. A Kleihauer-Betke acid elution test is performed and shows that 1.2% of red cells are positive. How many 300-μg doses of Rh immunoglobulin are recommended for administration?

a. 1 dose
b. 2 doses
c. 3 doses
d. 4 doses
e. 5 doses

87. What is the expected hematocrit when a 70 kg non-bleeding patient with a hematocrit of 25% receives two units of packed red cells?

a. 28%
b. 31%
c. 34%
d. 36%
e. 38%

88. Which of the following would result in the permanent deferral of a prospective blood donor?

a. Visited a malaria area
b. Received a tattoo
c. Intranasal use of cocaine
d. Positive test for syphilis but received treatment
e. Intake of etretinate (Tegison) for psoriasis

89. Transfusion-associated graft versus host disease has been identified in each of the following recipients after receiving nonirradiated cellular blood transfusion EXCEPT:

a. Hodgkin lymphoma
b. DiGeorge syndrome
c. Directed blood donation from blood relative
d. Neuroblastoma
e. AIDS secondary to HIV

90. All of the following statements regarding paroxysmal cold hemoglobinuria (PCH) are correct EXCEPT:

a. It is acute transient condition secondary to viral infections.
b. Occurs in children.
c. The antibody in PCH is IgM.
d. PCH diseases are most frequently positive for anti-P.
e. The antibody is a biphasic hemolysin.

91. Which of the following is true about the Lewis system?

a. Lewis system is intrinsic to red cells.
b. Lewis antigens are sensitive to trypsin.
c. Lewis B antigens is a product of two gene actions.
d. Anti-Lewis A and B are produced in Le (a-b-) recipients post transfusion.
e. Anti-Lewis causes neonatal hemolytic transfusion reaction.

92. What is the percentage of African American patients who may develop anti-U alloantibody after a transfusion?

a. 5%
b. 8%
c. 4%
d. 0%
e. 1%

93. An international sales person who has spent a month in London every year since 1985 is a regular United

Kingdom blood donor. He volunteers to donate blood in the United States. Which of the following statements is correct?

a. Since he donated in UK, he can donate in Manhattan.

b. The donor has to wait eight weeks after his London donation before donating in the United States.

c. The donor can donate only platelets in the United States.

d. The donor will be permanently deferred from blood donation in the United States.

e. The donor will be permanently deferred from blood donation in both the United States and the United Kingdom.

94. A patient with relapsed acute lymphoblastic leukemia (ALL) has been found to be platelet-refractory following multiple platelet transfusions. Which of the following is the proper technique to obtain proper platelet unit?

a. Perform platelet antigen phenotype

b. Perform platelet crossmatch

c. Perform autoimmune assay panel, including ANA, anti-DNA

d. Request HPA1 negative platelets

e. Request ABO matched platelets

95. Platelet refractoriness is best defined by performing which of the following?

a. Corrected Count Increment (CCI)

b. Post Platelet Recovery (PPR)

c. Platelet Surface Denisty (PSD)

d. Corrected Platelet Increment (CPI)

e. Percent Reactive Antibody (PRA)

96. Which product is LEAST likely to require crossmatch?

a. Red blood cells

b. Fresh frozen plasma

c. Granulocyte concentrate

d. A pheresis platelet

e. Platelet concentrate pool

97. Which of the following is LEAST likely to result in platelet refractoriness?

a. Fever

b. Splenomegaly

c. Amphotericin use

d. Cephalosporin use

e. Cyclosporin use

98. Provision of CMV "safe" products for indicated patients can be accomplished by:

a. First generation leukodepletion filter

b. 120 micron filter

c. Third generation leukodepletion filter

d. Irradiation at 2500 cgy

e. Irradiation at 5000 cgy

99. A patient with sickle cell disease is found to have a U antibody against high frequency antigen U. Which blood donor ethnicity will have U negative blood?

a. Blacks

b. Whites

c. Asians

d. American Indians

e. Arabs

100. Which of the antibodies identified on this panel (Table 15.1) could be a potential cause for hemolytic disease of the newborn?

a. Anti-Lewis^a

b. Anti-D

c. Anti-Kell

d. Anti-E

e. Anti-N

TABLE 15.1

Vial	D	C	E	c	e	Cw	f	K	k	Kpa	Jsa	Fya	Fyb	Jka	Jkb	Lea	Leb	p1	M	N	S	s	Xga		AHG
			Rh						**Kell**			**Duffy**		**Kidd**		**Lewis**		**P**		**MNSs**			**Xg**		
1	+	+	0	0	+	0	0	0	+	0	0	+	+	+	+	0	+	+	+	0	0	+	+	1	3+
2	+	+	0	0	+	+	0	0	+	0	0	0	0	+	0	0	0	+	+	+	+	0	+	2	3+
3	+	0	+	+	0	0	0	0	+	0	0	0	+	+	+	+	0	0	0	+	0	+	+	3	3+
4	0	+	0	+	+	0	+	0	+	0	0	+	0	+	0	0	+	+	+	0	+	+	+	4	0
5	0	0	+	+	+	0	+	0	+	0	0	0	+	0	+	0	+	+	0	+	0	+	+	5	0
6	0	0	0	+	+	0	+	+	+	0	0	+	0	0	+	0	+	+	0	+	0	+	+	6	0
7	0	0	0	+	+	0	+	0	+	0	0	0	+	+	0	0	+	+	+	+	+	0	0	7	0
8	+	0	0	+	+	0	+	0	+	0	0	0	0	0	+	0	0	+	0	+	0	0	+	8	3+
9	0	0	0	+	+	0	+	+	+	0	0	+	0	+	+	+	0	0	+	+	+	+	0	9	0
10	0	0	0	+	+	0	+	+	+	0	0	0	+	+	+	0	0	+	0	+	0	+	+	10	0
11	+	+	0	0	+	0	0	0	+	0	0	0	+	0	+	0	+	+	+	+	+	0	0	11	3+

TABLE 15.2

Vial	D	C	E	c	e	Cw	f	K	k	Kpa	Jsa	Fya	Fyb	Jka	Jkb	Lea	Leb	p1	M	N	S	s	Xga		AHG	Ficin
1	+	+	0	0	+	0	0	0	+	0	0	+	+	+	+	0	+	+	+	+	0	0	+	1	1+	0
2	+	+	0	0	+	+	0	0	+	0	0	0	0	+	0	0	0	+	+	+	+	+	0	2	0	0
3	+	0	+	+	0	0	0	0	+	0	0	0	+	+	+	+	0	0	0	+	0	+	+	3	2+	3+
4	0	+	0	+	+	0	+	0	+	0	0	+	0	+	0	0	+	+	+	0	+	+	+	4	2+	0
5	0	0	+	+	+	0	+	0	+	0	0	0	+	0	+	0	+	+	0	+	0	+	+	5	2+	2+
6	0	0	0	+	+	0	+	+	+	0	0	+	0	0	+	0	+	+	+	0	+	+	+	6	3+	0
7	0	0	0	+	+	0	+	0	+	0	0	0	+	+	0	0	+	+	+	+	+	0	0	7	0	0
8	+	0	0	+	+	0	+	0	+	0	0	0	0	0	+	0	0	+	0	+	0	0	+	8	0	0
9	0	0	0	+	+	0	+	+	0	0	0	+	0	+	+	+	0	0	+	+	+	+	0	9	3+	0
10	0	0	0	+	+	0	+	+	+	0	0	0	+	+	+	0	0	+	+	0	+	0	+	10	0	0
11	+	+	0	0	+	0	0	0	+	0	0	0	+	0	+	0	+	+	+	+	0	+	0	11	0	0

101. Which red cell antibody is destroyed after treatment with ficin (Table 15.2)?
a. Anti-Fy^a
b. Anti-JK^b
c. Anti-c
d. Anti-N
e. Anti-E

102. Prenatal testing on a woman at 20 weeks of gestation shows she is type group O, Rh positive, and her antibody screen is positive. What is the best interpretation of the antibody patient's panel (Table 15.3)?
a. Anti-D, anti-Kell, anti-Le^a
b. Anti-K, anti-Le^a, anti-s
c. Anti-K, anti-Le^a, anti-E
d. Anti-E, anti-K, and anti-Le^a
e. Anti-N, anti-K, and anti-Le^a

TABLE 15.3

Vial	D	C	E	c	e	Cw	f	K	k	Kpa	Jsa	Fya	Fyb	Jka	Jkb	Lea	Leb	p1	M	N	S	s	Xga		AHG
1	+	+	0	0	+	0	0	0	+	0	0	+	+	+	+	0	+	+	+	+	0	0	+	1	3+
2	+	+	0	0	+	+	0	0	+	0	0	0	0	+	0	0	0	+	+	+	+	+	0	2	3+
3	+	0	+	+	0	0	0	0	+	0	0	0	+	+	+	+	0	0	0	+	0	+	+	3	3+
4	0	+	0	+	+	0	+	0	+	0	0	+	0	+	0	0	+	+	+	0	+	+	+	4	0
5	0	0	+	+	+	0	+	0	+	0	0	0	+	0	+	0	+	+	0	+	0	+	+	5	0
6	0	0	0	+	+	0	+	+	+	0	0	+	0	0	+	0	+	+	+	0	+	+	+	6	4+
7	0	0	0	+	+	0	+	0	+	0	0	0	+	+	0	0	+	+	+	+	+	0	0	7	0
8	+	0	0	+	+	0	+	0	+	0	0	0	0	0	+	0	0	+	0	+	0	0	+	8	3+
9	0	0	0	+	+	0	+	+	0	0	0	+	0	+	+	+	0	0	+	+	+	+	0	9	4+
10	0	0	0	+	+	0	+	+	+	0	0	0	+	+	+	0	0	+	+	0	+	0	+	10	4+
11	+	+	0	0	+	0	0	0	+	0	0	0	+	0	+	0	+	+	+	+	0	+	0	11	3+

■ Answers

1. **d.** Blood products are irradiated to disable the T cell lymphocytes, which are the major cells causing transfusion-associated graft versus host disease (TAGVHD). Patients who require irradiated blood include low birth weight newborns, infants requiring *in utero* red cell exchange, congenital immunodeficiency, patients receiving granulocytes transfusions, patients with Hodgkin lymphoma, and patients who are receiving intensive immunosuppressive chemotherapy. There are no reports of TAGVHD in **HIV-infected** patients.

2. **e.** All blood products which contain viable lymphocytes need to be irradiated. There are no viable lymphocytes in **fresh frozen plasma** (FFP). Lymphocytes become nonfunctional when frozen and thawed. However, fresh plasma contains viable cells.

3. **d.** The FDA requires irradiation exposure to be a **minimum of 15 G** at the periphery of the irradiated field and 25 G at the center.

4. **e.** Most of irradiators have a Cesium or Cobalt as a source for irradiation. The intensity and dose of irradiation depends on the **half life of the source** and not on the time of exposure. Recently intensive X-ray has been used for the source to irradiate the lymphocytes.

5. **d.** The irradiation source (cesium) is **shielded** with lead; any person including pregnant women may use the irradiator.

6. **e.** AABB and FDA are the usual inspection agencies for Blood Banks. Recently Congress passed a bill allowing the NRC the right to inspect the security for any institute use radioactive sources.

7. **b.** The ABO antigens are carbohydrate antigen which can be attached to proteins, sphingolipid, or lipid carrier molecules. The basic structure of ABH antigen is a linear oligosaccharide chain composed of three monosaccharides, adding fucose will form H (O) antigens, further adding N-acetylgalactosamine or galactose to form group A or B antigen. So, **group A has N-acetylgalactosamine** and group B has galactose moiety.

8. **b.** The ABO blood groups are carbohydrate antigens while **IgM** is the immunoglobin isotype produced as anti-ABO antibody.

9. **e.** ABO antibodies are mostly **IgM** which do not cross the blood/placenta barrier.

10. **b.** **N-acetylgalactosidase** can split or remove N-acetylgalactosamine from group A antigen and convert A to O antigen. This technique was used to artificially produce O blood type which is then transfused to patients with no side effects. However, preparing this product is not cost-effective for wide use.

11. **c.** **Galactosidase** can break down or remove the galactose from B antigen and convert B to O.

12. **c.** **Type O plasma** contains anti-A and anti-B antibodies. O plasma with high titer of anti-A and anti-B antibodies can cause hemolytic transfusion reaction (HTR).

13. **e.** Patients with type A2 may have low level of clinically insignificant anti-A antibody. A2 type patient may receive either A1 or O red cells.

14. **c.** This is a case of micro angiopathy hemolytic anemia (**thrombotic thrombocytopenic purpura** [TTP]) which causes destruction of red cells. Lactate dehydrogenase (LD) is usually elevated in any destruction process in the body.

15. **b.** There are many causes that could cause thrombocytopenia accompanied with low hemoglobin and normal coagulation. Although TTP is the key disorder in the differential diagnosis, malignant hypertension must also be included. With normal blood pressure and normal coagulation, TTP is the most logical diagnosis.

16. **d.** In TTP, the main pathology is the presence of high molecular weight (MW) von Willebrand factor (vWF) with formation of microthrombi. The apheresis will remove the high MW vWF and in more than 50% of patients will remove the ADAMTS13 inhibitors (autoantibodies).

17. **d.** **Plasma** is the preferred replacement fluid in TTP with dual functions; pheresis removes high MW vWF, removes ADAMTS13 inhibitor, and increases ADAMTS13 level.

18. **c.** These symptoms are due to **citrate toxicity** secondary to decrease in ionized calcium.

19. **e.** **Calcium gluconate** may be given; the best route is intravenously. Oral calcium salt is acceptable but not effective in many patients.

20. **d.** Angiotensin-converting enzyme inhibitor may interact with the polymers of the plastic bags and activate the kallikrein system and produce severe hypotension.

21. **c.** Antibody against a high frequency antigen may produce positive reactions in all tested red cells; however, the DAT test is always negative in these cases.

22. **c.** **Citrate toxicity** is the most common side effect of plasmapheresis due to low plasma ionized calcium.

23. **d.** Plasma is the most common replacement fluid for TTP. FFP, 24-plasma, and thawed plasma can all be used. Plasma will remove high MW von Willebrand factor and ADAMTS13 inhibitor, and will increase the ADAMSTS13 level.

24. **d.** **Calcium citrate** is not part of the additive in red cell preservative solutions. Sodium citrate is added as anticoagulant, phosphate salts function as buffer, dextrose, and mannitol as source of carbohydrate for energy production, and adenine as source for ATP.

25. **d.** The shelf life is 42 days for all new red cell preservative solutions including AS-1, AS-3.

26. **d.** During red cell storage, both ATP and 2,3 diphosoglycerate are decreased by red cells metabolism, pH is decreased due to H ion production, and plasma hemo-

globin and potassium ions are elevated due to red cell hemolysis.

27. **b.** During red cells storage the red cells and the 2,3-diphosoglycerate concentration are reduced. The very low 2,3 DPG will shift the Hb-O association curve to the left.

28. **d.** Cryoprecipitated antihemophilic factor (AHF) is enriched with fibrogen, von Willebrand factor, factor VIII and factor XIII. Factor VII is present in low concentration in cryoprecipitate AHF.

29. **d. Cryoprecipitate AHF** is rich in fibrinogen, von Willebrand factor, factor VIII, and factor XIII.

30. **b.** Thawed Cryoprecipitate AHF will expire in 4 hours in an open system or pooled; 6 hours if thawed and not pooled.

31. **b.** Apheresis granulocyte function is time-dependent. Phagocytic functions deteriorate with time and a unit becomes unuseful after 24 hours and may be discarded.

32. **e. Anti-Ko antibodies** are known to suppress fetal bone marrow, causing intrauterine and postpartum severe anemic.

33. **d.** Duffy antigens are receptors for plasmodium vivax. In Africa, most of population are Duffy negative due elimination of infected Duffy positive population.

34. **e.** Anti-Kidd antibodies are high-affinity and high-avidity antibodies. Roughly, 72% of whites are Jk(a+,b+) and their antibodies can cause moderate to severe hemolytic transfusion reaction.

35. **e.** The **Lewis antigens** are not developed in newborn and are not intrinsic to red cells but rather adsorbed from the plasma onto the red cell membranes and become expressed on glycosphingolipid type I chain. Lewis antibodies do not usually cause hemolysis.

36. **d.** Low platelets and low ADAMT13 are the most reliable findings in **TTP**. In addition, elevated LDH, low hematocrit, and presence of ADAMTS13 inhibitors are present in most cases of TTP.

37. **e.** The binding of high molecular weight von Willebrand factor to the platelet and forming platelet thrombus is the main pathology in TTP.

38. **d.** All plasma preparation may be used for apheresis of TTP including only male plasma which is collected only from male donors to prevent TRALI. Plasma will increase the level of ADAMTS13. Several studies showed that human serum albumin is not suitable replacement fluid for TTP treatment.

39. **b.** The exact cause for the severity of TAGVHD is not known. However, several publications supported the notion that the bone marrow hemopoietic trilineage cells may be the target for TAGVHD.

40. **c.** TAGVHD may develop in patients with cellular immunodeficiency (especially deficiency of T cells) and those receiving high doses of potent immunosuppressors. Patients with IgA deficiency have an intact immune system with deficiency of IgA production and will not develop transfusion-associated graft versus host disease. These patients do not require irradiated blood products.

41. **c.** The leukoreduction filter is not sufficient to remove all of the lymphocytes which can cause TAGFHD. Leukocyte-reduced blood products have efficient lymphocytes to cause TAGVHD. All other choices may also lead to TAGVHD except irradiation, which prevents proliferation of the donor lymphocytes.

42. **a.** Donor T lymphocyte population is the cellular component responsible for TAGVHD. Lymphocyte number is implicated.

43. **c.** Transfusion-related acute lung injury (TRALI) may be caused by agglutinating patient granulocytes with donor anti-HLA or white cell antibodies in the small pulmonary arterioles and capillaries. All the mentioned agents could cause the TRALI except donor lymphocyte antibodies. No study has shown that anti-lymphocyte antibodies are responsible for TRALI.

44. **a.** Platelets carry ABO group and HLA class I antigens but not HLA class II antigens. HLA class II antigens are expressed on antigen presenting cells including B lymphocytes, monocytes/macrophages, dendritic cells, and activated T lymphocytes.

45. **d.** ITP is treated with intravenous immunoglobulin (IVIG), immunosuppressors, or splenectomy. In 2008, the FDA approved recombinant platelets growth factor for treatment of ITP.

46. **a. Anti-HPA-1a** is the most common antiplatelet antibodies in ITP.

47. **d.** Anti D antibody may be used to treat D positive patients and not D negative patients. Anti-D will bind to Rh D positive red cells; the coated cells will attract phagocytic cells and prevent the attack on platelets coated with antibody.

48. **b.** All of these conditions are indications for transfusion except non-bleeding patients with platelet count 20,000/μl or more. Several studies showed that 10,000/μl platelets have a reasonable haemostatic efficacy in non-bleeding patients.

49. **e.** All mentioned criteria are accepted for blood duties except tattoo done 1 month ago. For donor with recent **tattoo**, 12 months or more must relapsed before accepting the donor. There is no age limit for blood donation.

50. **c.** All the mentioned criteria cause donor deferral except receiving recombinant growth factor. Donors who in the past received animal source growth factor are permanently deferred.

51. **e. Post transfusion purpura** is a rare thrombocytopenia secondary to blood transfusion occurring 1 week to 9 days after red cell transfusion. It is characterized by abrupt onset of severe thrombocytopenia. Most patients have been previously transfused or pregnant. Fatal intracranial hemorrhage may occur. The mechanism of patient's platelets destruction by what appears to be platelets alloantibody is controversial. Treatment with IVIG or plasmapheresis is often helpful.

52. c. Screening for Cytomegalovirus by PCR is not a routine test for donor screening. It is not done routinely but upon request for patients whose immune system is suppressed such as in congenital immune deficiency, intrauterine blood exchange, or in those receiving high-dose immunosuppression.

53. c. Single unit of cryoprecipitated AHF may be, if not transfused immediately, stored for **6 hours at 20–24°C**.

54. c. Pooled cryoprecipitated AHF **expires within 4 hours** if kept at room temperature or 6 hours for a single unit.

55. c. **Dolichos biflorus** is a lectin which agglutinates A1 but not A2 red cells and may be used to differentiate between them.

56. c. **Lectins** are glycoproteins that may be bound to specific monosaccharides; either free monosaccharides or as part of glycoproteins.

57. d. **Posttransfusion purpura** is a rare post–red cell transfusion complication. It is characterized by severe thrombocytopenia occurring within an average 9 days (range of 1–24 days) after red cell transfusion. Most affected patients have been pregnant or transfused.

58. d. Transfusion-associated graft versus host disease may occur when nonirradiated blood is transfused from one relative to a related recipient due to similarities in the HLA of the donor and recipient. In homogenous populations such as the Japanese or Israelis, sharing of HLA is reported.

59. b. **IgA deficiency** is the most common congenital immunodeficiency affecting 1 in 700–800 persons of European descent. The production of IgE and anti-IgA may occur in these patients when receiving transfusion. Anaphylactic reaction may occur if these patients receive blood containing IgA. The cellular blood products must be washed to remove the plasma IgA or obtained from IgA-deficient donor.

60. d. Only 7% compatible units will be negative for Jka, E, and S (0.23 × 0.71 × 0.45).

61. b. The **AABB** publishes the *Standards for Blood Banks and Transfusion Services.*

62. c. Computer crossmatch does not require serologic crossmatch; the patient must have two ABO and Rh types performed in advance with negative antibody screen and no transfusion or pregnancy during the last 90 days.

63. b. Two independent unique identifiers and a method to identify the phlebotomist are required by AABB standard. These two unique identifiers may include patient's name, medical record, or social security number. Addresses and patient hospital room numbers are not unique identifiers.

64. c. Severe adverse reaction for patient or donor may be retained for **5 years** or more. In cases of infants and children, some hospitals require longer retention period.

65. a. Patient records with clinically significant antibody must be retained **indefinitely**.

66. d. Donors with increased risk of transmitting Hepatitis C virus (HCV) or HIV infection are included in Look Back policies. However, recent concern over vCJD and TRALI may result in change in those policies.

67. e. With the advancement of leukocyte-reduced filters and other methods of removing most of the white cells, **washed red cells** are not required for intrauterine exchange transfusion.

68. e. The combination of clinical evidence and hemoglobin concentration is the best tool to judge the need for red cell transfusion.

69. d. Plasma transfusion is used to replace coagulation factors in case of vitamin K-dependent coagulation factors deficiencies include liver disease and warfarin medication, and to increase ADAMTS13 in thrombotic thrombocytopenic purpura. It is not used to increase plasma albumin or as fluid replacement.

70. a. FDA requires that whole blood platelet units contain **5.5 × 10^{10}** or more in 75% of the units tested.

71. a. FDA requires that apheresis platelet unit may contain equal or less than **5 × 10^6 leukocytes**.

72. e. In Fisher and Race system, D-negative, C-negative and E-negative phenotypes are designated as **rr**.

73. b. The two highly homologous Rh genes are located on the short arm of **chromosome 1**.

74. e. In Fisher and Race system, the phenotype is **R^2R^2**.

75. c. The genes are located at **chromosome 9** (9q34.2).

76. b. There are two genes which control the production of Rh system, one gene for D and one gene for CE antigens.

77. a. MNS system is located on glycophorins A and B which are single-pass transmembrane glycoproteins.

78. c. The U antigen is a high-frequency antigen present in 100% of white population and present in 99% of black population. Blacks who are negative for U may develop anti-U antibody if they receive a U positive red blood cell unit. This antibody is capable of causing hemolytic transfusion reaction and hemolytic reaction of fetus and newborn.

79. d. **McLeod** phenotype lacks the Kell system and may show specific changes in red cell morphology such as shortened survival, reduced deformability, decreased permeability to water, and acanthocytic morphology.

80. e. A patient who is CDe is also designated **R^1R^1**.

81. c. This patient Rh type is D- - (Rh17); patient is not producing E, e, C, c antigens.

82. e. Le^a, Le^b, and I are not produced at birth.

83. d. The G antigen is present on red cells possessing either C or D antigens. Antibodies against G may be present with anti-C and D.

84. d. **TRALI** in most cases is caused by granulocyte agglutination in lung capillaries due to presence of anti-HLA/granulocytes antibodies in donor plasma.

85. c. **0.9% sodium chloride** (normal saline) is the only fluid permitted by FDA and AABB to be used simultaneously with blood products.

86. c. The 1.2% red cells acid resistance containing HbF is equivalent to 60 cc red cells. In an average pregnant fe-

male, 60 ml of whole blood needs 2 doses of anti-D antibody, and another dose is added (i.e., 3 of 300 μg
doses are required).

87. **b.** In a 70 kg non-bleeding person, each unit of packed
red cell should raise the hematocrit by **3% or 1 gm** of
hemoglobin.

88. **e. Etretinate** (Tegison) is a medication for psoriasis
and may cause fetal malformation. The user is permanently deferred.

89. **e.** HIV/AIDS does not cause TAGVHD due to dysfunction of T cells. It suggested that the virus infects
the donor T cells and becomes dysfunctional.

90. **c.** The autoantibody in PCH is **IgG** and in most cases
is **anti-P**. It reacts with red cells in colder areas of the
body causing irreversible complement (C3 or C4) binding which then dissociates from red cells at warmer
body temperature.

91. **c.** Individuals possessing Le and Se genes will have red
cells that express Le^b but not Le^a. The Lewis antigens
are not intrinsic to red cells but are expressed on glycosphingolipid type I chains, adsorbed from plasma
onto red cells. Lewis antigens are oligosaccharides and
trypsin has no effect on them. Anti-Lewis antibody
does not cause neonatal or fetal hemolytic reaction due
its inability to cross the placenta and its absence at
birth.

92. **e.** U antigen is high-frequency antigen with 100%
presence rate in whites and about 99% in black
populations. In heavily transfused sickle cell patients,
U negative patients may develop anti U.

93. **d.** According to FDA guideline, a donor who spends
more than three months cumulative period in the
United Kingdom is permanently deferred in the
United States.

94. **b. Platelet crossmatch** is the appropriate test to obtain platelets for this patient.

95. **a.** The Corrected Count Increment (CCI) will assist in
defining platelet alloimmunization versus consumption. The other tests are not helpful for this purpose.

96. **b.** Fresh frozen plasma does not usually require crossmatch. If more than 2 mL of red cells are present in a
platelet unit or granulocytes, crossmatching is
required.

97. **d.** The least likely cause of platelet refractoriness is
cephalosporin use. Others causes may suppress bone
marrow platelet production or increase the peripheral
destruction.

98. **c.** CMV safe products require a third generation
leukodepletion filter. The third generation filter may
reduce the number of leukocytes in red cells or platelet
components to less than 5×10^5, a level that reduces
the risk of the transmission of cytomegalovirus as well
as HLA alloimmunization.

99. **a.** U antigen is a high-frequency red cell antigen and is
present in 100% of all ethnic populations and in 99%
of black ethnicity.

100. **b.** The antibody is anti-D.

101. **a.** Two antibodies are not ruled out: anti-Fya and E
antibodies. Ficin destroyed Fya and enhance E antigens in the testing panel.

102. **a.** Anti-D, K, and Lea antibodies are not excluded.

■ Recommended Readings

Brecher ME, ed. *Technical manual,*15th ed. Bethesda, MD: AABB
Press, 2005.

Klein HG, Anstee DJ. *Mollison's blood transfusion in clinical medicine,*
11th ed. Oxford, England: Blackwell Publishing Ltd., 2005.

McLeod BC. *Apheresis principles and practice,* 2nd ed. Bethesda, MD:
AABB Press, 2003.

McPherson RA, Pincus MR. *Henry's clinical diagnosis and management
by laboratory methods,* 21st ed. Philadelphia: Saunders Elsevier, 2006.

16

Clinical Hematology and Coagulation

Edward Wong, Alison Huppmann, and David Zwick

■ Questions

1. In which of the following disorders is the bleeding time prolonged?
   a. Hemophilia A
   b. Hemophilia B
   c. von Willebrand disease
   d. Factor XIII deficiency
   e. Protein C deficiency

2. Which disorder is associated with a prolonged prothrombin time (PT)?
   a. Factor VIII deficiency
   b. von Willebrand disease
   c. Factor VII deficiency
   d. Factor XII deficiency
   e. Factor XIII deficiency

3. Which disorder is associated with a prolonged activated partial thromboplastin time (aPTT)?
   a. Bernard–Soulier syndrome
   b. von Willebrand disease
   c. Factor VII deficiency
   d. Idiopathic thrombocytopenic purpura (ITP)
   e. Thrombotic thrombocytopenia purpura (TTP)

4. Which of the following is NOT true regarding Waldenstrom macroglobulinemia?
   a. It usually involves bone marrow, lymph nodes, and spleen.
   b. The most common immunophenotype is CD5+, CD10-, CD23-, CD38+.
   c. Some cases are associated with t(9;14)(p13;q32) and *PAX-5* gene rearrangement.
   d. Serum monoclonal protein is usually of IgM type.
   e. The paraprotein may cause hyperviscosity and/or cryoglobulinemia.

5. The half-life of the polymorphonuclear neutrophil is:
   a. 2 to 5 days
   b. 1 to 2 days
   c. 5 to 20 hours
   d. 5 to 20 days
   e. 1 to 5 hours

6. All of the following are true regarding Kikuchi disease EXCEPT:
   a. It usually requires treatment with steroids.
   b. It has higher incidence in Asians.
   c. Lymph nodes display paracortical hyperplasia and areas of necrosis.
   d. It is most common in young females.
   e. It clinically presents as unilateral tender cervical lymph node enlargement.

7. High serum level of methylmalonic acid is characteristic of:
   a. Thalassemia minor
   b. Hereditary spherocytosis
   c. Aplastic anemia
   d. Folate deficiency
   e. Vitamin B12 deficiency

8. The formula for Bart's hemoglobin is:
   a. $\alpha_2\zeta_2$
   b. $\alpha_2\gamma_2$
   c. $\alpha_2\delta_2$
   d. β_4
   e. γ_4

9. Which of the following lymphomas is NOT associated with HIV infection?
   a. Burkitt lymphoma
   b. Primary effusion lymphoma

c. Nodular lymphocyte predominant Hodgkin lymphoma
d. Plasmablastic lymphoma of the oral cavity
e. Diffuse large B-cell lymphoma

10. Which of the following reactive lymph node disorders is NOT appropriately matched with its histologic description?
a. Toxoplasmosis – epithelioid histiocytes surround and encroach on follicles
b. Rheumatoid arthritis – florid follicular hyperplasia and sinus histiocytosis
c. Whipple disease – necrotizing granulomas
d. Dermatopathic lymphadenopathy – paracortical expansion with antigen-presenting cells
e. Kimura disease – infiltration of eosinophils, lymphocytes, plasma cells, and mast cells

11. Folic acid is absorbed:
a. In the stomach
b. In the duodenum
c. In the distal ileum
d. In the proximal jejunum
e. Throughout the entire small intestine

12. Ringed sideroblasts are formed by deposition of iron in:
a. The lysosomes of the erythroblasts
b. The endoplasmic reticulum of the normoblast
c. The nuclear membrane of the normoblasts
d. The mitochondria of bone marrow blasts
e. The mitochondria of the normoblasts

13. Inappropriate secretion of erythropoietin can be present in all the following disorders EXCEPT:
a. Hepatocellular carcinoma
b. Cerebellar hemangioblastoma
c. Uterine leiomyoma
d. Renal cyst
e. Sarcoidosis

14. In red blood cell (RBC) metabolism, ATP plays an essential role in:
a. Membrane lipid renewal
b. Maintaining hemoglobin in a functional state
c. Hemoglobin synthesis
d. Protecting hemoglobin from oxidative stress
e. Furnishing energy for the "membrane pump"

15. Total body iron content in an adult male is approximately:
a. 0.5 to 1 g
b. 1 to 3 g
c. 3 to 5 g
d. 5 to 7 g
e. 7 to 9 g

16. The proportion of the body's iron contained within hemoglobin represents:
a. 1% to 5%
b. 25% to 30%
c. 5% to 10%
d. 56% to 70%
e. 90% to 100%

17. A defect in hemoglobin synthesis is detected earliest by:
a. Decreased MCHC value
b. MCH greater than 30 pg
c. Hypochromia on peripheral smear
d. Decrease in RBC count
e. Decrease in hemoglobin

18. In the workup of Coombs-negative hemolytic anemia, which of the following tests is LEAST appropriate?
a. Sucrose hemolysis test
b. Serum haptoglobin levels
c. Hemoglobin electrophoresis
d. Antibody serology for mycoplasma
e. Osmotic fragility test

19. Which of the following drugs can cause a sideroblastic anemia?
a. Chloramphenicol
b. All-trans retinoic acid
c. Recombinant factor VIII
d. Gold salts
e. Pyramidon

20. In the workup of a patient with Hodgkin lymphoma, which of the following would indicate stage IV disease?
a. Bone marrow involvement
b. Splenic, hilar, celiac, or portal lymph node involvement
c. Involvement of lymph nodes on both sides of the diaphragm
d. Paraaortic, iliac, or mesenteric lymph node involvement
e. Splenic or thymic involvement

21. Which of the following set of laboratory findings is characteristic of thalassemia minor?

	Serum iron	Total iron-binding capacity	Soluble serum transferrin receptor	Bone marrow storage iron	RDW
a.	Low	High	High	Absent	High
b.	Normal	Normal	Normal	High	Normal
c.	Low	Low	Normal	High	Normal
d.	High	Low	Normal	High	Normal
e.	High	High	Low	Absent	High

22. All of the following disorders are associated with a ferritin level that is normal or elevated EXCEPT:
    a. Thalassemia minor
    b. Iron deficiency anemia
    c. B12 deficiency
    d. Sideroblastic anemias
    e. Repeated hemorrhages

23. Which of the following disorders is UNLIKELY to be associated with pancytopenia?
    a. Alcoholic cirrhosis
    b. Primary macroglobulinemia
    c. Hairy cell leukemia
    d. Thalassemia minor
    e. Folic acid deficiency

24. Which disorder is NOT associated with thrombocytosis?
    a. Iron deficiency anemia
    b. Post splenectomy state
    c. Hemophilia B
    d. Pyruvate kinase deficiency
    e. Pancreatic cancer

25. Which of the following is a poor prognostic factor in pediatric patients with precursor B lymphoblastic leukemia?
    a. Hyperdiploid chromosomes >50
    b. t(9;22)(q34;q11.2)
    c. Age 4–10
    d. t(12;21)(p13;q22)
    e. Low or normal leukocyte count at diagnosis

26. Ringed sideroblasts are seen in:
    a. Hairy cell leukemia
    b. Anemia of chronic disease
    c. Thalassemia minor
    d. Vitamin B12 deficiency
    e. Myelodysplasia

27. A leukoerythroblastic picture may be seen in all of the following disorders EXCEPT:
    a. Chronic idiopathic myelofibrosis
    b. Acute hemolytic anemia
    c. Metastatic cancer to bone
    d. Rh hemolytic disease of the newborn
    e. Anemia of chronic disease

28. In which of the following disorders is the platelet count decreased?
    a. von Willebrand disease
    b. Cytomegalovirus (CMV) disease
    c. Postsplenectomy
    d. Hypovitaminosis K
    e. Anemia of chronic disease

29. In which disorder is the thrombin time prolonged?
    a. Factor XI deficiency
    b. Factor VII deficiency
    c. Hemophilia A
    d. ITP
    e. Heparin therapy

30. Which test would confirm the diagnosis of hemoglobin H disease?
    a. Hemoglobin electrophoresis
    b. Osmotic fragility
    c. Direct antiglobulin test
    d. Heinz body test
    e. Search for Howell-Jolly bodies on blood smear

31. Which test would confirm the diagnosis of cold agglutinin disease?
    a. Hemoglobin electrophoresis
    b. Osmotic fragility
    c. Direct antiglobulin test
    d. Heat stability test
    e. Search for Howell-Jolly bodies on blood smear

32. CD30 (Ki-1) is sometimes or always positive in all of the following lymphoproliferative disorders EXCEPT:
    a. Histiocytic sarcoma
    b. Lymphomatoid papulosis
    c. Classical Hodgkin lymphoma
    d. Anaplastic large cell lymphoma
    e. Adult T-cell leukemia/lymphoma

33. Which test would confirm the diagnosis of hereditary spherocytosis?
    a. Hemoglobin electrophoresis
    b. Osmotic fragility
    c. Direct antiglobin test
    d. Heat stability test
    e. Search for Howell-Jolly bodies on blood smear

34. Which of the following is NOT a sign of extravascular hemolysis?
    a. Anemia
    b. Increase in indirect bilirubin
    c. Increase in urobilinogen
    d. Increase in fecal stercobilinogen
    e. Increase in plasma hemoglobin

35. Which of the following is NOT a sign of acute intravascular hemolysis?
    a. Increase in plasma hemoglobin
    b. Decrease or disappearance of haptoglobin
    c. Presence of methemoglobin
    d. Appearance of hemoglobinuria
    e. Increase in urobilinogen

36. Which of the following is NOT commonly seen with pyruvate kinase deficiency?
    a. Most commonly seen in frequency after G6PD deficiency
    b. Frequent in Europeans
    c. Autosomal recessive
    d. Osmotic fragility is normal
    e. Chronic, spherocytic hemolytic anemia

37. Excluding flow cytometry, which of the following is the best test for paroxysmal nocturnal hemoglobinuria?
    a. Sugar water test
    b. Kinetic studies with ^{51}Cr-labeled red cells
    c. Ham test
    d. Decreased red cell acetylcholinesterase
    e. Direct antiglobin test

38. Which of the following is NOT a cause or characteristic of methemoglobinemia?
    a. Hemoglobin M
    b. Deficiency of NADH reductase
    c. Neonatal ingestion of nitrates
    d. Cyanosis
    e. Dark- or brown-colored plasma

39. Which of the following is NOT characteristic of alpha thalassemia minor?
    a. 5% to 10% Hb Bart at birth
    b. Inheritance of homozygous or heterozygous genotype
    c. Microcytosis
    d. Elevated RBC count
    e. Elevated Hb A_2

40. What is the earliest marker of B-cell lineage?
    a. cCD22
    b. CD10
    c. CD19
    d. CD38
    e. CD79a

41. Hemoglobin H disease is NOT associated with:
    a. Normal Hb F level
    b. Tetramer of gamma chains at birth
    c. Hemolytic anemia
    d. <5% Hb Bart at birth
    e. Splenomegaly

42. Hemoglobin Lepore is NOT associated with:
    a. Elevated Hb A_2
    b. Crossover between β and δ genes
    c. Thalassemic indices
    d. Elevated Hb F
    e. Difficulty in detection early in life

43. Elevated hemoglobin F can be seen in all of the following EXCEPT:
    a. Pregnancy (first trimester)
    b. Juvenile myelomonocytic leukemia

    c. Myelofibrosis
    d. Trisomy 21
    e. Hemoglobin H disease

44. What ratio of Hb A to Hb S is seen in adult sickle cell trait patients?
    a. 30:70
    b. 40:60
    c. 50:50
    d. 60:40
    e. 70:30

45. Causes of elevated Hb A_2 are seen in:
    a. α Thalassemia minor
    b. δβ Thalassemia trait
    c. Iron deficiency
    d. Hereditary persistence of fetal hemoglobin
    e. β Thalassemia trait

46. Which of the following RBC abnormalities is NOT seen with myelofibrosis?
    a Anisocytosis
    b. Poikilocytosis
    c. Macrocytosis
    d. Schistocytes
    e. Acanthocytes

47. Which of the following RBC abnormalities is NOT seen with unstable hemoglobin?
    a. Heinz bodies
    b. Polychromasia
    c. Anisocytosis
    d. Microcytosis
    e. Poikilocytosis

48. Which of the following is NOT seen with impaired hemoglobin synthesis?
    a. Target cells
    b. Anisocytosis
    c. Schistocytes
    d. Microcytosis
    e. Basophilic stippling

49. Which RBC feature is characteristically seen with abetalipoproteinemia?
    a. Acanthocytes
    b. Polychromasia
    c. Anisocytosis
    d. Target cells
    e. Poikilocytosis

50. All of the following flow cytometry markers are expressed by hairy cell leukemia cells EXCEPT:
    a. CD25
    b. CD5
    c. CD19
    d. CD20
    e. CD11c

51. The megakaryoblast displays which of the following surface marker reactivity?
    a. CD34+, CD33−, HLA−DR+, CD41+, CD61+
    b. CD34+, CD33+, HLA−DR+, CD42+, CD36+
    c. CD34−, CD33+, HLA−DR−, CD42+, CD36+
    d. CD34+, CD33−, HLA−DR+, CD42+, CD36+
    e. CD34+, CD33−, HLA−DR−, CD42−, CD61−

52. The promonocyte displays which of the following surface marker reactivity?
    a. CD13+, CD33+, CD34+, HLD−DR+
    b. CD13+, CD33+, CD11b+, CD14+, HLA−DR+
    c. CD13+, CD33+, CD11b+, CD14+, HLA−DR−
    d. CD13+, CD33−, CD11b+, CD14+, HLA−DR−
    e. CD13+, CD33+, CD11b−, CD14−, HLA−DR−

53. Characteristics of acute promyelocytic leukemia include all the following EXCEPT:
    a. Bundles of Auer rods
    b. Intense MPO activity
    c. CD13+, CD33+, HLA−DR+, CD34− phenotype
    d. DIC
    e. t(15:17)(p21;q11)

54. Reactive megakaryocytic hyperplasia can be distinguished from neoplastic megakaryocytic hyperplasia by all of the following EXCEPT:
    a. Peripheral basophilia
    b. Leukoerythroblastic peripheral blood pattern
    c. Bone marrow fibrosis
    d. Packed bone marrow (90% cellularity)
    e. Spontaneous colony formation of megakaryocytic and/or erythroid precursors.

55. The 5q- syndrome associated with MDS has all the following features in an elderly female EXCEPT:
    a. Moderately increased platelet counts generally greater than $1000 \times 10^9/L$
    b. Regular RBC transfusions
    c. High risk to progression to AML
    d. Hypolobulated megakaryocytes
    e. Macrocytic anemia

56. Hematogones can be recognized using flow cytometry by all the following EXCEPT:
    a. Low forward scatter
    b. Low side scatter
    c. Heterogeneous CD20 intensity
    d. Strong CD34 expression
    e. CD10 expression that is often less bright than that expressed by ALL blasts.

57. The following is true of all natural killer cells EXCEPT:
    a. They comprise 10% to 15% of peripheral blood lymphocytes.
    b. Majority have a morphology of large granular lymphocytes.
    c. Maturation is thymic independent.

d. They are CD2+, CD7+, CD8+, CD16+, and CD56+.
    e. They can be distinguished using paraffin-resistant polyclonal CD3 antibodies.

58. All of the following are true of chronic myeloid leukemia EXCEPT:
    a. WBC count of at least $50 \times 10^9/L$
    b. Absolute basophilia greater than $0.2 \times 10^9/L$
    c. Marked granulocytosis with predominance of promyelocytes
    d. bcr-abl fusion
    e. NRBCs are present.

59. Pseudo Pelger-Huet cells can be seen in all of the following disorders EXCEPT:
    a. Iron deficiency
    b. Infectious/inflammatory processes
    c. Toxic intestinal disorders
    d. Chronic myeloid leukemia
    e. Myelodysplastic syndrome

60. Characteristics of mature T cells include all of the following EXCEPT:
    a. CD3+, CD4+ cells account for approximately 70% to 80% of peripheral blood T cells.
    b. CD3+, CD8+ cells account for approximately 20% to 35% of peripheral blood T cells.
    c. A subset of CD8+ cells expresses one or more NK-associated antigens, usually CD16 and CD57.
    d. Populations of CD4+/CD8+ and CD4-/CD8- cells are seen in very low percentages (approximately 1% to 2%).
    e. After chemotherapy, an increase of CD4-/CD8- cells in the 10% to 20% range can be seen.

61. Diagnostic criteria for monoclonal gammopathy of undetermined significance include all of the following EXCEPT:
    a. Serum monoclonal spike (<3.5 g/dL if IgG, <2 g/dL if IgA)
    b. Bone marrow plasmacytosis <10%
    c. No lytic bone lesions
    d. No symptoms associated with myeloma
    e. Increased serum calcium

62. Blast morphology of AML-M1 includes all of the following features EXCEPT:
    a. Nondescript cytology
    b. Round to irregular nuclear contours
    c. Absent nucleoli
    d. Scant to ample blue cytoplasm
    e. Rare to occasional Auer rods

63. Features seen in AML-M4E (AMML Eo) include all the following EXCEPT:
    a. Abnormal eosinophilic bone marrow precursors
    b. Abnormalities of chromosome 16

c. Decreased number of bone marrow neutrophils

d. Usually show peripheral blood eosinophilia

e. Positivity for nonspecific esterase staining in mono-cytic precursors

64. The AML–M3 microgranular variant may be distinguished from AML–M3 by all of the following EXCEPT:
    a. Blast morphology
    b. Higher WBC count
    c. Higher circulating numbers of malignant cells
    d. Down-regulation of HLA-DR
    e. Relapsed blast morphology after treatment with ATRA

65. Nonspecific esterase positivity in AML blasts indicates:
    a. Myeloid maturation
    b. Monocyte differentiation
    c. Decreased lysozyme in serum
    d. AML–M4 rather than AML–M5
    e. Predominance of promonocytes

66. AML–M6 leukemias are characterized by all of the following criteria EXCEPT:
    a. The presence of >20% myeloblasts with erythroid predominance
    b. Relation to therapy in most cases
    c. The presence of giant erythroid precursors with megaloblastic maturation
    d. The presence of erythroid precursors with prominent nuclear abnormalities such as binucleation, multinucleation, karyorrhexis, nuclear lobation, and vacuoles
    e. Another name is "Di–Guglielmo syndrome"

67. Normochromic, normocytic anemia without apparent reticulocytosis is usually seen in all of the following EXCEPT:
    a. Anemia of chronic disease
    b. Renal disease
    c. Liver disease
    d. Early iron or B12/folate deficiency
    e. Symptomatic G6PD deficiency

68. Spherocytes may be seen in all of the following conditions EXCEPT:
    a. Burn injury
    b. Hereditary elliptocytosis
    c. Hereditary spherocytosis
    d. Autoimmune hemolytic anemia
    e. Sickle cell disease

69. The following figure (Fig. 16.1) represents a sickling solubility test. All the following are true about the test EXCEPT:
    a. The test requires lysis of RBCs.
    b. The test depends on the solubility of deoxygenated sickle hemoglobin.

c. The test detects sickle cell disease only.

d. False positives are seen with hyperproteinemia.

e. In children younger than 6 months old, the test may be negative.

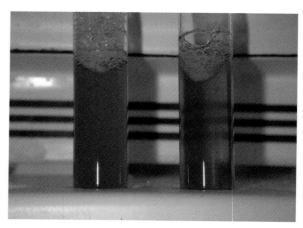

Figure 16.1

70. The following peripheral smear (Fig. 16.2) seen in hemoglobin SC below is different from the peripheral smear seen in sickle cell disease in all the following ways EXCEPT that hemoglobin SC:
    a. Shows more polychromasia
    b. Shows more target cells
    c. Shows irregularly shaped crystals
    d. Does not usually show Howell-Jolly bodies
    e. Shows "fat" sickle cells

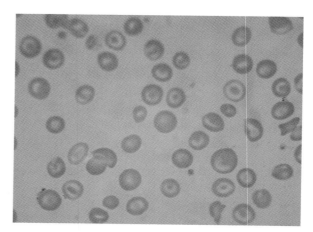

Figure 16.2

71. The blood smear (Fig. 16.3) was from a patient with the following hematologic data:
    RBC Count 5.81 [3.70–4.87] M/uL
    Hemoglobin 11.5 [10.6–13.5] g/dL
    Hematocrit 36.3 [32.9–41.2] %
    MCV 62.5 [77.7–93.7] fL
    MCH 19.8 [25.3–30.9] pg
    MCHC 31.7 [31.0–34.1] g/dL
    RDW 14.7 [12.4–15.1] %

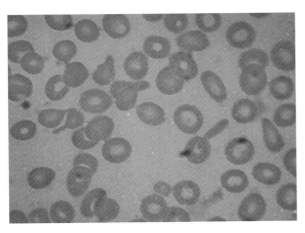

Figure 16.3

These data best represent:
a. Hemoglobin C trait
b. Homozygous C disease
c. Hemoglobin SC disease
d. Beta thalassemia trait
e. Homozygous E disease

72. Methodologies used for hemoglobin identification include all of the following EXCEPT:
    a. High-performance liquid chromatography
    b. Capillary zone electrophoresis
    c. DNA testing
    d. Sickle solubility testing
    e. Hemoglobin gel electrophoresis

73. The following figure (Fig. 16.4) best represents:

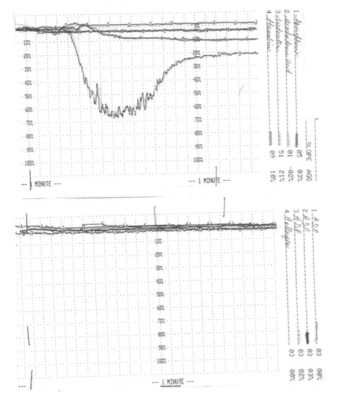

Figure 16.4

a. Platelet secretion defect
b. Bernard-Soulier disease
c. Glanzmann thrombasthenia
d. von Willebrand disease
e. May-Hegglin anomaly

74. Which of the following is NOT associated with a sickling disorder?
    a. Hemoglobin SS
    b. Hemoglobin SD
    c. Hemoglobin SG
    d. Hemoglobin SC$_{Harlem}$
    e. Hemoglobin SC

75. The following figure (Fig. 16.5) best represents:
    a. Glanzmann thrombasthenia
    b. May-Hegglin anomaly
    c. Bernard Soulier syndrome
    d. Gray platelet syndrome
    e. Hereditary elliptocytosis

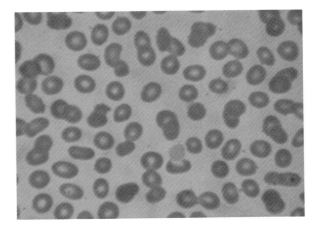

Figure 16.5

76. The following figure (Fig. 16.6) from a 32-year-old man with six-day history of coughing, emesis, and lymphocytosis best represents:
    a. Non-Hodgkin lymphoma
    b. Epstein-Barr infection

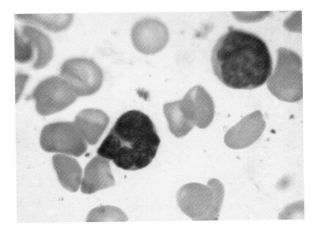

Figure 16.6

c. Congenital leukemia

d. RSV infection

e. *Bordetella pertussis*

77. The following figure (Fig. 16.7) best represents:
    a. *Plasmodium falciparum*
    b. *Plasmodium malaria*
    c. *Plasmodium vivax*
    d. *Plasmodium ovale*
    e. Babesiosis

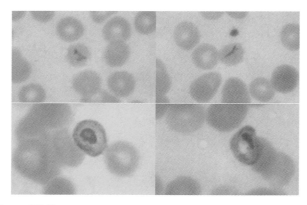

Figure 16.7

78. The picture (Fig. 16.8) is an iron stain of RBC inclusions that can be seen in:
    a. Functional asplenism
    b. Iron anemia
    c. Lead poisoning
    d. Beta thalassemia major
    e. Hereditary hemochromatosis

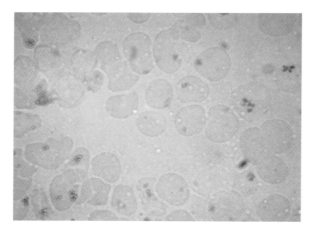

Figure 16.8

79. The following picture (Fig. 16.9) is an iron stain of an RBC inclusion that best represents all of the following EXCEPT:
    a. Sideroblast
    b. Nucleated RBC
    c. Iron deficiency
    d. Mitochondria iron staining
    e. Lead poisoning

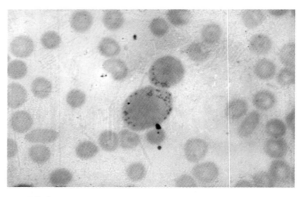

Figure 16.9

80. Which RBC abnormality seen with vitamin C overdose in an African American child is represented in the following picture (Fig. 16.10)?
    a. Methemoglobinemia
    b. Thalassemia major
    c. Hexokinase deficiency
    d. G6PD deficiency
    e. Pyruvate kinase deficiency

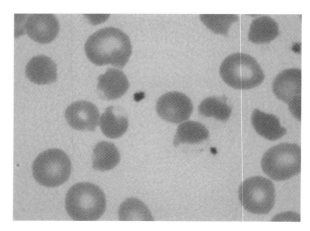

Figure 16.10

81. The following capillary zone electrophoresis (Fig. 16.11) demonstrates a very fast moving hemoglobin peak. All the following are true of this hemoglobin EXCEPT:
    a. Comprised of four beta globin chains
    b. Is an unstable hemoglobin
    c. Is detected early in life
    d. Carries oxygen
    e. Can be confirmed by Heinz body prep

82. Conditions that can give rise to spuriously low B12 levels include all the following EXCEPT:
    a. Drugs interfering with the microbiologic assay of vitamin B12
    b. Selenium deficiency
    c. Folate deficiency
    d. Pregnancy or birth control pills
    e. Transcobalamin I deficiency

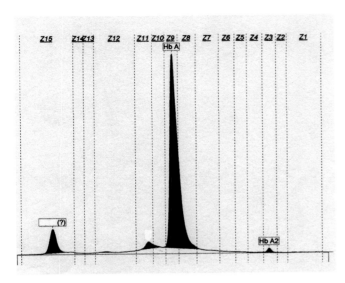

Figure 16.11

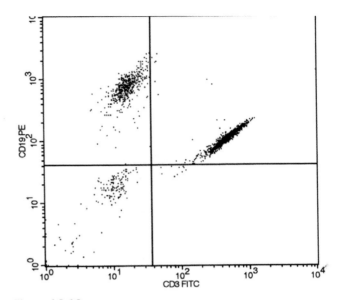

Figure 16.12

83. Peripheral blood findings of B12 deficiency include all the following EXCEPT:
   a. Hypersegmented neutrophils
   b. Macrocytosis
   c. Ovalocytosis
   d. Howell-Jolly bodies
   e. Reticulocytosis

84. In a patient receiving treatment with rituximab, which of the following markers may be altered or lost as result of treatment?
   a. CD10
   b. CD20
   c. CD5
   d. Surface light chains
   e. CD79a

85. Macrocytosis can occur in all of the following conditions EXCEPT:
   a. Dihydrofolate reductase deficiency
   b. Lesch–Nyhan syndrome
   c. Autoimmune hemolytic anemia
   d. Congenital dyserythropoietic anemia type I
   e. Deficiency of transcobalamin II

86. The following flow cytometry histogram (Fig. 16.12) from a peripheral blood two-color analysis of lymphoid cells:
   a. Indicates over compensation error with too high a proportion of the PE signal subtracted from the FITC channel
   b. Is consistent with biphenotypic B and T leukemia
   c. Indicates undercompensation error with too much spillover of FITC signals into the PE channel
   d. Indicates overcompensation error with too high a proportion of FITC signal subtracted from the PE channel

87. A laboratory records the daily mean peak fluorescent channel numbers (MPC) for a standardized fluorescent bead as a means of tracking instrument performance over time. The following chart (Fig. 16.13) depicts the results of this monitor for 1 month. Possible explanations for the observed results on day 18 include:
   a. Laser misalignment or degradation of laser output
   b. Photomultiplier tube or optical filter problem
   c. Deterioration of the beads
   d. Partial obstruction from a clog in the flow cell

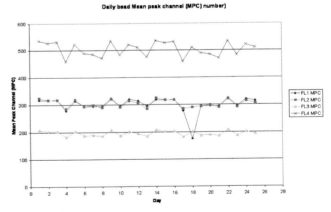

Daily bead Mean peak channel (MPC) number)

Figure 16.13

88. All of the following are hematologic causes of hydrops fetalis associated with increased red cell production EXCEPT:
   a. Pyruvate kinase deficiency
   b. $\delta\beta$ thalassemia trait
   c. Immune hemolysis: Rh and Kell
   d. Rare unstable α-chain variants
   e. G6PD deficiency

89. A 2-month-old male infant came for evaluation of cough and failure to thrive and was found to have a lymphocyte count of 1400/μL. Differential diagnostic considerations based on the depicted flow cytometry lymphocyte gated results (Fig. 16.14) include all the conditions EXCEPT:

a. DiGeorge syndrome
b. Severe combined immunodeficiency syndrome
c. Bruton agammaglobulinemia
d. CD3 delta-chain deficiency

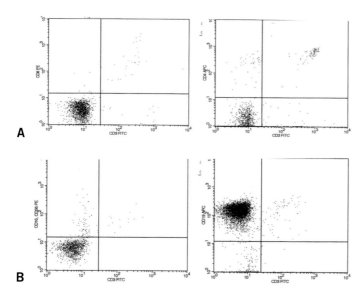

Figure 16.14

90. Characteristics of Kasabach-Merritt syndrome include all of the following EXCEPT:

a. Thrombocytosis
b. Anemia
c. Hypofibrinogenemia
d. Coagulopathy
e. Hemangioma formation

91. The following three histograms (Fig. 16.15) were acquired from a bone marrow sample of a 3-year-old boy with enlarged lymph nodes and elevated WBC with blasts in the peripheral blood. True statements regarding the histograms include:

a. The child has CD4-positive T-cell leukemia consistent with T precursor lymphoblastic leukemia.
b. The child has an increased number of immature B cells consistent with B-precursor lymphoblastic leukemia.
c. The findings are characteristic of *Bordetella pertussis* infection.
d. The histograms depict an unusual case of biclonal T- and B-cell lymphoblastic leukemia.

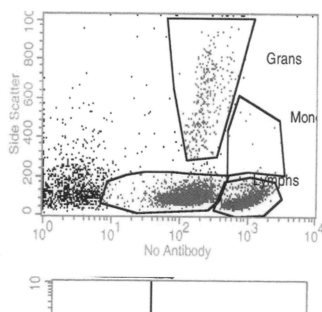

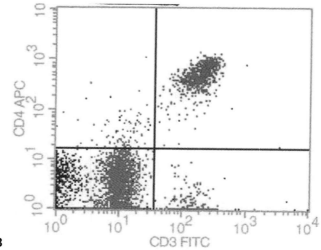

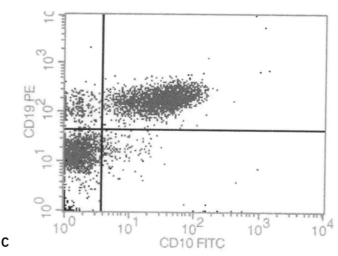

Figure 16.15

92. Characteristics of congenital dyserythropoietic anemia type II include all of the following EXCEPT:

a. Positive acidified ham test
b. Binuclear erythroblasts in the peripheral blood

c. Erythroid hyperplasia with binuclear to multinu-clear erythroblasts in the bone marrow
d. Failure of normal glycosylation of membrane proteins
e. RBC are agglutinated by anti-i.

93. An extensive panel of B and T lymphocyte and myeloid markers for the acute leukemia depicted below (Fig. 16.16) showed the blasts to express only CD19, CD10, Tdt, CD33, and CD13 (blue cell clusters). The leukemia is best classified as:
a. Bilineal B precursor and acute myeloid leukemia
b. Biphenotypic acute leukemia
c. Precursor acute lymphoblastic leukemia
d. Acute myeloid leukemia
e. Acute ambiguous undifferentiated leukemia

94. Characteristics of transient erythroblastopenia of childhood include all of the following EXCEPT:
a. Normocytic normochromic anemia
b. Reticulocytopenia

c. Normal RBC adenosine deaminase level
d. Clinical findings suggestive of a previous viral illness
e. Treatment with steroids

95. Characteristics of Diamond Blackfan anemia include all of the following EXCEPT:
a. Normocytic or macrocytic anemia
b. Reticulocytopenia
c. 25% of patients with mutations in ribosomal pro-tein S19
d. Elevated RBC adenosine deaminase activity
e. IVIG is the mainstay of treatment.

96. Characteristics of dyskeratosis congenita include all of the following EXCEPT:
a. Ectodermal abnormalities
b. Bone marrow failure
c. Cancer predisposition
d. Extreme telomere shortening
e. Autosomal dominance inheritance

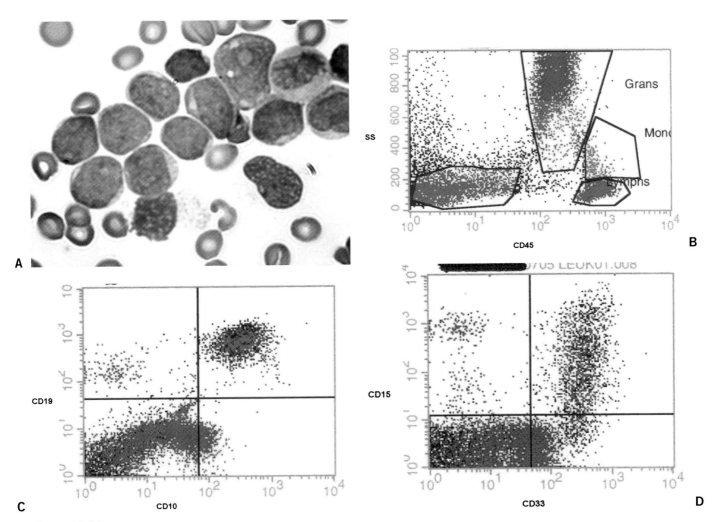

Figure 16.16

97. Characteristics of congenital amegakaryocytic thrombocytopenia include all of the following EXCEPT:
    a. Autosomal recessive inheritance
    b. Development of aplastic anemia in a high percentage of patients
    c. Mutations in the *c-mpl* gene
    d. Elevated thrombopoietin levels
    e. With time elevated MCV and hemoglobin F levels are seen

98. With respect to mature B-cell malignancies, which of the following statements are true?
    a. CLL cells characteristically express dim CD20, CD5, and CD10.
    b. Mantle cell lymphoma cells characteristically express bright CD20, CD5, and CD10.
    c. Follicular lymphoma cells characteristically express CD20 and CD10 but lack CD5.
    d. ALL the above are correct.
    e. Only a and b are correct.

99. Lymphoproliferative disorders that are sometimes or always associated with Epstein-Barr virus (EBV) include all of the following EXCEPT:
    a. Extranodal NK/T-cell lymphoma, nasal type
    b. Lymphomatoid granulomatosis
    c. Anaplastic large cell lymphoma
    d. Burkitt lymphoma
    e. Angioimmunoblastic T-cell lymphoma

100. Inherited bone marrow failure syndromes associated primarily with neutropenia include all of the following EXCEPT:
    a. Cyclic neutropenia
    b. Kostmann syndrome
    c. Myelokathexis
    d. WHIM syndrome
    e. Glycogen storage disease type Ia

101. MYH9-associated familial macrothrombocytopenia comprises all of the following syndromes EXCEPT:
    a. Thrombocytopenia with absent radii
    b. Alport syndrome
    c. Fechner syndrome
    d. May-Hegglin syndrome
    e. Sebastian syndrome

102. Which of the following is not a characteristic of mast cell disease?
    a. Bone marrow involvement is present in most patients.
    b. Cutaneous lesions may show the Darier sign.
    c. Cells stain with tryptase.
    d. Cells express CD45, CD33, CD68, and CD117.
    e. Point mutations in the KIT proto-oncogene may be observed.

103. Acquired sideroblastic anemias include all of the following EXCEPT:
    a. Macrocytic or normocytic RBCs
    b. Normal cytogenetics
    c. Ringed sideroblasts seen in early erythroblasts
    d. Increased RBC coproporphyrins
    e. Increased RBC porphyrins

104. Alder-Reilly granulation is usually seen in conjunction with:
    a. Mucopolysaccharidoses
    b. Chronic myeloid leukemia
    c. Hemochromatosis
    d. Aplastic anemia
    e. Reactive leukocytosis

105. A pathognomic finding in paroxysmal cold hemoglobinemia (PCH) includes:
    a. Positive DAT
    b. Cold reacting autoantibody
    c. Hemolytic anemia
    d. IgG autoantibody
    e. Neutrophils seen engulfing an RBC

106. Preparing a good quality peripheral blood smear depends on all of the following EXCEPT:
    a. The size of the drop
    b. Angle applied to the spreader
    c. The speed and steadiness in pushing the spreader
    d. Consideration of the hemoglobin level
    e. Consideration of the WBC count

107. For hemoglobinopathy evaluation by HPLC, isoelectric focusing, capillary zone electrophoresis, or hemoglobin acid/alkaline gel electrophoresis, the hemoglobin is in what state?
    a. Monomer
    b. Dimer
    c. Tetramer
    d. Combination of monomers and dimers
    e. Combination of dimers and tetramers

108. All the following are artifacts from suboptimal peripheral smear preparation EXCEPT:
    a. Cytoplasmic vacuolation in WBCs
    b. Naked lobulation in lymphocytes
    c. Crenated RBCs
    d. Vermilion red eosinophilic granules
    e. Water artifacts giving a false appearance of hypochromia

109. Children with precursor B acute lymphoblastic leukemia who manifest the following DNA ploidy pattern (Fig. 16.17):
    a. Have increased risk for relapse and shortened survival
    b. Have increased incidence of high risk chromosomal abnormalities, including t(4;11)

c. Harbor TEL;AML t(12;21) translocations with improved survival

d. Have decreased risk for relapse and improved survival

e. Require increased intensity of treatment but no difference in relapse and overall survival

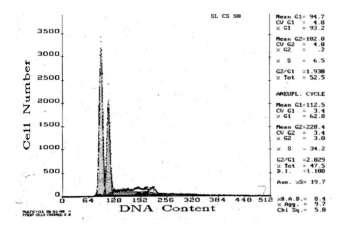

Figure 16.17

110. The following capillary zone electrophoresis (Fig. 16.18) demonstrates a very small, fast moving peak that is less than 1% of total hemoglobin in a 1-month-old infant who has microcytic indices. These findings are suggestive of:
   a. Beta thalassemia minor
   b. Alpha thalassemia minor
   c. Asymptomatic alpha thalassemia carrier state
   d. Degraded hemoglobin A
   e. Hemoglobin Lepore

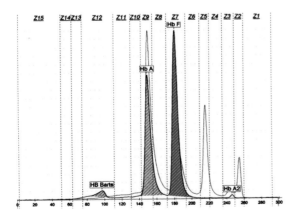

Figure 16.18

111. Characteristics of hairy cells in hairy cell leukemia include all of the following EXCEPT:
   a. "Fried egg" appearance
   b. Abundant pale cytoplasm
   c. Ovoid, reniform, or dumbbell-shaped nucleus
   d. Absent nucleoli
   e. High numbers of "hairy cells" seen in peripheral blood

112. Leukocyte adhesion deficiency (LAD) type I is associated with all of the following EXCEPT:
   a. Structurally abnormal or deficient expression of β2 integrin (CD18b)
   b. Deficiency of LFA-1 (preventing tight binding of neutrophils to vascular endothelium)
   c. Oxidative burst defect
   d. Severe recurrent bacterial infections
   e. Fungal infections

113. Chediak-Higashi syndrome is characterized by all of the following EXCEPT:
   a. Autosomal recessive inheritance
   b. Defect is due to mutations in the *CHS1* or *LYST* gene
   c. Fusion of heterogeneous lysosomes and formation of giant intracellular particles
   d. Multiple life-threatening bacterial and fungal infections
   e. No proven curative therapy

114. Chronic granulomatous disease (CGD) can be diagnosed by all of the following EXCEPT:
   a. Demonstration by flow cytometry of a defect in superoxide production
   b. Nitroblue tetrazolium test
   c. Western blot of a neutrophil protein lysate demonstrating the affected protein
   d. DNA confirmation of the mutation
   e. Demonstration of myeloperoxidase deficiency

115. Langerhans cell histiocytosis (LCH) is characterized by all of the following EXCEPT:
   a. Abnormal proliferation and accumulation of Langerhans cells that together with macrophages, lymphocytes, and eosinophils form granulomas.
   b. Expression by LCH cells of CD1a, S100, and CD207 (Langerin) but not markers of dendritic cells such as CD83, CD86, and DC-lamp.
   c. Multisystem organ involvement.
   d. Clonal proliferation of LCH cells.
   e. Predominant occurrence of older adults.

116. The molecular defect in Bernard Soulier syndrome is:
   a. Decreased von Willebrand factor activity
   b. Platelet secretion
   c. Abnormality of GPIb-IX-V complex
   d. Deficiency of GPIIb-IIIa
   e. Thromboxane A2 receptor deficiency

117. Pseudo-von Willebrand disease is characterized by all of the following EXCEPT:
    a. Abnormality in GPIbα
    b. Increased sensitivity to ristocetin-induced agglutination
    c. Absence of high molecular weight von Willebrand factor multimers
    d. Autosomal dominant inheritance
    e. Treatment with plasma-derived von Willebrand factor concentrates

118. Wiskott-Aldrich syndrome is characterized by all of the following EXCEPT:
    a. Clinically characterized by eczema, infections, and immunodeficiency
    b. X-linked inheritance
    c. Large platelets
    d. Mild to moderate bleeding syndrome
    e. Defect in the WASP protein

119. Basophilic stippling is found in all the following disorders EXCEPT:
    a. B12/folate deficiency
    b. Myelodysplastic syndrome
    c. Heavy metal poisoning
    d. Thalassemias
    e. Reactive leukocytosis

120. A dermatologist had been following this 54–year-old man for several years because of a persistent patchy, scaly skin rash over his trunk. He has recently developed generalized erythema and, because of an unexplained lymphocytosis, additional testing was done. Atypical lymphoid cells predominated in the peripheral blood with features as depicted below (Fig. 16.19). Cells from this condition are typically:
    a. CD8, CD7, and TCR gamma/delta chain positive
    b. CD4 and TCR alpha/beta positive, and CD7 negative

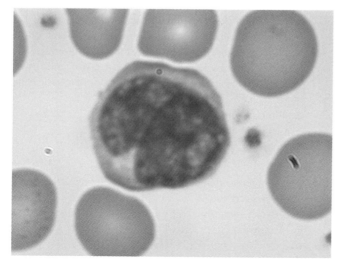

Figure 16.19

c. CD20 and CD25 positive with rearrangement of the IgH chain genes
    d. CD20 and CD23 positive with germline TCR and Ig chain genes

121. Hemophilia A must be differentiated from what type of von Willebrand disease?
    a. Type 2A
    b. Type 2B
    c. Type 2M
    d. Type 2N
    e. Pseudo von Willebrand disease

122. von Willebrand disease type 2A is characterized by all of the following EXCEPT:
    a. Decreased ristocetin cofactor activity compared to von Willebrand factor antigen level
    b. Decreased in high molecular weight von Willebrand factor multimers
    c. Increased sensitivity to ristocetin induced aggregation
    d. Defective dimerization and multimerization in the Golgi apparatus
    e. Abnormal proteolysis

123. von Willebrand disease type 2B is characterized by all of the following EXCEPT:
    a. Decreased ristocetin cofactor activity compared with von Willebrand factor antigen level
    b. Decreased in high molecular weight von Willebrand factor multimers
    c. Increased sensitivity to ristocetin-induced aggregation
    d. Defective dimerization and multimerization in the Golgi apparatus
    e. "Gain of function" mutation that stabilizes GPIb on platelets and the A2 domain of von Willebrand factor

124. von Willebrand disease type 3 is associated with a decrease in which organelle in endothelial cells?
    a. Mitochondria
    b. Golgi apparatus
    c. Weibel–Palade body
    d. Lysosome
    e. Nuclei

125. Acquired von Willebrand disease is associated with all of the following EXCEPT:
    a. Autoimmune clearance
    b. Proteolysis induced by increased fluid shear stress
    c. Increased binding to platelets
    d. Decrease synthesis
    e. Increased ADAMTS13 activity

126. The molecular basis for pseudo type von Willebrand disease is due to:
    a. Mutations in the platelet GPIbα subunit which enhance stability of the β-sheet conformation in this region upon binding to vWF

b. Mutations in the in the A1 domain that stabilize the binding of von Willebrand factor to GPIbα
c. Decreased binding to factor VIII
d. Increased proteolysis by ADAMTS13
e. Defective dimerization of the von Willebrand factor

127. Abnormalities in all of the following RBC proteins are associated with hereditary spherocytosis EXCEPT:
a. Protein 4.1
b. α-spectrin
c. β-spectrin
d. AE1
e. Ankyrin

128. Abnormalities in the following RBC proteins are associated with hereditary elliptocytosis EXCEPT:
a. α-spectrin
b. AE1
c. Ankyrin
d. Protein 4.1
e. Glycophorin C

129. The following phenotype (Fig. 16.20) is characteristic of:
a. AML–M0
b. AML-M1

c. AML-M3
d. AML-M6
e. AML-M7

130. Stomatocytosis is associated with the following EXCEPT:
a. Mild to moderate lifelong hemolytic anemia
b. Splenomegaly
c. Decreased osmotic fragility
d. Very high MCV
e. Low MCHC

131. Signs and symptoms of acute hepatic/neurovisceral porphyrias include all of the following EXCEPT:
a. Abdominal pain
b. Muscle weakness
c. Bulbar neuropathy causing respiratory paralysis

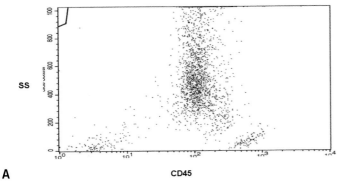
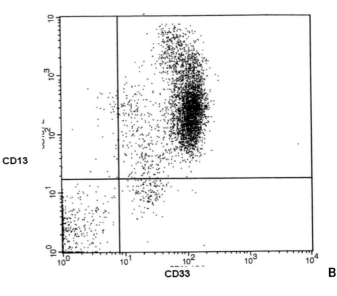
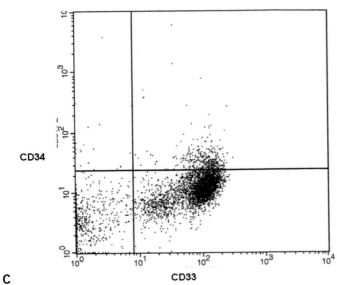
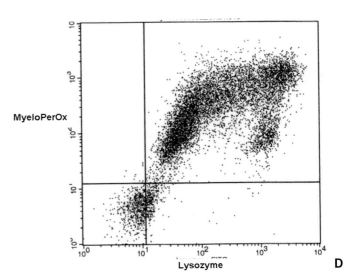

Figure 16.20

d. Psychiatric symptoms
e. Hemolytic anemia

132. A previously healthy five-month-old boy died suddenly from overwhelming *Staphylococcus aureus* septicemia. The following histograms (Fig. 16.21) display results of flow cytometric assessment of maternal granulocyte oxidative activity. The following conclusions can be drawn from the analysis:
   a. The mother is likely a carrier for chronic granulomatous disease (CGD).

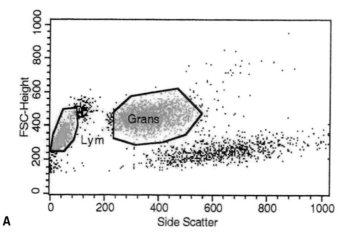

A

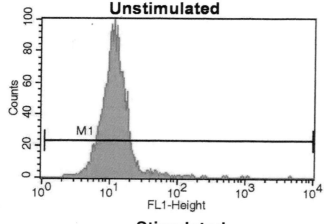

Unstimulated

B

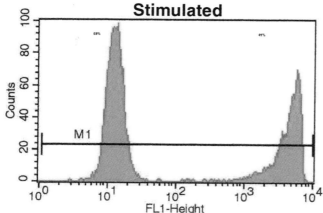

Stimulated

C

Figure 16.21

b. The mother has a subpopulation of granulocytes deficient in oxidase activity.
   c. The mother has autosomal recessive form of CGD.
   d. The son had CGD.
   e. Both a and b are correct.

133. All the following enzyme deficiency diseases are best matched with their clinical disorder EXCEPT:
   a. δ-aminolevulinic acid dehydratase and ALD deficiency porphyria
   b. Porphobilinogen deaminase and acute intermittent porphyria
   c. Uroporphyrinogen III synthase and congenital erythropoietic porphyria
   d. Coproporphyrinogen III oxidase and hereditary coproporphyria
   e. Ferrochelatase and variegate porphyria

134. Conditions that decrease δ-aminolevulinic acid dehydratase activity include all of the following EXCEPT:
   a. ALD deficiency porphyria
   b. Zinc deficiency
   c. Lead poisoning
   d. Acute renal insufficiency
   e. Diabetes mellitus

135. Characteristics of acute intermittent porphyria include all the following EXCEPT:
   a. Deficiency of porphobilinogen deaminase
   b. Increased porphobilinogen in urine
   c. Decreased aminolevulinic acid in urine
   d. Presentation of the disease after puberty
   e. Most attacks are caused by drugs

136. Characteristics of nodular lymphocyte predominant Hodgkin lymphoma include all the following EXCEPT:
   a. The nodules are closely packed and lack mantle zones.
   b. Most L&H cells are ringed by CD3+ T cells.
   c. Popcorn cells express CD45, CD20, and BOB.1.
   d. Involvement is usually widespread (stage III or IV) at the time of presentation.
   e. Mediastinal involvement is not common.

137. Characteristics of erythropoietic protoporphyria include all of the following EXCEPT:
   a. Deficiency of ferrochelatase
   b. Presents in early childhood
   c. Increased RBC protoporphyrin
   d. Increased free protoporphyrin in stool and plasma
   e. Decreased coproporphyrin I levels in urine

138. Hemoglobin variants with increased oxygen affinity have all the following features EXCEPT:
   a. Oxygen-binding curve shifted to the left
   b. Erythrocytosis
   c. Autosomal dominant inheritance

d. Patient may present with peripheral cyanosis or violaceous complexion

e. Are always detectable electrophoretically

139. Hemoglobin M variants are characterized by:
   a. Amino acid substitution in the heme iron–binding region that cause permanent and complete oxidation of the heme iron to the ferric form
   b. Instability
   c. Able to carry oxygen
   d. Heterozygotes are not cyanotic.
   e. Autosomal recessive inheritance

140. CSF findings in tuberculous meningitis include all of the following EXCEPT:
   a. Total WBC count seldom exceeding 1000 per mm³
   b. Neutrophil predominance in the first exudative stage
   c. Coexistence of many neutrophils, transformed lymphocytes, and plasma cells usually seen upon first admission
   d. Basophilic cytoplasm of the transformed lymphocytes and plasma cells
   e. Abundance of monocytes

141. Evidence of a cellular reaction to CSF hemorrhage can be seen as early as:
   a. 1 hour
   b. 2 hours
   c. 4 hours
   d. 24 hours
   e. 4 days

142. Plasma cells in the CSF have all the following characteristics EXCEPT:
   a. Are never normally seen in the CSF
   b. Presence indicates an inflammatory process
   c. Associated with viral diseases
   d. Associated with chronic infections such as syphilis and tuberculosis
   e. Seen in bacterial infections

143. Paroxysmal nocturnal hemoglobinuria has all the following characteristics EXCEPT:
   a. Clonal stem cell disorder

   b. Associated with a deficiency in glycosylphosphatidylinositol-linked surface proteins
   c. Negative acidified serum test (Ham test)
   d. Negative by flow cytometry for CD59 and CD55
   e. Unexplained chronic intravascular hemolysis

144. Warfarin skin necrosis is characterized by all of the following EXCEPT:
   a. Secondary to a drop in protein C after warfarin administration
   b. Congenital or acquired protein S deficiency as a risk factor
   c. More frequent in men
   d. Usually develops in areas where there is generous adipose tissue
   e. Best prevented by using starting doses that approximate the estimated maintenance dose

145. Aspirin affects platelet aggregation testing by all of the following EXCEPT:
   a. Decreased arachidonic acid induced aggregation
   b. Decreased secondary wave by ADP
   c. Decreased secondary wave by epinephrine
   d. Decreased low dose collagen-induced aggregation
   e. Decreased ristocetin-induced aggregation

146. Laboratory diagnosis of dysfibrinogenemia includes all of the following EXCEPT:
   a. Prolonged PT
   b. Prolonged PTT
   c. Prolonged thrombin time
   d. Lack of correction with 1:1 mix with normal pooled plasma
   e. Normal reptilase time.

147. Characteristics of factor XIII deficiency include all of the following EXCEPT:
   a. Factor levels are 10% to 20% normal.
   b. Can be seen in the neonatal period with umbilical stump bleeding.
   c. Intracranial bleeding occurs in 30% of patients.
   d. Diagnosis can be made by clot solubility test.
   e. Confirmation should be made by a factor XIII quantitative assay.

▧ Answers

1. **c. von Willebrand disease** causes prolonged bleeding time. The bleeding time is a test of primary hemostasis and is affected by platelet dysfunction and number and abnormal von Willebrand factor activity. Abnormalities in the extracellular matrix such as seen with Marfan syndrome can also prolong the bleeding time. Coagulation factor deficiencies do not affect the bleeding time.

2. **c. Factor VII** is part of the extrinsic coagulation pathway and its deficiency causes prolonged PT. The disorders in answers a, b, and d can prolong the activated partial thromboplastin time (aPTT). Factor XIII deficiency is not associated with prolongation of the PT or PTT.

3. **b. von Willebrand disease** is associated with prolonged aPTT. Bernard-Soulier syndrome, ITP, and TTP are associated with low platelet counts and not with disturbances in the PTT. Factor VII deficiency is associated with prolongation in the PT.

4. **b.** The neoplastic cells in Waldenstrom macroglobulinemia/lymphoplasmacytic lymphoma usually do not express CD5.

5. **c.** The **neutrophil's half-life** is 5 to 20 hours. This provides the basis for the daily granulocyte transfusions in patients who are febrile and not responding to broad spectrum antibiotics.

6. **a.** Most cases of Kikuchi disease are self-limiting and do not require treatment.

7. **e.** Increased methylmalonic acid is a sensitive test of cobalamin deficiency and is useful in early detection of vitamin B12 deficiency where levels of vitamin B12 are intermediate. Methylmalonic acid levels are normal in folate deficiency.

8. **e.** Bart hemoglobin, γ_4 is commonly seen in the neonates who have alpha thalassemia with the absence of two or more alpha globin chains.

9. **c. Hodgkin lymphoma** associated with HIV infection is of the classical subtype, most commonly of the mixed cellularity or lymphocyte-depleted forms, but occasionally the nodular sclerosis subtype. Almost all cases of Hodgkin lymphoma in HIV patients are associated with Epstein-Barr virus (EBV).

10. **c. Whipple disease** may be associated with peripheral and/or internal lymphadenopathy. The morphology is characterized by lipogranulomas with foamy histiocytes containing PAS+ cytoplasm. Nonnecrotizing (sarcoidal) granulomas may be present in some cases.

11. **d. Folic acid** is absorbed in the proximal jejunum.

12. **e.** The **mitochondria** in the developing erythrocytes are found in a perinuclear distribution resulting in a characteristic ring of staining by Prussian blue stain.

13. **e.**

14. **e.** RBCs carry out anaerobic glycolysis as they have no mitochondria in order to produce ATP, which, in turn, is necessary to maintain normal electrolyte composition in the intracellular compartment via Na^+/K^+ ATP-dependent pump activity.

15. **c.**

16. **d.**

17. **c.** Although a decreased MCHC can reflect a defect in hemoglobin synthesis, the **MCHC** is frequently normal in patients who have a microcytic anemia such as thalassemia minor. Defect in hemoglobin synthesis can therefore be seen in patients with MCH less than 27 pg or by the visual appearance of hypochromia. Decreased RBC count and hemoglobin level, although generally indicative of a hemoglobin synthesis defect, are usually late indicators of a synthesis problem and may not always reflect decreased hemoglobin synthesis such as in trauma or recent hemorrhage.

18. **d.** Coombs-negative anemia is nonimmune hemolytic anemia that should be investigated for possible glucose-6-phosphate dehydrogenase deficiency, paroxysmal nocturnal hemoglobinuria, red cell fragmentation, lead poisoning, hemoglobinopathy, and hereditary spherocytosis. Serum haptoglobin levels are helpful in determining if hemolysis is intravascular (undetectable haptoglobin level) or extravascular (normal haptoglobin level). Infection with mycoplasma may result in Coombs-positive hemolytic anemia.

19. **a. Acquired sideroblastic anemia** is associated with an abnormality in heme synthesis. Of the drugs listed above, only **chloramphenicol** interferes with heme synthesis via mitochondrial dysfunction.

20. **a. Staging of Hodgkin lymphoma** involves determining extent of lymph node and extralymphatic involvement along with clinical findings (weight loss, fever, night sweats). Radiographic studies are important for localization of disease. A minimum of two biopsies from each side of the iliac bones are required to evaluate bone marrow involvement.

21. **b.** Thalassemia minor may cause normal or increased iron with high iron stores. Iron-deficiency anemia will also result in low ferritin levels, while anemia of chronic disease will cause low iron and iron binding capacity with high ferritin and high bone marrow storage iron. RDW is usually normal in thalassemia minor. In comparison, sideroblastic anemia may have normal or increased RDW.

22. **b.** Thalassemia minor, repeated hemorrhages, and B12 deficiency although associated with anemia are not associated with decreased iron stores as reflected by normal ferritin levels. **Ferritin is almost always low in patients with iron deficiency anemia.** Sideroblastic anemias arise from secondary or primary mitochondrial defects, which cause abnormal heme synthesis and deposition of the iron in heme-containing cells. Prussian blue staining can demonstrate the deposition of iron in mitochondria. As a result of the formation of hydroxyl radicals through the Fenton reaction, cross-linking of the hydroxyl radicals to DNA, protein, and lipids takes

place, resulting in membrane and organelle damage and a resulting hemolytic anemia.

23. **d.** Of all the answers listed above, the disorder that is unlikely to have major deficit in cell lineage is **thalassemia minor**. Alcoholic cirrhosis is associated with B12 deficiency, and often macrocytic anemia, neutropenia, and thrombocytopenia can be present. Hematologically, folic acid deficiency can present in a similar fashion as B12 deficiency. Both hairy cell leukemia and primary macroglobulinemia are lymphoproliferative disorders and can affect the bone marrow, resulting in pancytopenia.

24. **c.** Thrombocytosis is associated with iron deficiency anemia in approximately 30% of cases, in nearly all postsplenectomy cases, and as a reactive process in pancreatic cancer. Because pyruvate kinase deficiency is often associated with splenomegaly, patients often have thrombocytopenia but can develop thrombocytosis postsplenectomy for life-threatening anemia.

25. **b.** Additional poor prognostic signs include age <1 year, hypodiploidy, and the translocations t(4;ll)(q21;q23) and t(1;19)(q23;p13.3).

26. **e.**

27. **e.** Any disorder that involves either bone marrow invasion or a brisk hemolytic process can result in a **leukoerythroblastic picture**; however, anemia of chronic disease (ACD), also called anemia of chronic inflammation, is usually associated with a mild to moderate normochromic normocytic anemia and variable presence of Pappenheimer and Howell-Jolly bodies. ACD is also associated with ineffective iron reutilization, which is evidenced by large deposits of iron in reticuloendothelial cells seen with Prussian blue staining. A recent key marker of ACD is hepcidin, which is produced in response to inflammatory cytokines. Hepcidin is thought to prevent ferroportin from releasing iron stores. However, in contrast to iron deficiency anemia, TIBC (total iron binding capacity) is usually low or normal with normal or high ferritin levels in ACD, whereas in iron deficiency anemia, TIBC is usually high with ferritin being low reflecting the bodies need to acquire iron.

28. **b. CMV disease** is the best answer, as viral suppression secondary to CMV can result in decreased platelet count. In all the other disorders, the platelet count is usually unaffected. Postsplenectomy usually results in a dramatic rise in platelet count.

29. **e. Heparin** accelerates the rate of inactivation of a number of activated clotting factors (such as IIa, Xa, IXa, XIa, and XIIa) by antithrombin III by causing a conformation change in antithrombin III. Thus, the presence of heparin in a citrated plasma specimen will inactivate thrombin, resulting in an apparent increase in the thrombin time.

30. **d.** Although high-performance liquid chromatography and isoelectric focusing or alkaline gel electrophoresis can demonstrate a fast-moving hemoglobin, the **Heinz body test** is required to demonstrate the unstable nature of hemoglobin H.

31. **c.** Patients with **cold agglutinin disease** commonly demonstrate a cold reactive IgM autoantibody, agglutination on peripheral smear, and a **direct antiglobulin test** that is positive for complement. Cold agglutinin disease comprises 16% to 32% of all autoimmune hemolytic anemias and is not associated with altered osmotic fragility, underlying hemoglobinopathy, or unstable hemoglobin. Howell-Jolly bodies are a sign of splenic dysfunction and are not seen in cold agglutinin disease.

32. **a.**

33. **b.** Patients with hereditary spherocytosis often demonstrate a compensated hemolytic anemia with increased reticulocytosis and increased indirect bilirubin. These patients may have an increased MCHC and increased number of spherocytes on peripheral smear. **Osmotic fragility testing** demonstrates osmotic fragility at higher sodium chloride concentrations upon immediate incubation of sample compared with controls. This difference in osmotic fragility is more marked upon 24-hour incubation.

34. **e. Increased plasma hemoglobin** is commonly seen in intravascular hemolysis.

35. **e.** Urobilinogen results from intrahepatic circulation of the breakdown products of bilirubin in the gut that is excreted by the kidneys and usually occurs as a result of chronic hemolysis. When **intravascular hemolysis** occurs, hemoglobin is released from red blood cells resulting in elevated plasma hemoglobin. Hemoglobinuria results when the hemoglobin (Hb) released into the plasma exceeds the binding capacity of plasma-binding proteins. Unbound Hb is reabsorbed into renal tubular cells, where iron is converted to hemosiderin. Hemosiderin appears in the urine when the renal tubular cells slough off and can be seen with chronic intravascular hemolysis. Elevated plasma hemoglobin causes marked decrease of haptoglobin because of the binding of hemoglobin to haptoglobin and subsequent rapid clearance and glomerular filtration and deposition of the hemoglobin in the proximal tubules. Plasma methemalbumin increases because there is increased release of oxidized heme from unbound plasma hemoglobin and binding to albumin.

36. **e. Pyruvate kinase deficiency** is associated with chronic, nonspherocytic hemolytic anemia.

37. **c. Paroxysmal nocturnal hemoglobinuria** (PNH) is suspected in patients who have unexplained normocytic anemia with intravascular hemolysis, especially if leukopenia or thrombocytopenia is present. The sugarwater test, which relies on the enhanced hemolysis of C3-dependent systems in isotonic solution of low ionic strength, is usually the first test performed and demonstrates high sensitivity. However, because this test is not specific for PNH, positive results require confirmation by flow cytometric testing or, alternatively, **the acid hemolysis test (Ham test)**, which demonstrates

hemolysis upon acidification of a blood specimen in the presence of a fresh source of complement.

38. b. **Methemoglobinemia** is a condition in which the iron within hemoglobin is oxidized from the ferrous (Fe^{2+}) state to the ferric (Fe^{3+}) state, resulting in the inability to transport oxygen and carbon dioxide. Clinically, this condition causes cyanosis and often results in dark or brown-colored plasma. In children, methemoglobinemia usually results either from exposure to oxidizing substances (such as nitrates or nitrites, aniline dyes, or medications) or is the result of inborn errors of metabolism (such as glucose-6-phosphate dehydrogenase [G6PD] deficiency and cytochrome b5 oxidase deficiency) or severe acidosis, which causes an acquired dysfunction of cytochrome b5 oxidase.

39. e. Elevated Hb A_2 is commonly associated with beta thalassemia trait. All the other answers are seen with alpha thalassemia minor.

40. a. The earliest B-cell precursors can be identified by **cCD22**. This is followed by the appearance of CD19 and CD10. The subsequent maturation and differentiation of the B-cell lineage is characterized by gradual decrease in CD10 together with gradual gain in CD20. CD38 is a lineage nonspecific marker of hematopoietic cells.

41. d. Hemoglobin H disease is associated with 20% to 40% Hb Bart at birth; however, by 1 year of age, there is only a trace of Hb Bart present.

42. a. Because hemoglobin Lepore is a result of an event that results in a crossover (knockout) of one of the β and δ genes, the expression of the hemoglobin A2 is decreased and not increased. Because the hemoglobin Lepore molecule is not well expressed in cells, it is difficult to detect early in life but does result in a microcytic anemia similar to beta thalassemia.

43. e. Hemoglobin F is a tetramer composed of two alpha chains and two gamma chains. Hemoglobin H disease involves a deletion of three of four alpha globin genes. The other diagnoses are not associated with a deletion of alpha globin genes. Elevated hemoglobin F is also seen in β thalassemia, sickle cell anemia, chronic myelomonocytic leukemia, and δβ thalassemia.

44. d. These numbers are important to remember because a ratio other than 60:40 may represent a transfused sickle cell disease patient or sickle beta (+) thalassemia.

45. e.

46. e. The RBC morphology in myelofibrosis includes all of the above except acanthocytes and also typically demonstrates teardrop cells. Acanthocytes are very rarely seen in normal peripheral smears and when seen in increased numbers, the diagnosis of abetalipoproteinemia should be entertained.

47. d. Unstable hemoglobins are associated with increased anisocytosis and poikilocytosis on peripheral smear. Because a hemolytic anemia is often involved, polychromasia (reticulocytosis) is often present. The Heinz body test is usually positive. Other tests that are used to evaluate the presence of an unstable hemoglobin include the isopropanol stability test and the heat stability test.

48. c. Schistocytes are usually associated with microangiopathic hemolytic anemia.

49. a.

50. b. Hairy cell leukemia cells have a specific phenotype that makes the detection of leukemic cells easier. Cells are positive for mature B-cell markers such as CD19, CD20, and CD22. CD25 and CD11c are also positive. They also show bright CD45 expression and expression of surface immunoglobulins. CD5 is typically negative.

51. c.

52. b. These markers are also seen on monocytes. Choice "a" could describe the phenotype of either a monoblast or myeloblast, while "c", "d", and "e" could describe a myelocytic, metamyelocyte/neutrophil, and promyelocyte phenotype, respectively.

53. c. The cells seen in acute promyelocytic leukemia are characteristically HLA-DR negative.

54. e. Most reactive disorders have a platelet count $<1000 \times 10^9$/L and a normocellular marrow. Occasionally some cases will have a more severe thrombocytosis and a hypercellular marrow simulating a myeloproliferative disorder. Peripheral basophilia, bone marrow fibrosis, extremely high cellularity (90% cellularity), and a leukoerythroblastic peripheral blood smear are features which favor a neoplastic megakaryocytic hyperplasia. Essential thrombocytosis (ET, also known as essential thrombocythemia) is a rare chronic myeloproliferative blood disorder characterized by the overproduction of platelets by megakaryocytes in the bone marrow in the absence of an alternative cause. In some cases this disorder may be progressive, and rarely may evolve into acute myeloid leukemia or myelofibrosis. Other supporting features for ET included enlarged hyperlobulated megakaryocytes, however, basophilia and bone marrow fibrosis are not typical features of ET. Appropriate clinical findings are also required for diagnosis. Using in vitro culture of hematopoietic precursors, approximately 75% of patients with ET will demonstrate spontaneous megakaryocytic and/or erythroid colony formation with the need for added growth factors. This is almost never seen in patients with reactive thrombocytosis.

55. c. The 5q- syndrome associated with MDS is primarily a cytogenetic and clinical entity with a favorable prognosis. The risk to progression to AML, concomitant infection, thrombosis, and anemia are low. In an elderly female the presence of elevated platelet counts (generally $>1000 \times 10^9$/L), hypolobulated megakaryocytes, and a macrocytic anemia suggest the 5q- syndrome. However, it should be noted that none of the above features are specific to the 5q- syndrome.

56. d.

57. e. NK cells are surface CD3−; however, these cells express CD3ε chains in the cytoplasm and therefore can-

not be distinguished on paraffin sections using paraffin resistant polyclonal anti-CD3 antibodies.

58. **c.** A predominance of myelocytes is seen in this disorder. All stages of the myeloid series are seen with peaks in the neutrophil and myelocytes stages.

59. **a. Pseudo Pelger-Hüet cells** can be seen in a variety of conditions, including trisomy 18, myxedema associated with panhypopituitarism, vitamin B12 and folate deficiency, multiple myeloma, malaria, muscular dystrophy, and leukemoid reactions secondary to bone metastases. This condition should be distinguished from the clinically innocuous Pelger-Hüet anomaly. **Iron deficiency** can be associated with thrombocytosis and often presents with a hypochromic microcytic anemia.

60. **a. CD3+, CD4+** cells account for approximately 55% to 65% of peripheral blood T cells.

61. **e.**

62. **c.** The nuclei in AML–M1 have one or more distinct nucleoli.

63. **d.** The peripheral blood findings are usually similar to other cases of AMML. Despite the presence of eosinophils in the bone marrow, only occasional cases display abnormal and increased eosinophils in the peripheral blood.

64. **d.**

65. **b.**

66. **a.** Greater than 30% myeloblasts are necessary to define AML–M6.

67. **e.** If the anemia is very mild or in the quiescent stage, the hemolytic anemia may present as a normocytic normochromic anemia with only mild RBC abnormalities.

68. **e.** The peripheral smear findings in sickle cell disease include anisocytosis, poikilocytosis, reticulocytosis, polychromasia, target cells, sickle cells, "boat-shaped" cells, and red cell fragments. However, because of the high level of hemoglobin F in the first months of life, these findings may not always be present.

69. **c.** The **sickle solubility test** detects the presence of a sickling hemoglobin and is positive in HbAS, HbSS, or HBS/$^{b+/0}$-thalassemia, where the level of hemoglobin S is greater than 10%. It is also positive in the rare sickling variants which have both the hemoglobin S beta globin gene mutation and other mutations such as hemoglobin C Harlem. False positives can occur in any

condition which results in increased plasma turbidity such as elevated WBC count, hyperproteinemia or hyperlipidemia. A positive sickling test needs to be confirmed by definitive testing.

70. **a.**

71. **d.** This is a molecularly confirmed **beta-thalassemia heterozygote.** Microcytosis, teardrop cells, and ovalocytes, rare target cells are most consistent with beta thalassemia.

72. **d.**

73. **c.** The table below describes the various platelet aggregation patterns seen in select disorders.

74. **c. Hemoglobin SG** can pose a diagnostic challenge since both an alpha and beta chain variant are seen. In the absence of significant levels of hemoglobin F, this should create four separate peaks or bands on HPLC, isoelectric focusing gel, capillary zone, or hemoglobin gel electrophoresis.

75. **d.**

76. **e.**

77. **b.** Answer b is the most correct because of the lack of enlargement of the infected RBCs and lack of Schüffner's stippling. This would eliminate *Plasmodium vivax* and *Plasmodium ovale.* The answer is most likely *Plasmodium malaria* because *Plasmodium falciparum* is usually associated with fine ring forms and the characteristic "banana" shaped gametocytes. Babesiosis would have many smaller ring forms infecting single RBCs, some demonstrating a "Maltese cross" formation.

78. **a.** The RBC inclusions are **Pappenheimer bodies,** which are iron-staining granules often seen as clumps at the periphery of the RBC. These are seen in sideroblastic and megaloblastic anemias, following splenectomy, alcoholism, and some hemoglobinopathies.

79. **c.**

80. **d.** The findings in Figure 16.10 demonstrate the "blister" and "bite" RBCs typically seen in G6PD deficiency, which is often seen in male patients of Mediterranean, Asian, or African descent. It should be noted that this picture is consistent with recent exposure to medications (including high dose vitamin C) that can create an overwhelming oxidative RBC stress. Bite cells, polychromasia, anisocytosis, and poikilocytosis can also be seen in a patient with methemoglobinemia. This can be

Disorder	Collagen	Epinephrine	1° ADP	2° ADP	Arachidonic acid
Glanzmann thrombocytopenia	↓ or absent	↓ or absent	↓ or absent	↓ or absent	↓ or absent
Aspirin, NSAID, and aspirin-like defects	↓ or absent	↓	Normal	↓↓	↓ or absent
Storage pool disease	↓ or absent	↓ or absent	Normal	↓	↓ or absent
Von Willebrand disease	Normal	Normal	Normal	Normal	Normal
Bernard Soulier disease*	Normal	Normal	Normal	Normal	Normal

* ↓ or absent ristocetin response

distinguished from G6PD deficiency by the appearance of brownish appearing blood, because of ingestion of medications that cause methemoglobinemia and cyanosis in the patient. Peripheral blood smear findings in pyruvate kinase deficiency (which is autosomal recessive in inheritance and commonly seen in patients of Northern European descent) include ovalocytes, elliptocytes and poikilocytosis prior to splenectomy and prominent echinocyte formation with a tendency toward macrocytosis after splenectomy. Patients with thalassemia major have marked anisocytosis, marked poikilocytosis, marked polychromasia, increased NRBCs, target cells and tear drop cells (especially beta thalassemia major). Hexokinase deficiency is also often seen in patients of Northern European decent with a peripheral blood picture indistinguishable from pyruvate kinase deficiency.

81. **d.** The very fast-moving peak is hemoglobin H (Hb H). Because it is composed of four beta globin chains, it has a very fast migration on alkaline gel electrophoresis, capillary zone electrophoresis, and HPLC. Hb H is the result of the loss of three alpha globin chains and can be detected using an assay such as a Heinz body test that detects unstable hemoglobin. Hb H has a high affinity for oxygen and is not subject to the Bohr effect; therefore, Hb H inadequately supplies oxygen to the tissues under physiologic conditions. Patients with significant levels of Hb H have a defect in oxygen-carrying capacity that is more than expected on the basis of the Hb concentration.

82. **b.** Megadose vitamin C is another spurious cause of low B12 levels.

83. **e.**

84. **b.** Rituximab is a chimeric antibody that recognizes the CD20 molecule and is used in the treatment of B-cell non-Hodgkin lymphoma. Anti-CD20 therapy may result in altered expression of CD20 in the tumor cells. Thus, CD20 cannot be used to identify B-cell populations. In this context, B cells can be identified by expression of CD19 and surface immunoglobulin. They may also retain expression of CD10, CD5, and CD23.

85. **c.** Other conditions that can be associated with a macrocytic anemia include Diamond Blackfan anemia, liver disease, postsplenectomy, and myelodysplastic syndrome.

86. **c.** The dual CD3+ and CD19+ events are displayed in a diagonal manner typical of excessive spillover and undercompensation of the FITC emission that spills over into the PE channel (i.e., there is too small a proportion of the FITC signal subtracted from the PE channel). Undercompensation errors often result in overestimating the frequency of dual positive cells. Diagonal clustering indicates that there is a fixed proportional relationship between PE and FITC emissions in the cluster of event that is seldom a natural phenomenon. In this case, the CD3 FITC positive events erroneously appear as if it also bound the CD19 PE antibody.

Correct compensation would have removed the proportion of CD3 FITC signal that spillover into the PE channel resulting in this population appearing in the CD3 only right lower quadrant of the histogram. In fact, careful inspection of the histogram reveals a second minor compensation error resulting from excess spillover of CD19 PE signal into the CD3 FITC channel (note the slight diagonal appearance of the CD19 only positive cluster in the upper left quadrant); this error was not of sufficiently magnitude to interfere with accurate enumeration of the B cells in this example. This illustration also reflects the fact that FITC emissions spillover into PE channel detector is proportionally greater than PE spillover into the FITC channel detector.

87. **b.** Day 18 shows a degradation of the signal detected by only one of the four detectors (FL-1) and hence does not reflect global excitation or emission problems that might arise from a misaligned or failing laser or from a clog in the flow cell that disrupts the sample stream – laser alignment. These types of problems would result in signal degradation in all four channels and not just one. Degraded beads or bead prepared in an improper manner may result in suboptimal excitation and emission characteristics and also would be the expected result in a drop in MPC in all four detectors, not just one. The low bead intensity in FL-1 on day 18 points to either a problem with the optic filters that are placed within the FL-1 collection pathway to block out secondary carryover signals coming from fluorochromes, or may be due to a problem with performance of the FL-1 PMT detector. In this particular case, someone forgot to remove a filter that was placed in front to the FL-1 PMT the evening before that used a special protocol and different fluorochrome.

88. **b.** Of all the above possibilities it would be very unusual for δβ **thalassemia** trait to cause the degree of anemia that would result in hydrops fetalis since the predominant hemoglobin during pregnancy and at the time of birth is hemoglobin F, which is composed of a tetramer of two alpha and two gamma chains. The amount of these globin chains would be near normal levels in δβ thalassemia trait. Hematologic causes of hydrops fetalis due to impaired red cell production include parvovirus B19 infection, Diamond-Blackfan anemia, congenital dyserythropoietic anemias, and α thalassemia major. These conditions markedly decrease red cell production to the point that high output cardiac failure with generalized edema and extramedullary hematopoiesis result.

89. **c.** One should be aware that a lymphocyte count below 3000/μL are abnormally low in newborns and infants and, if persistent, should lead to investigation of underlying immunodeficiency. Typically there are more T cells than B cells in the peripheral blood of infants just as in adults, albeit with a slightly high proportion of B cells; this is just the opposite of what is depicted in the

illustrations. Therefore, there is severe depletion of both T helper (CD3+ / CD4+) and T suppressor (CD3+ / CD8+) rather than an increased number of B cells. Even though B cells comprised over 90% of cells in the sample, the absolute number of B cells is actually in the normal range for infants. T lymphopenia may be seen in a number of conditions including malnutrition and chronic steroid treatment. T lymphopenia is also characteristic of severe combined immunodeficiency syndrome (SCIDS) and patients with the complete form of DiGeorge syndrome (i.e., thymic and parathyroid hypoplasia/aplasia with immunodeficiency, hypocalcemia and congenital heart disease). In contrast, Bruton agammaglobulinemia is associated with a decreased number of peripheral blood B cells and normal number of T cells. CD3 delta chain deficiency is one of the molecular causes of the SCIDS; this could have been surmised in view of the manner of typing T cells in this case (i.e., use of anti-CD3 antibodies). This patient actually presented with *Pneumocystis jiroveci* pneumonia and was subsequently found to have a variant of SCIDS due to a genetic mutation leading to deficiency of the common gamma chain that makes up a component of several cytokine receptors (IL-2, IL-7, IL-15).

90. **a.** As a result of the hemangioma formation, there is marked consumption or **sequestration** of coagulation factors and platelets. Thus "a" is the incorrect answer.

91. **b.** The findings are characteristic of phenotype of **common childhood ALL** with increased number of cells in the blast window of the CD45/SS histogram (i.e., weak CD45 expression and low side scatter depicted in blue) that co-express CD19 and CD10 (right histogram). It is fairly common to have some peripheral blood contamination that accounts for the increased number of mature CD4 positive T cells in marrow samples that are bright CD45 positive (depicted in red in middle histogram, upper right quadrant); this should not be construed as indicating biclonal disease. While *B. pertussis* infection is associated with a marked peripheral blood B cell lymphocytosis, the B cells are mature with bright CD45 and absent CD10.

92. **b.** Peripheral smears in congenital dyserythropoietic anemia (CDA) type II show anisocytosis, poikilocytosis, teardrop cells, and basophilic stippling, all nonspecific findings, this is despite the binuclear and multinuclear **erythroblasts seen in the bone marrow.** CDA type II cells are strongly agglutinated by anti-i more so in comparison to newborn cells. There is excess binding of C3 to these cells which is thought to be related to decreased N-acetylglucosaminyltransferase levels. Congenital dyserythropoietic anemia (CDA) type I is a macrocytic anemia with megaloblastic changes in the bone marrow. Nuclear chromatin bridging is occasionally seen in bone marrow erythroid precursors; however, unlike CDA type II, the Ham test is negative. Unlike congenital dysery-

thropoietic anemia (CDA) types I and II, CDA type III inheritance is autosomal dominant. Patients with CDA type III exhibit a mild macrocytic anemia, negative acidified ham test, gigantoblasts in the bone marrow and do show strong reactivity to anti-i. There is no association of monoclonal gammopathy with CDA type III.

93. **c.** This case highlights several important points including: (a) the need for integrating blast morphology with immunophenotyping results; (b) CD markers are not entirely lineage specific; and (c) there is often limited aberrant lineage marker expression in many cases of acute leukemia that should not be construed as indicating true biphenotypic acute leukemia. CD markers vary in their relative strength for assigning lineage. This led to the development of a grading system that recognizes some markers, such as intracellular myeloperoxidase (myeloid); cCD3 (T lymphocytic); and cCD22, cIgM, and surface CD79a (B lymphocytic) which are highly predictive of lineage. These makers are each assigned a score of 2.0 in a system that requires a minimal cumulative expression score of 2.5 or higher for conclusively assigning that lineage to the leukemia. Other B lymphocyte markers (e.g., CD19, CD10, CD20); T lymphocyte markers (e.g., CD2, CD5, CD8); and myeloid markers (e.g., CD117, CD13, CD33, and CD65) are less specific, and each assigned values of 1.0. Tdt (lymphoid); CD24 (B lymphocyte); CD7 and CD1a (T lymphocytic); CD14, CD15, CD64 (myeloid) markers have more limited specificity and each assigned scores of 0.5 in the scoring system. The morphology of the illustrated leukemia shows mainly **L1 type lymphoblasts.** The presence of CD19, CD10, and Tdt (cumulative score 2.5) and blast morphology are sufficient for assigning B precursor status to this case. Approximately 20% of B precursor ALL cases aberrantly coexpress myeloid markers such as CD33 and CD15 that together are not sufficient for meeting criteria for biphenotypic leukemia. Bilineal leukemia has two different cell lines, each of different lineage. Though the histograms are not displayed in a manner that shows coexpression of the myeloid markers CD15 and CD33 on the same cells as CD19 and CD10, it is clear that all the blasts express all four markers.

94. **e. Transient erythroblastopenia** of childhood is a self-limited normocytic normochromic anemia characterized by a history of a prior viral illness, reticulocytopenia, normal RBC adenosine deaminase levels. Platelet counts and WBC counts are usually normal in these patients. Median age at diagnosis is 40 months. Treatment is largely supportive with only RBC transfusions if cardiovascular compromise is imminent. **Steroids have no role** in the treatment. Prognosis is usually excellent in these patients.

95. **e.** Diamond Blackfan anemia is a congenital bone marrow failure syndrome characterized by a normo-

cytic, though often macrocytic, anemia associated with reticulocytopenia with thrombocytopenia and leukopenia often seen. Physical abnormalities are seen in approximately 24% of patients and largely involve the head and face. Approximately 25% percent of patients are noted to have a mutation in the DBA1 gene encoding ribosomal protein S19, and many patients are characterized by an elevated RBC adenosine deaminase activity. **Treatment largely involves RBC transfusions and steroids**, rarely bone marrow transplantation. Of concern is an increased risk of solid tumor and hematologic malignancies in those patients who reach adulthood.

96. **e. Dyskeratosis congenita** (DKC) is a rare form of ectodermal dysplasia and is characterized by dermatologic manifestations and nail dystrophies beginning in the first decade of life and leukoplakia in the second decade of life. Aplastic anemia occurs in one half of patients usually in the second decade of life with cancer developing in 10% by the third and fourth decades. From a hematologic view, thrombocytopenia or anemia is often first seen, followed by pancytopenia. Macrocytosis and elevation of hemoglobin F levels are commonly seen. Inheritance is primarily **X-linked**, although autosomal recessive and rarely autosomal dominant cases have been reported. Patients with DKC have reduced telomerase activity and abnormally short tracts of telomeric DNA compared with normal controls.

97. **e. Congenital amegakaryocytic thrombocytopenia** is a rare bone marrow failure syndrome expressed in infancy that is characterized by profound thrombocytopenia and megakaryocytopenia without physical abnormalities. Mutations in the *c-mpl* gene that result in incomplete formation of the thrombopoietin receptor are felt to be the molecular basis for the disease. Elevated thrombopoietin levels, although not specific to this disease, are typically elevated. Aplastic anemia may eventually develop in these patients. Bone marrow transplantation is the only cure for the disease, and patients require platelet transfusions for survival.

98. **c. CLL** cells characteristically express dim CD20 and CD5 but are negative for CD10. Similarly, mantle cell lymphoma cells express bright CD20 and CD5 but are also negative for CD10. Follicular center cell lymphomas characteristically express CD10 and CD20 but lack CD5.

99. **c.** Detection of EBV can be accomplished by immunohistochemical staining (latent membrane protein-1, LMP-1) or in situ hybridization (EBER).

100. **e.** Cyclic neutropenia is an autosomal dominant disorder characterized by 21-day cycles of repetitive neutropenia. Mutations of the *ELA2* gene usually occur at the active site of the neutrophil elastase and do not disrupt the enzymatic activity. However, the mutations affect the transmembrane domain and result in excessive granular accumulation of elastase and defective membrane localization. Myeloid precursors are associated with cycling increases in apoptosis. Kostmann syndrome is a congenital neutropenia associated with profound neutropenia, recurrent life-threatening infections and maturation arrest at the promyelocytic/myelocytic differential stage. Myelokathexis is a rare autosomal dominant disorder with recurrent bacterial infections caused by qualitative and quantitative defects of neutrophils. WHIM syndrome (warts, hypogammaglobulinemia, infections, and myelokathexis) is thought to be caused by mutation in the *CXCR4* gene which results in enhanced retention within the bone marrow. **Glycogen storage type Ib**, not Ia, is associated with an isolated neutrophils production defect.

101. **a. Thrombocytopenia with absent radii** is an inherited bone marrow failure syndrome that consists of hypomegakaryocytic thrombocytopenia and bilateral radial aplasia. Marrow CFU-Meg progenitors are for the most part reduced or absent. Thrombopoietin levels are consistently elevated. Almost all patients are diagnosed in the neonatal period. Diagnosis is based on physical findings, blood counts, and skeletal surveys. The MYH9-associated familial macrothrombocytopenia is characterized by autosomal dominant inheritance, large platelets, mild to moderate thrombocytopenia, normal megakaryocytic precursors, and variable platelet aggregation/secretion defects.

102. **a.** The majority of patients will only show skin involvement. 10% to 20% may have involvement of bone marrow (systemic mastocytosis). Any tissue may be involved, but the most commonly infiltrated organs include the lymph nodes, spleen, liver, and gastrointestinal tract.

103. **b.** Sideroblastic anemias can also be congenital and in this setting are **characterized by microcytosis**, ringed sideroblasts seen in late erythroblasts, normal RBC coproporphyrins and porphyrins, and normal chromosomes with defects often seen in relatives.

104. **a. Mucopolysaccharidoses** such as Hunter and Hurler syndromes often have extreme azurophilic granulation seen in the granulocytes, eosinophils and basophils. This granulation should be distinguished from the granulation seen commonly in cells of the myeloid series.

105. **e.** The serologic test that defines PCH is the **Donath-Landsteiner test** which allows detection of the biphasic hemolysin that is characteristic of this disease. Answers "a" through "d" are not unique to PCH.

106. **e.** The angle of the spreading must be modified depending on the hemoglobin level, especially if there is severe anemia or polycythemia. For example, a lower hemoglobin requires a higher angle of spreading.

107. **b.** This explains why there are four band/peaks with hemoglobin SG since both an alpha and beta chain variant are present.

108. **d.**

109. d. The DNA content histograms show 2 G0/G1 peaks indicative of a **DNA aneuploid leukemia with hyperdiploidy** (>1.16 DNA content). Hyperdiploidy is correlated with improved prognosis even when corrected for clinical risk categories of age and WBC. The ploidy pattern also correlates well with the presence of triple trisomies of chromosomes 4, 10, and 17 as well as other gains by cytogenetic karyotyping. New protocols have reduced intensity of treatment for patients with hyper diploid leukemia. The prognostically favorable TEL;AML t(12;21) and the very unfavorable t(4:11) translocations with MLL rearrangements are typically not found in hyperdiploid leukemias.

110. b. The picture demonstrates **hemoglobin Bart's,** which is composed of four gamma chains and is seen early on in life because of the abundance of hemoglobin F and the loss of alpha globin chains. Degraded hemoglobin A would be much closer to the parent hemoglobin peak. The following table describes the various percentages of hemoglobins seen in alpha thalassemia.

111. e. The typical clinical presentation is that of a pancytopenia, splenomegaly and 1–5% of "hairy cells" on peripheral smear. Flow cytometric immunophenotyping usually reveals strong CD20 and CD11c staining along with CD25 and CD103 positivity.

112. c. **Oxidative burst defect** is associated with chronic granulomatous disease. Diagnosis of LAD type I is made by flow cytometry. Because CD18b is a component of MAC-1, there is deficiency of C3bi receptor which prevents granulocytes and monocytes from binding C3bi opsonized particles.

113. e. **Stem cell transplantation** is the only known cure for this disease.

114. e. **Myeloperoxidase deficiency** is the most common inherited deficiency of neutrophil function and is seen in 1 in 2000 individuals with partial deficiency and complete deficiency in 1 in 4000 individuals. Myeloperoxidase deficiency can also be acquired and is rarely seen in AML-M2, M3, and M4. It is seen in 25% of patients with CML and myelodysplasia (with excess blasts). This disorder can be demonstrated by flow cytometry, and some cell counters may erroneously identify patients as being neutropenic because of the use of peroxide stain that is used to identify neutrophils. MPO-deficient neutrophils have increased respiratory burst in contrast to CGD. The mutations in CGD involve gp91^{PHOX} (64%); p22^{PHOX} (7%); p47^{PHOX} (23%); and p67^{PHOX} (6%) proteins.

115. e. Langerhans cell histiocytosis (LCH) is a **disease of young children** with a peak occurrence between 1 and 3 years of age with an incidence of approximately 0.9 per 100,000. At the time of diagnosis, a complete work-up should be performed to determine the full extent of the disease as the disorder can present in a multifocal manner.

116. c.

117. e. Because the defect is in the platelet GPIbα, treatment of bleeding disorders should include **platelet transfusions**.

118. c. Wiskott-Aldrich syndrome is characterized on peripheral smear by **small platelets**. Platelet aggregation studies demonstrate variable aggregation defects to a variety of agonists.

119. e.

120. b. The clinical history is typical of **mycosis fungoides** (MF) that has evolved to Sézary syndrome (SS)-like condition. The illustration depicts a cerebriform lymphocyte characteristic of this condition. MF/SS is a clonal T cell disorder with cells that typically express a helper phenotype (CD4+) with aberrant loss of CD7 and that express TCR alpha/beta protein on their surface; as such, cells have rearranged TCR α/β genes.

121. d. **von Willebrand disease type 2N** is characterized by abnormal binding of von Willebrand factor to factor VIII. This results in marked decreased in the circulatory half-life of factor VIII. Type 2N also has an autosomal recessive inheritance pattern. Thus, if family history is inconsistent with an X-linked pattern of inheritance, von Willebrand disease type 2N should be considered.

Clinical Syndrome	Genotype	Features	Hemoglobin Pattern-Newborn	Hemoglobin Pattern- >1 yr
Hydrops fetalis	−−/−−	Fetal or neonatal death	Hb Bart's >80%. Hb H, Hb Portland	
Hb H disease	−−/−α (−−/αα^{CS})	Chronic hemolytic anemia	Hb Bart's 20–40%. Hb CS present	5–30% Hb Bart's ± trace (Hb CS 2–3%)
Thalassemia minor	−−/αα −α/−α αα*/αα*	Little or no anemia. Thalassemic RBC		
Silent Carrier	−α/αα (αα/αα^{CS})	None	Hb Bart's 1–2 % (Hb CS present)	None (Hb CS 1%)
Normal	αα/αα	None	Hb Bart's 0-trace	None

*nondeletion α-thalassemia gene; CS, Constant Spring

122. c.
123. d.
124. c.
125. e.
126. a.
127. a. **Protein 4.1** is associated with hereditary elliptocytosis.
128. b. **AE1** is associated with hereditary spherocytosis and southeast Asian ovalocytosis.
129. c. The presence of MPO, Lysozyme, CD33, and CD13 are characteristic of **AML**. AML-M0 is, by definition, MPO negative. M1 AML characteristically has blasts with lower side scatter (fewer granules), and they are typically CD34+. AML-M6 will have a predominance of CD45 negative erythroid cells and fewer intermediate CD45 positive blasts. AML-M7 is MPO negative and will express megakaryocytic lineage markers CD41 and/or CD61.
130. c. **Increased osmotic fragility** can also be seen with hereditary spherocytosis but the two can be distinguished by morphology, red cell indices, and red cell monovalent cation content. The dominant abnormality is increased passive influx of sodium ion.
131. e. Other signs and symptoms include vomiting; constipation; polyneuropathy; tachycardia; diarrhea; fever; seizures; and head, neck, and chest pain. Signs and symptoms of *cutaneous* porphyrias include light-induced skin lesions, hemolytic anemia, splenomegaly, and keratoconjunctivitis.
132. e. This case illustrates a cell functional measurement of flow cytometry commonly used clinically for detection of **chronic granulomatous disease of childhood**. The assay is dependent on neutrophil fluorescent shift due to NADPH oxidase converting a weakly fluorescent rhodamine to strongly fluorescent oxidized rhodamine when stimulated. The mother has responding (41%) and nonresponding (59%) populations of granulocytes typical of carriers of X-linked CGD. The proportion of responding and nonresponding granulocytes reflects the frequency of random inactivation of the two X chromosomes that occurs in females: the X chromosome that harbors the mutant allele for CGD is inactivated in 41% of the mother's granulocytes while the X chromosome that harbors the nonmutant normal allele is inactivated in 59%. One cannot conclude that the child had CGD, though the chances are about 50:50 that he/she was affected based on the mother's results alone. Unfortunately, the patient died before testing could be done. Autosomal recessive forms of CGD exist but they display uniform reduced granulocyte oxidase activity rather than bimodal patterns seen in female carriers of the X-linked from of the disease.
133. e. Ferrochelatase deficiency is associated with erythropoietic porphyria. Porphyria cutanea tarda and hepatoerythropoietic protoporphyria is associated with uroporphyrinogen III decarboxylase deficiency. Variegate porphyria is associated with protoporphyrinogen oxidase.
134. d. **Chronic renal insufficiency** can decrease δ-aminolevulinic acid dehydratase activity. ALD deficiency porphyria can be determined by urine measurement of aminolevulinic acid where it will be 3 to 10 times higher.
135. c. There is an **increase in aminolevulinic acid** in urine with this disorder. The most common type of porphyria, porphyria cutanea tarda, is caused by a defect in uroporphyrinogen decarboxylase. Symptoms are initiated when 75% of the enzyme activity is inhibited, and blisters and erosion on light exposed areas are common. There is increased uroporphyrin I in urine and isocoporphyrin in stool
136. d. Most patients present with stage I or II disease. The lymph nodes most commonly involved are cervical, axillary, or inguinal.
137. e. **Increased coproporphyrin I** levels are seen in urine.
138. e. **Only 50%** are detected electrophoretically. The diagnosis is established by measuring the oxygen dissociation curve and by DNA analysis.
139. a. **Hemoglobin M variants** are unable to carry oxygen, are not unstable, and are inherited in an autosomal dominant fashion, although spontaneous mutations are common. Heterozygotes are cyanotic without physical impairment.
140. e. **Monocytes** are not predominant in tuberculous meningitis but may be present in the first exudative stage.
141. c. **Phagocytosis occurs 4 hours** after introduction of blood into the CSF. Histiocytes are seen in approximately 12–18 hours and about 4 days lapse until hemosiderin granules are first seen. Later, hematoidin crystals can be seen. Histiocytes can be seen weeks to months later with engulfed hematoidin crystals and hemosiderin granules and can indicate a remote hemorrhage.
142. e.
143. c. The **Ham test is positive** in paroxysmal nocturnal hemoglobinuria (PNH), which can be distinguished from congenital dyserythropoietic anemia type II by a positive sugar water test. The best way to determine if PNH is present is by flow cytometric studies and DNA confirmation of PIG-A (phosphatidylinositol glycan complementation group A) mutations. PNH can present in a variety of ways, and thus is it important to suspect the disease as definitive testing is available.
144. c. This disorder is **more frequent in women**. Because protein S is a cofactor for protein C, deficiency either acquired or congenital is risk factor for its development.
145. e. **Aspirin** not only inhibits the arachidonic acid pathway of generation of thromboxane A2, it also inhibits other thromboxane A2-dependent pathways such as seen in the secondary wave by ADP and epinephrine and low-dose collagen.

146. e. The **reptilase is often prolonged** in dysfibrino-genemia. Immunologic assay of fibrinogen may be normal, while decreased levels of fibrinogen may be noted upon use of functional assays. Other important diagnostic testing includes fibrinogen immunoelectrophoresis; however, definitive diagnosis may depend on DNA analysis or biochemical characterization such as protein sequencing.

147. a. Factor XIII deficiency occurs when factor **levels are less than 1% of normal**.

■ Recommended Readings

Arceci RJ, Hann IM, Smith OP (eds). *Pediatric hematology*, 3rd ed. Oxford, England: Blackwell, 2006.

Kitchens CS, Alving BM, Kessler CM (eds). *Consultative hemostasis and thrombosis*, 1st ed. Philadelphia: WB Saunders, 2002.

Kölmel HW (ed). *Atlas of cerebrospinal fluid cells*, 2nd ed. Berlin: Springer-Verlag, 1977.

Nguyen DT, Diamond LW (eds). *Diagnostic hematology: A pattern approach*. Oxford, England: Butterworth-Heinemann, 2000.

Petz LD, Garraty G (eds). *Immune hemolytic anemias*, 2nd ed. Philadelphia: Churchill Livingstone, 2004.

17

Clinical Chemistry

Jude Abadie and D. Robert Dufour

■ Questions

1. Based on a normal distribution of quality control (QC) data, which description of a QC rule best represents imprecision? For each case, assume that the same QC material is used in one run.
   a. Three sequential observations for a QC specimen that exceed 2 standard deviations from the target value in the same direction
   b. 10 sequential observations that fall between 3 and 4 standard deviations above the mean
   c. Eight sequential observations that exceed one standard deviation in the same direction from the target value
   d. Six sequential observations that all fall exactly one and a half standard deviation below the mean
   e. Two sequential observations with a range of four standard deviations between the two values

2. The following Levey-Jennings chart (Fig. 17.1) represents the "low" glucose quality control whose mean has been established at 80 mg/dL (represented by the solid horizontal line). Values for 3 consecutive days of the run are indicated by the three asterisks. The dotted lines represent standard deviations (SD) above and below the mean and are labeled with the corresponding glucose

value in mg/dL in parentheses. What is the probability that the event below occurred by chance alone?
   a. 1:64,000
   b. 1:32,000
   c. 1:16,000
   d. 1:8,000
   e. 1:4,000

3. Which of the following is the best statistical test to determine if the null hypothesis is correct in stating that no significant difference exists between the variances for two study groups?
   a. Chi-square test
   b. F-test
   c. Analysis of variance (ANOVA)
   d. T-test
   e. Sign test

4. In a chronic hepatitis study, serum alkaline phosphatase (ALP) levels were reported for patients with inactive and patients with active disease. The variances are not significantly different from one another. This data appears as follows:

	Inactive Disease	Active Disease
Mean (IU/L)	90	140
Variance	15	20
N	10	20

Which of the following is the best statistical test to determine if the means are different?
   a. Unpaired t-test
   b. Paired t-test
   c. Gap test
   d. Linear regression analysis
   e. Confidence interval test

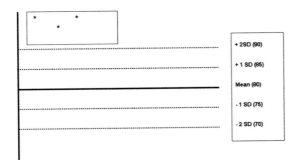

Figure 17.1

5. In Figure 17.2, the *x* axis represents results for a test, and the *y* axis represents frequency of individuals with the corresponding value. Changing the limit of normal values for the test from 10 to 20 (as indicated on the figure) would result in:
   a. Decreased specificity
   b. Increased negative predictive value and increased sensitivity
   c. Decreased false positives and decreased false negatives
   d. Increased false positives and decreased false negatives
   e. Decreased false positives and increased false negatives

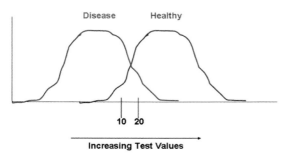

Figure 17.2

6. In which of the following common measurement variability would LEAST likely demonstrate a Gaussian statistical distribution?
   a. Aspiration volume
   b. Electronic noise in a measuring system
   c. Control material deterioration in storage
   d. Instrument temperature measurements over a 1-month period
   e. Precision study results

7. Which of the following statements regarding proficiency testing (PT) is considered to be an UNACCEPTABLE laboratory practice?
   a. PT should be used as a process of external evaluation of method performance.
   b. The laboratory should use an alternative approach to verify method performance when PT is not offered.
   c. PT data should be compared among laboratories using the same methods.
   d. If the primary facility analyzer is undergoing maintenance, PT surveys can be resulted and reported from testing conducted at a reference laboratory.
   e. PT allows for peer group evaluation.

Questions 8–10:

A new test is developed to test for an inherited metabolic disease. The disorder is found in 1 in 10,000 newborn infants. The test was evaluated in 300 healthy newborn infants, and 6 had results that were above the normal upper reference limits. Of a series of 100 banked samples from children with the disorder, 95 had results above the normal reference limits.

8. The sensitivity of this test for the metabolic disorder is:
   a. 2%
   b. 5%
   c. 25%
   d. 95%
   e. 98%

9. The specificity of this test for the metabolic disorder is:
   a. 2%
   b. 5%
   c. 25%
   d. 95%
   e. 98%

10. The positive predictive value of the test when used to screen all newborns for the disease is:
    a. 0.0001%
    b. 0.5%
    c. 5%
    d. 50%
    e. 95%

Questions 11–13:

A study is done to evaluate three tests for diagnosis of a disease, as illustrated in the ROC curve in Figure 17.3. Test A is the currently established screening test, Test B is another test that has been proposed, and Test C is a new test developed in the author's laboratory.

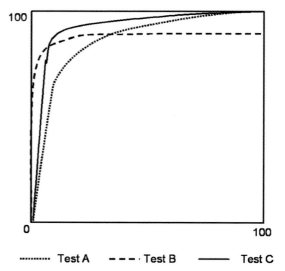

Figure 17.3

11. Which of the following statements is correct about this ROC analysis?
    a. False positive rate is displayed on the *y* axis.
    b. Predictive value is displayed on the *y* axis.
    c. Sensitivity is displayed on the *x* axis.
    d. Specificity is displayed on the *x* axis.
    e. True positive rate is displayed on the *y* axis.

12. In evaluating test performance, which of the following statements is correct?
    a. None of the tests appears to perform better than chance alone.
    b. Test A is more specific than either of the other two tests regardless of the decision level chosen.
    c. Test B would be a better choice for a screening test than the other two tests.
    d. Test B would be the best choice as a confirmatory test.
    e. Test C is more sensitive than the other two tests regardless of the decision level chosen.

13. Which of the following statements concerning use of ROC curves is INCORRECT?
    a. Area under the curve (AUC) is typically used to evaluate test performance, with higher numbers indicating better overall performance.
    b. For maximum diagnostic efficiency, the point closest to the upper left hand corner of the graph is used.
    c. If area under the curve is 0.60 (60%), this test is only slightly better than expected by chance alone.
    d. In comparing two tests, area under the curve is the best way to determine which test is better for screening or for confirmation of disease.
    e. ROC curves are prepared by determining the sensitivity and specificity of a given test at multiple cut-off points.

Questions 14–15:

A laboratory has purchased a new analyzer to measure α-fetoprotein (AFP). Thirty different samples are analyzed for AFP using the new analyzer and the old analyzer. The mean ± 1 SD for AFP using the new analyzer was 6.7 ± 0.7 ng/mL, and 6.1 ± 1.0 ng/mL using the old analyzer.

14. Which statistical test would be the best way to determine whether the means of the two methods were significantly different?
    a. Chi-square test
    b. F-test
    c. Kolmogorov-Smirnov test
    d. Paired t-test
    e. Unpaired t-test

15. Which statistical test should be used to determine whether the standard deviations of the two methods are significantly different?
    a Chi-square test
    b. F-test
    c. Kolmogorov-Smirnov test
    d. Paired t-test
    e. Unpaired t-test

16. To validate that a previously published reference interval is appropriate for the population served by a laboratory, which of the following criteria should be used?

    a. Ten apparently healthy individuals are studied; the range is appropriate if no more than one is outside of the published reference limits.
    b. 20 apparently healthy individuals are studied; the range is appropriate if no more than 2 are outside of the published reference limits.
    c. 30 apparently healthy individuals are studied; the range is appropriate if no more than 6 are outside of the published reference limits.
    d. 50 apparently healthy individuals are studied; the range is appropriate if no more than 10 are outside of the published reference limits.
    e. None of the above. Validation of reference intervals is not acceptable and a laboratory must always establish its own reference limits.

17. To establish a reference interval, assuming the results of the test have a Gaussian distribution (or can be transformed to a Gaussian distribution), how many individuals must be tested?
    a. 20
    b. 60
    c. 120
    d. 200
    e. None of the above. The exact number depends on the cost of the test reagents.

18. Upper reference limits for glucose and total cholesterol were established:
    a. As the 95th percentile of results from all apparently healthy individuals
    b. As the 97.5th percentile of results from all apparently healthy individuals
    c. As the 99th percentile of results from all apparently healthy individuals
    d. Based on outcomes data, at the point where risk of subsequent disease manifestations (diabetic complications, coronary artery disease) began to increase
    e. Separately by age (decades) at two standard deviations above the mean of individuals free from symptoms of coronary artery disease

19. For which of the following tests are reference intervals derived as the central 95% of results from apparently healthy individuals insensitive to disease-induced changes in a patient?
    a. Albumin
    b. BUN
    c. Free thyroxine
    d. Potassium
    e. Sodium

20. A test has reference intervals based on the central 95% of results from apparently healthy individuals. If a panel of 12 tests is run on a group of apparently healthy individuals, what is the approximate

likelihood that all 12 test results fall within the reference interval?
a. 5%
b. 25%
c. 50%
d. 80%
e. 95%

21. Which of the following tubes should be filled LAST during phlebotomy?
a. Blood culture tubes
b. EDTA (lavender top)
c. Nonadditive tubes (plain red top tubes)
d. Serum separator tubes
e. Sodium citrate (light blue top)

22. Prolonged use of a tourniquet would be expected to increase which of the following tests?
a. BUN
b. Calcium
c. Creatinine
d. Glucose
e. Sodium

23. Which of the following substances DO NOT show significant diurnal variation?
a. Creatinine
b. Glucose tolerance
c. Growth hormone
d. N-telopeptides of collagen
e. Osteocalcin

24. Which of the following tests should have lower reference limits during pregnancy?
a. Alkaline phosphatase
b. Creatinine
c. Estriol
d. Prolactin
e. Renin

25. During acute illness, increases occur in all of the following parameters EXCEPT:
a. Cholesterol
b. Cortisol
c. Glucose
d. Growth hormone
e. Triglycerides

26. Which of the following preanalytical variables is most likely related to specimen handling?
a. Drug regimen
b. Physical activity
c. Site preparation
d. Clotting
e. Body posture

27. Which of the following additives causes an increase in the corresponding analyte?

	Additive	Analyte
a.	EDTA	Iron
b.	Oxalate	Calcium
c.	Citrate	Amylase
d.	Fluorides	Alkaline phosphatase
e.	Heparin	Free thyroxine

28. Which of the following would have the highest inter- and intraindividual CV?
a. C-peptide
b. Calcium
c. Blood glycohemoglobin
d. Total protein
e. Plasma glucose

Questions 29–31:

A laboratory is evaluating a new method for measuring urea (BUN). A method (DXc) comparison study is performed comparing the new method (LXi) with an established method in the laboratory. The linearity of the two methods is up to 100 mg/dL.

29. The results of the two methods are compared using linear regression analysis, as illustrated in Figure 17.4. The equation for the regression line is y = 0.97 × + 2.9. Which of the following statements is correct concerning this correlation?

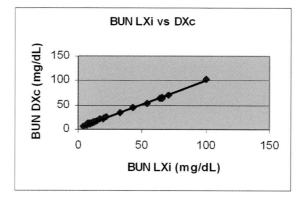

Figure 17.4

a. The correlation was done incorrectly; the new method should be plotted on the *x* axis, while the old method is plotted on the *y* axis.
b. The range of values indicated on the graph is inadequate to evaluate the performance of the new method.
c. The slope (0.97) indicates that there is no significant constant bias in the new method.

d. The spread of the points around the line is minimal, indicating that there should be a high correlation co-efficient for the data.

e. The y-intercept (2.9) indicates that there is no sig-nificant proportional bias between the two methods.

30. The correlation coefficient for the experiment, r, was 0.998. Which of the following statements is correct?
    a. The probability of a given X value accurately pre-dicting the corresponding Y value (within the range measured) is >99%.
    b. Since the r value was >0.9, it is not necessary to evaluate the method for constant or proportional bias.
    c. There is no significant difference between the re-sults using the two methods.
    d. The square of the r value, R, is a measure of average difference between the two methods.
    e. The low value for r (<1) indicates that there is poor agreement between the two methods.

31. The graph (Fig. 17.5) illustrates the difference between results of the old and new methods displayed as a func-tion of the value for BUN obtained using the current method using a bias (Bland–Altman) plot. Which of the following statements is correct?

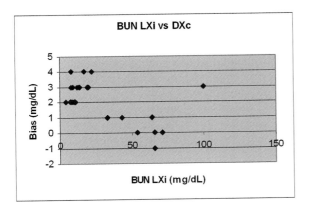

Figure 17.5

    a. There is a proportional bias between the new and old methods at values above 20 mg/dL.
    b. There is a constant bias of about 3 mg/dL at values below 20 mg/dL.
    c. There is a proportional bias of about 3% at values below 20 mg/dL.
    d. There is a constant bias of about 1 mg/dL at all values.
    e. There is a proportional bias of 2% at all values.

32. A clinician questions the results on an hCG value on a female patient. She had undergone D & C of a complete hydatidiform mole approximately six months previously, and had normal hCG levels at another

hospital; your lab reported an hCG of 240 IU/mL. The patient had gone to the other hospital for further treatment, but their laboratory had measured hCG as <0.5 IU/mL. A repeat sample in your laboratory one month later gave an hCG of 236 IU/mL, but was again negative at the other laboratory. By accident, a technol-ogist in your laboratory had also performed a PSA on the sample, and a value of 6.2 ng/mL was obtained. Which of the following is the most likely explanation for these values?
    a. Different calibrators are used by the two assays, and this represents common methodological differences in results.
    b. Heterophile antibodies are present and are causing false elevations of both PSA and hCG.
    c. The sample contains beta core fragment, which is not detected by all serum hCG assays.
    d. The sample contains free alpha subunits, a known cause for discrepant results in hCG assays.
    e. Tumor recurrence is present, and the tumor is also causing ectopic production of PSA.

33. Matrix effects:
    a. Are most commonly seen with chemical assays for substances such as glucose, urea, and electrolytes
    b. Are most commonly seen with tandem mass spec-trometric methods
    c. Can be prevented by using purified standards rather than calibrators for determining the relationship be-tween concentration and machine response
    d. Describes differences in measured concentration of a substance between samples of different composi-tion that actually have the same concentration
    e. Occur in most methods when aqueous controls are used to evaluate method performance

34. The Beer-Lambert law (Beer's law):
    a. Applies only to pure solutions and cannot be used in biologic samples
    b. Can be expressed by the formula A = abc, where A is absorbance, *a* is a constant for the compound, *b* is path length, and *c* is concentration
    c. Describes the direct relationship between amount of light transmitted through a solution and the concen-tration of a substance present
    d. Is used to determine the amount of current needed to produce adequate separation of compounds in an electrophoretic apparatus
    e. Represents the relationship between number of drinks and blood alcohol concentration

35. In evaluating method performance, which of the fol-lowing terms and corresponding method of determina-tion is defined INCORRECTLY?
    a. Carryover – running a low sample before and after a very high sample

b. Linearity – use of samples with known concentration and comparison of measured concentration to known concentration

c. Precision – multiple measurements of the same sample

d. Sensitivity – multiple measurements of the zero calibrator or standard

e. Within-run variation – comparison of results from the same sample over the course of 2 weeks, using the same calibrators

36. Coefficient of variation:
   a. Can be calculated by measuring samples from multiple persons used for reference range studies
   b. Defines the variation observed in a person over a period of time
   c. Is calculated as (standard deviation * 100)/mean value
   d. Should typically be about 5% for serum sodium
   e. Should typically be about 10% for serum glucose

37. Comparing nephelometry and turbidimetry, which of the following statements is INCORRECT?
   a. Both are most often used in the laboratory to measure antigen-antibody complexes to determine the amount of an antigen present.
   b. Both are typically performed on large analyzers used for routine clinical chemistry testing.
   c. In nephelometry, the detector is at an angle to the incident light.
   d. In turbidimetry, the detector is in a straight line with the incident light.
   e. Triglycerides are a major source of interference with both measurement principles.

38. A patient with metastatic prostate cancer has an initial PSA measurement of 345.7 ng/mL. After his first course of chemotherapy, a repeat sample has a PSA result of 952 ng/mL. The oncologist questions the initial PSA result. When the initial sample is retrieved (it had been stored frozen) and run in dilution, the PSA result on the 1:10 dilution is 1157 ng/mL, yielding an apparent PSA concentration in the initial sample of 11,570 ng/mL. The second sample is also run in a 1:10 dilution, with a result of 96.3 ng/mL. What is the most likely explanation for the initial result on the first sample?
   a. A high-dose hook effect was present, causing falsely low formation of antigen-antibody complexes in the presence of very large amounts of antigen.
   b. An inhibitor of PSA's enzymatic activity was present, but was removed by dilution.
   c. Heterophile antibodies were present in the initial sample, causing falsely low results, but the antibody was removed by sample dilution.
   d. The high enzymatic activity of PSA caused substrate depletion, which resulted in a falsely low activity measurement.

e. The technologist performing the initial run mixed-up the samples, and ran the wrong patient.

39. Which scenario is LEAST helpful in determining that a sample being tested for prostate specific antigen (PSA) is falsely elevated due to the presence of human anti-mouse antibodies (HAMA)?
   a. A 1:2 sample dilution gives linear and proportional PSA results.
   b. The PSA results from the sample are 10 times above the upper reference limit when using one method and not detectable when using another method.
   c. The use of an antibody blocking agent gives an undetectable PSA result on a sample that was previously elevated without the blocking agent.
   d. The sample is positive for interference using a PSA HAMA specific immunoassay.
   e. Medical records consistently indicate the patient's PSA is elevated due to HAMA.

40. Which instrumentation principle or use is INCORRECTLY described?
   a. Nephelometry is used to measure large particle concentrations.
   b. The principle of freezing point osmometry is related to the heat of fusion.
   c. Crystal scintillation is primarily used to detect beta radiation using sodium iodide crystals that contain thallium.
   d. Nuclear magnetic resonance spectroscopy is a technique for determining inorganic compound structures in a process that, like mass spectroscopy, destroys the compound.
   e. Capillary electrophoresis is a separation technique using a high voltage and electro-osmotic flow to move excess positive ions toward the cathode.

41. Which of the following statements about electrochemistry is FALSE?
   a. An ideal reference electrode should exhibit a potential that is constant with time.
   b. The calomel electrode makes use of sodium bicarbonate buffer and a gas-permeable membrane.
   c. The pH electrode is a glass electrode that measures hydrogen ion activity.
   d. The ion-selective electrode is an electrochemical transducer capable of responding to one specific ion.
   e. The polypropylene membrane is often associated with the PO_2 electrode and is effective in preventing blood constituents other than oxygen from passing through.

42. The phenomenon of electroendosmosis:
   a. Describes the faster migration of substances when increased osmotic activity buffers are used.
   b. Is the cause for the more anodal migration of immunoglobulins in serum protein electrophoresis.

c. Is caused by hydronium ions in solvents, attracted to the negative charge on the electrophoretic medium, moving toward the negatively charged pole in the system.

d. Occurs with all types of electrophoretic media.

e. Should be prevented by use of low osmotic activity solutes and nonaqueous buffer solutions to avoid artifacts of separation.

43. When proteins are denatured (such as by sodium dodecyl sulfate), polyacrylamide gel primarily separates them on the basis of:
a. Charge
b. Charge density
c. Degree of folding
d. Molecular length
e. Molecular weight

44. In agarose gel electrophoresis, all of the following are important in affecting the separation of substances EXCEPT:
a. Ionic strength of the buffer
b. pH of the buffer
c. Temperature of the system
d. Time of electrophoresis
e. Voltage applied to the gel

45. Which of the following is NOT a feature or benefit of point-of-care testing (POCT)?
a. Improved turnaround time for laboratory results
b. Less traumatic and less blood (for fingerstick systems)
c. Decreased manpower requirements in the central laboratory
d. Ease of use for serum or plasma
e. Built-in quality control systems

46. Which of the following is NOT a synonym or alternate name meaning point-of-care testing?
a. Ancillary testing
b. Decentralized testing
c. Distributed testing
d. Platform testing

47. Which statement LEAST describes point-of-care testing (POCT)?
a. The driving forces behind the use of POCT differ distinctly depending on the setting.
b. A significant potential benefit of POCT in the hospital setting is more rapid and (ideally) more effective assessment and management of critically ill patients.
c. POCT analyzers have less disposables and lower reagent costs than traditional laboratory systems and are therefore less expensive to operate.
d. The use of POCT systems is subject to regulations associated with the clinical laboratory testing.
e. Ultimate responsibility and control of POCT reside within an accreditation agency and require at least one laboratorian to be responsible for each POC program.

48. Which statement regarding clinical enzymology is FALSE?
a. Enzyme reactions generally proceed at zero order kinetics immediately following the lag phase.
b. When plotting a Lineweaver-Burk plot of a Michaelis-Menten enzyme in the presence of a competitive inhibitor, the value for 1/Vmax is constant for different concentrations of inhibitor.
c. In uncompetitive inhibition, the inhibitor binds only to the free enzyme and not to the enzyme-substrate complex.
d. ATP can serve as the rate-limiting step for coupled enzyme reactions.
e. When plotting a Lineweaver-Burk plot of a Michaelis-Menten enzyme in the presence of a noncompetitive inhibitor, lines of different slope correspond to different values of inhibitor concentration.

49. Which of the following statements regarding a specific enzyme is FALSE?
a. Acid phosphatase in serum is generally stable at all temperatures as long as the pH is above 7.
b. Lactate dehydrogenase is an example of an enzyme whose presence in plasma may indicate cellular damage.
c. The reference range for alkaline phosphatase is generally higher for children than it is for adults.
d. Alcohol dehydrogenase levels in the gastric mucosa of males are generally higher than in females.
e. Patients who have been at complete bed rest for several days generally have significantly lower values for creatine kinase.

50. Which of the following enzymes has the LOWEST red cell:serum activity ratio?
a. Aspartate transaminase
b. Alanine aminotransferase
c. Lactate dehydrogenase
d. Creatine kinase

51. Which of the following cholinesterase statements is FALSE?
a. Pseudocholinesterase can be used to monitor exposure to cholinesterase inhibitors.
b. Organophosphate insecticides are irreversible inhibitors of both pseudocholinesterase and acetylcholinesterase.
c. Pseudocholinesterase measurement can provide a good assessment of liver injury.
d. Acetylcholinesterase can be identified in amniotic fluid from pregnancies with neural tube defects.
e. Pseudocholinesterase testing can be used to recognize genetic variants in individuals demonstrating apnea during succinyl choline administration.

52. A 34-year-old who is taking prescribed oxycodone for pain has a positive drug screen for opiate and

methadone. The confirmatory test is performed by a reference laboratory via gas chromatography mass spectrometry. This confirmatory test for opiates is positive for oxycodone, hydromorphone, and hydrocodone only (negative for methadone). The clinician taking care of the patient is concerned about possible interferences with the positive results and calls the laboratory to ask if the patient is taking other narcotics besides the prescribed OxyContin. Which of the following would be an INCORRECT statement about this case?

a. It is possible that methadone is not reported on the confirmation test because the scanning ion monitoring method is used, and a separate method may be used for methadone confirmation.
b. Methadone is likely the cause of the positive test result and is not likely interfering.
c. Hydrocodone and hydromorphone are metabolites of oxycodone.
d. Hydrocodone and hydromorphone are not likely to interfere with the methadone assay.
e. The patient is taking another drug besides oxycodone.

53. An 18-year-old man was admitted with multiple broken bones, a punctured lung, and a ruptured spleen after an automobile accident. He was driving the car. A passenger in his car was also admitted to the emergency room; however, he died from multiple injuries shortly after admission. The police are waiting for the driver to recover because their intent is to arrest him for manslaughter for being under the influence of alcohol and drugs at the time of the accident. A serum alcohol obtained at the time of admission was 11 mg/dL (110 mg/L), and a urine drug screen was positive for cannabinoids. Of the following, the best statement that can be made about the driver is that he is:

a. Under the influence of alcohol and marijuana
b. Under the influence of alcohol but not marijuana
c. Under the influence of marijuana but not alcohol
d. Under the influence of neither alcohol nor marijuana
e. None of the above

54. Which of the choices listed is the best method for collecting and storing a sample for forensic analysis to determine the possibility of ethanol and cocaine use? Assume proper chain of custody procedures is followed.

a. Whole blood collected in a red-top tube (no preservative) and refrigerated (4°C) for 2 months
b. Adipose tissue immediately fixed in formalin
c. Whole blood collected in a grey-top tube (NaF) at the time of death and frozen for 2 months
d. Whole blood collected in a red-top tube and stored at room temperature for 3 days
e. Serum or plasma that is immediately separated and frozen at the time of autopsy

55. Which of the following pharmacokinetic parameters is defined as the amount of an administered dose that gains entry into the systemic circulation?
a. Dose
b. Bioavailability
c. Volume of distribution
d. Clearance
e. Steady state

56. Which of the following drugs of abuse could be classified best as a tranquilizer?
a. Morphine
b. Diazepam
c. Phenobarbital
d. Cocaine
e. Phencyclidine

57. Which statement regarding a specific cardiotropic agent is INCORRECT?
a. Toxic effects of procainamide can include reversible lupus erythematous-like syndrome.
b. Digoxin slows AV node conduction.
c. Lidocaine is highly protein bound and therefore has a relatively long half-life compared with other cardiotropic agents.
d. Digoxin is an active metabolite of digitoxin.
e. Amiodarone functions mainly by blocking potassium channels in cardiac muscle.

58. Which of the following drugs can be monitored by inference through the measurement of caffeine?
a. Acetylsalicylic acid
b. Valproic acid
c. Carbamazepine
d. Primidone
e. Theophylline

59. Which of the following systemic effects (therapeutic or adverse) is matched INCORRECTLY for an opioid action?
a. Nervous – Euphoria
b. Pulmonary – Respiratory depression
c. Gastrointestinal – Constipation
d. Cardiac – Tachycardia
e. Endocrine – Increased ADH secretion

60. Which of the following compounds is most appropriate to detect cocaine use in a sweat sample?
a. Cocaine
b. Ecgonine methyl ester
c. Norcocaine
d. Benzoylecgonine
e. Ecgonine

61. Which of the following elements is INCORRECTLY matched with the corresponding toxicity description?
a. Aluminum – Proper kidney function plays a significant role in aluminum levels, returning to normal once exposure has ended.

b. Arsenic – Elemental arsenic (As°) is quite toxic.

c. Iron – Iron toxicity can include hepatic necrosis.

d. Lithium – Lithium toxicity can be associated with thyroid enlargement.

e. Lead – Lead toxicity often leads to inhibition of the ferrochelatase enzyme converting protoporphyrin IX to Heme.

62. Which of the following is NOT an ADH-deficient cause of polyuria due to water diuresis?
    a. Central diabetes insipidus
    b. Dipsogenic diabetes insipidus (excessive water intake)
    c. Gestational diabetes insipidus (excessive vasopressinase)
    d. Pituitary or hypothalamic infection
    e. ADH receptor mutation causing congenital nephrogenic diabetes insipidus

63. Which of the following neuroendocrine tumors would most likely be associated with gallstones, diabetes, diarrhea, and hypochlorhydria?
    a. Carcinoid
    b. Gastrinoma
    c. Insulinoma
    d. VIPomas
    e. Somatostatinoma

64. Which of the following assays generates the highest sensitivity for diagnosing a pheochromocytoma?
    a. Plasma-free metanephrines
    b. Plasma catecholamines
    c. Urine catecholamines
    d. Urine total metanephrines
    e. Urine vanillylmandelic acid

65. Which of the following disorders is associated with increased renin levels?
    a. Cushing syndrome
    b. Liddle syndrome
    c. Addison disease
    d. Primary hyperaldosteronism
    e. Dexamethasone-suppressible hyperaldosteronism

66. Which of the following causes of congenital adrenal hyperplasia is most likely to result in increased levels of 11-deoxycortisol?
    a. 21-hydroxylase deficiency
    b. 11 beta-hydroxylase deficiency
    c. 3 beta-hydroxylase deficiency
    d. 3 beta-hydroxysteroid dehydrogenase deficiency
    e. 17 alpha-hydroxylase deficiency

67. A 24-hour urine sample was submitted to the laboratory from a 32-year-old man who is being evaluated for a possible pheochromocytoma. The catecholamines that were ordered were determined to be 145 μg/day (reference range = 90–150 μg/day). The printout indicated that the creatinine was 0.5 g/day. Which of the following is most appropriate for the technician to take?
    a. Check the urine pH to verify that it has been acidified correctly (pH < 2).
    b. Report the catecholamines as grams of creatinine.
    c. Measure metanephrines and cancel the order for catecholamines.
    d. Request a plasma sample to obtain corresponding plasma catecholamine levels.
    e. Cancel the order and request a new 24-hour urine sample.

Questions 68–72:

For these questions, use the following reference limits: Total T4, 4.5–12.5 mcg/dL, Total T3 80–220 ng/dL, Free T4 0.7–1.7 ng/dL, T3 uptake 22% to 33%, TSH 0.45–4.8 mIU/L, thyroglobulin 2.0–35 ng/mL. Anti-thyroglobulin and anti-thyroid peroxidase <1.0 relative units, thyroid-stimulating immunoglobulin 70% to 130%.

68. A 53-year-old woman is admitted with hypotension, fever, and abdominal pain and is found to have a perforated colon. Because of concerns for coexisting thyroid disease, a full panel of thyroid tests was ordered, including total T4 6.7 mcg/dL, total T3 45 ng/dL, T3 uptake 28%, and TSH 4.4 mIU/L. The surgeon is concerned and has called for your assistance in interpreting these results. The correct interpretation would be:
    a. No interpretation is possible, since thyroid tests are always misleading in the setting of acute illness.
    b. The high ratio of T4 to T3 suggests early hyperthyroidism, and could be due to a TSH-producing tumor, since TSH is not suppressed.
    c. These results are typical for "euthyroid sick syndrome," or nonthyroidal illness, and do not indicate underlying thyroid disease.
    d. This patient likely has early hypothyroidism, and should have measurement of TPO antibodies.
    e. This patient likely has a decreased level of thyroid binding proteins due to the surgery, which causes the observed results.

69. A 35-year-old woman complained of feeling tired, and so had thyroid function tests ordered. Results included total T4 14.3 mcg/dL, total T3 280 ng/dL, T3 uptake 18%, TSH 2.5 mIU/L. Her primary care physician asked for your input in interpreting these results. The correct interpretation would be:
    a. A heterophile antibody is likely present, causing falsely increased T4 and T3 and falsely low T3 uptake.
    b. These results are typical for euthyroid sick syndrome, or nonthyroidal illness, and do not indicate underlying thyroid disease.
    c. These results indicate increased thyroid-binding proteins, most likely due to increased estrogenic effect; you are told the woman is taking oral contraceptives.

    d. This patient is hyperthyroid and further testing is required to determine the cause.

    e. This patient has hyperthyroidism that is likely due to a TSH-producing pituitary tumor.

70. A 75-year-old man presents with acute shortness of breath and is found to be in atrial fibrillation with a rate of 150 beats/minute. Thyroid function tests include free T4 of 1.6 ng/dL, Total T3 of 530 ng/dL, TSH <0.01 mIU/L. Thyroid peroxidase antibodies are 25.3 units, and thyroid stimulating antibodies are 420%. The most likely diagnosis is:

    a. Euthyroid sick syndrome (nonthyroidal illness)

    b. Euthyroid with increased thyroid-binding globulins due to medications

    c. Hyperthyroidism due to Graves disease

    d. Hyperthyroidism due to thyroid adenoma

    e. Hyperthyroidism from thyroid damage in Hashimotos thyroiditis

71. A 56-year-old woman was diagnosed with hypothyroidism after presenting with tiredness, cold intolerance, and weight gain; her initial thyroid function test results included free T4 of 0.3 ng/dL and TSH 75 mIU/L. She has started on thyroxine therapy and has repeated thyroid function tests performed 10 days later; free T4 is 0.5 ng/dL and TSH is 56 mIU/L. What is the most likely interpretation for these results?

    a. The patient is hypothyroid, but an inadequate dose of thyroid hormone was given, and the dose should be increased with repeat thyroid function tests performed in another 10 days.

    b. The patient is hypothyroid, but free T4 is not the correct thyroid function test to monitor treatment, since it is not the active hormone; free or total T3 should be followed instead.

    c. The patient is hypothyroid, but TSH is falsely elevated because of a heterophile antibody, and only free T4 should be used to guide treatment.

    d. The patient is hypothyroid, but repeat thyroid function tests were performed too soon after starting treatment; at least 5 to 6 weeks is needed to reach steady state on replacement hormone.

    e. These results indicate a high likelihood of interference from heterophile antibodies in both TSH and free T4 assays, and a repeat analysis after incubation with neutralizing mouse serum would likely result in normal results for both tests.

72. A 56-year-old man with papillary thyroid carcinoma had a thyroglobulin level (measured by competitive immunoassay) of 5.7 ng/mL after total thyroidectomy. A therapeutic dose of radioactive iodine is administered, and a repeat thyroglobulin measurement is performed 4 weeks later and is 5.6 ng/mL. A postablation radioactive iodine scan had been done after the treatment, and

no foci of iodine uptake were identified. What is the most likely interpretation of these results?

    a. An ectopic source of thyroglobulin is likely present; a search for another tumor should be performed.

    b. No residual thyroid carcinoma is present; these values are within the reference range.

    c. Residual thyroid cancer is likely present, and the tumor does not take up iodine indicating a poorly differentiated carcinoma.

    d. There was a remnant of normal thyroid tissue present after surgery that was not destroyed by the administered radioactive iodine.

    e. The persistent increase in thyroglobulin suggests the presence of thyroglobulin antibodies; if confirmed, thyroglobulin levels should not be done to follow the patient in the future.

73. Which of the following cardiac markers would best be used to identify plaque destabilization?

    a. Interleukin 6

    b. Soluble CD40 ligand

    c. Myeloperoxidase

    d. NT-proBNP

    e. Cardiac troponin I

74. Which of the following cardiac injury markers would remain elevated longest after an acute myocardial infarction?

    a. Myoglobin

    b. CK-MB

    c. Troponin C

    d. Troponin I

    e. Troponin T

75. Which of the following has the greatest CK-MB activity (i.e., IU/g)?

    a. Skeletal muscle

    b. Heart

    c. Brain.

    d. GI tract

    e. Lungs

76. Which of the following is the most accurate statement describing the recommended use of CK-MB or cardiac troponin (cTn) to evaluate patients presenting to the ER with chest pain?

    a. CK-MB is the reference biomarker for myocardial infarction detection and risk stratification in acute myocardial infarction diagnosis.

    b. In an acute coronary syndrome patient, three consecutive, nonfluctuating, elevated cTn results are diagnostic of acute myocardial infarction.

    c. The 99th percentile of troponin values from healthy adults is the generally accepted cutoff level used by most hospitals.

    d. CK-MB values greater than the 20% CV of the assay defines the reference range for a "normal" population.

e. cTn values greater than the 20% CV of the assay defines the reference range for a "normal" population.

77. Which statement regarding B-type natriuretic peptide (BNP) is most accurate?
   a. NT-proBNP and BNP are released from the cardiac myocyte in a 1:1 ratio.
   b. The circulating levels of NT-proBNP are generally lower than circulating BNP.
   c. NT-ProBNP is significantly more accurate in predicting heart failure than BNP.
   d. BNP levels are about equal for population-matched men and women.
   e. Measuring serum Prepro-BNP is a good predictor of heart failure within the subsequent six months for patients diagnosed with congestive heart failure.

78. Which of the following is directly measured/detected by the ischemia modified albumin assay?
   a. Albumin
   b. Copper
   c. Ascorbic acid
   d. Cobalt
   e. Superoxide dismutase

79. Which statement is FALSE regarding cardiac troponin I (cTnI) assays?
   a. The signal is determined by using a microparticle that fluoresces and sends a signal read by the instrument.
   b. Capture antibodies are designed to detect specific epitopes of cTnI.
   c. Capture antibodies are attached to the manufacturer's microparticles.
   d. Manufacturers use capture antibodies to improve cTn assay sensitivity.

80. Which of the following markers is present in skeletal but not cardiac muscle and can be used as a "negative" cardiac injury marker?
   a. Creatine kinase MB_2
   b. Heart fatty acid-binding protein
   c. Glycogen phosphorylase
   d. Myosin
   e. Carbonic anhydrase III

81. Which of the following would be best for assessing risk of coronary heart disease?
   a. Homocysteine
   b. High sensitivity C-reactive protein
   c. Cardiac natriuretic peptides
   d. Cardiac troponin
   e. Lipid profile

82. A 47-year-old motor vehicle accident victim with a history of hypertension is seen in the emergency room complaining of leg pain (due to crush injury), severe chest pain, nausea, and vomiting. ST elevation is seen in the lateral leads. He is noted to be hypotensive and

develops evidence of intestinal infarction. Which of the following creatine kinase (CK) isoenzymes would NOT be found in his blood?
   a. CK MM
   b. CK MB
   c. CK BB
   d. All of these would be present to some extent.

83. Figure 17.6 illustrates a tube of plasma after ultracentrifugation. Which of the following lipoproteins settles at the density indicated by 1.063 g/mL?

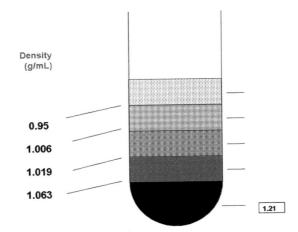

Density (g/mL)

0.95

1.006

1.019

1.063

1.21

Figure 17.6

   a. Chylomicrons
   b. IDL
   c. HDL
   d. LDL
   e. VLDL

84. In the figure of lipoprotein electrophoresis (Fig. 17.7), which letter correctly indicates the location of the lipoprotein with the shortest half-life?

   a. A
   b. B
   c. C
   d. D
   e. E

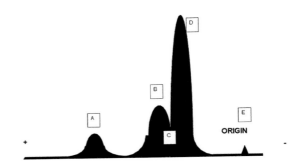

Figure 17.7

85. Which of the following apolipoproteins is associated with the largest lipoprotein and has also been associated with increased risk of coronary heart disease?
    a. A-I
    b. C-I
    c. D
    d. (a)
    e. E

86. Which of the following characteristics is true of Lp(a)?
    a. Prothrombotic lipoprotein that is homologous to plasminogen.
    b. Deficiencies are associated with reduced clearance of triglyceride-rich lipoproteins.
    c. Carboxy-terminal recognition signal targets LDL to the LDL receptor.
    d. Activates lecithin cholesterol acyltransferase, which esterifies cholesterol in plasma
    e. Associated with a risk of Alzheimer disease

87. Which of the following additives is best for assessment of lipid and lipoprotein levels using electrophoresis studies?
    a. Citrate
    b. Heparin
    c. EDTA
    d. Sodium fluoride

88. Which statement is FALSE regarding assessment of lipids?
    a. Cholesterol levels increase with age starting in early adulthood in both men and women.
    b. The levels of calculated LDL cholesterol and HDL cholesterol are not reliable after consuming a meal.
    c. The presence of chylomicrons after a 12-hour fast is considered abnormal.
    d. The National Cholesterol Education Program Adult Treatment Panel III recommends that patients be seated for 5 minutes prior to lipid sampling.
    e. Total cholesterol and HDL levels are always significantly altered in nonfasting (compared to fasting) individuals.

89. According to the Adult Treatment Panel III guidelines, at what LDL-cholesterol level should drug therapy be considered in an otherwise healthy individual whose risk category contains zero or one risk factors?
    a. 70 mg/dL
    b. 100 mg/dL
    c. 130 mg/dL
    d. 160 mg/dL
    e. 190 mg/dL

90. Which of the following best represents a disorder in which patients have both high cholesterol and high triglycerides?
    a. Diabetic dyslipidemia
    b. Familial combined hyperlipidemia (type 2B)
    c. Familial hypertriglyceridemia

    d. Lipoprotein lipase deficiency (hyperlipoproteinemia type I)
    e. Apolipoprotein C-II deficiency

91. Which of the following is FALSE with respect to testing for gestational diabetes?
    a. A 50-g glucose load is given for the screening test performed between the 24th and 28th weeks of pregnancy.
    b. A glucose level of 120 mg/dL 1 hour after initiation of the screening test indicates the need for the diagnostic test.
    c. A 100-g or 75-g glucose load can be given for the diagnostic test after a period of fasting.
    d. The diagnostic test is diagnostic for gestational diabetes if the fasting glucose level is 115 mg/dL and the 2-hour glucose level is 180 mg/dL.
    e. The diagnostic test is diagnostic for gestational diabetes if the 1-hour glucose level is 195 mg/dL and the 3-hour glucose level is 160 mg/dL.

92. All of the following statements about albuminuria are true EXCEPT:
    a. An albumin to creatinine ratio can be determined from an untimed "spot" urine.
    b. Microalbuminuria is an important clinical marker that is associated with risk of progressive renal disease in diabetics.
    c. Macroalbuminuria can be defined by the molecular weight of excreted albumin rather than the urinary excretion rate.
    d. Microalbuminuria can be defined as a urinary excretion rate between 30 and 300 mg/24 hours.
    e. The development of assays to detect total urinary albumin levels may lead to earlier identification of individuals at risk for diabetic nephropathy and cardiovascular disease.

93. Which statement about HbA1c is INCORRECT?
    a. Iron deficiency anemia is generally associated with decreased HbA1c values.
    b. The glycation process inside the red blood cell forms HbA1c without the use of enzymes.
    c. The Amadori rearrangement describes an irreversible reaction that forms glycated hemoglobin.
    d. The first step in forming HbA1c involves glucose reversibly binding to hemoglobin.
    e. Ketoamine (glycated hemoglobin) undergoes a spontaneous conformational change to for a cyclic glucose structure at physiologic pH.

94. Which of the following is more commonly associated with type 2 than with type I diabetes mellitus?
    a. Age of onset is most common in young children and young adults.
    b. Risk factors are more related to race/ethnicity.
    c. The pathogenesis is autoimmune beta cell destruction.

d. No known therapy or medications to prevent onset of diabetes.

e. Associated with very low or undetectable C-peptide levels

95. A 35-year-old man whose percent hemoglobin A1c (HbA1c) was 6.0% 2 years ago is reevaluated. It is determined that his current level is 8.0%. If his average plasma glucose level was 135 mg/dL when his HbA1c was 6.0%, what is his approximate current average plasma glucose level?
   a. 150 mg/dL
   b. 180 mg/dL
   c. 195 mg/dL
   d. 215 mg/dL
   e. 240 mg/dL

96. Which of the following is a ketone body present in the greatest proportion in diabetic ketoacidosis (DKA) but is NOT detected by laboratory techniques using nitroprusside reagents?
   a. Beta-hydroxybutyric acid
   b. Acetone
   c. Acetoacetic acid
   d. Fructosamine

97. A defect in which of the following enzymes can result in an X-linked glycogen storage disease (GSD) affecting hepatic glycogenoses?
   a Glucose-6-phosphatase
   b. GLUT-2
   c. Glycogen branching enzyme
   d. Glycogen phosphorylase
   e. Phosphorylase kinase

98. Which of the following statements is LEAST correct regarding hypoglycemia?
   a. Whipple triad refers to symptoms consistent with hypoglycemia associated with low plasma glucose levels and relief of symptoms when hypoglycemia is corrected.
   b. Pentamidine used for the treatment of *Pneumocystis carinii* pneumonia can cause hypoglycemia by damaging pancreatic beta cells.
   c. Individuals with autoimmune insulin syndrome demonstrate very low insulin levels after consuming a meal.
   d. Non-islet cell tumor hypoglycemia is mostly of mesenchymal origin.
   e. Widespread hepatic disease as well as severe cardiac failure can result in hypoglycemia.

99. In general, which of the following statements regarding tumor markers is FALSE?
   a. Knowledge that a tumor marker is present may cause worry and can therefore decrease the patient's quality of life.

b. A biomarker may be widely expressed in different tissue; however, serum concentrations may be elevated in only one or a limited number of malignancies.

c. Tumor markers can be described as the biochemical or immunologic serum counterparts that can represent differentiation of tumor states.

d. If the half-life of the tumor marker after treatment is longer than the expected half-life, it is likely that the treatment has not been successful in removing the tumor.

e. When establishing reference values for tumor markers, it is better to use the nondiseased healthy population rather than using a corresponding benign disease-based population.

100. In the following graph table, open symbols represent patient 1, a 42-year-old woman with a 1-cm, node-negative, well-defined, estrogen receptor-rich breast cancer. The closed symbols represent patient 2, a 42-year-old woman with a 1-cm mass, 3 of 15 positive axillary lymph nodes, poorly differentiated estrogen receptor-poor breast cancer.

Prognostic risk of development of recurrent or metastatic disease:	Local Therapy	Tamoxifen	Chemotherapy
Poor >40%	●	●	
Moderate 10% to 40%			●
Good <10%	○	○	○

Given the above information, which of the following statements is LEAST correct?
   a. Chemotherapy likely decreases the relative risk for patient 1.
   b. Chemotherapy significantly improves the prognosis for patient 1.
   c. Patient 2 is likely at a higher risk of recurrence and may have a lower chance of benefit from tamoxifen.
   d. For patient 2, the benefits of adjuvant chemotherapy likely outweigh the risks associated with treatment.

101. Which statement about cancer antigen (CA) 125 is FALSE?
   a. CA125 lacks sensitivity for ovarian cancer detection.
   b. In a patient previously diagnosed with ovarian cancer, doubling of CA125 levels in serum above baseline at any interval should prompt physical examination, sonography, and a computerized tomography scan.
   c. In postmenopausal women, CA125 may be useful in the differential diagnosis between benign and malignant pelvic masses.

d. Postmenopausal women have an elevatedCA125 level when compared with premenopausal women.

e. Serum CA125 may be elevated in other conditions including the first trimester of pregnancy and severe hepatic disease.

102. Which of the following serum assays is the best one to use as a screening tool for early cancer detection?
a. Prostate specific antigen
b. Carcinoembryonic antigen
c. Cancer antigen 15-3
d. BR27.29
e. Human chorionic gonadotropin

103. The National Academy of Clinical Biochemistry and the European Group on Tumor Markers established recommendations for using tumor markers to measure prognostic classification of metastatic germ cell tumors. Which of the following markers would LEAST likely be used as such an initial assessment of a germ cell tumor?
a. Alpha-fetoprotein
b. Human chorionic gonadotropin
c. Lactate dehydrogenase
d. Placental alkaline phosphatase
e. Carcinoembryonic antigen

104. Which of the following statements is true regarding the following two cases?

Case 1: A 25-year-old woman presented with irregular menstrual bleeding. Her hCG laboratory result was 175 U/L (upper limit of reference range = 5 U/L). Scans showed no indication of a tumor; however, she was diagnosed with cancer and started on chemotherapy. During the subsequent 4 months, her hCG levels from the same laboratory fluctuated between 175 and 200 U/L. Hysterectomy was performed, but the tissue indicated no malignancy. Levels of hCG remained elevated postsurgery. A suspicious spot was observed on a lung scan, and additional surgery revealed no evidence of cancer. A recheck of hCG was 180 U/L. This same sample was sent to a reference laboratory that used a different immunoassay, and the reported result was <5 U/L.

Case 2: The laboratory received a sample for CEA measurement from a 60-year-old woman. No clinical information was provided with the sample. CEA measured by an immunoassay was 4.8 μg/L (normal range <5μg/L). At a 1:2 dilution, the result was 17.3 mg/L. The result was reported as "appears normal but fails to dilute correctly." A further confirmatory test that was requested indicated with a second sample that indicated "known liver metastases" on the order form. The sample was further diluted and reported as 325,500 μg/L. The same sample was sent to a reference laboratory using a different method. Their report was 365,250 μg/L.

a. Case 1 likely indicates metastatic cancer to the lung, and Case 2 likely indicates metastatic cancer to the liver.
b. Case 1 and Case 2 both likely represent noncancerous conditions.
c. Case1 likely indicates a high-dose hook effect and Case 2 likely indicates a heterophilic antibody.
d. Case 1 likely indicates a heterophilic antibody and Case 2 likely indicates a high-dose hook effect.
e. Case 1 likely indicates a heterophilic antibody and Case 2 likely indicates a human mouse antibody.

105. A mutation in which of the following is considered the most frequent known genetic alteration in all human cancers?
a. p53
b. erbB2
c. Tropomyosin
d. dsDNA
e. MUC1

106. Which of the following is LEAST likely to increase serum levels of prostate specific antigen?
a. Physical activity
b. Benign prostatic hyperplasia
c. Prostatitis
d. Ejaculation
e. Finasteride

107. Which of the following intracranial germ cell tumors is associated with a cerebrospinal fluid increase in the corresponding marker?
a. Teratoma – Alpha-fetoprotein
b. Choriocarcinoma – Beta-human chorionic gonadotrophin
c. Endodermal sinus tumor – Placental alkaline phosphatase
d. Germinoma – Alpha-fetoprotein
e. Embryonal carcinoma – Placental alkaline phosphatase

108. A 28-year-old woman delivered a 9.5-pound infant. The infant was in the 95th percentile for weight and length. Shortly after birth, the infant became lethargic and flaccid. Upon further investigation, it was determined that the mother did not receive regular medical care during pregnancy; therefore, her history was incomplete. However, during week 26 of pregnancy, the mother's whole blood glucose was 130 mg/dL and her plasma glucose was 140 mg/dL. These two results were exactly reproduced during week 27 of pregnancy. Which of the following statements is LEAST correct about this case?
a. The mother is diabetic.
b. The neonate had stimulated insulin secretion.
c. The infant developed hypoglycemia after the cord was cut.
d. The mother has a 50% increased lifetime risk for developing diabetes.

e. The whole blood and plasma glucose should be retested due to the discrepancy between them.

109. A 29-year-old woman in her 33rd week of pregnancy presents with hypertension, proteinuria, and pitting edema. She experienced a 5-pound weight gain in the past week. Her blood pressure was about 145/95 mm Hg on three separate readings. A 2+ proteinuria was determined by dipstick and sulfosalicylic acid precipitation. No casts or RBCs were noted in the urine. Her laboratory results were as follows:

Analyte/Units	Patient's Result	Reference Range for Healthy Nonpregnant Women
Serum BUN (mg/dL)	18	7–18
Creatinine (mg/dL)	1.2	0.5–1.2
Uric acid (mg/dL)	6.5	3–8
AST (U/L)	100	8–20
ALT (U/L)	150	8–20
Alk Phos (U/L)	150	20–70
GGT (U/L)	30	3–35
Bilirubin	Normal	

Which of the following statements is LEAST correct about this case?
a. The BUN, creatinine, and uric acid values are normal for pregnancy.
b. There may be mild periportal (zone 1) necrosis.
c. The patient has preeclampsia.
d. Albumin is mainly being lost in the urine.
e. The elevated alkaline phosphatase is expected and does not indicate liver disease.

110. Of the following individuals seen in clinic on one given day, who should NOT be screened for gestational diabetes at this time?
a. A 22-year-old obese woman in her 25th week of pregnancy
b. A 23-year-old athletic woman in her 22nd week of pregnancy with a family history of gestational diabetes
c. A 25-year-old athletic woman in her 27th week of pregnancy whose mother developed gestational diabetes
d. A 35-year-old woman in her 25th week of pregnancy who is a racial group normally experiencing a high degree of gestational diabetes
e. A 28-year-old white athletic woman in her 25th week of pregnancy with no family history of gestational diabetes

111. A sample of amniotic fluid is obtained from a 25-year-old woman who is 26 weeks into a pregnancy. The

sample is free from hemolysis and the OD450 is 0.170. The baseline OD450 for a bilirubin-free sample is 0.015. Using the modified Liley graph in Figure 17.8, which of the following statements is most correct?

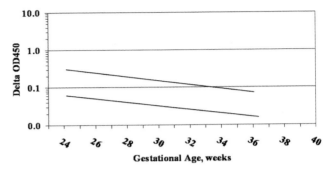

Figure 17.8

a. The fetus is at high risk for hemolytic disease of the newborn.
b. The fetus is at moderate risk for hemolytic disease of the newborn.
c. The fetus is at low risk for hemolytic disease of the newborn.
d. The presence of hemoglobin could not alter interpretation of risk assessment for these analyses.
e. If the laboratory values remain the same, increasing gestational age corresponds to an increased risk for hemolytic disease of the newborn.

112. In which of the following methods would the presence of red blood cells or hemolysis demonstrate the LEAST interference with testing interpretation of fetal lung maturity?
a. Lecithin-to-sphingomyelin ratio
b. Fluorescence polarization assay
c. Lamellar body count
d. Phosphatidylglycerol
e. Fetal fibronectin

113. Which of the following set of serum results most likely indicates Edwards syndrome (trisomy 18)?
a. Normal levels of hCG; normal levels of unconjugated estradiol; elevated levels of alpha-fetoprotein
b. Low levels of hCG; low levels of unconjugated estradiol; elevated levels of alpha-fetoprotein
c. Low levels of hCG; low levels of unconjugated estradiol; low levels of alpha-fetoprotein
d. High levels of hCG; low levels of unconjugated estradiol; low levels of alpha-fetoprotein; high levels of inhibin A
e. High levels of hCG; low levels of unconjugated estradiol; low levels of alpha-fetoprotein; low levels of inhibin A

114. Which of the following mutations found in Noonan syndrome is most1 associated with hypertrophic cardiomyopathy?

a. PTPN11 (protein-tyrosine phosphatase, nonreceptor-type, 11)

b. RAF1 (V-RAF-1 murine leukemia viral oncogene homolog 1)

c. SOS1 (son of sevenless homolog 1)

d. KRAS (V–Ki-Ras Kirsten rat sarcoma 2 viral oncogene homolog)

115. Which of the following statements is FALSE regarding dielectrophoresis for tumor cell isolation?

a. Dielectrophoresis takes advantage of cellular atypical morphologies in tumor cell identification.

b. The dielectrophoresis method uses cellular dielectric properties that generate a force to physically move cells.

c. One limitation of dielectrophoresis is that cells of identical size and density cannot be differentiated from one another.

d. In general, if there are microscopic differences between two cells' cytoplasmic membrane organization, then dielectrophoresis can separate them.

e. Ion species in different cellular compartments may take different amounts of time to respond to the applied electrical field.

116. Which of the following apoptosis-related genes is a tumor suppressor whose function in healthy cells promotes apoptotic death of excessive or harmful cells and contributes to cell homeostasis?

a. BAX

b. BCL-2

c. BCL-X

d. BCL-W

e. A1/BFL-1

117. Which of the following would be LEAST useful in studies using tissue banking for proteome analysis?

a. Collection of clinical information linked to specific specimens

b. Collection of paired sera and other body fluid

c. Ability to link laboratory results with genomic data

d. Institutional Review Board approval and explicit patient consent

e. Tissue harvested within 30 minutes of resection and stored at 4°C

118. Which of the following statements is most correct regarding the use of array-based comparative genomic hybridization (CGH) for genome survey?

a. CGH targets chromosomes in anaphase.

b. CGH is limited in that it is able to screen only specific parts of the genome.

c. CGH can be coupled with microarray technology to identify DNA sequences on a glass slide.

d. CGH technique is unable to detect cDNA.

119. Which of the following in vivo events is/are essential for an effective anti-tumor T cell response to occur?

a. Expression of tumor-specific antigens

b. Processing and presentation of tumor antigens with HLA molecules by antigen-presenting cells

c. Tumor antigen recognition by T cells followed by clonal expansion of the antigen-specific T cell population

d. Differentiation of tumor-specific T cells into cytotoxic effector cells

e. All of the above

120. Which of the following is a melanin-related metabolite that can be used as an advanced melanoma marker and detected in the urine or serum?

a. 5-S-Cysteinyldopa (5SCD)

b. CD44 (Pgp-1, HCAM)

c. Melanoma cell adhesion molecule (MCAM)

d. Alphavbeta 3

e. Melanoma antigen recognized by T cells (MART-1)

121. A 39-year-male actor is experiencing vertigo, headache, weakness, and some sensory loss. His CSF was clear, colorless, free from debris, and showed no growth. The CSF lactate, WBCs, and protein were within the reference ranges. The CSF glucose was 60 mg/dL compared with a serum level of 90 mg/dL. The IgG:albumin ratio was 1.7 and IgG oligoclonal banding was evident in the CSF electrophoresis, but it was not present in the serum. Which of the following statements is the most accurate about this case?

a. The difference between CSF and plasma glucose suggests hyperglycemia.

b. The increased protein is due to rhinorrhea.

c. Myelin basic protein is the most specific test needed to make the diagnosis.

d. The prealbumin band on the electrophoresis will likely be decreased.

e. The electrophoresis results and increased CSF IgG without increased albumin are most suggestive of the diagnosis.

122. Which of the following proteins, if detected in fluid draining from the ear, is most likely to indicate trauma of the blood-brain barrier?

a. Beta-1-transferrin

b. Beta-2-transferrin

c. Alpha-transferrin

d. Carbohydrate deficient transferrin

e. F2-isoprostanes

123. Which of the following is NOT consistent with pleural fluid exudate?

a. Pleural fluid cholesterol 100 mg/dL

b. Pulmonary infarction

c. Rheumatoid arthritis

d. Breast cancer

e. Low levels of pleura fluid lactate dehydrogenase

124. Which of the following conditions would most likely be associated with high pleural fluid glucose levels?
     a. Hyperglycemia
     b. Rheumatoid arthritis
     c. Malignancy
     d. Empyema
     e. Tuberculosis

125. Each of the following choices lists an analyte in ascitic fluid and a corresponding possible function for assessing the analyte in the fluid. Which choice states a function that is INCORRECTLY matched to the corresponding analyte?
     a. Fibronectin – Differentiate malignant from sterile ascites
     b. Lactate – Used with pH to differentiate spontaneous bacterial peritonitis from uncomplicated ascites
     c. Bilirubin – Useful for diagnosing choleperitoneum (ruptured gallbladder)
     d. Cholesterol – Differentiating malignant form cirrhotic ascites
     e. CA125 – Useful in diagnosing gastric carcinoma

126. Each of the following choices lists an analyte in pleural fluid and a corresponding possible function for assessing the analyte in the fluid. Which choice states a function that is INCORRECTLY matched to the corresponding analyte?
     a. Tuberculostearic acid – Facilitates diagnosis of pulmonary tuberculosis
     b. C-reactive protein – Elevated values in parapneumonic infections
     c. Triglyceride – Facilitates identification of chylous effusions
     d. Interferon gamma – Facilitates diagnosis of melanoma
     e. Rheumatoid factor – Facilitates diagnosis of rheumatic pleuritis

127. An infant who appeared normal at birth began to develop lethargy, hypothermia, and apnea within 24 hours. These problems were traced to a deficiency of ornithine transcarbamylase. Which of the following laboratory results will most likely indicate the disorder?
     a. High blood levels of urea
     b. Low blood levels of citrulline
     c. Low blood levels of ammonia
     d. High blood levels of arginine
     e. High urine levels of orotic acid

128. Which of the following amino acids is LEAST affected by transport defects in someone with cystinuria?
     a. Cystine
     b. Lysine
     c. Arginine
     d. Ornithine
     e. Valine

129. A newborn in the neonatal intensive care unit on total parenteral nutrition for the past 2 weeks is being evaluated for maple syrup urine disease (MSUD). An increase in which of the following amino acids would be the most definitive indicator of MSUD in this patient?
     a. Alloisoleucine
     b. Isoleucine
     c. Leucine
     d. Proline
     e. Valine

Questions 130–143:

For all hepatic questions, assume the following reference intervals (even though reference intervals should be distinct for males and females): aspartate aminotransferase (AST) 5–40 IU/L; alanine aminotransferase (ALT) 3–33 IU/L; alkaline phosphatase (ALK) 45–130; total bilirubin (T Bil) 0.3–1.3 mg/dL; direct bilirubin (D Bil) 0–0.2 mg/dL; total protein (TP) 6.3–8.0 g/dL; albumin (Alb) 3.7–4.8 g/dL; prothrombin time 12.3–14.2 sec; ceruloplasmin 18–35 mg/dL; serum iron 44–160 mcg/dL; iron binding capacity 200–380 mcg/dL; ferritin 20–240 mcg/L.

130. A 57-year-old woman presents with a history of itching, bone pain, and recurrent yellow plaques over the extensor surfaces of her arms. Laboratory findings include AST 35, ALT 21, ALK 370, T Bil 1.2, D Bil 0.5, TP 7.2, ALB 3.9. Imaging studies showed normal bile ducts, and liver biopsy showed marked portal inflammation, reduction in bile ducts, and granulomas involving bile duct radicals. Which of the following additional findings would NOT be consistent with the diagnosis?
     a. Decreased levels of 25-hydroxyvitamin D
     b. Elevated cholesterol with presence of abnormal lipoprotein on electrophoresis
     c. Elevated IgM on quantitative immunoglobulins
     d. Increased risk of development of cholangiocarcinoma in long-term follow-up
     e. Positive antibodies to the dihydrolipoamide acyltransferase component of pyruvate decarboxylase

131. A 34-year-old woman presents with fever, jaundice, and loss of appetite for the past several weeks. She denies exposure to anyone with hepatitis or yellow skin. She denies any risk factors for viral hepatitis. Laboratory tests include AST 720 IU/L, ALT 1250 IU/L, ALK 82 IU/L, total bilirubin 7.8 mg/dL, direct bilirubin 5.2 mg/dL, total protein 8.5 g/dL, albumin 3.2 g/dL. HBsAg, anti-HCV, and IgM anti-HAV are all negative; total anti-HBc and anti-HBs are positive, but IgM anti-HBc is negative. Ceruloplasmin is 45 mg/dL, and antinuclear antibody is positive at 1:1280. The diagnosis is most likely:
     a. Acute alcoholic hepatitis
     b. Acute viral hepatitis
     c. Autoimmune hepatitis

d. Cirrhosis

e. Wilson disease

132. A 54-year-old man presents with fever, jaundice, and loss of appetite for approximately 5 days. He has a past history of alcohol abuse, but says he has not had any alcohol for the past 2 months. Laboratory tests include AST 280 IU/L, ALT 125 IU/L, ALK 125 IU/L, total bilirubin 13.7 mg/dL, direct bilirubin 8.6 mg/dL, total protein 7.2 g/dL, albumin 3.8 g/dL, prothrombin time 12.8 sec., HBsAg, anti-HCV, and IgM anti-HAV, and IgM anti-HBc are all negative. Ceruloplasmin is 38 mg/dL, and antinuclear antibody is negative. The most likely diagnosis is:
   a. Acute alcoholic hepatitis
   b. Acute viral hepatitis
   c. Autoimmune hepatitis
   d. Cirrhosis
   e. Wilson disease

133. A 17-year-old boy with no prior medical history is admitted with jaundice of 5-day duration accompanied by weakness and lethargy. His urine output has also been low over the past 2 days. One of his friends recently was hospitalized for acute hepatitis as well. Physical examination was significant for pale mucous membranes as well as jaundice. A slit lamp examination was negative for Kayser-Fleischer rings. Laboratory tests include AST 370 IU/L, ALT 650 IU/L, ALK 25 IU/L, total bilirubin 12.4 mg/dL, direct bilirubin 4.6 mg/dL, total protein 6.9 g/dL, albumin 3.7 g/dL. HBsAg, anti-HCV, IgM anti-HBc, and IgM anti-HAV are all negative. Ceruloplasmin is 24 mg/dL, and anti-nuclear antibody is negative. Other laboratory findings include LDH 890 IU/L (reference interval 90–210 IU/L), hemoglobin 9.4 g/dL, BUN 75 mg/dL, and creatinine 4.8 mg/dL. The diagnosis is most likely:
   a. Acute alcoholic hepatitis
   b. Acute viral hepatitis
   c. Autoimmune hepatitis
   d. Cirrhosis
   e. Wilson disease

134. A 54-year-old man presents for routine physical examination. He admits to occasional abdominal discomfort and has no other problems except for chronic pain in his knees on exertion. Laboratory tests include AST 68 IU/L, ALT 112 IU/L, ALK 91 IU/L, total bilirubin 1.1 mg/dL, direct bilirubin 0.1 mg/dL, total protein 7.6 g/dL, albumin 4.2 g/dL. HBsAg, anti-HCV, and IgM anti-HAV are all negative; total anti-HBc and anti-HBs are positive. Iron is 125 mcg/dL, TIBC is 220 mcg/dL, and ferritin is 2,480 mcg/L. Antinuclear antibody is positive at a titer of 1:40. The diagnosis is most likely:
   a. Autoimmune hepatitis
   b. Chronic hepatitis B
   c. Chronic hepatitis C

d. Cirrhosis

e. Hemochromatosis

135. A 61-year-old man is found to have abnormal liver-related tests as part of a routine physical examination. On eliciting history, he indicates that he experimented with drugs in his teens, including injecting drugs on "two or three occasions," but denies other risk factors for hepatitis. There is no family history of liver disease. Laboratory tests include AST 57 IU/L, ALT 83 IU/L, ALK 87 IU/L, total bilirubin 0.9 mg/dL, direct bilirubin 0.1 mg/dL, total protein 7.2 g/dL, albumin 3.9 g/dL. Anti-HCV and total anti-HBc are positive, while HBsAg and anti-HBs are negative. Iron is 62 mcg/dL, TIBC is 295 mcg/dL, and ferritin is 320 mcg/L. Antinuclear antibody is negative. The likely diagnosis is:
   a. Autoimmune hepatitis
   b. Chronic hepatitis B
   c. Chronic hepatitis C
   d. Cirrhosis
   e. Hemochromatosis

136. A 69-year-old man presents for routine physical examination. He is obese and has a history of hypertension and type 2 diabetes that is controlled by glyburide, but has no other major health problems. Laboratory tests include AST 74 IU/L, ALT 25 IU/L, ALK 118 IU/L, total bilirubin 1.9 mg/dL, direct bilirubin 0.3 mg/dL, total protein 7.6 g/dL, albumin 3.1 g/dL, and prothrombin time is 15.1 sec. Anti-HCV, HBsAg and total anti-HBc are negative. Iron is 81 mcg/dL, TIBC is 253 mcg/dL, and ferritin is 166 mcg/L. Antinuclear antibody is negative. The most likely diagnosis is:
   a. Autoimmune hepatitis
   b. Chronic hepatitis B
   c. Chronic hepatitis C
   d. Cirrhosis
   e. Hemochromatosis

137. Which of the following statements concerning bilirubin assays is correct?
   a. Accelerants such as caffeine are not needed in the direct bilirubin assay.
   b. Biliprotein (delta-bilirubin) is typically included in the indirect bilirubin calculation.
   c. Conjugated bilirubin is the only form that is measured in the direct bilirubin assay.
   d. Total bilirubin is measured by direct spectrophotometry in most assays.
   e. Unconjugated bilirubin becomes less water soluble when exposed to ultraviolet light.

138. Which of the following is a correct statement about ammonia?
   a. Levels can be increased by drugs, most notably valproic acid.
   b. Ammonia is detoxified by converting pyruvate to alanine.

c. It is a sensitive and specific marker of hepatic encephalopathy.

d. It is produced in the liver by the action of alanine aminotransferase.

e. The most common congenital cause of increase is deficiency of the enzyme arginosuccinic acid dehydratase.

139. Which of the following statements concerning hereditary hemochromatosis is correct?

a. Hepcidin, an iron regulatory hormone, is produced by the liver in response to iron deficiency.

b. Hepcidin stimulates iron transport across cell membranes by the iron transport protein ferroprotein.

c. Increased transferrin saturation is seen in most persons homozygous for the C282Y mutation, but iron overload is seen in only about one fourth of males.

d. The HFE gene is located on the long arm of chromosome 11.

e. The most common genetic defect causing this is the H63D mutation in the HFE gene product.

140. The MELD score is typically used in patients with cirrhosis to evaluate the priority for transplantation and in some forms of acute hepatitis to predict prognosis. Which of the following combinations of laboratory tests is used to calculate the MELD score?

a. Albumin, bilirubin, and platelet count

b. AST/ALT ratio, bilirubin, and albumin/globulin ratio

c. Bilirubin, creatinine, and INR

d. Bilirubin, INR, and platelet count

e. INR, NH3, and platelet count

141. Which of the following findings would favor a diagnosis of primary biliary cirrhosis over primary sclerosing cholangitis in a person with chronically increased alkaline phosphatase?

a. Association with ulcerative colitis

b. Development of cholangiocarcinoma as a late complication

c. Involvement of only intrahepatic ducts

d. Male gender

e. Positive atypical perinuclear antineutrophil cytoplasmic antibodies

142. Which pair of analytes will be most likely elevated with biliary obstruction?

a. AST, albumin

b. ALT, LD

c. ALK, bilirubin

d. Bilirubin, TP

e. LD, TP

143. Which of the following is LEAST correctly matched?

a. Carbohydrate deficient transferrin – Specific marker of ethanol consumption

b. HbA1c – Related to the lifespan of a red blood cell

c. Fructosamine – Related to the half-life of albumin

d. Delta bilirubin – Related to the half-life of albumin

e. Ischemia-modified albumin – Specific marker of myocardial injury

144. Which of the following statements concerning hepatitis B e antigen is INCORRECT?

a. It is associated with high viral load levels and infectivity.

b. During treatment, its loss (and development of anti-HBe) is associated with sustained response after withdrawal of therapy.

c. It is typically present during acute hepatitis B.

d. It may be spontaneously lost in chronic hepatitis B (about 5% to 10% of cases/year).

e. When absent, indicates lack of circulating HBV DNA.

145. In chronic hepatitis C, which of the following laboratory tests is the best predictor of likelihood of response to treatment?

a. Anti-HCV positive

b. AST level

c. HCV genotype

d. HCV RIBA positive

e. HCV RNA level

146. Which of the following tests for HBV would typically be NEGATIVE at the time of presentation with acute hepatitis B?

a. Anti-HBc total

b. Anti-HBs total

c. HbeAg

d. HBsAg

e. HBV DNA

147. A 52-year-old woman has been treated with glucocorticosteroids for autoimmune hemolytic anemia. Approximately 2 months after treatment is completed, her hematocrit and hemoglobin remain stable, but she develops jaundice, right upper quadrant tenderness, and low-grade fever. Laboratory tests include AST 270 IU/L (ref 5–40 IU/L); ALT 470 IU/L (ref 3–33 IU/L); ALK 77 IU/L (ref 45–130 IU/L); LDH 185 IU/L (ref 90–220 IU/L); total bilirubin 7.4 mg/dL (ref 0.3–1.3 mg/dL); direct bilirubin 4.9 mg/dL (ref 0–0.2 mg/dL). While previously she had been negative for HBsAg and positive for anti-HBs and anti-HBc, repeat testing showed positive HBsAg and negative anti-HBs, and positive total and IgM anti-HBc. Which of the following answers is the best interpretation of these results?

a. Acute infection by hepatitis B

b. Chronic hepatitis B with mutant strain causing previous false-negative HBsAg

c. False-positive HBsAg due to interference from autoantibody causing hemolytic anemia

d. Reactivation of hepatitis B due to immunosuppression

e. Superinfection with hepatitis D

148. With acute exposure to HIV, which of the following statements concerning laboratory testing is correct?
    a. Anti-HIV is the first marker to appear, usually 1 to 2 weeks after exposure.
    b. Combination tests with p24 antigen and anti-HIV increase sensitivity for detection.
    c. HIV RNA levels are barely detectable, but rise markedly after stimulation of the immune system to produce anti-HIV.
    d. Rapid point-of-care anti-HIV assays are significantly more likely to be negative at this time than are central laboratory assays.
    e. Because Western blot results are often negative with acute exposure, so confirmatory testing is not required in this setting.

149. Which of the following tests is LEAST helpful in detecting response to treatment of *Helicobacter (H.) pylori* infection?
    a. Antibody to *H. pylori*
    b. Biopsy with PCR for *H. pylori*
    c. Biopsy with urease test (Clo test)
    d. Stool *H. pylori* antigen
    e. Urea breath test

Questions 150–152:

For each of the following questions, select the correct autoantibody association with the disease.
    a. Anti-actin
    b. Anti-CPY2C21
    c. Anti-GAD65
    d. Anti-Hu
    e. Anti-topoisomerase

150. Type I diabetes mellitus

151. Autoimmune hepatitis type I

152. Small cell carcinoma associated polyneuropathy

Questions 153–163:

In these questions, assume the following reference intervals: Na − 136–144 mmol/L; K − 3.5–5.0 mmol/L; Cl 100–108 mmol/L; total CO_2 content (CO_2) − 22–30 mmol/L; anion gap − 4–11 mmol/L; BUN − 8–21 mg/dL; creatinine: 0.6–1.4 mg/dL; glucose: 75–100 mg/dL; pH − 7.37–7.43; pCO_2 − 36–44 mm Hg; pO_2 − 88–105 mm Hg; lactate: 0–1.2 mmol/L.

Questions 153–156:

For each of these questions, select the pathophysiologic condition from the list below that is most likely present in the clinical scenario discussed in the questions.
    a. Anion gap metabolic acidosis
    b. Non-anion gap metabolic acidosis
    c. Metabolic alkalosis
    d. Respiratory acidosis
    e. Respiratory alkalosis

153. A 55-year-old man presents with acute mental status changes. Electrolytes: Na 137 mmol/L, K 5.1 mmol/L, Cl 87 mmol/L, CO_2 42 mmol/L, BUN 18 mmol/L, creatinine 1.3 mg/dL, glucose 92 mg/dL, pH 7.37, pCO_2 75 mm Hg, pO_2 65 mm Hg.

154. A 23-year-old woman passed out at work. Electrolytes: Na 139 mmol/L, K 2.1 mmol/L, Cl 90 mmol/L, CO_2 39 mmol/L, BUN 21 mmol/L, creatinine 1.0 mg/dL, glucose 75 mg/dL, pH 7.46, pCO_2 51 mm Hg, pO_2 91 mm Hg.

155. A 61-year-old man is admitted with tense ascites and jaundice; asterixis is present. Electrolytes: Na 125 mmol/L, K 2.7 mmol/L, Cl 103 mmol/L, CO_2 18 mmol/L, BUN 14 mmol/L, creatinine 1.8 mg/dL, glucose 82 mg/dL, pH 7.46, pCO_2 21 mm Hg, pO_2 75 mm Hg.

156. A 24-year-old man with a history of depression is found unconscious. Electrolytes: Na 140 mmol/L, K 6.3 mmol/L, Cl 105 mmol/L, CO_2 11 mmol/L, BUN 35 mmol/L, creatinine 2.3 mg/dL, glucose 89 mg/dL, pH 7.16, pCO_2 24 mm Hg, pO_2 94 mm Hg.

157. A 54-year-old woman with no prior medical problems is seen for weakness. Electrolytes: Na 137 mmol/L, K 2.5 mmol/L, Cl 111 mmol/L, CO_2 17 mmol/L, BUN 15 mmol/L, creatinine 0.9 mg/dL, glucose 86 mg/dL. Urine electrolytes: Na 21 mmol/L, K 7 mmol/L, Cl 75 mmol/L. The most likely diagnosis is:
    a. Anion gap metabolic acidosis due to starvation ketoacidosis
    b. Non-anion gap metabolic acidosis due to type 4 renal tubular acidosis
    c. Non-anion gap metabolic acidosis due to type 2 renal tubular acidosis
    d. Non-anion gap metabolic acidosis due to GI losses of bicarbonate
    e. Respiratory alkalosis due to chronic hyperventilation from anxiety

158. A 75-year-old man has a history of diabetes and hypertension. He presents with weakness and lethargy, and peaked T waves are noted on his ECG. Laboratory results include: Na 135 mmol/L, K 7.2 mmol/L, Cl 109 mmol/L, CO_2 16 mmol/L, BUN 45 mmol/L, creatinine 3.2 mg/dL, glucose 246 mg/dL. The most likely diagnosis is:
    a. Anion gap metabolic acidosis due to diabetic ketoacidosis

b. Non-anion gap metabolic acidosis due to type 4 renal tubular acidosis

c. Non-anion gap metabolic acidosis due to type 2 renal tubular acidosis

d. Non-anion gap metabolic acidosis due to GI losses of bicarbonate

e. Respiratory alkalosis due to chronic hyperventilation from anxiety

159. A 49-year-old man with no prior medical history presented in a coma. Laboratory findings included Na 143 mmol/L, K 5.9 mmol/L, Cl 102 mmol/L, CO2 9 mmol/L, BUN 24 mmol/L, creatinine 1.6 mg/dL, glucose 92 mg/dL. Serum osmolality was 336 mosm/kg. Urine dipstick was negative. The most likely cause of this picture is:
    a. Diabetic ketoacidosis
    b. Ethylene glycol ingestion
    c. Lactic acidosis
    d. Starvation ketoacidosis
    e. Uremia

160. A 63-year-old woman is admitted with severe shortness of breath and hypotension. She is noted to have a respiratory rate of 32 and cyanosis. Laboratory findings include Na 135 mmol/L, K 6.1 mmol/L, Cl 94 mmol/L, CO2 23 mmol/L, BUN 18 mmol/L, creatinine 1.4 mg/dL, glucose 116 mg/dL, pH 7.21, pCO2 65, pO2 71, osmolality 281 mosm/kg. The most likely cause of this laboratory picture is:
    a. Diabetic ketoacidosis plus respiratory alkalosis
    b. Lactic acidosis plus respiratory acidosis
    c. Lactic acidosis plus metabolic alkalosis
    d. Metabolic alkalosis plus respiratory alkalosis
    e. Uncompensated respiratory acidosis

161. Which of the following would be the likely diagnosis in a patient with an acidosis accompanied by hypochloremia?
    a. Diabetic ketoacidosis
    b. Diarrhea
    c. Lactic acidosis
    d. Renal tubular acidosis
    e. Respiratory acidosis

162. In a patient with metabolic alkalosis, which of the following findings would suggest mineralocorticoid excess as its cause?
    a. Decreased potassium
    b. Hypernatremia
    c. Increased bicarbonate
    d. Increased BUN and creatinine with high BUN/creatinine ratio
    e. Urine chloride of 45 mmol/L

163. An increase in which of the following would cause the oxyhemoglobin dissociation curve to shift to the left?

a. 2,3 DPG
b. Bicarbonate
c. pCO2
d. pH
e. Temperature

164. Which of the following would most likely be associated with a low 24-hour urinary sodium?
    a. Diuretics
    b. SIADH
    c. Adrenal failure
    d. Psychogenic polydipsia
    e. Diabetic hyperosmolarity

165. All of the following should be considered in the differential of a patient with the syndrome of inappropriate antidiuresis EXCEPT:
    a. Cirrhosis
    b. Meningitis
    c. Phenothiazine usage
    d. Small cell carcinoma of lung
    e. Tuberculosis

166. A 56-year-old with a history of type 2 diabetes presents with blurred vision and abdominal pain. A sample was run on the Vitros in the stat laboratory, and sodium was reported at 138 mmol/L; a second tube, drawn at the same time, was run on the Beckman analyzer in the main laboratory and the sodium was 123 mmol/L. The second tube was re-run on the Vitros and the result was 139 mmol/L. What is the cause of the discrepant results between the two instruments?
    a. Dilution of sodium due to high glucose, falsely decreasing results on the Beckman
    b. Expected difference between the two instruments, since the Vitros uses whole blood, which contains less sodium than plasma
    c. Hyperkalemia due to insulin deficiency and interference of potassium in the sodium assay on the Vitros, falsely increasing results
    d. Osmotic effect of glucose on measurement of sodium by ion selective electrodes, falsely increasing results on the Vitros
    e. Pseudohyponatremia on the Beckman due to the presence of severe lipemia

167. All of the following are causes for artifactual hyperkalemia EXCEPT:
    a. Delayed centrifugation of blood stored at 4°C
    b. Fist pumping during tourniquet application
    c. Hemolysis
    d. Recentrifugation of blood collected in serum separator tubes
    e. Use of heparinized plasma in a patient with extreme thrombocytosis

Questions 168–169:

In these questions, assume the following reference intervals: Na − 136–144 mmol/L; K − 3.5–5.0 mmol/L; Cl 100–108 mmol/L; total CO2 content (CO2) − 22–30 mmol/L; anion gap − 4–11 mmol/L; BUN − 8–21 mg/dL; creatinine: 0.6–1.4 mg/dL; glucose: 75–100 mg/dL

168. A 64-year-old man was admitted with severe acute chest pain and was found to have ST-segment elevation on his ECG; thrombolysis was begun using tissue plasminogen activator. His chest pain resolved, but 12 hours later he developed severe headache progressing rapidly to coma, requiring intubation and respirator support. Routine laboratory results that morning included Na 137 mmol/L, K 3.9 mmol/L, Cl 103 mmol/L, CO2 25 mmol/L, BUN 14 mg/dL, creatinine 1.1 mg/dL, glucose 103 mg/dL. Results the next morning included Na 167 mmol/L, K 4.1 mmol/L, Cl 130 mmol/L, CO2 27 mmol/L, BUN 19 mg/dL, creatinine 1.2 mg/dL, glucose 114 mg/dL. What is the most likely explanation for these different results?
   a. Administration of sodium bicarbonate during resuscitation
   b. Artifactual increase due to drawing blood through IV containing normal saline
   c. Diabetes insipidus due to massive cerebral hemorrhage
   d. Movement of water into cells due to mannitol administration to reduce cerebral edema
   e. Severe dehydration due to excessive administration of diuretics

169. A 35-year-old overweight woman is evaluated for hypertension and electrolyte disturbances. She has two children following otherwise uncomplicated pregnancies at ages 22 and 26, and her menstrual periods have been normal. She has had elevated blood pressure for 8 years, and her blood pressure has been difficult to control; currently, it is 152/102, despite treatment with metoprolol, clonidine, felodipine, and lisinopril. Laboratory results include Na 142 mmol/L, K 2.6 mmol/L, Cl 98 mmol/L, CO2 34 mmol/L, BUN 12 mg/dL, glucose 89 mg/dL. Urine electrolytes include Na 25 mmol/L, K 38 mmol/L, Cl 50 mmol/L. The most likely cause of this clinical picture is:
   a. Congenital adrenal hyperplasia due to 11-hydroxylase deficiency
   b. Cushing syndrome
   c. Hyperaldosteronism
   d. Previous diuretic treatment for hypertension
   e. Renal tubular acidosis type 2

170. In the measurement of creatinine, which of the following statements is correct?
   a. Creatine ingestion can increase creatinine regardless of method used.

   b. Different methods must be used to measure creatinine in urine and in serum due to the buffering present in urine.
   c. Enzymatic assays are subject to interferences from ketone bodies.
   d. The most widely employed method is an enzymatic method using creatininase.
   e. Unless an extraction step is used, the Jaffe reaction is too unreliable for routine use in estimation of serum creatinine.

171. Which of the following can be used to evaluate renal tubular function?
   a. BUN
   b. Creatinine
   c. Cystatin C
   d. Fractional excretion of sodium
   e. Urine glucose

172. A 5-year-old boy presents with anasarca and is found to have 4+ proteinuria. All of the following would also be expected findings in a child with this condition EXCEPT:
   a. Decreased serum albumin
   b. Decreased C3 component of complement
   c. Increased serum low-density lipoprotein cholesterol
   d. Increased serum BUN with high BUN/creatinine ratio
   e. Oval fat bodies in the urine

173. Urine protein electrophoresis showed the findings in Figure 17.9 (compared with normal serum protein illustrated above the urine). Which of the following would be the most likely cause of this finding?
   a. Diabetic nephropathy
   b. Lupus nephritis
   c. Multiple myeloma
   d. Renal tubular injury from drugs
   e. Rhabdomyolysis

174. Which of the following tests would be falsely decreased by the presence of ascorbic acid?
   a. Bilirubin
   b. Glucose
   c. pH
   d. Protein
   e. Urobilinogen

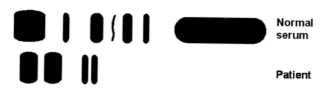

Normal serum

Patient

Figure 17.9

175. A urine sample is yellow, but on standing overnight becomes black. This indicates the likely presence of:
    a. Blood
    b. Homogentisic acid
    c. Melanin
    d. Myoglobin
    e. Peroxidase

176. A 54-year-old man is admitted in a coma with an increased anion gap, and has two types of crystals seen in the urine sediment: square pyramidal nonpolarizable and ovoid crystals with flattened ends that polarize. This indicates likely toxicity due to:
    a. Acetaminophen
    b. Ethanol
    c. Ethylene glycol
    d. Methanol
    e. Paraldehyde

177. Which of the following crystals, when found in urine, are always considered pathologic?
    a. Calcium oxalate (dihydrate)
    b. Cystine
    c. Triple phosphate (magnesium ammonium phosphate)
    d. Urates (amorphous)
    e. Uric acid

178. Which of the following, when found in urine sediment, should always be considered evidence of disease?
    a. Hyaline casts (1–2 per high-power field)
    b. Red blood cells (15–20 per high-power field)
    c. Transitional epithelial cells (10–15 per high-power field)
    d. Waxy casts (1–2 per high-power field)
    e. White blood cells (2–5 per high-power field)

179. A patient presenting with partially compensated respiratory alkalosis would produce urine with a pH of about:
    a. 4
    b. 5
    c. 6
    d. 7
    e. 8

180. All of the following are expected findings in Zollinger-Ellison syndrome EXCEPT:
    a. Diarrhea
    b. Duodenal tumor as the source of gastrin production
    c. Gastrin levels over four times the upper reference limit
    d. Hyperparathyroidism
    e. Multiple gastric ulcers

181. A 35-year-old man presents with fatigue and is found to have iron deficiency anemia. A bleeding site is not found in the intestinal tract on endoscopy. Which of the following tests would be helpful to suggest the disorder that most commonly causes iron deficiency not due to blood loss?
    a. Amylase clearance ratio
    b. Anti-mitochondrial antibody
    c. Fecal fat excretion
    d. HFE gene mutation analysis
    e. IgA antitissue transglutaminase

182. The test most commonly used to screen newborn infants for cystic fibrosis is:
    a. Genetic analysis for the $\Delta F508$ mutation
    b. Immunoreactive trypsin in serum
    c. Lipase in serum
    d. Meconium analysis for elastase
    e. Urinary amylase excretion

183. In comparing screening for colorectal cancer using guaiac-based tests with those using immunochemical detection of hemoglobin, which of the following statements is correct?
    a. Bleeding from the upper gastrointestinal tract commonly gives positive results for both tests.
    b. Both tests are highly sensitive for detection of both adenomas and carcinomas of the colon.
    c. Dietary restrictions on meat ingestion are required for guaiac-based tests, but not for immunochemical tests.
    d. Rehydration of test strips before adding the detection reagent is recommended to improve test sensitivity for guaiac-based tests.
    e. While sampling from three stools is recommended for guaiac-based tests, this is not needed with immunochemical tests due to their superior sensitivity.

184. All of the following proteins are typically increased as part of the acute phase response EXCEPT:
    a. Alpha-1 antitrypsin
    b. Ceruloplasmin
    c. C3 component of complement
    d. Haptoglobin
    e. Transferrin

185. Decreased levels of transthyretin (prealbumin) are typically seen in:
    a. Acute inflammation
    b. Cirrhosis
    c. Malnutrition
    d. Nephrotic syndrome
    e. All of the above

186. A unit of cryo-poor plasma is noted to develop an intense pale blue-green color while sitting on the shelf in the blood bank. The donor most likely:
    a. Has Gilbert syndrome
    b. Has hemochromatosis

c. Has Wilson disease
d. Is on oral contraceptives
e. Should be permanently deferred for advanced liver disease

187. A serum protein electrophoresis shows the findings displayed on the tracing in Figure 17.10 (tracing with white background, compared with normal on left with gray background) from a patient with a total protein of 5.1 g/dL (normal 6.7–8.0 g/dL). What is the most likely diagnosis?
    a. Cirrhosis
    b. Chronic inflammation
    c. Heavy chain disease
    d. Monoclonal gammopathy
    e. Nephrotic syndrome

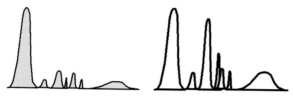

Figure 17.10

188. A serum protein electrophoresis shows the findings displayed on the tracing in Figure 17.11 (tracing with white background, compared with normal on left with gray background) from a patient with a total protein of 6.5 g/dL (normal 6.7–8.0 g/dL). What is the most likely diagnosis?
    a. Cirrhosis
    b. Chronic inflammation
    c. Heavy chain disease
    d. Monoclonal gammopathy
    e. Nephrotic syndrome

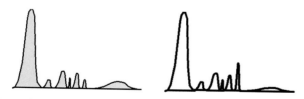

Figure 17.11

189. The most common cause of chronic hypercalcemia in ambulatory individuals would be confirmed by finding:
    a Decreased serum phosphate
    b. Increased intact PTH
    c. Increased 1,25-dihydroxyvitamin D
    d. Increased PTH-related peptide
    e. Lytic bone lesions on skeletal survey

190. A low calcium level may be seen in all of the following EXCEPT:
    a. Hypoparathyroidism
    b. Magnesium deficiency

c. Pseudohypoparathyroidism
d. Pseudopseudohypoparathyroidism
e. Vitamin D deficiency

191. "Intact" PTH immunoassays typically measure:
    a. Intact (1–84) PTH plus large metabolic fragments (such as 7–84)
    b. Intact (1–84) PTH plus large and small (such as 35–84) fragments
    c. Intact (1–84) PTH plus small (such as 35–84) fragments, but not large metabolic fragments (7–84)
    d. Intact (1–84) PTH plus PTH-related peptide
    e. Only intact (1–84) PTH

192. Features that should suggest a cause of hypercalcemia other than primary hyperparathyroidism include all of the following EXCEPT:
    a Increased serum phosphate despite normal renal function
    b. Increased serum alkaline phosphatase bone isoenzyme
    c. Markedly increased (>13 g/dL) serum calcium
    d. Monoclonal IgG band of 3.5 g/dL on protein electrophoresis
    e. Rapid rise in calcium over 3-week period

193. Of those listed, the tumor most commonly associated with PTH-related peptide production and hypercalcemia is:
    a. Bladder transitional cell carcinoma
    b. Gastric adenocarcinoma
    c. Head and neck squamous cell carcinoma
    d. Hepatocellular carcinoma
    e. Lung small cell carcinoma

Questions 194–196:

For each of the following conditions, use the answer key below to select the expected changes in serum iron, iron binding capacity, and ferritin.
    a. Decreased iron, decreased iron binding capacity, decreased ferritin
    b. Decreased iron, decreased iron binding capacity, increased ferritin
    c. Decreased iron, increased iron binding capacity, decreased ferritin
    d. Decreased iron, increased iron binding capacity, increased ferritin
    e. Increased iron, decreased iron binding capacity, increased ferritin

194. Iron deficiency anemia

195. Anemia of chronic disease (chronic inflammation)

196. Hemochromatosis

197. In a patient with hemolytic anemia, all of the following findings would be expected EXCEPT:
   a. Decreased serum haptoglobin
   b. Decreased serum iron
   c. Increased unconjugated bilirubin
   d. Increased urine urobilinogen
   e. Positive urine hemosiderin

198. Which of the following statements related to methemoglobinemia (metHb-emia) is FALSE?
   a. In metHb-emia, one or more iron atoms that is bound to hemoglobin is incapable of binding oxygen because it is in the ferric (+3) oxidation state.
   b. MetHb-emia is associated with a left shift in the oxyhemoglobin dissociation curve.
   c. MetHb levels approaching 15% (normal is ~1.5%) are associated with a high mortality.
   d. Methylene blue treatment will likely increase MetHb levels in an individual who has a glucose 6-phosphate dehydrogenase genetic deficiency.
   e. Cytochrome b5 reductase (NADH-dependent methemoglobin reductase) facilitates conversion of MetHb to physiologically functional hemoglobin.

199. Which statement about vitamin B12 (cobalamin) is INCORRECT?
   a. Serum B12 levels can be elevated in myeloproliferative disorders and hepatic tissue damage.
   b. Methylmalonic acid can be used as an early indicator to detect B12 deficiency.
   c. Folate can correct anemia but not neurologic symptoms in individuals who are B12 deficient.
   d. Decreased folate leads to both increased homocysteine and increased methylmalonic acid while decreased B12 only leads to increased homocysteine.
   e. B12 is involved in both methylmalonic acid and homocysteine synthesis while tetrahydrofolate is only involved in homocysteine synthesis.

200. A defect in which of the following enzymes results in the only autosomal recessive porphyria? This porphyria is also the only one whose tissue expression is in erythroid cells.
   a. Uroporphyrinogen III synthase
   b. Protoporphyrinogen oxidase
   c. Ferrochelatase
   d. Porphobilinogen deaminase
   e. Coproporphyrinogen oxidase

201. Which statement about zinc protoporphyrin is LEAST correct?

   a. Zinc protoporphyrin, measured as free erythrocyte protoporphyrin, provides an assessment of iron available for hemoglobin production.
   b. Free erythrocyte protoporphyrin is usually decreased in response to both iron deficiency (absolute lack of iron) and chronic disease (impaired use of iron).
   c. Lead's interference with ferrochelatase usually results in increased free erythrocyte protoporphyrin.
   d. The zinc protoporphyrin heme ratio reflects iron status within bone marrow because zinc can substitute for iron within the marrow.
   e. Zinc protoporphyrin regulates heme catabolism via competitive inhibition of heme oxygenase.

202. Which of the following is LEAST correct about fecal porphyrins?
   a. Fecal porphyrins can be used to distinguish variegate porphyria from coproporphyria.
   b. Increases in fecal porphyrin excretion up to threefold the upper reference limit may be seen in healthy individuals.
   c. Fecal porphyrins are usually increased in acute intermittent porphyria.
   d. The main components of fecal porphyrins are coproporphyrin and protoporphyrin.
   e. Diet can influence the amount of fecal porphyrin excretion.

203. Which of the following is a laboratory-related governmental agency?
   a. American Society of Clinical Pathology (ASCP)
   b. College of American Pathologists (CAP)
   c. Clinical and Laboratory Standards Institute (CLSI)
   d. Joint Commission (JC)
   e. Centers for Medical and Medicaid Services (CMS)

204. Which financial management-related term best describes the condition or diagnosis of a patient?
   a. International Classification of Disease, 9th Revision with Clinical Modifications (ICD-9-CM)
   b. Current Procedural Terminology (CPT) codes
   c. Diagnostic Related Groups (DRGs)
   d. Healthcare Financing Administration Common Procedural Coding System (HCPCS)

205. Which of the following expenses incurred by the clinical laboratory is BEST classified as both a direct and a variable cost?
   a. Analyzer purchase
   b. Salaries for laboratory staff performing the tests
   c. Proficiency testing materials
   d. Reagents
   e. Utility expenses

■ Answers

1. **e.** Choice A represents systematic bias. Choices B and C represent both systematic bias and a trend. Choice D represents a shift and demonstrates excellent precision. Choice E represents a system demonstrating poor precision.

2. **a.** Another way of asking the same question is: "What is the probability that three consecutive values will fall greater than 2 SD above the mean or greater than 90 mg/dL?" This question can be viewed as a normal (Gaussian) distribution with a 95% confidence interval. The probability that one value will fall outside of this 95% confidence interval is 5%. However, the probability of one value falling greater than 2 SD above the mean is 2.5% (1/40). Therefore, the probability that three consecutive values will all fall greater than 2 SD above the mean is the product of each of the individual probabilities or $(1/40)(1/40)(1/40)$ or 1 in 64,000. This event is not likely to occur by chance alone.

3. **b.** Chi-squared analysis evaluates observed and expected observations to determine if populations are related. ANOVA is a method for testing the hypothesis that three or more groups with normal distributions are the same. The sign test is similar to the t-test except that it uses the median rather than the mean. The F-test (aka: variance ratio test) is used to determine if standard deviations of two data sets are statically different. The F-test statistic is calculated by dividing the square of the larger variance by the square of the smaller variance. This value is evaluated using degree of freedom and an appropriate table.

4. **a.** The unpaired (student) t-test is used to compare two groups of observations that are unrelated to each other, such as diseased and non-diseased groups. The sample sizes do not have to be different. The paired t-test evaluates data derived from a single group (samples, patients) in which two different procedures or treatments are evaluated for differences.

5. **e.** With this change, fewer healthy individuals will be called positive. As you move to the right, the positive predictive value increases and negative predictive value decreases.

6. **c.** Choice C would likely demonstrate a shift or a drift. All others should demonstrate a Gaussian distribution. This distribution type is also known as a normal distribution wherein the population of data clusters symmetrically around a central value such that the mean, median, and mode of the data set are all identical.

7. **d.** CLIA-88 prohibits survey material to be shared among different facilities and laboratories. The PT survey should be used only for its intended facility and platform. Peer group evaluation allows a laboratory to verify that it is using a method according to manufacturer's specifications. Furthermore, it demonstrates that patient results are consistent with those of other laboratories.

8. **d.** Sensitivity is defined as the percentage of individuals with a disease who have an abnormal result. Of the 100 children with the disease, 95 (95%) had an abnormal result.

9. **e.** Specificity is defined as percentage of normal results in individuals without the disease. Of the 300 children without the disease, 294 (300–6, or 98%) had a normal result.

10. **b.** When tested in a screening program, one must use the prevalence of disease to evaluate the predictive value. When calculating predictive value problems for the boards, approximations will allow you to determine the correct answer. If the test has 95% sensitivity, then it is likely that the one infant with disease will have a positive result. Of the 10,000 (actually 9,999) without disease, 2% would be expected to have an elevated value; this represents 200 individuals. The positive predictive value is calculated as the true positive results (1) divided by total positive results (201), multiplied by 100 to report it as a percent, or in this case 0.5%. It is not appropriate to use the 300 persons without disease and 100 persons with disease initially tested to calculate positive predictive value, because this does not represent the true frequency of disease in the population tested.

11. **e.** In an ROC curve, true positive rate or sensitivity is plotted on the y axis, and false-positive rate (100–specificity) is plotted on the x axis. In some versions of the plot, specificity is plotted on the x axis, but in that case the numbers on the x axis go from 100 on the left to 0 on the right.

12. **c.** In evaluating an ROC curve comparing more than one test, several features of the graph can be used to compare test performance against expectations. In viewing the graph, tests A and B reach sensitivity of approximately 100%; however, test A clearly has better specificity for any level of sensitivity chosen. In screening programs, sensitivity is the most important characteristic of test performance. On the other hand, test C has high specificity, but never reaches over approximately 80% sensitivity. Confirmatory tests require high specificity, so test C would be a good choice for a confirmatory test. Chance alone would be depicted by a straight line running from the lower left-hand corner to the upper right-hand corner of the graph. All of the tests perform significantly better than chance alone.

13. **d.** ROC curves are prepared by calculating sensitivity and specificity of a test at a number of different cutoff points. Inspection of the graphs is the best way to determine tests that may perform better as screening tests (high sensitivity) or confirmatory tests (high specificity). Area under the curve (i.e., the proportion of the square below and to the right of the ROC curve) is a common way to evaluate overall test performance; the higher the number (with 1.0 being a perfect test), the better. Since a straight line from the lower left to upper right corners (performance of chance alone) will in-

clude an AUC of 0.50, an AUC of 0.6 is only slightly better than chance alone. Efficiency refers to the proportion of all persons who are correctly classified by a test (true positive + true negative/total tested). Efficiency will be highest at that point closest to the upper left-hand corner of the graph.

14. **d.** (See discussion below in question 15.)

15. **b.** The t-test is a statistical evaluation of whether the means of two sets of observations (which have a gaussian distribution of results) are significantly different. There are several versions of the t-test, but the ones that cause the most confusion (and are often asked about on exams) are paired and unpaired t-tests. Basically, if the same samples or individuals are studied using two different drugs or two different tests, the paired t-test would be used. If different individuals or samples are studied, then the unpaired t-test would be used. The chi square test is typically used for evaluating differences in proportions between two groups. For example, consider a treatment for a disease. If 24/75 persons treated with drug A responded, while 10/57 treated with drug B responded, the response rates could be evaluated using the chi square test. The Kolmogorov-Smirnov test is used to determine whether a set of data follows a gaussian distribution.

16. **b.** According to the Clinical and Laboratory Standards Institute (CLSI), a laboratory is allowed to use a published reference interval, providing that it has validated that the reference interval is appropriate for its population. The approved protocol for performing this is to take 20 representative individuals and test their samples; if no more than two of the results are outside the published reference interval, it is said to be validated. If more than two are outside the interval, a second series of 20 can be tested, and the same criterion used to make sure the first observation was just by chance. Practically speaking, one would not wish to repeat this experiment if, say, half of the results were outside the published reference interval. If the published figures cannot be validated, then the laboratory must establish its own reference interval.

17. **c.** According to the CLSI standards, to achieve statistical reliability in determining limits for a reference interval, 120 individuals must be tested. The data should be inspected for outliers, and calculations repeated after excluding any such outlier data points.

18. **d.** In contrast to most other tests, upper reference limits for cholesterol and glucose are based on subsequent risk of developing clinical evidence of disease. By analyzing results of prospective studies, and analyzing test results at baseline, the values above which risk began to increase were chosen as the upper reference limits of healthy or desirable. In the case of cholesterol, this was at values markedly lower than would have been derived from studies of apparently healthy individuals, while for glucose it is at values markedly higher than from such studies.

19. **c.** For many tests, results within a person are kept within extremely narrow limits, while varying considerably from one person to the next. For such tests, population-based reference limits are insensitive to the presence of disease. Among common tests with small individual variation are alkaline phosphatase, calcium, and free thyroxine. On the other hand, individual variation is similar to population variation for the other tests listed here, along with phosphate.

20. **c.** This can be calculated similarly to calculating the odds that all 12 coin flips would turn up heads or tails. In that case, the likelihood of one flip resulting in a head is 0.5 (50%); the odds that all 12 would be heads is $(0.5)^{12}$. Assuming all tests are independent variables, then the likelihood that all 12 would be within the reference interval is the likelihood of 1 (0.95) to the 12th power. The exact answer is 54%. This type of question commonly appears on the boards.

21. **b.** According to the CLSI guidelines on blood collection, the suggested order of collection is blood culture tubes first, followed (in order) by plain tubes, coagulation (sodium citrate) tubes, serum separator tubes, and tubes with additives. For plastic tubes, however, "plain" tubes often contain additives to accelerate coagulation; when plastic tubes are used, sodium citrate tubes should be filled before the "plain" tubes.

22. **b.** Prolonged use of a tourniquet causes hemoconcentration, which can increase the concentration of proteins and substances bound to proteins (calcium, iron, lipids, protein-bound hormones, and drugs).

23. **a.** While diurnal variation is best known for cortisol, there is significant diurnal variation for many other substances as well. Most pituitary hormone levels are lowest at bedtime and rise significantly during sleep to peak in the morning. Substances regulated by pituitary hormones (including many bone markers, such as osteocalcin, and collagen degradation fragments, such as N-telopeptides) also have marked diurnal variation. Glucose tolerance is affected by cortisol and growth hormone levels and is significantly better in the afternoon than in the morning.

24. **b.** During pregnancy, there is an increase in glomerular filtration rate of approximately 50%, resulting in a significant decrease in BUN and creatinine. It is important to consider this decrease in interpreting renal function tests during pregnancy. Increases in reference limits are needed for each of the other tests. Alkaline phosphatase levels increase to two–three times the nonpregnant reference limits, both from placental alkaline phosphatase and an increase in bone isoenzyme. During the second trimester, third spacing of fluid increases renin and aldosterone production. A number of hormones increase during pregnancy, including estriol (a marker of the fetal-placental unit) and prolactin.

25. **a.** Acute illness causes a number of changes in physiology. Cytokines lead to increased production of several pituitary hormones, including cortisol, growth hormone,

and prolactin; however, gonadotropins are typically decreased. Increased cortisol causes increases in glucose and worsens glucose tolerance. Cytokines appear to increase uptake of cholesterol by macrophages; with acute illness, cholesterol often falls by up to 40%, and the decrease begins within 24 hours of onset of illness. Similar decreases occur in LDL-cholesterol, with lesser decreases in HDL-cholesterol, while triglycerides and VLDL increase by up to 35%.

26. **d.** Drug regimen and physical activity are more related to subject preparation. Site preparation and body posture are more related to specimen collection. Clotting is the only choice most likely related to specimen handling.

27. **e.** Heparin causes increases in laboratory testing such as thyroid hormone, PT, PTT, Li (Li-Heparin tubes), and sodium (Na-Heparin tubes). EDTA decreases iron; oxalate decreases calcium levels; citrate decreases amylase, and fluorides inhibit alkaline phosphatase activity.

28. **a.** C-peptide has about a 65% inter- and a 30% intra-individual CV. Calcium, glycohemoglobin, total protein, and glucose demonstrate at most ~10% CV for either inter- or intraindividual CV.

29. **d.** Comparison studies are typically graphed using the current (or, ideally, a reference) method on the x axis and the new or comparison method on the y axis. Correlation coefficient is reflective of two things: the spread of points around the line and the range of values measured. High correlation coefficients occur when an adequate range of samples is tested and when the points are closely fit to the resulting line. Slope is a measure of proportional bias, while y intercept is a measure of constant bias.

30. **a.** Correlation coefficient is only a measure of fit of points to the line and an indicator of the range of the values measured. A perfect positive correlation would occur with an r value of 1, while a perfect negative correlation would be indicated by an r of -1. A value of 0 indicates that there is no correlation between the two methods. The square of r (also called R), when expressed as a percentage, indicates the likelihood of predicting the value of y for a given x value. For method comparison studies, values of r should ideally be >0.97, and for most methods will be >0.99 unless there are significant problems with the comparison study. The square of the r value indicates how much of the individual value for y can be explained by the x variable; for method comparison studies, this should therefore be a very high number. The correlation coefficient does not indicate that values are equal; for example, a new method for an enzyme could give results three times those of the old method, but as long as that relationship always held, the r value would be high; as a consequence of this fact, correlation coefficient cannot be used to evaluate methods for bias.

31. **b.** Bias (Bland-Altman) plots are the most sensitive way to detect biases, particularly those that occur only in part of the measurement range. Bias plots can use either the absolute difference or the percent difference. When using either, the goal is to have the points centered on the zero line, with about half above and half below. Values that are consistently on one side of the zero line represent bias in that part of the measurement range.

32. **b.** Heterophile antibodies are a common cause of erroneous results in sandwich immunoassays, which are used to measure most tumor markers, peptide hormones, cardiac markers, and a number of other compounds. These antibodies react with immunoglobulins from other species, which may generate a signal in the immunoassay that is read as the presence of the analyte. While manufacturers take steps to minimize heterophile antibody interference, they vary in their effectiveness (even within different assays from the same manufacturer), so discrepant results are common in samples containing high titer heterophile antibodies. While fragments of hCG may also cause discrepant hCG results, they would not explain the positive PSA in a female, and ectopic PSA production has not been reported in trophoblastic tumors. Use of different calibrators may also cause slight differences between assays, but not to this degree.

33. **d.** Matrix effects are defined as differences in apparent concentration between samples with different composition (e.g., serum and urine). Matrix effects are common for substances that are poorly soluble in water (such as lipids) or in which there is a complex interaction between the sample and the reagents (such as enzyme assays and immunoassays). This creates problems in use of pure standards, which often have a very different matrix than serum samples. The solution to matrix effects is to use calibrators, solutions similar in composition to the samples being tested in which the concentration has been determined. Either calibrators or standards are used to prepare a standard (calibration) curve, in which the signal (e.g., amount of light absorbed) generated by the instrument on samples of known concentration is used to interpolate concentrations in unknown samples by measuring their generated signal in the assay.

34. **b.** The Beer-Lambert law is the basis for photometric measurement, which is the underlying principle for most chemical assays. It describes a linear relationship between amount of light absorbed and the concentration of a compound in a solution. While biologic samples have a variety of other compounds within them, use of chemical reactions specific for the compound of interest allows use of this relationship in the clinical laboratory. Transmittance has an inverse relationship to absorbance (light that was not absorbed is transmitted through a solution), so there is an inverse relationship between transmittance and concentration.

35. **e.** Within-run variation is a measure of repeatability of results over a single set-up of an instrument, typically

during the course of a single shift, when a single operator sets up the instrument and performs a group of tests. The description given would apply to between-run variation, which is generally a larger number.

36. c. Coefficient of variation is a measure of the repeatability for a test, calculated as the percentage of the mean represented by the standard deviation of measurement. It is calculated by making multiple measurements of the same sample, either a control or a single patient. Coefficient of variation should be for electrolyte measurements, and in general is in the range of 2% to 5% for most tests. However, it may be as much as 10% for enzyme activity measurements, measurement of substances in very low concentrations, and for some immunoassays. For very complicated assays, it may be even higher. It is ideal that measurement variation be significantly lower than the variation within a person over time, so that changes in condition can be detected as changes in laboratory test results.

37. b. Turbidimetry and nephelometry are often used to measure the amounts of antigens (often proteins) that are present in concentrations of mg/dL or higher by measuring the number of antigen-antibody complexes present. The complexes form particles that prevent light from traveling in a straight line to a detector, instead causing the photons to be sent off at an angle to the incident light. This produces turbidity in a solution. Turbidimetry measures the decrease in light in the straight line path from the light source to the detector, while nephelometry places a detector at an angle to the incident light and measures the amount reaching the detector. Common applications are measurement of immunoglobulins, C-reactive protein, haptoglobin, and hemoglobin A1c. Anything else that causes turbidity in a sample, most commonly triglycerides, will interfere with measurement. Turbidimetry can be run using the same instrumental setup as spectrophotometry, which is used for most routine chemistry tests; nephelometry requires an instrument with a detector at an angle to the light source and is commonly done on dedicated instruments.

38. a. High-dose hook effect is seen in immunometric assays for substances that have very large ranges of concentration, most commonly tumor markers. When the range of assay concentration seen in samples exceeds 4–5 logs (for PSA, from <0.05 to over 5000, for example), there is the possibility of such an effect occurring. Since what is measured in immunometric assays is the number of antigen-antibody complexes, and this decreases with great antigen excess, a falsely low concentration results. Such samples can have extremely low apparent concentrations when the result is 6–7 logs above the usual measured concentration (e.g., for hCG measurements). PSA is not measured by its enzymatic activity, so those choices could not be correct. Heterophile antibodies typically cause falsely increased results, and would not be expected to disappear in the

short period of time between diagnosis and first round of chemotherapy. While sample mix-up is always a possibility, it would be unusual to have another patient with the very high PSA value seen in the initial result.

39. a. Some reports indicate that as many as 50% of HAMAs are likely to dilute linearly. Therefore, the lack of proportional results with dilution provides useful information. However, proportional results alone are uninformative. Single dilutions should not be used to make decisions regarding the presence or absence of a heterophilic antibody. A more robust determination would consider a multipronged approach using blocking agents, measuring specifically for HAMA, and assaying the sample on more than one analytical platforms that use different antibodies.

40. d. NMR determines structures of organic compounds and, unlike MS, is not destructive. The other statements correctly describe each corresponding instrumentation principle.

41. b. The PCO_2 electrode uses sodium bicarbonate buffer and a gas-permeable membrane. The calomel electrode is made of mercury that is in contact with a mercury (I) chloride-saturated solution. This solution is referred to as "calomel" and contains a known concentration of potassium chloride. The other choices correctly describe each of the corresponding electrodes.

42. c. Electroendosmosis describes the paradoxical migration of charged molecules (such as immunoglobulins) in a direction contrary to what would be expected. When support media with a negative surface charge (such as cellulose acetate or agarose) are used, hydronium ions (as H_3O^+) are attracted to the surface and migrate toward the cathode (negatively charged) pole. The weak negative charge on proteins such as immunoglobulins causes them to be carried along with the solvent toward the cathode, instead of the expected migration toward the anode. Electroendosmosis does not occur with uncharged support media such as polyacrylamide gel or starch gel. It improves separation of proteins, and thus is helpful in analysis of serum proteins.

43. e. SDS-PAGE separates the denatured proteins primarily on the basis of molecular weight. Charge density is the most important factor in electrophoresis with nondenatured proteins. Degree of folding is irrelevant when proteins are denatured.

44. c. Temperature does not directly affect separation of compounds in electrophoresis; however, cooling is often used to prevent protein denaturation, which may affect migration of proteins. All of the other variables can be adjusted to improve separation of compounds in electrophoresis.

45. d. Whole blood would have to be centrifuged to assay serum or plasma. Centrifugation is not a feature consistent with the use of point-of-care testing devices. Sampling volumes are often smaller and are less traumatic for the patient, and built-in quality control checks lend to the ease of use.

46. **d.** Testing done on an analytical platform or bench-top analyzer would likely be a test performed in the main laboratory and would therefore not be a point-of-care test.

47. **c.** POCT analyzers generate more disposables, and reagent costs are usually more expensive than traditional laboratory systems. One of the main drawbacks of POCT systems is the expensive price.

48. **c.** In classic noncompetitive inhibition, the inhibitor binds only to the free enzyme and not to the enzyme-substrate complex. In uncompetitive inhibition, the inhibitor binds only to the enzyme-substrate complex and not to the free enzyme. Therefore, no enzyme-inhibitor complex will form, and binding of the substrate will lead to a conformational change that will create an inhibitor binding site.

49. **a.** Acid phosphatase is unstable at all temperatures unless the pH of the serum is reduced to between 5 and 6.

50. **d.** Red cells do not contain creatine kinase. The highest ratio would be seen with lactate dehydrogenase (around 500:1). The ratio of AST is about 15:1, while that of ALT is about 7:1.

51. **c.** In contrast to other hepatocyte enzymes, pseudo-cholinesterase production by the liver reflects hepatic synthetic function rather than hepatocyte injury.

52. **c.** Very little interferes with screening tests for methadone. It is possible that methadone does not show up on confirmation because of the specific method used in the laboratory. Also, many reference laboratories such as the Mayo Clinic identify methadone separately, and it is not part of their screen to confirm opiates. Hydrocodone and hydromorphone are not metabolites nor do they interfere with methadone or oxycodone detection. Because both were found on gas chromatography mass spectrometry confirmation, a third drug is indicated. Methadone is likely the cause of the positive test result.

53. **e.** The legal limit for alcohol is 80 mg/dL (equivalent to "blowing" a 0.08 on a breathalyzer). Additionally, only whole blood (not serum) analyzed by head space gas chromatography from a chain-of-custody sample can be used to define a legal/forensic alcohol level. The driver's measured level of 11 mg/dL (equivalent to blowing a 0.011) does not indicate impairment. Impairment is reported to begin at 40 mg/dL. Blood alcohol levels between 0.02 and 0.03 are associated with slight euphoria and loss of shyness but are not usually associated with loss of coordination. Depressant effects are not apparent at these levels. The presence of marijuana indicates past exposure and does not prove that an individual is under the influence of the drug. Urine immunoassays are screening tests, not confirmatory tests.

54. **c.** NaF is preferred for collecting samples from individuals who are suspected of cocaine use. Cocaine is metabolized by hydrolysis of ester linkages. In blood, cocaine is hydrolyzed to ecgonine methyl ester via cholinesterase. This reaction is dependent on the concentration of cocaine and may be inhibited by freezing or addition of fluoride or cholinesterase inhibitors. At 4°C 1 mg/L of cocaine will loose 100% of the parent drug after 21 days.

55. **b.** The dose is the amount of drug given. Bioavailability is the amount of an administered dose that enters the systemic circulation. The bioavailability of an intravenous dose is generally 100%. Volume of distribution is the apparent volume into which the administered drug has distributed. Clearance is the amount of serum completely cleared of drug in a unit of time (e.g., mL/min or L/hr). Steady state is achieved when the net rate of drug input is exactly matched by the rate of elimination. The rate going in equals the rate going out. The rate going out equals clearance. Steady state is the level achieved and maintained in the therapeutic range.

56. **b.** Diazepam (Valium) is a tranquilizer. Morphine is an opiate. Phenobarbital is a barbiturate. Cocaine is a stimulant (dopaminergic pathway). Phencyclidine is a hallucinogen.

57. **c.** Lidocaine is neither highly bound to protein nor is it appreciably stored in tissue. It has a relatively short half-life of about 2 hours. The other statements correctly state a function of the indicated cardiotropic agent.

58. **e.** About 90% of theophylline is metabolized by the liver, with caffeine being one of the major metabolites in children. In adults, caffeine is argued to be undetectable with theophylline use.

59. **d.** Opioids are associated with feelings of euphoria that are often accompanied by respiratory depression and bradycardia. Constipation and increased ADH secretion are other common associations with opioid ingestion.

60. **a.** In sweat, cocaine is primarily excreted as the parent drug. This offers an added advantage of simple gas chromatography analysis.

61. **b.** Aluminum phosphide is a grain fumigant that has been orally ingested in both suicides and accidents. Blood levels of aluminum rise during exposure and subsequently return to normal, unless kidney function is impaired. In increasing levels of toxicity, common forms of arsenic exist as arsenate (As^{+5}), arsenite (As^{+3}), and arsine (AsH_3) gas. Elemental arsenic is relatively not toxic. Effects of excess iron ingestion can include hepatic necrosis after 4 days and has also been associated with GI obstruction after 4 weeks. Patients taking Li_2CO_3 for manic-depressive disorders sometimes develop thyroid enlargement. Lead toxicity leads to inhibition of several mitochondrial enzymes in heme synthesis; ferrochelatase is directly affected.

62. **e.** Choices A–D all describe ADH-deficient causes of polyuria due to water diuresis. Choice E is not related to this pathogenesis.

63. **e.** Somatostatin inhibits a number of intestinal and pancreatic hormones. It causes diabetes through inhibition

of insulin and hypochlorhydria due to inhibition of gastrin. Diarrhea is at least partially due to inhibition of pancreatic enzyme production, and gallstones may be due to inhibition of CCK production. While diarrhea can be seen with carcinoid and gastrinoma, the other findings are rare, while insulinomas only cause hypoglycemia and none of the other manifestations.

64. **a.** Measurement of plasma-free metanephrines is between 97% and 99% sensitive for diagnosing hereditary and sporadic pheochromocytomas and has the highest sensitivity among the choices listed for diagnosing a pheochromocytoma; however, specificity is relatively low (85%). Specificity is highest for measurement of fractionated metanephrines or catecholamines in urine.

65. **c.** Addison disease is associated with elevated levels of renin. Primary hyperaldosteronism and Cushing and Liddle syndromes are conditions associated with decreased renin levels. Additionally, decreased renin levels are associated with dexamethasone-suppressible hyperaldosteronism.

66. **b.** 11 beta-hydroxylase converts 11-deoxycortisol to cortisol in the glucocorticoid pathway (*zona fasciculata*) in the adrenal cortex. Congenital adrenal hyperplasia (CAH) associated with elevated levels of 11-deoxycortisol will likely be caused by a deficiency in 11 beta-hydroxylase. This enzyme defect represents approximately 5% of all cases of CAH, while 21-hydroxylase deficiency represents almost all of the remaining 95% of CAH cases. Much rarer causes include deficiencies of enzymes further "upstream" in the glucocorticoid and mineralocorticoid cascade.

67. **e.** A urine creatinine much less than 0.9 g/day likely means that the sample collection was incomplete. These values would lead to a misinterpreted catecholamine result.

68. **c.** The normal T4, T3 uptake, and TSH with low T3 are typical of "euthyroid sick syndrome," or nonthyroidal illness. In acute illness, peripheral conversion of T4 to T3 (by the type I monodeiodinase) is impaired, while pituitary conversion of T4 to T3 (by the type 2 monodeiodinase) is normal, preventing an increase in TSH. Those who are acutely ill may actually have abnormal TSH due to the effects of a number of factors (cortisol, dopamine, cytokines) that impact TSH production, often making it hard to evaluate actual thyroid status in acute illness.

69. **c.** These results, with increased levels of total thyroid hormones, low T3 uptake, and normal TSH, are typical of increased levels of thyroid-binding proteins, especially TBG. Common causes for this are pregnancy, use of oral contraceptives, exposure to other drugs that increase TBG (such as phenothiazines, antidepressants, and opiates), and active liver injury. Hyperthyroidism should cause increases in both thyroid hormones and T3 uptake, as well as suppressed TSH. Euthyroid sick syndrome should cause low T3 but normal T4, T3 uptake,

and TSH. Heterophile antibodies typically interfere in sandwich assays (such as are used for TSH measurement) and should not increase T3 and T4 (which are measured by competitive immunoassays) and would not affect T3 uptake (which is not an immunoassay at all).

70. **c.** The normal free T4 with even increased T3 and suppressed TSH is typical for hyperthyroidism, particularly that due to Grave disease. The overactive thyroid cells in this state tend to produce proportionally more T3 and proportionally less T4 per cell, resulting in earlier increases in T3 than in T4, and earlier return of T4 to normal with treatment. This impression is confirmed by the presence of thyroid-stimulating immunoglobulins (TSI), which are highly specific for Grave disease. While thyroid peroxidase antibodies are used as a test for Hashimoto thyroiditis, they are present in 85% of those with Grave disease. Thyroid adenoma can cause hyperthyroidism, as can Hashimoto disease, but in both conditions T4 is increased to a greater extent than T3 and TSI should be absent. In euthyroid sick syndrome, T3 should be low, not high; while TSH may be lower than normal, it is not undetectable. With increased TBG, total thyroid hormones are increased while free hormone levels are normal; however, TSH would be normal and thyroid autoantibodies would be absent.

71. **d.** These results are typical of primary hypothyroidism at baseline. Thyroxine (thyroid hormone) has a half-life of 1 week, and it takes five half-lives to reach about 95% of steady-state levels for any drug. It is common for nonspecialist physicians to repeat thyroid function tests too soon after beginning treatment and to incorrectly modify therapy based on those results. While heterophile antibodies may cause falsely increased TSH, one would expect results to be similar on repeat testing rather than decrease as observed; heterophile antibodies do not typically affect free T4 measurements, since these are not measured using sandwich assays. T3 is not monitored in hypothyroidism because it is not a sensitive test of thyroid dysfunction, and since most T3 comes from metabolism of T4, levels reflect thyroxine levels closely.

72. **e.** Thyroglobulin antibodies are common in the general population and are even more common in persons with thyroid cancer; some studies suggest as many as one third of those with differentiated thyroid cancer have thyroglobulin antibodies. These antibodies cause falsely increased thyroglobulin with competitive immunoassay and falsely decreased results with the more commonly used sandwich immunoassays. The presence of thyroglobulin antibodies invalidates its measurement, preventing its use to monitor residual thyroid cancer; however, with successful destruction of all thyroid tissue, thyroglobulin antibody titers should fall over time and ultimately disappear in many cases, so that decrease in titer indicates a good prognosis. After total thyroidectomy, and especially destruction of any

thyroid remnant by radioactive iodine, thyroglobulin levels should be undetectable; reference ranges from persons who have intact thyroid glands are inappropriate comparison ranges for monitoring a person following total thyroidectomy. The negative scan indicates that there was no significant residual thyroid tissue, either normal or neoplastic, remaining. Ectopic production of thyroglobulin is extremely rare and generally only occurs in teratomas (which actually have thyroid tissue within them).

73. **c.** IL-6 is an indicator of proinflammatory cytokines. Soluble CD40 ligand indicates plaque rupture. NT-proBNP is a good indicator of myocardial dysfunction, and cardiac troponins T and I indicate myocardial necrosis. Myeloperoxidase is a granulocyte enzyme that converts hydrogen peroxide into hyporchlorus acid (bleach) and is a good indicator for plaque destabilization.

74. **e.** Myoglobin is cleared by the kidney and remains elevated only about 24 hours. CK MB has a half-life of about 12 hours and generally remains elevated 24–36 hours. Troponin C is not measured, as it is not cardiac specific. Because detection limits are lower for troponin T than for troponin I, it generally remains elevated for up to 10 to 14 days (depending on the size of the infarct), several days longer than that for troponin I.

75. **b.** The distribution of total CK is significantly grater in skeletal muscle than any in other tissue. However, CK-MB activity represents only 1% to 2% of skeletal muscle and is even greater in neonates. Cardiac muscle contains, on average, 10% to 20% CK MB. The brain, GI tract, and lungs have predominantly CK BB.

76. **c.** Cardiac troponin is the reference biomarker for myocardial infarction (MI) and risk stratification in acute MI. A rise and fall in troponin is considered diagnostic of myocardial infarction. The cutoff value used to diagnose MI is the 99th percentile of values from healthy individuals, or where the CV of the assay is 10%, whichever value is higher. If cTn values remain constant, the elevated result may be due to an interfering antibody or to another condition, such as renal failure (which causes chronic elevation in troponin). CK MB is less sensitive and less specific than troponin, and is no longer considered the reference marker for diagnosis of myocardial infarction; however, it is still used if troponin is not available.

77. **a.** The following figure (Fig. 17.12) illustrates release of BNP from a cardiac muscle cell. Inside the cardiac myocyte, pre-pro-BNP (a 134 amino acid peptide) is cleaved to a signal peptide (a 26 amino acid peptide) and pro-BNP (a 108 amino acid peptide). Pro-BNP is cleaved and released into the blood as equal molar amounts of NT-pro-BNP (amino acids 1 through 76 of pro-BNP) and BNP (amino acids 77 through 108 of pro-BNP). Once in the blood, NT-pro-BNP has a longer half-life and is therefore present at higher levels than BNP. The utility of both analytes is about equal in predicting heart failure, and the major differences are

manufacturer specific with respect to reagents, reference ranges, and proprietary rights. Other differences include: BNP is lower in obese individuals, and NT-proBNP is higher in the presence of renal failure.

Release of BNP from Cardiac Myocytes

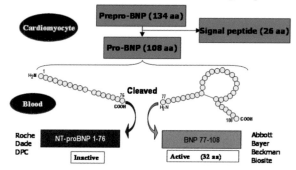

Figure 17.12

78. **d.** This assay is also called the albumin–cobalt binding test. Exogenous cobalt used in the reagent is unable to bind to modified albumin in the location where copper can also bind. During the assay procedure when modified albumin is removed from the analytical reaction cell, all unbound cobalt remains and is spectrophotometrically measured. Because all cobalt bound to non-modified albumin is no longer present, the level of modified albumin is calculated from the remaining unbound cobalt.

79. **a.** The signal is generated by acridinium ester that directly binds to cTnI via another antibody. Figure 17.13 illustrates possibilities of how different components of cTnI can generate signal in an assay.

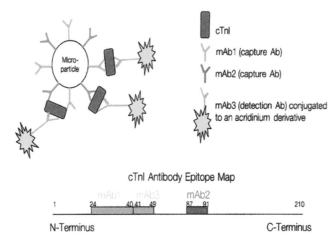

Figure 17.13

80. **e.** Carbonic anhydrase III (CAIII) is an enzyme present in skeletal but not cardiac muscle. It is released from damaged muscle at a fixed ratio to myoglobin. Therefore, myoglobin is a more specific indicator of myocardial damage when its ratio to CAIII is also ele-

vated. Glycogen phosphorylase is a ubiquitous enzyme that catalyzes the first step in glycogenolysis. Heart fatty acid binding protein is a low molecular weight (15 kD) protein that can be an early marker of myocardial damage with kinetics similar to myoglobin (18 kD).

81. **e.** High sensitive C-reactive protein (CRP) is used to assess low-grade inflammation (associated with vascular lesions). Cardiac natriuretic peptides are markers of congestive heart failure. Troponins and lactate dehydrogenase may indicate cardiac injury. Risk assessments for coronary artery disease and treatment choices are based on lipid levels. While CRP, homocysteine, and natriuretic peptides have been found to indicate risk of coronary heart disease, they are much weaker predictors than LDL-cholesterol.

82. **d.** Skeletal muscle contains about 99% CK MM, about 1% CK MB, and no CK BB. Cardiac muscle contains about 79% CK MM, 20% CK MB, and no CK BB. Smooth muscle (as found in the intestine) contains mainly CK BB. The patient in the example has cardiac (myocardial infarction), skeletal muscle (crush injury), and smooth muscle (intestinal infarction) injury. Therefore, all of the CK isoenzymes listed (CK MM, CK MB, and CK BB) would be present in the sample to some extent.

83. **d.** Figure 17.14 explains the density and ultracentrifugation relationships.

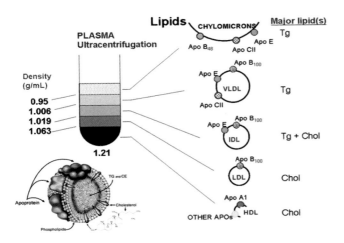

Figure 17.14 (Adapted with permission from Dr. Carmen Wiley at the Marshfield Clinic)

84. **e.** The half-life of chylomicrons is about 15 minutes. Figure 17.15 illustrates the lipoprotein electrophoresis migration pattern, with chylomicrons at the origin.

85. **d.** Lp(a) is the major lipoprotein containing apolipoprotein (a) and ranges from 350 to 700 kDa. The others listed are much smaller, ranging from about 6.5 to 34 kDa. Lp(a) is similar to LDL in terms of density and composition. Increased levels can be familial, showing autosomal dominant inheritance and are

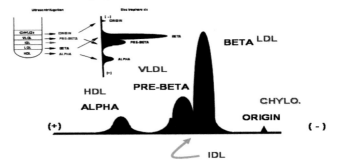

Figure 17.15

associated not only with coronary heart disease but also cerebrovascular disease and stroke.

86. **a.** Lp(a) is homologous to plasminogen and may be prothrombotic. It is bound to apolipoprotein B–100 by disulfide linkage. Choice B refers to apolipoprotein C–II that is mainly distributed in chylomicrons and VLDL and is responsible for activating lipoprotein lipase. Choice C describes apolipoprotein B–100. Choice D describes apolipoprotein A–I in HDL. Choice E describes apo E4.

87. **c.** Citrate can exert significant osmotic effects that can lead to falsely low plasma lipid and lipoprotein levels. Because of its high molecular weight, heparin will have little effect on plasma volume; however, it can alter electrophoretic mobilities of lipoproteins. Even though EDTA plasma cholesterol and triglyceride concentrations are about 2% to 4% lower than in serum, EDTA prevents oxidative and enzymatic alterations that occur in lipoproteins during storage.

88. **e.** Generally, the concentrations of total cholesterol and HDL cholesterol can be measured in nonfasting individuals. This fact greatly facilitates screening. LDL cholesterol itself does not change following meals, but the Friedewald formula (which is usually used to estimate LDL cholesterol) is affected by the presence of chylomicrons, which will be found in nonfasting individuals, and HDL cholesterol assays can be affected by high triglycerides (depending on the assay used). Direct measurement of LDL cholesterol is used by some laboratories to measure LDL cholesterol when the patient is not fasting.

89. **e.** With zero or one risk factors, therapeutic lifestyle changes are recommended for LDL cholesterol levels ≥160 mg/dL. It is recommended to consider drug therapy for levels ≥190 mg/dL.

90. **b.** Familial combined hyperlipidemia (type 2B) is the only condition among the choices that demonstrates both high cholesterol and high triglycerides. The other choices all represent conditions with high triglycerides; however, cholesterol levels for each of these disorders are typically within the reference range.

91. **b.** The screening test involves a 50-g load of glucose usually administered between the 24th and 28th week

of pregnancy. At 1 hour, glucose values greater than 140 mg/dL indicate the need for the diagnostic test. After an approximate 10-hour fast, 100-g glucose load is given for the diagnostic test. In general, measurements are taken every hour for 3 hours. The test is diagnostic for gestational diabetes if two or more results are as follows: fasting >95 mg/dL; 1 hour >180 mg/dL, 2 hour >155 mg/dL, 3 hour >105 mg/dL.

92. c. Macroalbuminuria has proved quite valuable as a marker associated with risk of progressive renal disease and is defined as an albumin excretion rate between 30 and 300 mg per 24 hours (or 30–300 mg per g creatinine). Early detection of microalbuminuria can provide early identification of individuals who are at risk for diabetic nephropathy and cardiovascular disease. Macro- and microalbuminuria are not defined based on size or molecular weights.

93. a. Iron deficiency anemia leads to increased lifespan of the red blood cell. Therefore, HbA1c levels in these individuals will generally be increased. Increased HbA1c values are also seen in individuals who had a splenectomy. HbA1c values will be lower with hemolytic anemia. The other choices describe the three-step, nonenzymatic glycation formation of HbA1c inside the red blood cell. Note that the aldimine structure is converted to the ketoamine, glycated hemoglobin via the Amadori rearrangement.

94. b. Type 2 diabetes can be related to genetics, obesity, sedentary lifestyle, and race/ethnicity. Early onset, childhood, type 1 diabetes can be caused by islet cell destruction from an autoimmune process that may not be prevented with medications or drug therapy. These individuals have little to no detectable associated C-peptide.

95. c. A general rule of thumb is that every 1% increase in HbA1c corresponds to a mean plasma glucose increase of 29 mg/dL. Therefore, a HbA1c of 8% likely represents a plasma glucose level that would be approximately 60 mg/dL higher than a HbA1c value of 6%. In this patient, this rule of thumb would put the projected glucose at 135 + 60 = 195 mg/dL.

96. a. Beta-hydroxybutyric acid and acetoacetic acid are normally present in a 1:1 ratio. However, this ratio is greatly increased in DKA. Beta-hydroxybutyric acid is not detected by conventional assays that use a sodium nitroprusside reagent. To quantitate beta-hydroxybutyric acid, some tests employ enzymatic, electrochemical, chromatographic, electrophoretic, or colorimetric methods. Because beta-hydroxybutyric acid levels fall and acetoacetic acid and acetone levels rise during DKA treatment, these tests are not useful for monitoring therapy. Furctosamine is a glycated albumin at the e-amino lysine, and it is used to assess short-term (about 3 weeks) glycemic control, which is directly related to the half-life of albumin.

97. e. Choice A represents Type Ia GSD (aka: von Gierke disease); choice B represents Type XI (aka: Fanconi-Bickel syndrome); choice C represents Type IV (aka:

Andersen disease); choice D represents Type VI (aka: Hers disease). Choice E represents Type IXa and is the only choice that is X-linked; the others (A-D) are all autosomal recessive.

98. c. Individuals with autoimmune disease or recent ingestion of sulfhydryl drugs are at increased risk for autoimmune insulin syndrome. After a meal, excessive amounts of insulin are secreted but are bound to antibodies. This insulin becomes unavailable to target tissues. Subsequently, the insulin dissociates from the antibodies and results in hyperinsulinemia and hypoglycemia. Such insulin levels can be dangerously high, even higher than an insulinoma.

99. e. Knowledge of increased levels of tumor markers can cause worry and therefore decrease quality of life. One example illustrating truth in choice B is human kallikrein 6. It is expressed in many tissues; however, its serum concentration is increased only in ovarian cancer. While the magnitude of tumor marker reduction may reflect the degree of treatment success or extent of disease involvement, a longer half-life often indicates unsuccessful treatment. In most cases, it is more appropriate to use patients with benign disease to represent the nondisease group. Such a group would be a better estimation of the reference range than would be represented in a healthy population.

100. b. Although chemotherapy decreases the relative risk for patient 1, her prognosis is so good that only 1% to 2% of such patients have been shown to benefit. For this patient, the toxicity of adjuvant systemic chemotherapy likely outweighs the benefits. Studies demonstrated that for women with estrogen-rich breast cancer, treatment with tamoxifen has a 40% reduction in risk of recurrence and death. In contrast, females with estrogen-poor cancer have a small benefit (about 5%).

101. d. The European Group on Tumor Markers guideline states that the use of CA125 cannot be recommended for general population screening to detect sporadic forms of ovarian cancer. CA125 is not a specific marker for ovarian cancer and may be elevated in adenocarcinoma of the fallopian tubes, endometrium, cervix, pancreas, colon, breast, and lung. About 95% of healthy adult premenopausal women have CA125 values of 35 U/mL or less. Postmenopausal women tend to have lower values (less than 20 U/mL in 99% of apparently healthy women).

102. a. Despite limitations, PSA is currently one of the best screening modalities available for the detection of early stage prostate cancer, for which there is the greatest potential for successful treatment. The other markers are too insensitive in localized disease to be used to screen for cancer.

103. e. Survival and prognosis in germ cell cancer are highly dependent on staging and initial concentrations of AFP, HCG, LDH, and PALP. Pretreatment serum concentrations of these markers all can influence choice

of therapy. CEA is more frequently suggested as a marker for GI, breast, and lung cancers.

104. d. Case 1 is an example that no single immunoassay is perfect in all clinical situations and that laboratory results that do not correlate with a clinical picture should be considered highly suspect. For Case 2, evidence is shown for the use of a two-step assay that includes a sequential wash, using solid phase antibodies of higher binding capacity, or by assaying specimens at two different dilutions.

105. a. The p53 gene is mutated or deleted in up to half of breast carcinomas and in many other types of cancer. Most biologically significant mutations limit p53 ability in maintaining genomic stability. P53 alterations and protein accumulation (determined immunohistochemically) are usually related to shorter disease-free survival time.

106. e. 5-alpha-reductase inhibitors, such as finasteride, used for treatment of symptomatic bladder outlet obstruction, are known to decrease serum PSA levels up to 50%. However, the ratio of free to total PSA is not changed significantly. PSA levels rise with prostatitis, benign prostatic hyperplasia, and after ejaculation. PSA levels are higher in ambulatory individuals than during hospitalization, suggesting that physical activity may increase PSA.

107. b. Beta-human chorionic gonadotrophin CSF levels are significantly increased in choriocarcinoma. All other markers listed are not increased in the CSF associated with the other listed germ cell tumors.

108. e. The infant's large size is likely due to the mother being diabetic. Because of gestational diabetes, the fetal insulin secretion is stimulated; however, when the infant is born and the cord is cut, the infant's oversupply of glucose is terminated. This leads to hypoglycemia in the infant. One major complication is a lifetime risk of type 2 diabetes that is at least 50%. The whole blood and plasma glucose discrepancy is normal because there is more water in plasma (93%) than whole blood (80%) and therefore, fasting glucose is about 15% less than plasma glucose.

109. a. Preeclampsia is common in the third trimester. The increased alkaline phosphatase is normal for pregnancy and is likely of placenta origin and does not indicate liver disease because the GGT is normal. The transaminases increase in preeclampsia and are from hepatic necrosis and usually increase only in severe preeclampsia. Dipstick detects albumin but not globulins. Sulfosalicylic acid test detects both albumin and globulins. Therefore, since both are equal, then it can be concluded that albumin is being lost in the urine. Proteinuria in preeclampsia may sometimes be in the nephrotic range (>3.5 g/24 hr). In that case, there would likely be fatty casts in the urine and more advanced pitting edema would result from hypoalbuminemia and loss of plasma oncotic pressure. During pregnancy, the plasma volume increases greater than the RBC mass. There is also an increase in clearance of creatinine, urea, and uric acid. Therefore, the values are likely abnormal for BUN, creatinine, and uric acid.

110. b. It is recommended to screen for gestational diabetes between the 24th and 28th week of pregnancy in women who are older than 25 years old or less than 25 years and obese. The recommendation also applies to women who have a first-degree relative/family history of gestational diabetes or if they are from a racial group associated with a high prevalence of the disease. The female in choice B will need to be screened at the appropriate time.

111. b. From the figure (Fig. 17.16), 0.155 is the absorbance determined for use on the modified Liley graph. Area above the top line indicates high risk; area between the two lines indicates moderate risk, and area below the bottom diagonal line indicates low risk for hemolytic disease of the newborn. If hemoglobin were present in the sample, another peak would have been generated at OD410 on the graph below. In such cases, 5% of this peak's absorbance from baseline would be subtracted from the OD450 peak to determine the absorbance value to be used with the Liley graph. Therefore, the interference of hemoglobin in the sample could alter interpretation of risk assessment.

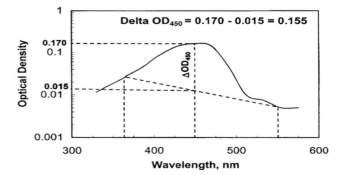

Figure 17.16

112. d. Contamination of samples with blood tends to produce falsely elevated values for very immature samples and falsely lowered values for very mature samples when using the L:S ratio. Meconium, vaginal secretions, and maternal urine contamination can also produce false results. FPIA results >50 mg/g are generally considered mature. Values near this cutoff may be sensitive to contamination. Lamellar bodies are produced from type II pneumocytes and are about the same size as platelets. Therefore, lamellar body counts can be determined using the platelet channel of a hematology analyzer. Blood contamination would cause interference. PG values are generally not affected by blood contamination. Fetal fibronectin is used to monitor women at risk of preterm labor.

113. c. Choice A represents open spina bifida; choice B represents anencephaly; choice D represents trisomy 21. The quad screen measures hCG, unconjugated estradiol, alpha-fetoprotein, and dimeric inhibin A.

114. **b.** As many as 78% of individuals with a clinical diagnosis of Noonan syndrome are expected to have a mutation in 1 of 4 genes encoding proteins of the RAS-ERK signaling pathway, PTPN11, RAF1, SOS1, and KRAS. Germline mutations in PTPN11 have been found in half of individuals with a clinical diagnosis of Noonan syndrome. Genotype-phenotype correlations suggest that PTPN11 mutations are often associated with pulmonic stenosis (70%), while association with hypertrophic cardiomyopathy is rare (6%). In contrast, about 76% to 80% of Noonan syndrome patients with a mutation in the RAF1 gene can be expected to develop hypertrophic cardiomyopathy. Certain RAF1 mutations that cluster in two mutational hot spots in exons 7 (encoding the CR2 domain) and exon 17 almost invariably appear to result in hypertrophic cardiomyopathy.

115. **c.** Two cells of identical size and density can be moved by dielectrophoresis in opposite directions or, if desired, in the same direction with different forces if they have different dielectric properties. Ion species in different cellular compartments may take different amounts of time to respond to the applied electrical field.

116. **a.** BCL-2, BCL-X, BCL-W, and A1/BFL-1 are genes that are all unfavorable in cancer states and have anti-apoptotic properties. The BAX gene functions in healthy cells to promote apoptotic death to maintain homeostasis.

117. **e.** When banking for proteome analysis, tissue should be immediately snap-frozen in liquid nitrogen to preserve proteins and should be maintained at -70°C. Choices A-D describe good laboratory practices for banking tissue for proteome analysis.

118. **c.** CGH targets chromosomes in metaphase and has a unique advantage of being able to screen the entire genome for changes in copy number. CGH is readily carried out on cDNA arrays.

119. **e.** All of the choices listed are essential to give an effective antitumor T cell response.

120. **a.** 5SCD is a very specific marker of melanin metabolism that can be detected in urine or serum from patients with advanced stages of melanoma. Choice B is a membrane glycoprotein with cellular receptors for hyaluronic acid that is expressed on leukocytes and erythrocytes and allows lymphocyte adhesion to endothelial veins. Choice C represents another membrane glycoprotein that corresponds to melanoma thickness and may be related to metastatic potential. Choice D is an integrin vitronectin receptor with angiogenic properties that may be related to melanoma invasiveness. Choice E is a protein whose expression is limited to melanocytes of skin and retina. In melanoma, its detection is via immunohistochemical stains.

121. **e.** Albumin is only made in the liver, and any albumin in the CSF gets there via membrane transport. CSF IgG can arise by local plasma cell synthesis. Albumin is measured in CSF and in serum to normalize the IgG values from each matrix to determine the source of

IgG. The CSF index is generally less than 0.85. Here, a IgG:albumin ratio of 1.7 in conjunction with the banding is one criteria for diagnosis of multiple sclerosis. In general, CSF glucose is about two thirds of the corresponding plasma value. Decreased prealbumin banding can indicate spinal blockage, while increased banding can indicate cerebral atrophy. Myelin basic protein is a dated testing that is not considered specific for multiple sclerosis.

122. **b.** Beta-2-transferrin (aka tau protein) is present only in the central nervous system and is synthesized by the catalytic conversion of beta-1-transferrin by neuraminidase. F2-isoprostanes levels are increased in diseased areas of the brain in individuals with Alzheimer's.

123. **e.** Pulmonary infarction and breast cancer are characterized by inflammation with increases in protein, WBCs, and lactate dehydrogenase. Exudates are also characterized by pleural fluid cholesterol levels greater than 40 mg/dL and pleural fluid lactate dehydrogenase greater than about 70% of the serum reference range.

124. **a.** In general, pleural fluid and plasma glucose levels are about the same. The only condition associated with high pleural fluid glucose is hyperglycemia. In some conditions, pleural glucose fluid can be very low. For example, when rheumatoid disease affects the lungs, pleural fluid glucose levels can be as low as 25 mg/dL.

125. **e.** Ascitic fluid CA125 can be elevated in several non-malignant conditions and may be elevated in cardiovascular and chronic liver disease. Generally, CA125 lacks specificity as a marker for malignancy. Very high CA125 levels have been associated with epithelial carcinomas of the ovary, fallopian tubes, or endometrium. High levels of carcinoembryonic antigen, not CA125, measured in peritoneal fluid indicate a poor prognosis in gastric carcinoma.

126. **d.** Interferon gamma levels are significantly increased in pleural fluid in patients with tuberculosis pleuritis. The other choices illustrate an example of an analyte in ascetic fluid that can be effectively used to facilitate the corresponding diagnosis.

127. **b.** Ornithine transcarbamylase (OTC) deficiency leads to impaired condensation of carbamyl phosphate and ornithine to form citrulline. This impairment leads to reduced ammonia incorporation, which, in turn, causes symptomatic hyperammonemia and excess of both substrates for the reaction. OTC deficiency is the most common of the urea cycle disorders.

128. **e.** Valine can be found in the urine from someone with maple syrup urine disease. The other amino acids listed (COAL or COLA) demonstrate transport problems in individuals with cystinuria.

129. **a.** D-Alloisoleucine (allo-Ile) is the only pathognomonic marker of MSUD. Increased concentrations of Leu, Ile, and Val are considered indicative of MSUD; however, abnormal levels of these amino acids are often seen in newborns who are receiving TPN.

130. d. This is a typical description of primary biliary cirrhosis, which occurs most commonly in young to middle-aged women. It is commonly associated with antimitochondrial antibodies of the M2 type, which react with the dihydrolipoamide acyltransferase component of the pyruvate decarboxylase complex, and with increased total IgM. Deficiencies of fat soluble vitamins can occur, particularly involving vitamin D, and can lead to osteomalacia. Increased cholesterol with development of the abnormal lipoprotein X can occur in any chronic cholestatic disorder. Patients with this disease are at increased risk to develop hepatocellular carcinoma, but not cholangiocarcinoma.

131. c. Autoimmune hepatitis most commonly presents as a chronic disorder, but in about 25% of cases has an acute presentation. The low albumin with markedly increased globulins and positive antinuclear antibody in high titer all point to this diagnosis. Hepatitis B markers indicate previous exposure to the virus, but are not consistent with acute viral hepatitis.

132. a. The high ratio of AST/ALT ($>$2:1) and relatively mild enzyme elevations in the setting of acute hepatitis is strongly suggestive of alcoholic hepatitis. Viral serologies are negative, and markers for other causes are also negative. While AST/ALT ratio is also greater than one in cirrhosis, the normal total protein, albumin, and prothrombin time are against this diagnosis.

133. e. This is a classical presentation of acute hepatic injury due to Wilson disease. Typical diagnostic findings such as Kayser-Fleischer rings and low ceruloplasmin are absent in most cases of acute hepatitis due to Wilson disease, making the diagnosis more difficult. The markedly increased copper levels that result from the hepatic injury typically cause hemolytic anemia from copper toxicity, and acute tubular necrosis often results from the toxic effects of copper as well. Very high copper levels typically cause very low alkaline phosphatase activity as well.

134. e. Initial laboratory results of moderately increased AST and ALT are typical for chronic hepatitis, but viral serologies show only previous exposure to HBV and no active viral infection. Prothrombin time, total and direct bilirubin, and total protein and albumin are normal, indicating normal liver function. A weakly positive antinuclear antibody is common in older adults and of no significance. The markedly elevated ferritin along with high transferrin saturation (Fe divided by TIBC; values over 50% in males are considered elevated) are consistent with iron overload. Hemochromatosis is often first detected as chronic liver injury, but mild intermittent abdominal pain and degenerative joint disease are common findings in hemochromatosis as well.

135. b. Chronic hepatitis C is often detected as asymptomatic elevations in aminotransferases, usually only slightly elevated and often fluctuating between normal and increased. While anti-HCV alone is not proof that he is currently infected, 85% of those with positive anti-HCV (and 95% of those with positive anti-HCV and elevated liver enzymes) turn out to be HCV RNA positive, so the diagnosis is highly likely. HCV exposure typically occurred in most due to injection drug use; only brief exposure in the 1960s and 1970s is common in many chronically infected with HCV. Most persons with HCV have evidence of previous exposure to HBV, but for some reason often have only anti-HBc and lack other HBV markers. Mild increases in ferritin are common in those with chronic hepatitis and are considered nonspecific.

136. c. The laboratory findings including AST being higher than ALT, increased bilirubin (predominantly indirect reacting), normal total protein but low albumin, and prolonged prothrombin time are all typical of persons with cirrhosis. In this case, the etiology would need further investigation, but is clearly not viral hepatitis or hemochromatosis given negative viral markers and normal iron studies. While autoimmune hepatitis is a possible diagnosis, the negative anti-nuclear antibody would argue against that diagnosis. The most likely etiology is nonalcoholic fatty liver disease, given the presence of the metabolic syndrome.

137. a. The total bilirubin assay includes accelerants, such as caffeine or methanol, to allow all forms to react; these are not needed in the direct bilirubin assay. Total bilirubin is typically measured by the diazo reaction; direct spectrophotometry is used in neonatal transcutaneous bilirubin measurements, but not in laboratory methods. Conjugated bilirubin, biliprotein (delta-bilirubin), and a small but variable amount of unconjugated bilirubin are included in the direct bilirubin assay, while the indirect bilirubin calculation is primarily an indication of unconjugated bilirubin. Exposure of unconjugated bilirubin to ultraviolet light, detergent, or acidic pH allows more water soluble isomers to predominate, allowing more to be measured in the direct reaction.

138. a. Valproic acid commonly causes increased ammonia. Ammonia is detoxified through the urea cycle; the most common deficiency in this cycle is that of ornithine transcarbamylase. While ammonia is a liver function test, and is often increased in hepatic encephalopathy, there is little correlation between blood ammonia and changes in degree of encephalopathy.

139. c. Hemochromatosis is most commonly caused by mutations in the HFE gene, located close to the HLA complex on the short arm of chromosome 6. The most common mutation causing the disease is homozygosity for the C282Y mutation, which occurs in about 1:200 person of northern European ancestry; while the overwhelming majority have high transferrin saturation, only about one fourth of males and less than 5% of females develop iron overload from the mutation. Hepcidin, a hormone produced by the liver, inhibits iron movement across cell membranes mediated by the iron transport protein ferroprotein. In hemochromatosis, despite high

iron stores, hepcidin is suppressed, leading to continued iron absorption and recycling from body stores and accumulation in inappropriate locations such as the liver.

140. **c.** While a number of other groupings of tests have been used in persons with chronic hepatitis to detect likelihood of significant fibrosis, the MELD score uses total bilirubin, creatinine, and INR to evaluate prognosis.

141. **c.** Primary sclerosing cholangitis is a presumably autoimmune destructive disorder mainly affecting the extrahepatic bile ducts. It is associated with ulcerative colitis in over 80% of cases, and (like that disorder) is often associated with positive atypical perinuclear anti-neutrophil cytoplasmic antibodies (not directed against myeloperoxidase, but against a variety of other antigens including lactoferrin). It is a male predominant disease, and often results in cholangiocarcinoma as a late complication.

142. **c.** Biliary obstruction is characteristically associated with increases in canalicular enzymes such as alkaline phosphatase, gamma-glutamyl transferase, leucine aminopeptidase, and 5'-nucleotidase. If obstruction is complete, total and direct bilirubin will be increased as well. While AST and ALT may also be increased in bile duct obstruction, LDH, albumin, and total protein are not increased.

143. **e.** Carbohydrate deficient transferrin is a marker used to detect ethanol consumption during the past two–three weeks. Hemoglobin A1c is linked to the life span of the red blood cell and is a good indicator of glucose levels during the past 90 days, while fructosamine is bound to albumin and is a good indicator of glucose control during the past 19–21 days (the half-life of albumin). Delta bilirubin is bilirubin bound to albumin. Ischemia modified albumin is a marker of ischemia, not injury. Injury markers include troponins, CKMB, and myoglobin.

144. **e.** Hepatitis B e antigen is a protein produced during viral gene transcription, but is not part of the complete viral particle. It is usually present at times of high infectivity, such as in acute hepatitis B, and is usually associated with high viral loads (>1 million copies/mL). During treatment, it is an important marker; if lost and anti-HBe develops, response is often sustained after discontinuation of treatment. In chronic hepatitis B, it is lost in about 5% to 10% of cases per year. The majority of untreated persons who are e antigen negative actually have circulating HBV DNA; this may either be due to relatively low levels of virus (most common in the US and northern Europe) or the presence of mutant strains that do not make HBeAg (so-called pre-core mutants), often with high viral loads.

145. **c.** Essentially all patients with chronic HCV will have positive anti-HCV and positive HCV RIBA, so these tests are useless for predicting likelihood of treatment response. The response rate is similar in those with normal and increased AST (or ALT). While there is a weak correlation between likelihood of treatment

response and viral load, the most important predictor is genotype. Genotypes 2 and 3 typically respond to lower doses of ribavirin and shorter duration of treatment with higher rates of treatment response, while genotype 4 has higher rates of response but requires the same treatment doses and duration as does therapy for the most common genotype 1.

146. **b.** At the time of presentation with acute hepatitis B, viral replication is typically high, so markers of virus (HBsAg, HbeAg, and HBV DNA) are typically positive. Anti-HBc is a later marker to appear, but is present in 100% of those with acute hepatitis B at the time of presentation. Since total anti-HBc is also present with chronic hepatitis and with past exposure to HBV, IgM anti-HBc is usually used to indicate recent exposure; however, it may also be present with flares of activity in chronic HBV.

147. **d.** The majority of persons with acute exposure to hepatitis B spontaneously clear HBsAg and develop protective titers of anti-HBs, along with anti-HBc (and anti-HBe), which is not protective. While new exposure to hepatitis B could occur, the positive anti-HBs previously demonstrated should still provide protection. Superinfection with HDV requires the presence of HBsAg, so alone could not explain these findings. False-positive results for HBsAg are rare, and would not explain the rise in enzymes. While there are mutant strains of HBV that can be missed by some HBsAg assays, this would also not explain the acute rise in enzymes and jaundice, nor the loss of anti-HBs. The likely explanation is reactivation of HBV from immunosuppression. After "clearance" of HBsAg, the virus is typically still present in hepatocytes and replicates at low levels, controlled by the host immune response. With immune suppression (especially that using glucocorticosteroids and rituximab [anti-CD20]), reactivation of HBV is relatively common and can cause severe flares of activity and even death.

148. **b.** After acute infection, viral markers such as p24 and HIV RNA are the first markers to appear, typically within a few weeks of exposure. Levels are quite high at this time, but fall after development of antibody, and for p24 may become very low to undetectable, so use of combination tests markedly increases likelihood of detection of acute infection. Rapid HIV tests and Western blot have similar sensitivity to central laboratory tests in the acute setting.

149. **a.** After successful treatment of *H. pylori* infection, antibody titers fall very slowly and are not helpful for monitoring treatment response. Tests that detect bacterial antigens or nucleic acids are helpful, but may be positive for some time after successful treatment. The most rapidly responsive tests are the urea breath test, which is noninvasive, and the Clo test, which requires a repeat biopsy; for this reason, the former is typically preferred for monitoring patients.

150. c. Type I diabetes is typically associated with multiple autoantibodies in children, including antibodies against glutamic acid decarboxylase (GAD65), tyrosine phosphatase (IA-2), and insulin. In adults with autoimmune diabetes, more commonly anti-GAD65 is the only autoantibody found.

151. a. Autoimmune hepatitis has several types described based on autoantibody patterns. Type I is the only form commonly seen in the United States, and is associated with anti-nuclear antibodies and antibodies to actin, often formerly detected as anti-smooth muscle antibodies. Type 2 is associated with antibodies to liver-kidney microsomes (anti-LKM1), while type 3 is associated with antibodies to soluble liver antigen–liver/pancreas.

152. d. Small cell carcinoma is associated with many paraneoplastic manifestations. Small cell tumors, as neuroendocrine tumors, commonly produce large amounts of the Hu antigen family, a marker also found in all cells of the nervous system. The vast majority of patients with small cell carcinoma express this antigen, although autoantibodies are not as common. Most commonly, the antibodies produce a polyneuropathy, but may also produce an encephalitis. Treatment of the tumor may lead to regression of the syndrome.

153. d. This is a typical panel of tests in a patient with chronic obstructive lung disease leading to respiratory acidosis that is fairly well compensated, although pH is at the low end of normal.

154. c. These results indicate a metabolic alkalosis, accompanied by hypokalemia; compensation is not complete, so pH is above normal. Rarely, as in this case, a person with bulimia may have severe enough alkalosis and hypokalemia to require medical attention.

155. e. Persistent respiratory alkalosis occurs in persons with chronic hypoxemia when there is either impaired oxygen exchange across the alveolar wall (interstitial fibrosis, inflammation, or edema), or with right to left shunting of blood (intrinsic cardiac defects, pulmonary hypertension, cirrhosis). In this case, the clinical presentation is typical for decompensated chronic liver disease with portal hypertension.

156. a. The anion gap is 24 mmol/L in the presence of a significant decrease in bicarbonate and pH. The history of depression with an anion gap metabolic acidosis should suggest the possibility of a suicide attempt; common agents to produce metabolic acidosis include ethylene glycol, methanol, and salicylates.

157. d. The laboratory results indicate a low bicarbonate and high chloride and a normal anion gap (9 mmol/L), which could either represent non-anion gap metabolic acidosis or respiratory alkalosis. Hyperventilation due to anxiety does not cause chronic respiratory alkalosis, and respiratory alkalosis does not typically cause hypokalemia. Type 4 renal tubular acidosis (RTA) causes hyperkalemia, and can be excluded. While both type 2 RTA and GI losses of bicarbonate can cause non-anion gap metabolic acidosis with hypokalemia, the urine

electrolytes are conclusive: the urine anion gap (the difference between the sum of [Na + K] and Cl) is typically a positive number in RTA (and respiratory alkalosis) reflecting increased bicarbonate loss, while in GI losses of bicarbonate the urine anion gap is strongly negative, as in this case. This woman, on further questioning, had chronic diarrhea and was found to have a large villous adenoma of the colon.

158. b. The laboratory results indicate a low bicarbonate and high chloride and a normal anion gap (10 mmol/L), which could either represent non-anion gap metabolic acidosis or respiratory alkalosis. While diabetes can cause ketoacidosis, the anion gap should be increased. Hyperventilation due to anxiety does not cause chronic respiratory alkalosis, and respiratory alkalosis does not typically cause hyperkalemia. Type 2 renal tubular acidosis and GI bicarbonate losses would be expected to produce hypokalemia. Type 4 renal tubular acidosis is common in persons with moderate renal insufficiency, particularly that due to diabetes, where production of renin is often decreased. In this patient, hypertension was treated by an ACE inhibitor (which is also indicated in diabetes to minimize progression of diabetic nephropathy), but which may exacerbate hyperkalemia and metabolic acidosis in a few patients.

159. b. The basic metabolic panel shows a low bicarbonate and an anion gap of 22 mmol/L, which is diagnostic for a metabolic acidosis. All of the choices could cause an increased anion gap, but not an increased osmotic gap. The combination suggests ingestion of ethylene glycol, methanol, or paraldehyde. Uremia is ruled out by the only minimally increased BUN, while diabetic ketoacidosis is ruled out by the normal glucose. Starvation ketoacidosis is ruled out by the negative urine dipstick (no ketones are present). Lactic acidosis does not produce an increased osmotic gap.

160. b. The pH indicates acidemia is present. The increased anion gap (18 mmol/L) indicates the presence of a metabolic acidosis, while the high pCO2 in an acidemic patient indicates a respiratory acidosis. While a variety of conditions may cause increased anion gap, the normal glucose rules out diabetic ketoacidosis, while normal osmolality and osmotic gap would rule out an ingestion (except for salicylates) as a cause. In the setting of hypotension, lactic acidosis is likely. Looked at another way, uncompensated respiratory acidosis would have low pH, high pCO2, and normal bicarbonate, as seen in this case, but would not give an increased anion gap.

161. e. In all acid-base disorders except for anion gap acidosis, chloride changes in the opposite direction to bicarbonate, but by the same amount. In metabolic acidosis with a normal anion gap (such as caused by diarrhea or renal tubular acidosis), chloride would be increased. In anion gap acidosis, chloride is typically normal. The only acidosis with a high bicarbonate, and low chloride, is respiratory acidosis.

162. **e.** The most common causes of metabolic alkalosis are vomiting and dehydration. In these disorders, urine chloride is typically quite low (below detection limits or <10 mmol/L), while mineralocorticoid excess is usually associated with high urine chloride. Low potassium and increased bicarbonate are seen in all forms of alkalosis. Hypernatremia is rare in mineralocorticoid excess and most commonly occurs with dehydration, as would increased BUN and creatinine with a high BUN/creatinine ratio.

163. **d.** A shift of oxyhemoglobin dissociation curve to the left causes increased binding of oxygen to hemoglobin and decreased oxygen delivery to tissues. A decrease in pCO2, 2,3 DPG, and temperature would shift the curve to the left, while an increase in pH does the same thing. Bicarbonate has no direct effect on the oxyhemoglobin dissociation curve.

164. **d.** Diuretics, SIADH, and adrenal failure are all associated with elevated levels of 24-hour urinary sodium. Diabetic hyperosmolarity does not elevate 24-hour urinary sodium, as levels in this condition will likely be within the reference range.

165. **a.** The syndrome of inappropriate antidiuresis, or SIADH as it is often called, is a common cause of chronic hyponatremia in adults. There are four major associations with SIADH: medications (particularly psychiatric medications such as phenothiazines and other antipsychotics), pulmonary diseases, cerebral disorders, and tumors (especially small cell carcinoma of the lung). While cirrhosis causes hyponatremia, it is due to third spacing of fluid and not to SIADH.

166. **e.** The presentation of a diabetic patient with abdominal pain and discrepant results between the Vitros (which uses direct reading ion selective electrodes) and other instruments (which use indirect or diluted ion selective electrodes) is typical for pseudohyponatremia, which is usually caused by markedly elevated triglycerides. The high triglycerides are a common problem in diabetics with poor control and can cause abdominal pain and pancreatitis. With diluted ion selective electrode assays, a known volume of plasma is tested; when increased lipids (or proteins) are present, a given volume of plasma contains less water and, thus, less sodium. With direct reading ion selective electrodes, sodium activity (directly related to sodium concentration in water) is measured, and so increased lipids or proteins do not affect results. Accurate sodium measurement can be obtained in lipemic samples by removing lipids by ultracentrifugation prior to testing.

167. **e.** Artifactual hyperkalemia is the most common artifact in laboratory testing. Common causes include: leakage of potassium from red blood cells (hemolysis; delayed separation of serum from cells, particularly if stored under refrigeration; recentrifugation of blood in serum separator tubes); tube contamination (especially from EDTA tubes); leakage from muscle (fist pumping during tourniquet application); leakage from platelets (serum, but not plasma potassium); and leakage from white blood cells (leukemia). In thrombocytosis, serum potassium is increased by up to 0.15 mmol/L for every 100,000/mm^3 increase in platelet count (potassium is released from platelets when they clot).

168. **c.** The most common cause of hypernatremia is loss of fluid without its replacement. Most commonly, this is due to common causes of dehydration such as diarrhea, excessive sweating, or diuretic administration. These are usually accompanied by intravascular volume depletion and reflected by an increase in BUN/creatinine ratio, as seen in prerenal azotemia. Diabetes insipidus can also cause fluid losses and dehydration, but does not cause a high BUN/creatinine ratio. The mechanism of the increase in ratio is reabsorption of urea along with water absorption mediated by ADH, which does not occur in diabetes insipidus. Administration of normal saline would not change sodium, since it is isotonic with plasma. Administration of sodium bicarbonate during resuscitation could cause increased sodium, but would also cause increased CO2 and not chloride. Mannitol causes water to move out of cells, decreasing serum sodium.

169. **c.** Primary hyperaldosteronism is a common cause of refractory hypertension and is often not considered by clinicians, despite the fact that it may cause 5% to 10% of hypertension. Key features to recognizing hyperaldosteronism, in addition to the refractory hypertension, are hypokalemia (seen in over half of cases), metabolic alkalosis, and inappropriate potassium wasting in urine. In most other causes of metabolic alkalosis, urine chloride is below 10 mmol/L. Serum sodium is usually normal in hyperaldosteronism. Renal tubular acidosis would produce low bicarbonate and high chloride, and does not cause hypertension. Cushing syndrome could cause obesity and hypertension, as well as low potassium and metabolic alkalosis, but usually causes hyperglycemia and menstrual irregularities, and is much less common than hyperaldosteronism. Congenital adrenal hyperplasia due to 11-hydroxylase deficiency can cause hypertension, hypokalemia, and metabolic alkalosis, but is associated with androgen excess, ambiguous genitalia, and amenorrhea. Diuretic administration can cause hypokalemia, but would resolve after the drug is discontinued, and would not cause continuous potassium losses in urine unless dehydration had occurred (in which case urine chloride would be <10 mmol/L).

170. **a.** Creatinine is a breakdown product of creatine, found in skeletal muscle. Creatine, which is used by many body builders, is also metabolized to creatinine, increasing serum creatinine. The most commonly used creatinine assay for both serum and urine is the Jaffe reaction, which uses an alkaline solution of picrate; this method is subject to interferences, most commonly from ketone bodies and cephalosporins. While extraction steps are available, these are not needed for routine measurements. Enzymatic

assays are less widely used, but are seldom subject to interferences.

171. **d.** The first three tests measure substances cleared by glomerular filtration, and are not useful as tests of tubular function. Urine glucose is affected by tubular function, but is primarily related to serum glucose concentration. Fractional excretion of sodium reflects the percentage of filtered sodium reabsorbed by the renal tubules. While it is also affected by the intake of sodium and by levels of hormones such as aldosterone and the natriuretic peptides, fractional excretion of sodium is the most widely used test to determine whether oliguria is due to tubular dysfunction such as seen in acute tubular necrosis.

172. **b.** The clinical scenario indicates nephrotic syndrome, which in a child is usually associated with minimal change nephropathy. A decreased C3 would suggest another cause for nephrotic syndrome. Low albumin, increased LDL-cholesterol, and oval fat bodies are found in all causes of nephrotic syndrome. While high BUN/creatinine ratio is often thought to indicate prerenal azotemia, it is also seen in any condition with third spacing of fluid, as occurs with nephrotic syndrome.

173. **d.** The urine shows the presence of albumin, plus a band migrating between albumin and the normal serum alpha-1 band, along with two bands in the alpha-2 region. This is typical of the pattern seen with tubular injury. In diabetic nephropathy, there would typically be albumin plus, in many cases, smaller serum proteins such as alpha-1 antitrypsin and transferrin (which migrates in the beta globulin region). While both myeloma and rhabdomyolysis could also cause tubular injury, there should be an abnormal band in the beta or gamma globulin region (myoglobin in rhabdomyolysis, light chain in myeloma).

174. **b.** Glucose is measured in urine using the glucose oxidase method, which typically measures the ability of the generated hydrogen peroxide to oxidize a dye to a visible form by the action of peroxidase. Ascorbic acid reacts with hydrogen peroxide to produce a colorless product. This is also a problem for urine tests for leukocyte esterase and blood, which also involve oxidized dyes. The other mentioned tests use different principles and are not affected by ascorbic acid. Some dipstick manufacturers include a pad for ascorbic acid to detect levels that may interfere with test interpretation.

175. **b.** Homogentisic acid, the metabolic product that accumulates in the disease alkaptonuria, shows this characteristic change in color after urine is allowed to stand. This may be the initial finding that calls attention to the disease, which may otherwise be undiagnosed into later adult life. Alkaptonuria most commonly causes degenerative joint damage, but may also lead to damaged heart valves.

176. **c.** The crystals are two different forms of calcium oxalate. The square, "envelope-shaped" crystals of cal-

cium oxalate dihydrate are a common finding in urine sediment, and are of no clinical significance by themselves. The ovoid calcium oxalate monohydrate crystals often predominate in ethylene glycol poisoning, and are the form that deposits in tissues.

177. **b.** Most urine crystals are of no clinical significance; they typically form as urine cools, and are therefore more commonly seen in urine that has been refrigerated before analysis. The common crystals that are encountered in urine sediment are uric acid and calcium oxalate, which are found in acidic urine, and triple phosphate, which is found in alkaline urine. Amorphous urates are also common and can be found in either type of urine pH; they often give an orange-pink appearance to urine after they crystallize. Cystine crystals are never found in normal urine. These hexagonal crystals, however, may be mimicked by crystals of sulfonamides.

178. **d.** Waxy casts (wide, brittle casts that often show horizontal fissures) are considered pathognomonic of chronic renal failure; their presence should always be noted. While a large number of red blood cells would be considered pathologic in a male or an older female, large numbers of red blood cells are often present in women during the menstrual cycle. A few white blood cells and hyaline casts can be considered normal, while increased numbers would be more significant. Transitional epithelial cells are a normal finding in urine sediment; cytology or detection of abnormal transitional cells using tumor markers (including FISH analysis) would be needed to recognize pathologic transitional cells reflecting urothelial neoplasia.

179. **e.** Acid-base balance, water balance, diet, and renal function play key roles in determination of urine pH. In the acid base disorder presented here, the kidneys are reabsorbing less bicarbonate, resulting in lower net acid excretion. The urine pH is alkaline because bicarbonate loss helps to compensate for the alkalosis.

180. **e.** Zollinger-Ellison syndrome is caused by gastrin-producing tumors; although originally described as produced by islet cell tumors of the pancreas, the majority of cases actually have duodenal tumors. Diarrhea is present in about half of patients, while hyperparathyroidism is found in about 20% (even without other evidence of MEN-1 syndrome). Gastrin levels are often markedly elevated, but are less than 4 times the upper reference limit in 30% to 40% of cases. Ulcers are mainly duodenal, but may be located in atypical places such as the jejunum; however, gastric ulcers are rare in this syndrome.

181. **e.** An increasingly commonly recognized cause of iron deficiency is celiac sprue. This disorder is much more frequent than previously recognized; most studies suggest about 1% to 2% of adults of northern European ancestry have this disease. In contrast to presentations in children, in adults the disease may present as irritable bowel syndrome or iron deficiency anemia; some

studies suggest that 5% to 10% of iron deficiency anemia in men is due to celiac sprue. While fecal fat excretion may be abnormal in celiac sprue, it is also abnormal in pancreatic insufficiency and in biliary tract dysfunction and is not a diagnostic test for any cause. Although HFE mutations are associated with iron overload, they are not linked to iron deficiency. Primary biliary cirrhosis and pancreatic disease are not linked to iron deficiency.

182. **b.** While a number of states do genetic analysis, this is performed using a panel of mutations in the *CFTR* gene on chromosome 7, and usually as a follow-up test for infants who have increased serum immunoreactive trypsin, which is the most widely used screening test for cystic fibrosis. The other mentioned tests have inadequate sensitivity to be used for screening for the disease.

183. **c.** Dietary restrictions are not needed for immuno-chemical tests, since they only detect intact human hemoglobin, while guaiac detects the peroxidase activity of heme, which typically persists even after degradation of the protein chain. Dietary restrictions on ingestion of meat and peroxidases in foods (such as cauliflower and horseradish) are needed when guaiac tests are used. For similar reasons, upper intestinal bleeding is usually not detected using immunochemical tests. Both tests are similarly sensitive for detecting colon cancer, but are insensitive to the presence of colonic adenomas. Use of three bowel movements is needed for adequate sensitivity with both tests. Although rehydration of stool samples increases sensitivity of guaiac tests, it significantly increases the likelihood of false positive results and so is not recommended.

184. **e.** Cytokines (particularly IL-6 and IL-1) stimulate the production of a number of inflammatory response modifiers, including protease inhibitors (such as alpha-1-antitrypsin), ceruloplasmin, complement, fibrinogen, factor VIII, and haptoglobin. In contrast, there is generally a fall in a number of other proteins, including albumin and transferrin.

185. **e.** While transthyretin (prealbumin) is often touted as a nutritional marker, it is also decreased by a number of other conditions. It is a small protein, so is often lost in nephrotic syndrome. Like a number of other proteins, its levels fall in acute inflammation. It is produced by the liver, so will be decreased in cirrhosis.

186. **d.** The blue-green color of plasma is likely due to ceruloplasmin, which is significantly increased by estrogens. The copper in this enzyme is oxidized on standing, giving the blue-green color. While persons with Wilson's disease have increased free copper, their ceruloplasmin and total copper levels will be decreased. Gilbert's syndrome might cause a more intense yellow-green color, but this would not change on standing. Similarly, increased bilirubin in advanced liver disease may cause a yellow-green color. While iron stains blue in the Prussian blue reaction, it does not turn blue on standing, so hemochromatosis would cause no visible change in plasma.

187. **e.** In protein electrophoresis, the band with the highest amount is automatically adjusted to fill the tracing from top to bottom. In the patient's tracing, the alpha-2 globulins appear to be present in as high concentration as albumin; there is also an increase in beta-1 globulins. Because the largest molecular weight proteins (alpha-2 macroglobulin, haptoglobin, and low-density lipoprotein) migrate in these two regions, these proteins are often markedly increased in nephrotic syndrome. It is difficult from such a tracing to appreciate that the other proteins are actually decreased, because of the artifact induced by adjusting the gain.

188. **d.** The tracing illustrates a decrease in gamma-globulins and a band of restricted mobility that migrates in the beta-2 globulin region. The combination of these two findings is strongly suggestive of a monoclonal gammopathy, most likely due to a monoclonal IgA. Other monoclonal proteins may also migrate in this location, including free heavy or light chains, as well as monoclonal IgG or IgM.

189. **b.** The most common cause of chronic hypercalcemia in ambulatory individuals is primary hyperparathyroidism, which would be confirmed by finding elevated PTH (typically using the intact assay). Persons with primary hyperparathyroidism often have low phosphate and increased 1,25-dihydroxyvitamin D as well.

190. **d.** The most common causes of hypocalcemia include low serum albumin (with low total calcium but normal free or ionized calcium) and chronic renal failure. About 10–15% of hypocalcemia, however, is due to less common causes. The most frequent of these are hypoparathyroidism, malabsorption or other causes leading to vitamin D deficiency, and magnesium deficiency. Pseudohypoparathyroidism is an inherited disease in which PTH is produced, but its receptors are defective. It is accompanied by a number of dysmorphic features. Pseudopseudohypoparathyroidism is a disorder with the same phenotypic features but normal calcium, phosphate, and PTH. Both disorders seem to involve impaired signaling through G protein-coupled pathways.

191. **a.** While termed "intact" PTH assays, most use antibodies that recognize larger metabolic fragments. While for many years it was felt that PTH fragments were inactive, it is now recognized that there are additional receptors that recognize PTH fragments, and that these receptors mediate actions opposite to those of PTH. In persons with normal renal function, large metabolic fragments represent only a small portion of what is measured in intact PTH assays, but PTH fragments accumulate in renal failure. In some individuals with renal failure, 7–84 PTH may be the dominant form detected by PTH assays. Newer "1–84" or "biointact" PTH assays detect only 1–84

PTH, but do not seem to be any better in evaluating degree of parathyroid dysfunction. Because there are two antibodies that detect opposite ends of the molecule in all intact PTH assays, PTH-related peptide (which is similar to PTH only at its N-terminus) is not measured.

192. **b.** Because alkaline phosphatase is produced in response to PTH (as well as to other factors that stimulate osteoblastic activity), increased bone alkaline phosphatase does not distinguish primary hyperparathyroidism from other causes of hypercalcemia. Primary hyperparathyroidism typically causes chronic, mild hypercalcemia that is stable untreated over long time periods. The other common cause of hypercalcemia, malignancy, is often associated with rapid rises in serum calcium to markedly increased levels. The most common mechanism of hypercalcemia of malignancy is production of PTH-related peptide, but lytic bone lesions (particularly those due to multiple myeloma) can also be responsible. Both PTH and PTH-related peptide block phosphate reabsorption by the kidney, reducing serum phosphate; an increase in phosphate suggests another mechanism of hypercalcemia.

193. **c.** Three tumors that commonly make PTH-related peptide are squamous cell carcinomas (of any site), renal cell carcinoma, and breast carcinoma. These three tumors are responsible for about 80% of hypercalcemia in malignancy, and between one fourth and one third of those having one of these tumors will develop hypercalcemia, often as a late complication. While hepatocellular carcinomas can produce PTH-related peptide, they do so in less than 5% of cases. The other tumors listed rarely cause hypercalcemia unless extensive bone metastases are present. Small cell carcinomas often make other hormones, however, and can cause Cushing's syndrome and SIADH.

194. **c.** In iron deficiency, body stores of iron (reflected by ferritin) are decreased, while serum iron is low. In response to depleted iron stores, transferrin (which is estimated by iron binding capacity) will be increased.

195. **b.** In chronic inflammation, iron stores (reflected by ferritin) are increased; however, mobilization of iron from stores is reduced because of increased hepcidin, which inhibits actions of ferroprotein in moving iron across cell membranes; this leads to decreased serum iron. The increased iron stores decrease synthesis of transferrin (which is estimated by iron binding capacity).

196. **e.** In hemochromatosis, iron stores (reflected by ferritin) are increased, and the inappropriately low hepcidin levels lead to increased transport of iron across cell membranes, causing increased serum iron levels. The increased iron stores decrease synthesis of transferrin (which is estimated by iron binding capacity).

197. **b.** Release of hemoglobin from red cells leads directly to formation of increased amounts of unconjugated bilirubin. The increased processing of bilirubin by the liver increases intestinal bilirubin, which increases urobilinogen production; its enterohepatic circulation causes increased urine urobilinogen excretion. Hemoglobin binds to haptoglobin, and the complex is rapidly (minutes) removed from the circulation. Iron released from red cells increases iron filtration; the reabsorbed iron is converted to hemosiderin within renal tubular cells. These are eventually shed, and can be detected using iron stains on urine sediment. If any changes are seen in serum iron, it tends to be increased.

198. **c.** Adult hemoglobin contains four polypeptide chains each with a heme group containing an iron atom in the ferrous ($+2$) state that facilitates binding of oxygen. In metHb, the iron oxidation state is ferric ($+3$). Additionally, the presence of ferric iron inhibits oxygen release by the remaining heme groups containing the ferrous iron. These events lead to a functional anemia, decreased oxygen release, and a subsequent left shift of the oxyhemoglobin dissociation curve. Reference levels of metHb are $<2\%$ with levels of 15% associated with an asymptomatic cyanosis. Levels approaching 20% are associated with dyspnea, fatigue, nausea, dizziness, headache, and syncope. Symptoms are exacerbated as levels increase, and levels or 60% to 70% or more are associated with a high mortality. Methylene blue is an oxidant, however, the reduced leucomethylene blue formed in vivo by NADPH-dependent methemoglobin reductase is responsible for reducing the metHb ferric iron to the ferrous state. This enzyme is produced by the hexose monophosphate shunt pathway and requires adequate levels of G6PD. In metHb-emia, dextrose infusion is often administered in conjunction with methylene blue to serve as substrate to form the reduced leucomethylene blue substrate. Patients with genetic deficiencies of G6PD may not produce enough NADPH for this conversion; therefore, methylene blue will increase metHb levels in these individuals. Every day about 3% of hemoglobin is converted to metHb; however, cytochrome b5 reductase prevents metHb accumulation.

199. **d.** A decrease in B12 will lead to increased homocysteine and increased methylmalonic acid levels; however, decreased folate will only lead to increased homocysteine levels. The reason is given in choice E. B12 is needed to convert homocysteine into methionine with the help of methionine synthase. Methyltetrahydrofolate is demethylated during this reaction. Propenyl CoA is converted to methylmalonic-CoA which is subsequently converted to succinyl CoA via methylmalonic-CoA synthase and B12 as the cofactor. Tetrahydrofolate is not involved in this reaction.

200. **a.** Congenital erythropoietic porphyria is the result of an enzyme defect in uroporphyrinogen III synthase and is the only porphyria with an autosomal recessive mode of inheritance. The others are autosomal

dominant. A defect in protoporphyrinogen oxidase results in variegate porphyria. A defect in ferrochelatase results in erythropoietic protoporphyria. A defect in porphobilinogen deaminase results in acute intermittent porphyria. A defect in coproporphyrinogen oxidase results in hereditary coproporphyria. Tissue expression for protoporphyria can be both erythroid cells and liver; congenital erythropoietic porphyria is the only one with only erythroid cell expression. Tissue expression for the other porphyrias are liver only.

201. **b.** Free erythrocyte protoporphyrin is often used as a screen for iron deficiency because it usually increases in both iron deficiency and chronic disease. Zinc protoporphyrin level increases in response to decreased iron and is often measured as free erythrocyte protoporphyrin. Lead interferes with ferrochelatase, the final step in heme synthesis. Zinc protoporphyrin regulates heme catabolism by competition with heme oxygenase, the rate limiting enzymatic step in heme degradation to biliverdin followed by biliverdin reductase conversion of biliverdin to bilirubin. Because zinc protoporphyrin can assess bilirubin formation, it may also be used to monitor hyperbilirubinemia in neonates.

202. **c.** Coproporphyrin, protoporphyrin, and other dicarboxylic porphyrins make up fecal porphyrins. One of the most important applications of fecal porphyrins is to distinguish between variegate porphyria (coproporphyrin and protoporphyrin) and coproporphyria (coproporphyrin only). Fecal porphyrins are usually increased in all of the porphyrias except acute intermittent porphyria. The amount of fecal porphyrins excreted is a function of diet and the anaerobic flora of the colon. Therefore, healthy individuals may demonstrate variability in fecal porphyrin excretion as much as three times the upper reference limit.

203. **e.** Choices A–D are all considered non-governmental organizations. The ASCP offers certification for various specialties. JC is a non-profit organization based on setting quality standards and may substitute for federal Medicare and Medicaid surveys. JC meets licensure and insurers' requirements. CAP provides a proficiency survey program that is accompanied with a peer-surveyed laboratory accreditation program that has CLIA-deemed status and is recognized by JC as meet-

ing laboratory standards. CLSI (formerly known as NCCLS) is a professional peer group with standard criteria directed laboratory practices (retrieved from: http://www.clsi.org). CMS (formerly known as HCFA) sets quality standards and reimbursement rates for laboratory tests and services that are considered standards for use by third-party payers.

204. **a.** Before medical claims are paid, the claim must describe the patient's medical condition or diagnosis in addition to the list of services and/or tests performed. This information is translated to a standard coding system recognized by all government and non-government organizations. HCPCS codes provide a description of the tests or services performed. The ICD-9-CM codes describe the patient's condition or diagnosis. These standards facilitate communication between health care providers and third-party organizations. CPT codes are a component of HCPCS that are used to identify clinical laboratory tests and medical services. DRGs classify patients to facilitate reimbursement of hospital costs for Medicare patients. The DRG does not cover physician services.

205. **d.** Variable costs change proportionately with the test volume. Reagent costs grow with increasing number of tests performed. Fixed costs are considered constant and therefore do not vary with the volume of tests performed. Except for reagents, all of the expenses listed are fixed costs. Direct costs can be directly linked to an end product (i.e., billable test). Reagents and technologist time are examples of direct costs. While indirect costs are not directly linked to a billable test, they are essential for laboratory function. Indirect costs are also known as overhead

■ Recommended Readings

Burtis CA, Ashwood ER, Bruns DE. *Tietz textbook of clinical chemistry.* 4th ed. Philadelphia: Elsevier Saunders, 2006.

Clarke W, Dufour DR. *Contemporary practice in clinical chemistry.* Washington, DC: AACC Press, 2006.

Diamandis EP, Fritsche HA, Lilja H, et al. *Tumor markers: physiology, pathobiology, technology, and clinical applications.* Washington, DC: AACC Press, 2002.

Mahon CR, Fowler DG. *Diagnostic skills in clinical laboratory science.* New York: McGraw-Hill, 2004.

Price CP, Christenson RH. *Evidence based laboratory medicine: from principles to outcomes.* Washington, DC: AACC Press, 2003.

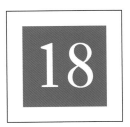

18

Molecular Pathology and Genetics

Ronald M. Przygodzki

■ Questions

1. The missense mutation Ser810Lys in the mineralocorticoid receptor results in:
   a. Neoplastic processes unresponsive to hormonal therapy
   b. Dominant form of pseudohypoaldosteronism
   c. Early-onset hypertension that is exacerbated by pregnancy
   d. Early-onset hypertension that is not accelerated by pregnancy
   e. A constitutively activated receptor with abnormal activation by aldosterone

2. Which of the following NAT1 gene variants retains normal enzyme activity?
   a. NAT1*1
   b. NAT1*2
   c. NAT1*8
   d. NAT1*14
   e. NAT1*15

3. An increased level of *S*-warfarin, under standard anti-coagulant drug dosage, would be expected in a patient with which of the following polymorphisms?
   a. CYP2C9*2
   b. CYP2C9*3
   c. CYP2C19*2
   d. All of the above
   e. Only a and b are correct.

4. Which of the following does NOT support the Hardy-Weinberg law of population genetics?
   a. It enables one to have the ability to take information about the frequency of alleles in the population and make predictions about the frequency of genotype in the population.
   b. Individuals with all genotypes are equally capable of mating and passing on their genes (there is no selection against any particular genotype).

   c. Rate of mutation will not have an appreciable effect.
   d. The population tested is large and matings are expected to be random with respect to the locus in question.
   e. There is no significant immigration of individuals from a population with allele frequencies markedly different from the endogenous population.

5. What type of structural chromosomal abnormality is identified in Figure 18.1?
   a. Insertion
   b. Duplication

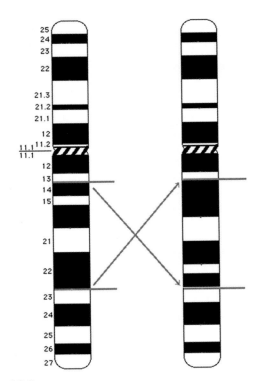

Figure 18.1

369

c. Derivative chromosome
d. Isochromosome
e. Paracentric inversion

6. A stillbirth is presented to you at autopsy. The family is worried that another birth might yield a child with similar phenotypic features. The mother is noted to lack a superior labial frenulum. Given the facial features of this child (Fig. 18.2) and the family history, which of the following molecular and genetic findings are correct?
   a. The nonsyndromic form of this disease is exclusively autosomal recessive.
   b. It occurs with an equal male:female distribution.
   c. Most common gene alteration is a gain-of-function mutation.
   d. You should have the family members evaluated for Sonic Hedgehog mutation.
   e. Patients exclusively present with marked facial dysmorphism, cyclopia, and marked central nervous system malformations.

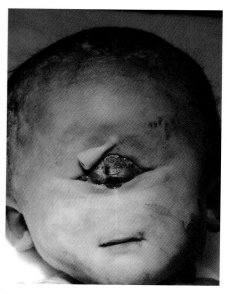

Figure 18.2

7. Which of the following statements pertaining to Prader-Willi syndrome (PWS) is correct?
   a. Hypogonadism is present in both males and females.
   b. Maternal deletions of 15q11–q13 accounts for approximately 70% to 80% of alterations.
   c. The estimated prevalence of PWS is 1/500,000.
   d. Spontaneous mutations account for approximately 15% of alterations.
   e. Paternal uniparental disomy of chromosome 15 accounts for approximately 25% of alterations.

8. Which of the following antibody against tumor antigen/tumor antigen combinations is INCORRECT?
   a. Bevacizumab (Avastin)/VEGF
   b. Rituximab (Rituxan)/CD52 lymphocyte surface antigen

c. Cetuximab (Erbitux)/EGFR
d. Trastuzumab (Herceptin)/HER2 receptor
e. Panitumumab (ABX-EGF)/EGFR

9. Which of the following is correct with respect to myotonic dystrophy type I?
   a. It is the least common dystrophy presenting in adults.
   b. Involves an expansion of the CCG triplet repeat.
   c. It is a disease of chromosome 16.
   d. May cause sudden death and myocardial fibrosis.
   e. The triplet repeat expansion involves the 5′ untranslated region.

10. Which of the following in NOT valid for Kerns-Sayre syndrome (KSS)?
    a. It is a mitochondrial myopathy.
    b. It is very rarely inherited maternally.
    c. Mitochondrial homoplasmy is present.
    d. Mitochondria with the alteration are more localized to muscle and CNS.
    e. Onset of disease is in infancy/early childhood.

11. Which of the following is NOT deemed a tumor suppressor gene?
    a. *RON*
    b. *Rb*
    c. *APC*
    d. *VHL*
    e. *P53*

12. You decide to identify whether you have loss of heterozygosity by PCR using one fluorescently labeled and a second unlabeled oligonucleotide primer set in a particular tumor and nontumor sample. You further know that the primers span a region of AT repeats. The PCR of the tumor reveals a single band, similar to that found in the nontumor sample. The positive and negative control samples produced appropriate results. Which of the following statement is correct?
    a. LOH is informative in the tumor sample.
    b. The sample may or may not have LOH.
    c. The sample does not have LOH and is informative.
    d. Direct sequencing may be required to identify LOH.
    e. You require the use of a new set of primers.

13. Which of the following genes may be inactivated by hypermethylation?
    a. *BRCA1*
    b. *MLH1*
    c. *KRAS*
    d. *Rb*
    e. *P16*

14. Which of the following is correct with respect to herpes simple virus?
    a. Two type are identified – HSV1 with genital and HSV2 with orofacial lesions.
    b. No FDA-approved methods are available for HSV PCR-based molecular testing.

c. Direct detection by Tzanck stain is superior to all detection methods.

d. RT-PCR is not possible on CSF samples.

e. Acute necrotizing encephalitis associated with HSV is localized to the base of the brain.

15. Which of the following is INCORRECT with respect to familial adenomatous polyposis (APC)?
   a. Most APC alterations are simple missense point mutations.
   b. APC has an integral function with beta-catenin.
   c. MLPA and gene sequencing are used for APC mutation detection.
   d. APC is a tumor suppressor gene.
   e. Protein truncation testing is useful in detecting alterations.

16. Which of the following statements is INCORRECT?
   a. Tumor suppressor genes are inactive when both genes are inactivated or deleted.
   b. Short tandem repeats are lethal.
   c. Oncogenes are activated when amplified, mutated, or translocated.
   d. Knudsen's "two-hit" hypothesis pertains to tumor suppressor genes.
   e. Polymorphisms are not lethal.

17. Which is INCORRECT regarding telomerase?
   a. It is a reverse transcriptase.
   b. It adds a specific RNA sequence (TTAGGG) to the 3′ end of DNA strands.
   c. It consists of two molecules each of TERT, TERC, and dyskenin.
   d. Its activity may be identified by RT-PCR or the TRAP assay.
   e. Stem cells maintain an active telomerase enzyme.

18. Which of the following statements regarding the brain mass in Figure 18.3 are INCORRECT?
   a. Primary method to assess for chromosomal loss is by FISH and LOH.
   b. 1p and 19q loss if fairly specific for this tumor; unfortunately, sensitivity is below 100%.
   c. Patients with chromosomal losses of 1p and 19q have longer survival times than those without this change.

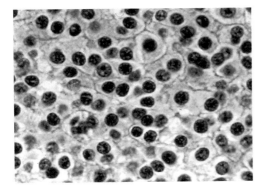

Figure 18.3

d. Patients with chromosomal losses of 1p and 19q respond worse to therapy than those without this change.

e. 19q loss alone will not enable exclusion of an astrocytoma or mixed oligo/astrocytoma.

19. Which of the following statements is INCORRECT with respect to alpha-1-antitrypsin (A1AT) phenotypes?
   a. ZZ accounts for nearly all clinically recognized A1AT deficiencies.
   b. SS patients have a minimal risk for development of emphysema.
   c. Detection by genotyping is superior to isoelectric focusing electrophoresis.
   d. Lung disease is associated with either S or Z alleles, whereas liver disease is associated with the Z allele.
   e. A1AT is a member of the SERPIN family.

20. You are reviewing the autopsy liver sample from a 40-year-old man. You identify a brown pigmented material that strongly stains with Prussian blue (Fig. 18.4). All of the following statements about this disease are correct EXCEPT:
   a. It may be associated with diabetes insipidus.
   b. Cirrhosis and hepatocellular carcinoma may be a feature.
   c. Homozygous C282Y mutation is often the cause in hereditary (primary) type.
   d. Clinical penetrance of the disease is not 100%.
   e. The genes that could produce this disease are autosomal dominant as well as recessive.

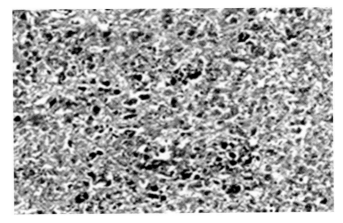

Figure 18.4

21. When is routine testing for factor V Leiden NOT indicated?
   a. Patient with venous thrombosis at age <50
   b. Patient with recurrent thrombosis
   c. Strong family history of thrombotic disease
   d. Patient with family history of arterial thrombosis
   e. Patient with thrombosis present in unusual sites (e.g., mesenteric or hepatic vein)

22. All of the following are true regarding analyte specific reagents (ASRs) EXCEPT:
   a. ASRs are considered active ingredients used in diagnostic testing for identification and/or quantification of a chemical substance, ligand, or biologic target in patient specimens.
   b. Companies that sell ASRs must register their establishments and list their reagent(s) with the FDA.
   c. The user assembles the clinical assay using the ASR; however, is not required to validate the performance of the new assay in the intended population.
   d. Most ASRs are class I devices and thus exempt from premarket approval or notification requirement.
   e. An ASR is a single reagent, such as nucleic acid probe, that can be used by laboratories in developing a functional clinical assay.

23. All of the following statements regarding multiplex ligation-dependent probe amplification (MLPA) are true EXCEPT:
   a. Permits multiple targets to be amplified with only a single primer pair.
   b. Each probe consists of a pair of primers that needs to be PCR-amplified for detection.
   c. Only the ligated sequences are amplified.
   d. One of the MLPA primer pairs has the target sequence as well as a predefined length of "stuffer sequence."
   e. Is useful in determining presence of duplications and deletions.

24. The following pedigree (Fig. 18.5) is representative of which of the following?
   a. Autosomal dominant
   b. X-linked recessive
   c. Mitochondrial
   d. X-linked dominant
   e. Partial/reduced penetrance

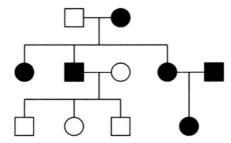

Figure 18.5

25. Which of the following is INCORRECT regarding BRAF?
   a. It is one of three subtypes of similar serine/threonine kinases.
   b. V600E (exon 15) is the most common mutation.
   c. Somatic mutation is identified in primary melanomas.

   d. Mutation leads to massive induction of the ERK signaling pathway.
   e. Mutation of BRAF is an integral component of HNPCC colorectal carcinomas.

26. Using conventional gene nomenclature, please identify which of the following regarding the fictitious gene (abc) represents the accurate nomenclature for a human gene product (protein)?
   a. abc
   b. ABC
   c. *abc*
   d. *ABC*
   e. v-*abc*

27. Which of the following is NOT true with respect to EGFR?
   a. It encodes for a receptor tyrosine kinase.
   b. Small molecule inhibitors include Gefitinib (Iressa) and Erlotinib (Tarceva).
   c. EGFR amplification detected by FISH is superior to IHC.
   d. Mutations associated with resistance to EGFR inhibitors include exon 20 (T790M).
   e. The FDA has not approved the use of EGFR inhibitors for use in patients with lung carcinoma who failed to respond to chemotherapy.

28. Which of the following answers is NOT correct with respect to patients with Li-Fraumeni syndrome?
   a. The *P53* tumor suppressor gene is mutated.
   b. Triplet repeat deletions are typically identified in the coding region of the gene.
   c. Alterations involve the binding domain of the gene.
   d. Germline mutations are the rule.
   e. LOH of the *P53* gene is present.

29. You are asked to perform PCR testing on a patient with a history of renal transplantation. You are asked to evaluate whether a urine sample has BK virus present. Which of the following facts regarding BK virus is INCORRECT?
   a. BK virus testing should be performed on a urine sample.
   b. Renal transplant patients with BK infection have graft failure in nearly half of the cases.
   c. Can be secondary to tacrolimus, sirolimus, or mycophenolate mofetil therapy.
   d. H&E-stained kidney biopsy tissue may reveal the organism.
   e. Develops in less than 5% of renal transplant recipients.

30. The RAS protein product is normally active:
   a. As an intercellular factor
   b. At the cell membrane
   c. Intracellularly at the juxtamembrane region
   d. In the nuclear membrane
   e. In the nucleoplasm

31. Which of the following is true about *CKIT*?
    a. Capillary electrophoresis of fluorescently labeled PCR product will detect all alterations possible in gastrointestinal stromal tumors.
    b. Autosomal recessive piebaldism may be found among patients with germline inactivating mutations.
    c. Exon 11 deletions are associated with good prognosis.
    d. Tumors with exon 17 mutation respond well to Imatinib.
    e. The most prevalent mutation in mastocytosis is D816V (A2648T).

32. You performed a PCR on an archival (formalin-fixed, paraffin-embedded) tissue (Fig. 18.6). Which action is most accurate in order for you to optimize the reaction?
    a. Increase the annealing temperature.
    b. Increase the annealing time.
    c. Increase the amount of MgCl2 in the reaction.
    d. Increase amount of template DNA.
    e. Increase amount of oligonucleotide primer.

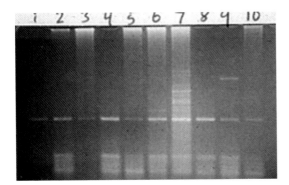

Figure 18.6

33. You have performed a traditional Sanger sequencing gel from the gene of your choice (Fig. 18.7). Which of the following statements is INCORRECT?

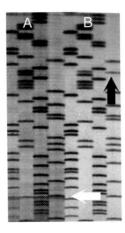

Figure 18.7

a. Sequence A and B are from the same exon.
b. Sequence A displays extensive mutation as evidenced by the white arrow.
c. Sequence B displays a heterozygous mutation.
d. Four sequencing reactions with ddATP, ddGTP, ddCTP, and ddTTP separately placed into each reaction allow determination of the sequence present.
e. Current technologies use dye terminators instead of unlabeled dideoxynucleotides and can be run in a single lane.

34. Which of the following is INCORRECT regarding DNA methylation?
    a. CpG islands are DNA regions that mark the start of many exons.
    b. Cytosine is methylated.
    c. Promoter regions of cancers cells may be hypermethylated or hypomethylated.
    d. Sodium bisulfite treatment is used in determining the presence or absence of methylation by PCR techniques.
    e. Methylation of maternal or paternal alleles is random.

35. You are reviewing a slide (Fig. 18.8) of an intra-abdominal mass from a young child. The cells are positive for CD20, CD79a, CD10, and BCL6 but negative for BCL2. MIB-1 reveals positively in all of the cells. Which translocation is most consistent with this tumor?
    a. t(11;18)
    b. t(3;14)
    c. t(11;14)
    d. t(14;18)
    e. t(8;14)

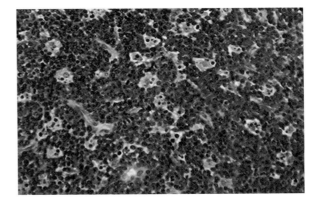

Figure 18.8

36. All of the tumors stemming from the following translocations/mutations will respond to Imatinib mesylate EXCEPT:
    a. *BCR-ABL1*
    b. *FIP1L1-PDGFRA*
    c. *STIL-TAL1*
    d. *ETV6-PDGFRB*
    e. *KIT* exon 11 mutation

37. The approximate carrier rate of Gaucher disease in Ashkenazi Jewish people is:
    a. 1:5
    b. 1:18
    c. 1:30
    d. 1:80
    e. 1:128

38. Which gene is affected in patients with Niemann Pick type A disease?
    a. HEXA
    b. MCOLN1
    c. SMPD1
    d. MFTHR
    e. FOXO1A

39. An HIV viral load change must be greater than what for it to be considered clinically relevant?
    a. 0.1 log units
    b. 0.2 log units
    c. 0.3 log units
    d. 0.4 log units
    e. 0.5 log units

40. A blood sample is taken from a patient for molecular-based testing. You realize that the sample was delivered the night before and that the sample was kept at room temperature. Which of the following substances is most likely to be degraded in this sample?
    a. DNA
    b. RNA
    c. Amino acids
    d. Protein
    e. Lipids

41. Which of the following probes will be most appropriate in an assay in which you target the DNA sequence 5′ – TTTCCCTATGCGAAAAGGG –3′?
    a. 5′ – AAAGGGATACGCTTTCCC –3′
    b. 5′ – GGGTTTTCGCTACCCAAA –3′
    c. 5′ – CCCTTTTCGCATAGGGAAA –3′
    d. 5′ – AAATTTTGCGTAGGGAAA –3′
    e. None of the above

■ Answers

1. **c.** Patients with the **Ser810Lys mutation** have severe **hypertension**, which present mostly before age 20. The mutation is not associated with neoplastic formation. The dominant forms of pseudohypoaldosteronism are secondary to the following inactivating mutations: ΔG1226, ΔT1597, C/T1831stop, and ΔA intron splice site. The mutation results in a constitutively activated mineralocorticoid receptor; however, it retains its normal activation by aldosterone.

2. **a.** All polymorphisms with a "star" *1 are considered to be wild-type by convention. Hence, all other variants are altered, leading to either excess, depressed, or absent production.

3. **e.** Individuals **with CYP2C9*2 and CYP2C9*3** have an impaired metabolism of *S*-warfarin, which leads to an increased plasma concentration of the drug despite standard dosing. Hence, such patients will experience an increased risk for serious or life-threatening bleeding complications despite obtaining a standard dose of medication. The VKORC1 polymorphism likewise has a role in warfarin therapy.

4. **c.** Genetic equilibrium is a basic principle of population genetics. Violations of the **Hardy-Weinberg law** can cause deviations from expectation. Among such deviations are inbreeding/co-sanguinuity (increases homozygosity for all genes), small population size (can cause random change in genotypic frequency – also known as genetic drift), and assortative mating (causes an increase of homozygosity only of those genes involved in the trait). The law further assumes that there is no appreciable rate of mutation; changes in this manner would affect the allelic frequencies, which are assumed to be constant.

5. **e. Paracentric inversion** consists of an inversion within a given arm of the chromosome. Insertions "insert" additional chromosome, whereas duplication inserts a portion of duplicated chromosome. Isochromosomes lose one of the chromosome arms and contains a duplicate inverted other chromosome arm (e.g., 2p arms in mirror image at centromere).

6. **d.** The picture depicts a child with **holoprosencephaly**. Nonsyndromic forms of holoprosencephaly are predominantly autosomal dominant, with an incidence of 1 in 10,000 to 1 in 12,000 births. Autosomal recessive and X-linked recessive forms do occur, however are rare. It affects twice as many girls as it does boys. The facial dysmorphisms occur as a spectrum, with mild alterations including lack of frontal incisor, lack of superior labial frenulum, hypotelorism or hypertelorism, bifid uvula all the way to marked CNS alterations, including alobar holoprosencephaly. Sonic Hedgehog (*SHH*) mutations are loss-of-function mutations and account for nearly 40% of familial nonsyndromic autosomal dominant holoprosencephaly. Other genes implicated in this disease include *ZIC2*, *PTCH*, and *TGIF*.

7. **a.** Loss of the paternal allele of the PWS/AS region on chromosome 15 accounts for the syndrome; maternal uniparental disomy (~25%) and paternal deletion of 15q11–q13 (~70% to 80%) account for the brunt of alterations. An additional however small component (<5%) imprinting defects are noted; however, mutations, per se, do not occur in PWS. The prevalence of PWS is 1/10,000 to 1/15,000. **Hypogonadism** is present in both males and females, with most individuals unable to reproduce.

8. **b. Rituximab** is directed against **CD20** B-cell surface antigen and is used for therapy in non-Hodgkin lymphoma. The CD52 lymphocyte surface antigen antibody used for treatment of CLL and T-cell lymphomas is alemtuzumab (Campath).

9. **d. Myotonic dystrophy type I** is the most common muscular dystrophy presenting in adults. It is characterized by myotonia, progressive weakness, and atrophy of skeletal muscles, as well as systemic manifestations including cardiac involvement. The cardiac involvement initially manifests as asymptomatic ECG abnormalities, prolonged PR and QRS duration leading to arrhythmia, progressive heart block, and trial/ventricular fibrillation. **Sudden death** may occur as a consequence of myocardial fibrosis and degeneration of the cardiac-conduction system. The CTG triplet repeat expansion is found in the 3′ untranslated region of the *DMPK* (dystrophia myotonica protein kinase) gene.

10. **c.** KSS by rule is **heteroplasmic**. KSS is exceedingly rarely inherited maternally and if present, it is due to mtDNA duplication. Spontaneous mtDNA rearrangements/deletions are noted in ~80% of cases. The most common deletion (~30%) is 4.9kb in size.

11. **a.** *RON* (macrophage-stimulating 1 receptor, MST1R) is a member of the receptor tyrosine kinase gene family that includes the MET **oncogene**.

12. **b. LOH testing** required that a sample have two DNA strands of varying length of the region being amplified in the non-tumor sample in order to be informative. In this way, PCR amplification reveals two bands, both of different sizes, in this case in Nx2 bp difference. LOH would be considered when two bands were to be present in the non-tumor sample and one band to be present in the tumor sample. Because the normal sample in this question reveals a single band, it might be assumed that both strands are of the same length therefore uninformative; however, the region being testing may be missing from one of the chromosome arms, therefore producing a single PCR product. Neither sequencing nor new primer sets for the region will resolve such questions; however, testing on the level where chromosome copy number is determined (e.g., comparative genomic hybridization, karyotyping, copy number variant testing) should resolve such cases more definitively.

13. **c. KRAS**, an oncogene, is typically activated by mutation - methylation does not play a role in activating oncogenes. Hypermethylation of MLH1 (colon, endometrial cancer), P16 (esophageal, lung cancer), RB, and BRAC1 (breast ovarian cancer) are tumor suppressor genes that may either be inactivated by mutation or hypermethylation. Either path to inactivation leads to detrimental outcomes in these genes.

14. **b.** Indeed, no molecular based **HSV** testing is currently (2008) approved by the FDA. HSV1 is associated with orofacial lesions, whereas HSV2 is associated with genital lesions. HSV encephalitis typically affects the neurons of the temporal lobe. Tzanck skin tests are rarely used to identify viral inclusions from a vesicle base and are considered obsolete. RT-PCR, with numerous ASRs available, is the easiest qualitative test for this infection.

15. **a.** The most common (70% to 90%) mutations and alterations is the FAP gene are **nonsense/frameshift mutations**, producing premature stop codons. APC controls beta-catenin, which prevents cell division from being turned. Protein truncation testing is useful because of the premature stops introduced by the gene mutations. MLPA is useful in detecting deletion by PCR methodology. APC is a tumor suppressor gene.

16. **b. Short tandem repeats** are repeats of various lengths of di-, tri-, tetra-, or pentanucleotides which occur naturally within DNA. The two-hit hypothesis of Knudsen refers to the mutation of one and deletion of the second copy of a tumor suppressor gene. Hence, alteration of both tumor suppressor gene copies is required for detrimental effect, because their effect if to retard action – lack of the "brake" causes deregulation of the cell. In contrast, unique point mutation(s) of an oncogene usually will active it, as will amplification or translocation of a downstream portion of the gene onto an activated second gene. Polymorphisms are not lethal because they constitute the usual genetic variety present in humanity.

17. **b. Telomerase** is a reverse transcriptase that adds specific DNA sequence repeats to the **3′ end of DNA strands**. It consists of two molecules each of TERT (telomerase reverse transcriptase) and TERC (telomerase RNA), as well as dyskenin. Assays that may be used for telomerase activity include RT-PCR as well as the TRAP (telomerase repeat amplification protocol) assay. Usually, telomerase is inactive. Stem cells and cancer cells are immortal due to their ability to activate the telomerase enzyme and thereby maintain telomere length.

18. **d.** The photo is that of the glial tumor **oligodendroglioma**. Losses of chromosome **1p and 19q** have been strongly associated with oligodendroglioma; however, loss of 19q alone has been noted among astrocytomas and mixed oligo/astrocytoma tumors. Patients with oligodendroglioma with loss of 1p and 19q survive longer and respond better to therapy. Not all of these

tumors will display the chromosomal alteration; hence, such testing at this time should be pursued as an adjunct to histologic assessment.

19. **c. A1AT (SERPIN1A)** is a member of the serine protease inhibitor family. Although genotyping may be easier to interpret than isoelectric focusing electrophoresis, it is deficient in finding all possible mutations in this highly polymorphic gene. **Genotyping** identifies Z, S, and "non-Z, non-S" genotypes, the latter including several M subtypes. The S allele affects lung alone, whereas the Z allele affects lung and/or liver.

20. **a.** The H&E reveals an autopsy liver sample with **hemochromatosis**. Several clinical features may be seen in advanced disease, including iron deposition in skin, liver, and pancreas, the latter yielding **diabetes mellitus**. Long-standing damage of the liver will also produce cirrhosis and an increased propensity for hepatocellular carcinoma. Homozygous **HFE C282Y** mutation is the most common mutation associated with primary (heritable) hemochromatosis; however, compound heterozygotes (C282Y/H63D) are likewise associated. The clinical penetrance, that is, the fraction of patients with a particular genotype that manifest the disease, is low even for compound C282Y homozygotes, and much less for the compound heterozygotes. The genes associated in hemochromatosis include HFE, HJV, AMP, and TFR2 that are all inherited in an autosomal recessive fashion. SCL40A1 (ferroprotein) is however inherited in an autosomal dominant fashion.

21. **d.** Valid recommendation presented also include patients with myocardial infarction in female smokers <50 age. The test is not recommended in case of **arterial thrombosis** or as random screening tests.

22. **c.** All clinical assays assembled by the user are required to be validated for their performance in the intended population. All remaining statements are valid.

23. **b.** Each probe consists of a primer pair that straddles the target site of interest and is subsequently ligated into a complex target sequence. The ligated sequences are amplified, not the original target DNA. Stuffer sequences allow the identification of particular amplicons at particular positions along the electrophoresis. This methodology is particularly useful in determining the presence or absence of deletion as well as duplications of sequence.

24. **c.** The pedigree is that of **mitochondrial inheritance**. The maternal proband disseminates the alteration, whereas the male (son) does not. Partial/reduced penetrance would display a skip in presence of disease.

25. **e. BRAF** is one of three serine/threonine kinases (ARAF, BRAF, CRAF) that act on the RAS/RAF/MEK/ERK/MAPK signal transduction pathway. Somatic mutations of BRAF are found in primary melanomas, papillary thyroid carcinomas, ovarian

carcinomas, as well as colorectal cancers. BRAF mutations are **not found in HNPCC colorectal cancers**, however are associated with sporadic tumors with MLH1 loss, hence BRAF mutation is associated with colorectal tumors of sporadic origin.

26. **b.** Recommendations of the International Standing Committee on human genes nomenclature are as follows: capital letter = human; lower case letters = animal (e.g., mouse). The gene's product is non-italicized, whereas the gene is italicized. Therefore, *ABC* is a human gene, however **ABC is the genes product**. Viral oncogenes are referred usually with "v-" before the gene.

27. **e.** EGFR inhibitor use is in fact approved for use in patients with non-small cell lung carcinoma (NSCLC) who failed chemotherapy response. Of note, EGFR mutations with sensitivity to EGFR inhibitors include exon 19 (delE746–750), and exon 21 (L858R).

28. **b.** Li-Fraumeni syndrome involves germline mutation of the binding domain regions (exons 5–8) of the *P53* gene in one DNA strand and loss of heterozygosity of the other DNA strand in the *P53* gene region. **Triplet repeat deletions are not noted** in this syndrome.

29. **a.** **BK virus** can be excreted at high levels **into the urine** even without illness, whereas exceedingly high levels are noted in active infection ($>10^{10}$ genome copies/mL). Renal transplant patients with BK infection have graft failure in up to 50% to 70% of cases. The main risk factor is their immunosuppressive therapy for their transplant, which includes the drugs listed. It is readily identifiable by H&E or immunohistochemistry on renal biopsy sample.

30. **c.** **RAS** functions at the **juxtamembrane region** just beneath the cell membrane and functions as a signaling protein shuttling activation signals from tyrosine kinases within the cell membrane downstream to other proteins.

31. **e.** The most prevalent mutation in mastocytosis is the mutation noted. Capillary electrophoresis will detect deletion/insertion mutations, however will not detect point mutations within such tumors. Piebaldism, an autosomal dominant disorder or melanocytic development requires germline inactivating mutations of *CKIT*. Exon 11 deletions portend bad prognosis, however good response to Imatinib. Exon 17 as well as exon 13 mutations do not respond to Imatinib.

32. **a.** The PCR gel demonstrate the presence of a unique band present in all reaction; however, additional random bands are likewise noted making the reaction not "clean." Increasing the annealing time may increase the chance for mispriming of oligonucleotides in this reaction. An increase in MgCl2 will lower the specificity of the priming; in this case a decrease might be useful. An increase in template may actually reduce the product yield. Moreover, lanes 2, 3, and 5–7 and 10 demonstrate smearing of DNA throughout the length of the gel run, which is indicative of overloading of template. Numerous primer-dimer bands are noted in the lower portion (leading end) of the gel. An increase of primers would only make a greater primer-dimer band, robbing primers from the reaction. **An increase of the annealing temperature** may eliminate the primer-dimer band, as well as at the other spurious bands due to an increased specificity of the primer-template binding.

33. **b.** The band crossing all four lanes of case A is a **compression band** which is formed by inadequate denaturation of template prior to loading the sequencing gel. Similar alterations may be seen in current fluorescent sequencing techniques. The dark arrow demonstrates a heterozygous mutation because two bands can be seen at the same level, as well as the original band is fainter (compare A second column to B second column). Homozygous mutations would present as a band in a different column with the original band missing. This radiolabeled sequencing gel requires four separate reactions in order to determine the sequence in question. Current technologies allow the reaction to be performed in a single reaction because the dideoxynucleotides (e.g., ddCTP, etc.) are themselves fluorescently tagged.

34. **e.** Methylation of maternal and paternal alleles, or **imprinting, is not random**, rather is conserved and crucial. Alterations in maternal/paternal allele methylation can lead to diseases like Angelman syndrome, Beckwith-Wiedemann syndrome, or Prader-Willi syndrome due to such methylation alterations.

35. **e.** The diagnosis is **Burkitt lymphoma**, which typically displays near 100% Ki-67 (MIB-1) staining. Translocation of *MYC* (chromosome 8) and *IGH* (chromosome 14) is the most frequent breakpoint partner. Other possible translocations include the t(2;8) and t(8;22) fusing MYC with *IGK* or *IGL*. The following association between translocation/ B cell tumor are presented: t(3;14) – diffuse large cell lymphoma, t(11;14) – mantle cell lymphoma, t(14;18) – follicular lymphoma, and t(11;18) – MALT.

36. **c.** Gleevec responsive tumors include CML (*BCR-ABL1*, *ETV6-PDGFRB*), ALL (*BCR-ABL1*), Chronic eosinophilic leukemia (*FIP1L1-PDGFRA*), and *KIT* mutations in exon 11. *STIL-TAL1* is present in **T cell ALL**, and is not responsive to Gleevec.

37. **b.** The carrier rate is 1:18.

38. **c.** Sphingomyelin phosphodiesterase 1. HEXA is associated with Tay-Sachs disease. MCOLN1 is associated with mucolipidosis type IV. MFTHR converts homocysteine to methionine. FOXO1A is a transcription factor associated with alveolar rhabdomyosarcoma when translocated with PAX3.

39. **e.** At least a threefold change is required for this to be valid.

40. **b.** **RNA is exceedingly heat labile.** Samples that will entail RNA testing should be kept on ice and brought to the clinical diagnostic lab as soon as possible.

41. **c.** Pairing occurs in an antiparallel fashion, that is, 5′–3′ over-riding 3′–5′. In essence, one needs to read the antisense code from the 3′ to 5′ (right to left) in order to identify the 5′ to 3′ probe.

■ Recommended Readings

Leonard DGB. *Molecular pathology in clinical practice,* 1st ed. New York: Springer, 2007.

Nussbaum RL, McInnes RR, Willard HF. *Thompson & Thompson genetics in medicine,* 7th ed. Philadelphia: Saunders, 2007.

O'Leary TJ. *Advanced diagnostic methods in pathology,* 1st ed. Philadelphia: Saunders, 2003.

Pfeifer JD. *Molecular genetic testing in surgical pathology,* 1st ed. Philadelphia: Lippincott Williams & Wilkins, 2006.

Runge MS, Patterson C. *Principles of molecular medicine,* 2nd ed. Totowa, NJ: Humana Press, 2006.

Index